Cranial Osteopathy
for **INFANTS, CHILDREN** and **ADOLESCENTS**

Commissioning Editor: Sarena Wolfaard
Senior Associate Editor: Claire Wilson
Development Editor: Claire Bonnett
Project Manager: Frances Affleck
Designer: Gene Harris/Stewart Larking
Illustration Manager: Merlyn Harvey
Illustrator: Oxford Illustrators

Cranial Osteopathy

for INFANTS, CHILDREN and ADOLESCENTS

A PRACTICAL HANDBOOK

Nicette **Sergueef** DO (France)

Adjunct Assistant Professor, Department of Osteopathic Manipulative Medicine, Chicago College of Osteopathic Medicine, Midwestern University, Chicago, IL, USA

Foreword by
Harold **Magoun** Jr., DO, FAAO, DO Ed (Hon)

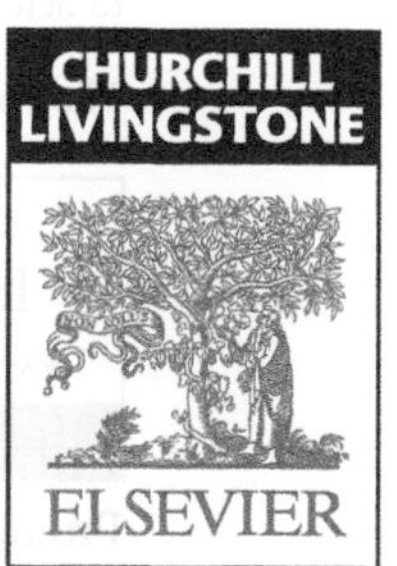

Edinburgh London New York Oxford Philadelphia St Louis Sydney Toronto 2007

Transferred to Digital Print 201[illegible]

CONTENTS

FOREWORD

William Garner Sutherland as a child was encouraged to 'dig on' in the family potato patch. He found that the more he dug, the more rewarding the digging became. He carried that philosophy throughout his whole life. Dr Sutherland observed a disarticulated skull in osteopathic school and was struck with the idea that the adjacent surfaces were designed for motion. He could find no substantiation for that, so with a great deal of bravery he experimented with his own head, dug on and proved his 'skull motion'. He initially dealt only with adults, but with his great success was subsequently asked to treat infants and children. He provided many clinical cases by volunteering to work at an institute for handicapped children, and again met with great success. Dr Sutherland minimized his contribution by saying he had 'only pulled aside a curtain.' But what a tremendous vista that curtain has revealed!

Cranio-sacral osteopathy has made a tremendous contribution to health care and has probably had a greater impact in helping infants and children realize their full potential, than in correcting the many adult problems which occur. This is not to minimize its benefit in that area.

Osteopathy has spread throughout much of the world, and is particularly strong in France. My father, author of *Osteopathy in the Cranial Field*, was one of the first to teach in France over 40 years ago, and was gratified to see his efforts bear fruit. These French osteopaths have a keen understanding of the teachings of both Still and Sutherland, and in turn have dug on. They not only practice osteopathy, they teach it, and contribute to osteopathic literature. Nicette Sergueef has been practicing and teaching osteopathy for almost 30 years, both in Europe and at the Chicago College of Osteopathic Medicine. She is the author of a number of French osteopathic texts, several of which have been translated into German and Italian.

Cranial Osteopathy for Infants, Children and Adolescents is Nicette Sergueef's first text in English. She has covered the whole spectrum from the birth process, the development of the child, the cranial concept and how it applies to our young patients, and goes beyond the usual limited cranio-sacral consideration to cover the many clinical problems which can affect the whole body when its various components are not in harmony. This will be a valuable addition to osteopathic literature.

Harold Magoun Jr, DO, FAAO, FCA, DO Ed (Hon)

PREFACE

This text is intended to provide the reader with an organized approach to the osteopathic treatment of infants, children and adolescents. The contents represent 30 years of clinical practice supplemented by a thorough review of the scientific literature. I have tried to provide the anatomic basis that helps explain somatic dysfunction in order that the reader understands the logical processes that lead to the effective application of osteopathic manipulative procedures in the treatment of the pediatric patient.

Osteopathy expounds a whole-body approach to the care of the patient, and this book, although focused upon the principles of cranial osteopathy, employs this philosophy: all of the tissues of the body are functionally linked. Consequently, the practitioner does not just simply treat the skull. The practitioner must treat every part of the body where somatic dysfunction is identified.

Many different models for manipulative treatment have been developed and taught. There is but one truth, however, and that truth is the truth of the body, and it is based upon anatomy. There exist a plethora of manipulative models, but careful analysis reveals that the different models represent descriptions of the same process. The interesting point about the pediatric patient is that children demonstrate basic functional and dysfunctional patterns that are not yet perturbed by the multiplicity of dysfunctions, traumas and compensatory patterns that life brings to us all. Therefore, the patterns in these youngsters are easier to understand than patterns encountered in adults where time has permitted the accumulation of layers of added dysfunctions. If the practitioner understands what happens with children, they can then more easily understand the body of the adult.

The use of cranial osteopathy for the treatment of infants, children and, to a lesser degree, adolescents is particularly appropriate. Anatomically, these patients are still dynamically growing. Their sutures are not fused; their bones are not completely ossified, they are still pliable. Their anatomy is in such a vital state that somatic dysfunction can not only be alleviated, but the impact that it has had upon the individual may often be reversed. Consequently, the long-term outcome of proper treatment for pediatric patients is of particular importance. The tremendous potential for the growth of bones, joints and myofascial structures must begin on good foundations in order for the individual to be optimally functional during their childhood and the rest of their life. Further, as patients, infants and children are psychologically unique. They are not simply smaller versions of adults. They have not yet developed expectations as to what the healthcare practitioner may provide. They feel their discomfort and are very much aware of what is being attempted to alleviate it. Instinctively, they feel what is right, and, consequently, they are the best teachers when the practitioner is willing to pay attention to their responses.

Nothing in this book is intended to be a replacement for sound medical advice and the established medical treatment of specific disease processes. Osteopathy is not a panacea. Osteopathic manipulation treats somatic dysfunction and somatic dysfunction only. The elimination of dysfunction allows the self-healing properties of the human body to function optimally. When effectively treated, the response is rapid and unequivocal. Failure of the patient to respond after an appropriate trial of osteopathic manipulation should indicate to the practitioner that they reconsider their diagnosis and seek appropriate consultation and treatment.

Osteopathic manipulation works well when treating young patients, because they respond rapidly. It is this quality, however, that requires that the non-responding individual be re-evaluated post-haste, to prevent the sequelae of failure to diagnose. This having been said, it must be recognized that osteopathic manipulation may be employed to treat the somatic dysfunction that often complicates the status of individuals with specific, and often chronic, medical conditions. Here, however, the treatment of somatic dysfunction must be considered to be adjunctive to established standards of care.

It is my hope that this text will facilitate the understanding of the significant impact that somatic dysfunction has upon the pediatric population, and that its content will assist the reader in caring successfully for these young patients. Osteopathy offers our patients the ability to respond most effectively to their illnesses and to go on to develop optimally into healthy functional adults.

NS
Chicago, 2007

ACKNOWLEDGEMENTS

I wish to express my thanks to Kenneth E. Nelson, DO, for his tremendous help in producing the English version of this text, and to Tom Glonek, PhD, for his mastery and ability to explain the secrets of the English language.

I should also like to thank Elsevier for permission to reproduce the following figures:

From Williams PL et al (eds) Gray's Anatomy, 38th edition, 1999: Figures 1.1, 1.2, 2.1–2.10, 2.13, 3.10, 3.11, 7.3.3, 7.3.5–7.3.7, 7.3.15, 7.3.21, 7.7.1, 7.7.4.

From Drake RL et al (eds) Gray's Anatomy for Students, 2005: Figures 1.12–1.14, 1.18, 1.19, 2.12, 3.1–3.9, 3.12, 7.1.1, 7.2.1, 7.2.3–7.2.6, 7.2.9, 7.3.1, 7.3.2, 7.3.4, 7.3.8–7.3.14, 7.3.16–7.3.20, 7.4.1, 7.5.1–7.5.5, 7.6.1, 7.7.2, 7.7.3.

ABBREVIATIONS

AIS – adolescent idiopathic scoliosis
ANS – autonomic nervous system
AOM – acute otitis media
AP – anteroposterior
ASIS – anterior superior iliac spine
CMT – congenital muscular torticollis
CN X – cranial nerve X
CNS – central nervous system
COME – chronic otitis media with effusion
CRF – corticotropin-releasing factor
CRI – cranial rhythmic impulse
CSF – cerebrospinal fluid
CTEV – congenital idiopathic talipes equinovarus
DDH – developmental displacement of the hip
DT – dilatator tubae
ENS – enteric nervous system
ENT – ears, nose, throat
EOM – extraocular muscles
ET – Eustachian tube
GALT – gut-associated lymphoid tissue
GER – gastroesophageal reflux
GERD – gastroesophageal reflux disease
GH – growth hormone
GI – gastrointestinal
GEJ – gastroesophageal junction
HEENT – head, eyes, ears, nose, throat
HPA – hypothalamic–pituitary adrenal (axis)
Ig – immunoglobulin
LES – lower esophageal sphincter
LM – left mentum
LO – left occiput
LOA – left occiput-anterior
LOP – left occiput-posterior
LS – left sacrum
LVP – levator veli palatini
MRI – magnetic resonance imaging
NNS – non-nutritive sucking
NO – nitric oxide
NSP – non-synostotic plagiocephaly
NTS – nucleus tractus solitarius
OM – otitis media

OMT – osteopathic manipulative treatment
OSA – obstructive sleep apnea
PRM – primary respiratory mechanism
PSIS – posterior superior iliac spines
PT – pharyngotympanic tube
RM – right mentum
RO – right occiput
ROA – right occiput-anterior
ROM – range of motion
ROP – right occiput-posterior
RS – right sacrum
RSV – respiratory syncitial virus
RTM – reciprocal tension membranes
RVA – rib–vertebra angle
SBS – sphenobasilar synchondrosis; today, spheno-occipital synchondrosis
SCM – sternocleidomastoid
SDB – sleep-disordered breathing
SI – sacroiliac (joint)
SIDS – sudden infant death syndrome
TLESR – transient lower esophageal sphincter relaxation
TMJ – temporomandibular joint
TVP – tensor veli palatini

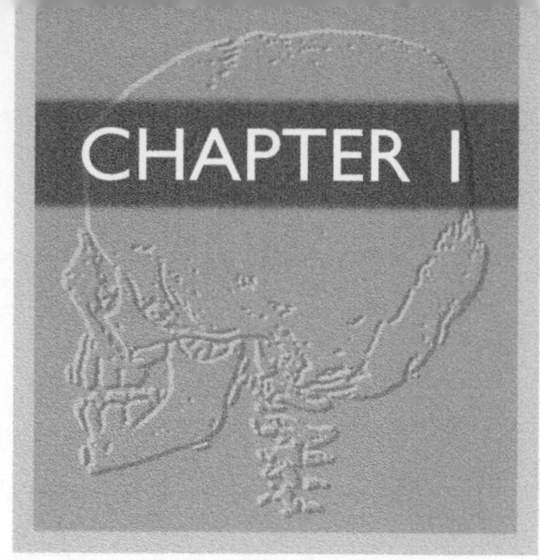

THE BIRTH PROCESS AND THE NEWBORN

'The baby of today represents the man of tomorrow.' —BE ARBUCKLE[1]

Birth is obviously one of the most important events of one's life. It is also a time when some of the primary dysfunctions that an individual must contend with throughout life are established. A review of the various characteristics of the fetus at term, of the maternal pelvis, the environment where the fetus evolves with its potential to contribute to fetal dysfunction, and lastly, the description of birth process, is necessary to understand pediatric somatic dysfunction, its diagnosis and treatment.

Fetus at term

FETAL HEAD

At 40 weeks from the onset of the last menstrual period, term is reached and the fetus is completely developed. Its weight is about 4000 g and its crown–rump length averages 36 cm. From the point of view of cranial osteopathy, as well as an obstetrical point of view, the fetal head is of particular significance. The facial part of the head – the viscerocranium – is much smaller than the neurocranium. It represents one-eighth of the total volume of the skull compared with one-half in an adult.

The bones of the cranial base are separated by cartilaginous spaces named synchondroses; the bones of the vault are separated by membranous spaces named sutures. The junctions between several sutures of the calvarial bones are the sites of fontanelles. At birth, six fontanelles are present: the anterior and posterior fontanelles are medial and unpaired; the sphenoid and mastoid fontanelles are lateral and paired. Little accessory fontanelles may also be present in the sagittal and metopic sutures.

The anterior (or greater or bregmatic) fontanelle is a lozenge-shaped space, located at the junction of the sagittal and the coronal sutures. It is the largest fontanelle, with a diameter, at birth, of about 25 mm. The posterior (or lesser or lambdatic) fontanelle is shaped like a small triangle, located at the junction between the sagittal and lambdoid sutures. They overlie the superior sagittal dural venous sinus and pulsations are palpable through these fontanelles. The anterolateral or sphenoid fontanelles are located between the greater wing of the sphenoid, the frontal bone and the parietal bone. The posterolateral (or mastoid) fontanelles are between the parietal bone, the occipital bone and the mastoid portion of the temporal bone (Figs 1.1, 1.2).

The two sagittal fontanelles are significant landmarks during labor, allowing palpatory assessment of

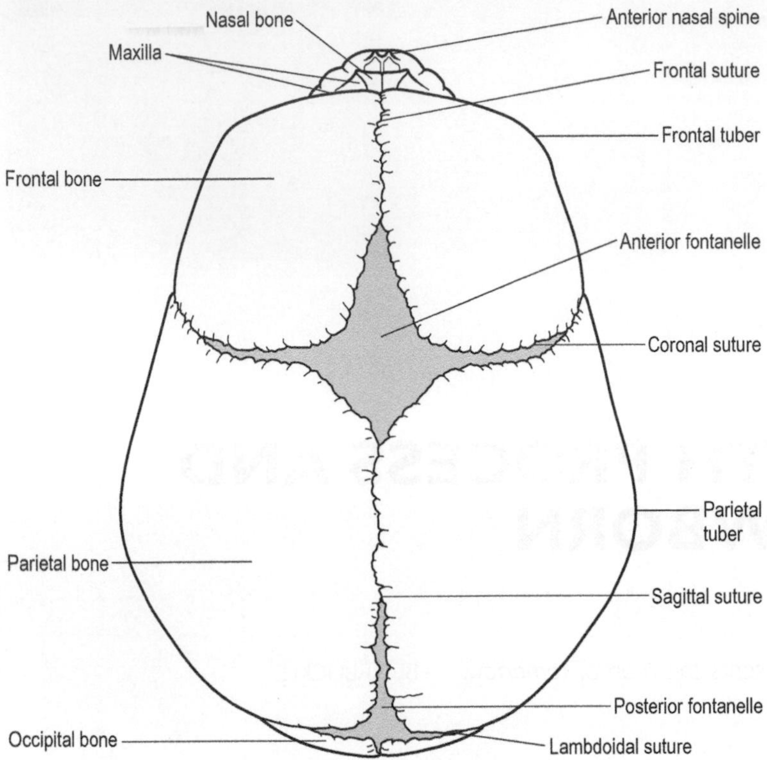

Figure 1.1. *Superior aspect of the full-term neonatal skull.*

the position of the fetal head. In the months following birth, the size of the fontanelles may be monitored to evaluate the progressive ossification of the calvaria. Normally, the posterior and sphenoid fontanelles are obliterated by 6 months of age, and the anterior and mastoid are obliterated by the second year.[2]

Diameters and circumferences of the fetal head are usually measured. The diameters are as follows:

- occipitofrontal (11.5 cm), between a point located on the frontal bone above the root of the nose and the occipital protuberance
- biparietal (9.5 cm), from one parietal to the other, the greatest transverse dimension of the head
- occipitomental (12.5 cm), from the chin to the most prominent part of the occipital bone
- suboccipito-bregmatic (9.5 cm), from the most anteriorly palpable part of the occipital bone to the anterior fontanelle (Figs 1.3, 1.4).

The occipitofrontal diameter corresponds to the plane of the greater circumference of the head that is normally too large to pass through the maternal pelvis. Therefore the fetal head must be oriented differently. The head may bend upon the child's chest so that the chin contacts the sternum, inducing a complete flexion, thereby presenting a smaller diameter for passage through the maternal pelvis (Figs 1.5, 1.6). The bones of the cranium accommodate the size and shape of the maternal pelvis by sliding and overlapping each other at the level of the sutures. This process is referred to as molding. It results in different head shapes postpartum, depending on the presentation of the fetal head and characteristics of the maternal pelvis. When fetopelvic disproportion is signifi ant, cesarean delivery is indicated.

FETAL TRUNK

Although the bulkiest part of the fetus, the trunk – because it is more compressible – is actually smaller than the head during the passage of the fetus through the pelvis. The bisacromial diameter (12 cm; Fig. 1.7) is the greatest distance between the acromial processes and may be compressed to 9.5 cm. The dorsosternal diameter (9.5 cm) is the anteroposterior (AP) distance at the level of the shoulders.

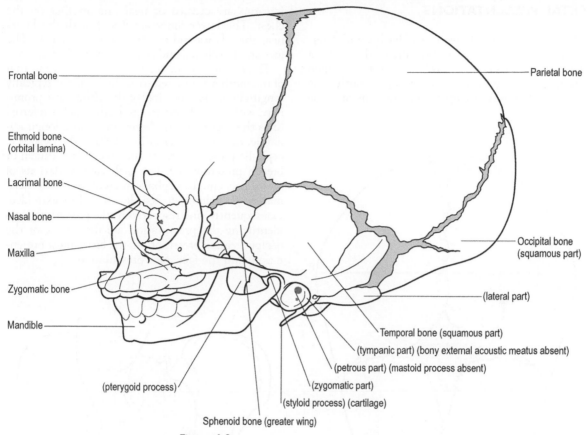

Frontal bone
Parietal bone
Ethmoid bone (orbital lamina)
Lacrimal bone
Nasal bone
Maxilla
Zygomatic bone
Mandible
Occipital bone (squamous part)
(lateral part)
Temporal bone (squamous part)
(tympanic part) (bony external acoustic meatus absent)
(petrous part) (mastoid process absent)
(zygomatic part)
(styloid process) (cartilage)
(pterygoid process)
Sphenoid bone (greater wing)

Figure 1.2. *Lateral view of the full-term neonatal skull.*

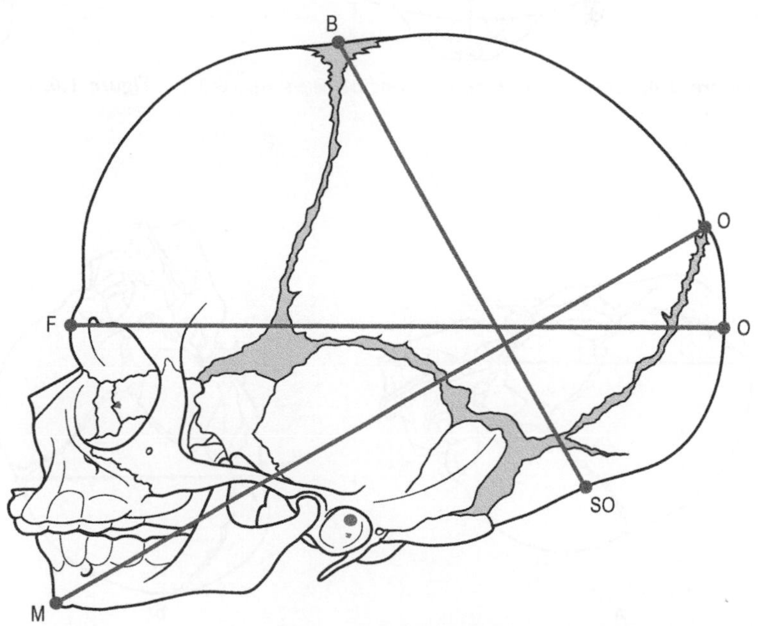

Figure 1.3. *Lateral view of the fetal head diameters: occipitofrontal, 11.5 cm; occipitomental, 12.5 cm; suboccipito-bregmatic, 9.5 cm.*

FETAL PRESENTATIONS

The fetal position relative to the birth canal determines the relative ease or difficulty of the route of delivery. Typically, the fetal body is flexed upon itself, causing the back to be convex posteriorly. The head is bent forward upon the sternum and the forearms are crossed or near one another on the chest. The lower limbs are flexed, with the knees near the elbows and the feet near the breech. The feet are dorsiflexed and slightly inverted (Fig. 1.8).

The relation of the fetal long axis relative to that of the mother is referred to as the lie and is typically longitudinal. The portion of the child most prominent within or closest to the birth canal is referred to as the presentation. Accordingly, in a longitudinal lie, the fetal presentation is either the head (i.e. cephalic presentation) or the breech (i.e. caudal or breech presentation). For each case, variations of position occur. In cephalic presentations the head may be completely flexed, less flexed or extended. Consequently, and respectively, the presenting parts identifying the presentation are the vertex or the occiput, vertex presentation; the brow, brow presentation; and the face, face presentation.

Figure 1.4. *Superior view of the fetal head diameters: biparietal, 9.5 cm.*

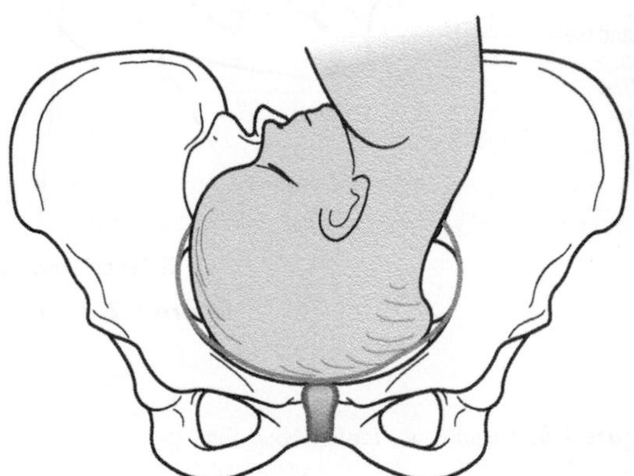

Figure 1.6. *Fetal head orientation during engagement with cervical flexion.*

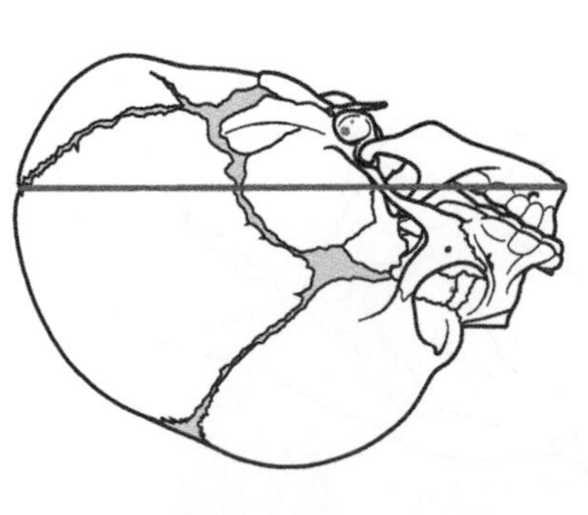

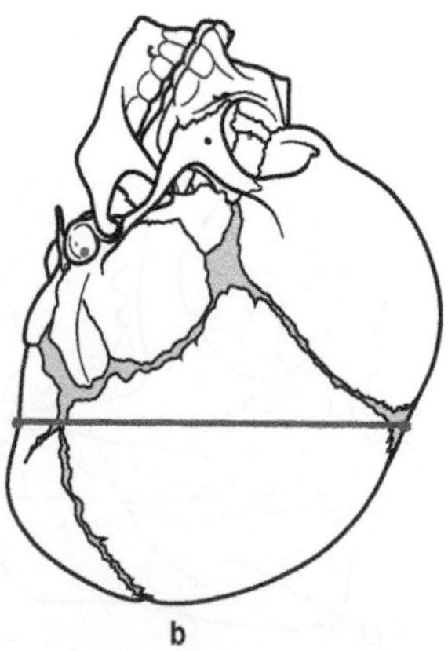

Figure 1.5. *Fetal head orientation during engagement: (a) without cervical flexion; (b) with cervical flexion.*

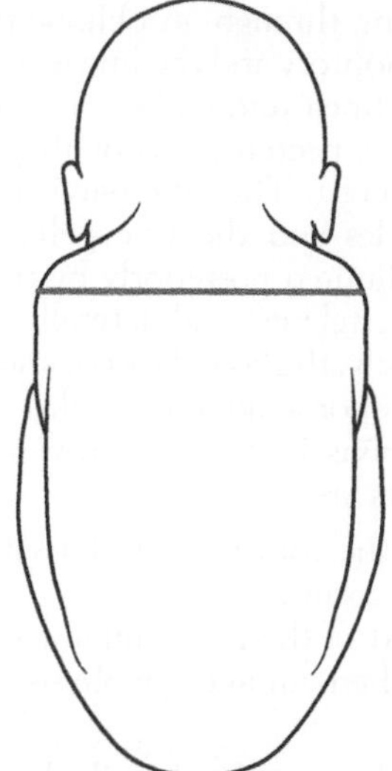

Figure 1.7. *Posterior view of the fetal trunk: bisacromial diameter, 12 cm.*

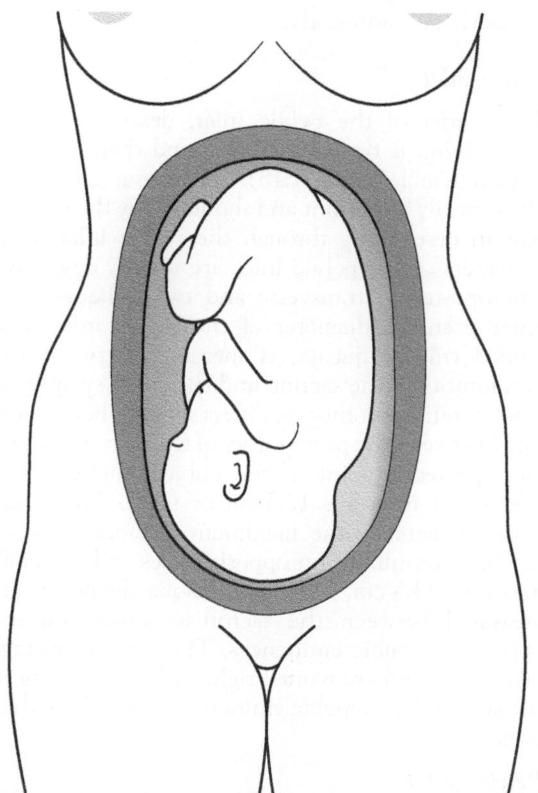

Figure 1.8. *Typical fetal position: head bent forward on the sternum, forearms crossed on the chest, lower limbs flexed.*

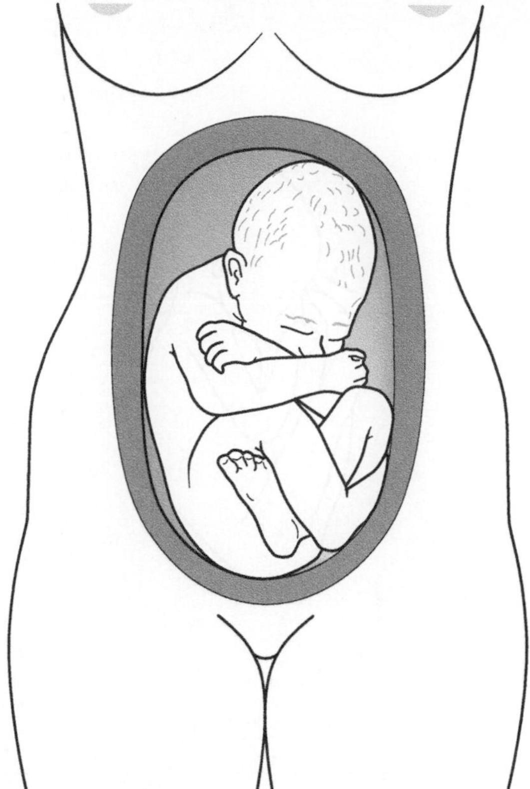

Figure 1.9. *Breech presentation: complete presentation with the legs flexed upon the thighs.*

Breech presentations are classified according to the position of the fetal legs. A complete breech presentation occurs when both lower limbs are flexed at the hip joints and the legs flexed upon the thighs (Fig. 1.9). An incomplete breech presentation occurs when the thighs are flexed but the knees extended (Fig. 1.10).

The term fetal presentation is used to define the relationship between conventional parts of the fetus relative to the maternal pelvis. The point of reference for the presenting part is the occiput in occipital presentations, the chin (or mentum) in face presentations and the sacrum in breech presentations. The occiput, mentum or sacrum may be located on the maternal right or left side, named right or left occiput (RO, LO), right or left mentum (RM, LM) or right or left sacrum (RS, LS). On each side, it can be located transversely (T), anteriorly (A) or posteriorly (P). Accordingly, a left occiput-anterior is abbreviated LOA (Fig. 1.11). Cephalic or vertex presentations are the more frequent (96%), followed by breech (3%), face (0.3%) and shoulder

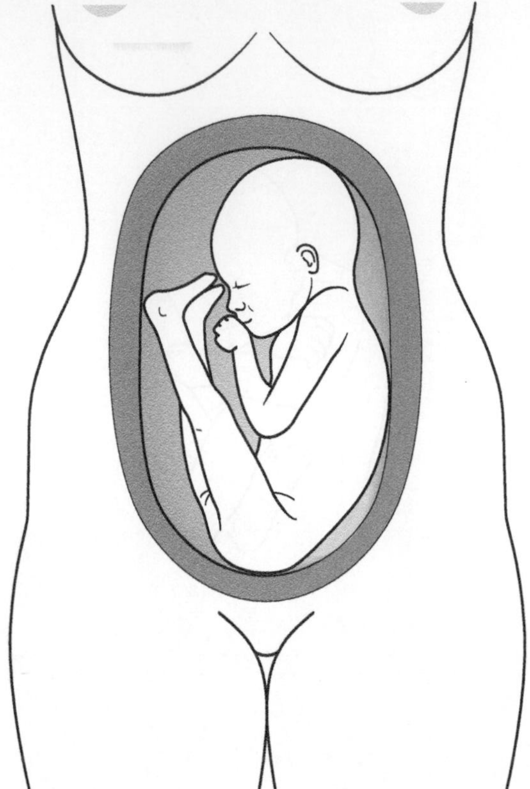

Figure 1.10. *Breech presentation: incomplete presentation with extended knees.*

(0.4%). Among vertex presentations, LOA is the most frequent (57%).[3]

The maternal pelvis

BONY PELVIS

The pelvis is composed of four bones: the two pelvic bones, the sacrum and the coccyx. The pelvic bones articulate with the sacrum at the sacroiliac joints, and with one another at the pubic symphysis, while the coccyx articulates with the sacrum at the sacrococcygeal joint. Very strong ligaments contribute to pelvic stability, particularly the posterior sacroiliac ligament and the pubic symphyseal ligaments[4] (Fig. 1.12).

The term pelvis also applies to the cavity within the bony skeletal ring, and in obstetrics the difference between the true (or lesser) and false (or greater) pelves is of consideration. The division is arbitrary, passing through an oblique plane joining the sacral promontory and the lineae terminales. On each side, the linea terminalis consists of the iliac arcuate line, the pecten pubis or iliopectineal line and the pubic crest. The false pelvis lies above the lineae terminales and the true pelvis below. The false pelvis is limited posteriorly by the sacral base and lumbar vertebrae, and laterally by the iliac fossae. Anteriorly, the boundary consists of the lower part of the anterior abdominal wall.

The true pelvis is in continuity with the false pelvis. Its limits are:

- posteriorly, the concave anterior surface of the sacrum and coccyx
- laterally, part of the fused ilium and ischium
- anteriorly, the rami and symphysis of the pubic bones.

The true pelvis can be described as a truncated cylinder with a superior opening, the pelvic inlet, and an inferior opening, the pelvic outlet. This cylinder is bent, following the anterior concavity of the sacrum and coccyx. In the anatomic position, the upper portion of the pelvic canal is directed inferiorly and posteriorly and the lower part curves inferiorly and anteriorly.

Pelvic inlet

The border of the pelvic inlet, described as the pelvic brim, is typically more round than ovoid in human females (Fig. 1.13). Its measurements are obstetrically important and should allow the head to pass in descending through the pelvic inlet. Four diameters of the pelvic inlet are usually described: anteroposterior, transverse and two obliques. The anteroposterior diameter of the pelvic inlet, also named true conjugate, is measured between the promontory of the sacrum and the pubic symphysis. The obstetrical conjugate differs slightly, being measured between the promontory of the sacrum and the most posterior point of the pubic symphysis. On average, it measures 10.5 cm or more. The transverse diameter is the maximum distance between the linea terminalis on opposite sides and normally measures 13.5 cm. The two oblique diameters are measured between the sacroiliac joints and the opposite iliopubic eminences. They are an average of 12.5 cm and are named right or left according to the side of the iliopubic eminences from where they originate.

Pelvic outlet

The pelvic outlet is diamond shaped (Fig. 1.14). It consists of the sacrum and tip of the coccyx posteriorly,

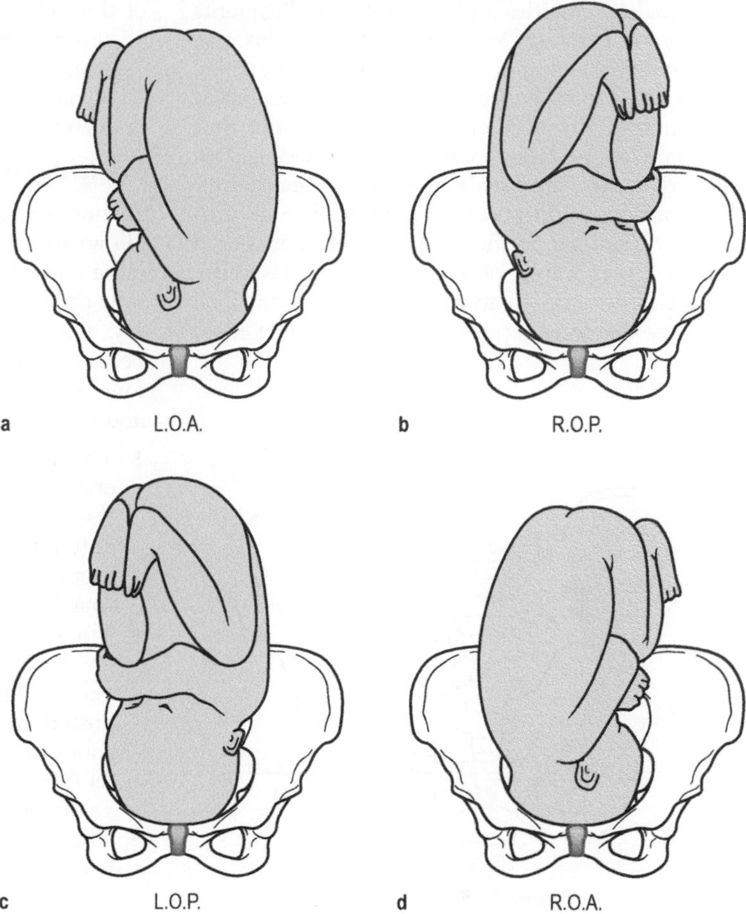

Figure 1.11. *Cephalic presentations: (a) LOA, left occiput-anterior; (b) ROP, right occiput-posterior; (c) LOP, left occiput-posterior; (d) ROP: right occiput-posterior.*

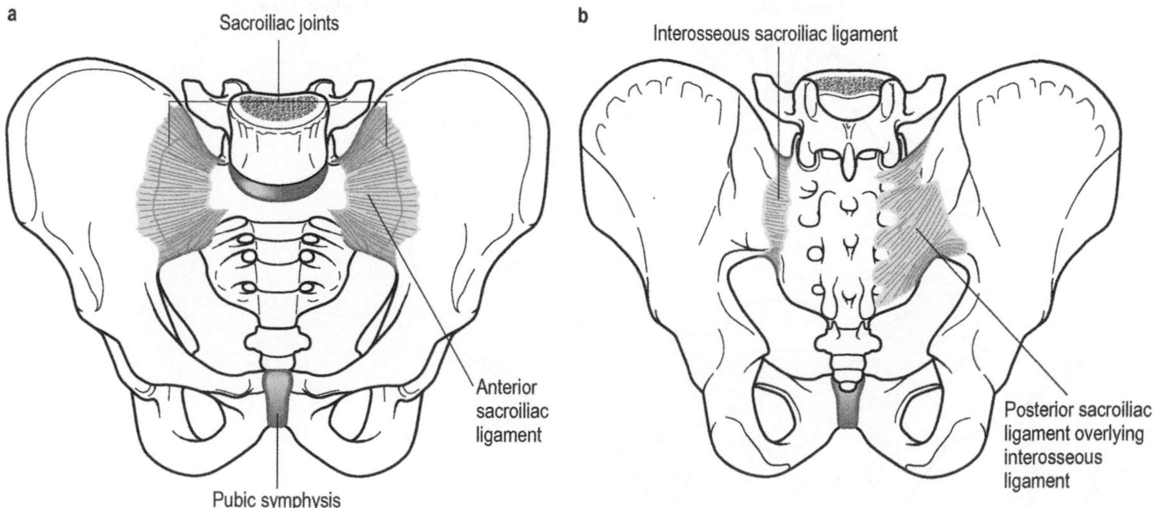

Figure 1.12. *Bony pelvis: (a) anterior view; (b) posterior view.*

the ischial tuberosities and sacrotuberous ligaments laterally, and the inferior ramus of the pubis and pubic symphysis anteriorly. The pelvic outlet may vary in shape according to the position of the coccyx. Furthermore, the elasticity of the ligaments that contribute to the lateral part reduces pelvic rigidity. Three diameters are usually described: anteroposterior, transverse and posterior sagittal. The anteroposterior diameter of the pelvic outlet is measured from the lower margin of the pubic symphysis to the coccygeal apex and is between 9.5 and 11.5 cm. The transverse diameter extends between the inner edges of the ischial tuberosities and averages 11 cm. The posterior sagittal diameter, normally greater than 7.5 cm, is the distance between the tip of the sacrum to a right angle intersection with the transverse diameter.

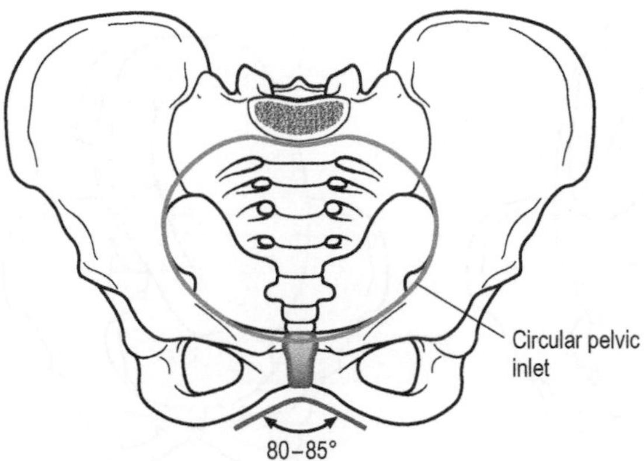

Figure 1.13. *Pelvic inlet.*

Pelvic shapes

A thorough knowledge of the anatomy of the pelvis allows for the understanding of the physiology of labor and how structure affects function, in this case how the pelvic shape determines the route of delivery. Caldwell and Moloy's 1933 classifi cation of pelvic shape, which is still in use today, identifies four variations of the female pelvis: gynecoid, android, anthropoid and platypelloid:[5]

- The gynecoid type is the most frequently encountered. Its transverse pelvic inlet diameter is either equal to or slightly greater than the anteroposterior diameter, and, therefore, the shape of the inlet is either somewhat oval or round.
- The android type, the second most frequently encountered type, presents with an anterior pelvis that is narrow and triangular. The posterior sagittal pelvic inlet diameter is much shorter than the anterior, with less space for the fetal head. This type has a poor prognosis for vaginal delivery.
- The anthropoid type has a more oval shape, with an anteroposterior pelvic inlet diameter that is greater than the transverse diameter.

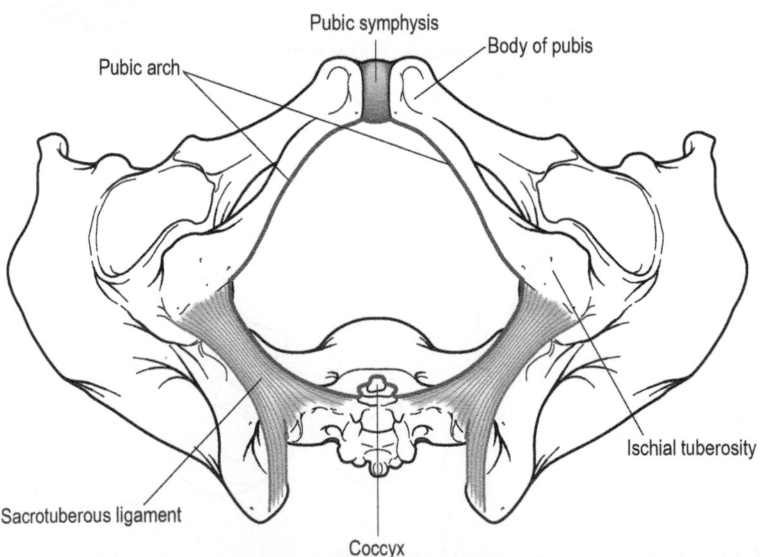

Figure 1.14. *Pelvic outlet.*

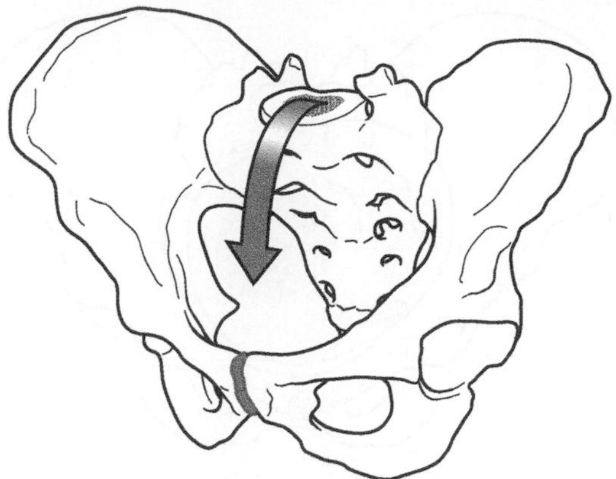

Figure 1.15. *Pelvic movements. Anatomic flexion (craniosacral extension): the sacral base moves anteriorly and the sacral apex moves posteriorly.*

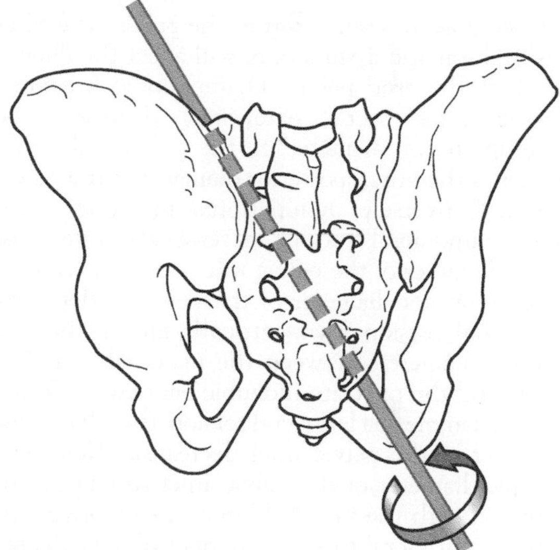

Figure 1.16. *Pelvic movements. Left sacral torsion: sacral rotation to the left on the left oblique axis.*

- The platypelloid type is less frequently encountered and presents a wide transverse pelvic inlet diameter and a short anteroposterior diameter.

Interestingly, the shape of the female pelvis, in addition to the genetic predisposition, appears to be influenced by athletic activities of adolescence, when strenuous physical activities predispose to the android type of pelvis.[6]

Contemporary methods of fetal cephalometry and pelvimetry, as done by MRI, provide a more precise measurement of pelvic dimensions and configuration. This allows the detection of pelvic abnormalities and cephalopelvic disproportion which are risk factors for dystocia.[7] These methods of detection, no matter how sophisticated, augment, but do not replace, the skills of a good osteopathic obstetrician.

Pelvic movements

Pelvic motions have been identified in the general medical literature.[8,9] Sacral motion within the pelvis has been described as nutation and counternutation, motions that in the osteopathic literature are also referred to, respectively, as anatomic flexion (craniosacral extension) and anatomic extension (craniosacral flexion). This opposition of terms between anatomic and craniosacral nomenclature for movement of the sacrum is unfortunate, but it is the terminology that is currently in use; therefore, in order to communicate, in this chapter the anatomic terms employed will be followed, when appropriate, by the respective craniosacral terms in parentheses.

The hypothetical axis of motion for anatomic flexion–extension of the sacrum is a horizontal transverse axis said to pass through the anterior aspect of the sacrum at the level of the second sacral segment.[10] The exact location of such an axis is open to debate, and more than likely altered by the changes in weight distribution that occur during pregnancy.[8]

During anatomic flexion (craniosacral extension), the sacral base moves anteriorly and the sacral apex moves posteriorly (Fig. 1.15). During anatomic extension (craniosacral flexion), the sacral base moves posteriorly and the sacral apex moves anteriorly. The coccygeal bones follow the movement of the sacrum.

The other motions demonstrated by the sacrum are sacral torsions that occur as motion around a hypothetical oblique axis passing from the superior aspect of the sacroiliac articulation on one side to the inferior aspect of the opposite sacroiliac articulation.[11] The oblique axis is named as left or right, determined by the side of its superior point of origin. Sidebending of the spine above establishes the side of the oblique axis. Therefore, spinal sidebending to the right engages the sacral right oblique axis. Sacral torsions – sacral rotation on the oblique axes – are named for the side toward which sacral rotation occurs. Sacral rotation to the left is, therefore, a left torsion. In the absence of dysfunction, the pelvic bones follow the motion of the sacrum. Consequently, following a left sacral torsion, the left pelvic bone exhibits internal rotation while the right pelvic bone externally rotates (Figs 1.16, 3.24).

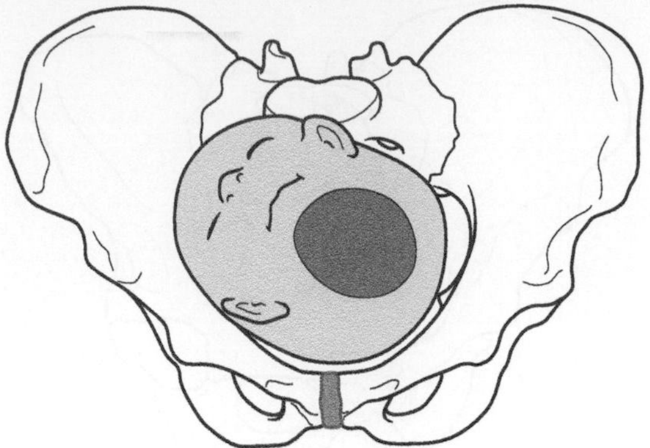

Figure 1.17. *Fetal head entering the pelvic inlet in the left pelvic oblique diameter.*

Craniosacral dysfunction of the pelvis, as well as postural somatic dysfunction, will affect the dimensions of the true pelvis. Dysfunctional anatomic flexion (craniosacral extension) decreases the anteroposterior diameter of the pelvic inlet and increases the anteroposterior diameter of the pelvic outlet. Conversely, dysfunctional anatomic extension (craniosacral flexion) increases the anteroposterior diameter of the pelvic inlet and decreases the anteroposterior diameter of the pelvic outlet. Dysfunctional torsion asymmetrically affects the two oblique diameters between the maternal sacroiliac joints and the opposite iliopubic eminences. In the above example of a left sacral torsion, the left oblique diameter of the pelvic inlet decreases. (*Note*: The oblique diameter of the pelvic inlet should not be confused with the sacral oblique axis.) Conversely, with a right sacral torsion, the right oblique diameter of the pelvic inlet decreases.

This is of great importance in obstetrics, in that it contributes to the ease, or difficulty, of the second phase of labor, and consequently impacts the infant. When the fetal head enters the pelvic inlet, it most commonly does so with its anteroposterior orientation in one of the two pelvic oblique diameters (Fig. 1.17). A sacral torsional dysfunction that decreases one of the oblique diameters will make orientation of the fetal head in that diameter, and consequently the birth process, more difficult.

During pregnancy, relaxation of the pubic symphysis and sacroiliac joints occurs as a result of hormonal changes that peak for relaxin at the 10th to 12th week of gestation.[12] Therefore, motions of the pubic symphysis and sacroiliac joints are facilitated to adapt for stresses caused by the growing uterus, altered weight-bearing mechanics of pregnancy and the impending birth process. In the presence of sacral and lumbar somatic dysfunction, these adaptive changes are restricted and may be the sources of pain during pregnancy and delivery. Anything that impacts the wellbeing of the mother affects the wellbeing of the infant. Osteopathic practice is holistic and must consider the environment of the child, i.e. in this case, the mother.

SOFT TISSUES

The true bony pelvis, when completed by the soft tissues of muscles and fasciae, forms a 'basin'. The pelvic walls and the pelvic floor are parts of the 'basin' and are important guides in the process of engagement and descent of the fetus. Two groups of muscles arise from within the pelvis: the piriformis and obturator internus (Fig. 1.18), and the levator ani and coccygeus (Fig. 1.19).

On each side, the piriformis forms part of the posterolateral wall of the lesser pelvis. It originates from the anterior surface of the sacrum and passes out of the pelvis through the greater sciatic foramen to insert on the greater trochanter of the femur. The two obturator internus muscles form part of the anterolateral wall of the lesser pelvis. They arise from the surface of the obturator membrane and the surrounding parts of the obturator foramen. The fibers converge toward the lesser sciatic foramen and reflect at a right angle around the ischium to insert on the greater trochanter of the femur.

In the absence of somatic dysfunction, the sacrum can be seen as balanced between the two piriformis muscles. During pregnancy, because the position of the developing fetus is asymmetric, the uterus enlarges in an oblique manner. This places asymmetric tension on the sacrum which tends to accommodate by moving into a torsional position. This, in turn, results in greater stress being placed on the piriformis muscle, on the side toward which the sacrum has rotated. Any increase in tension of the piriformis may affect the sciatic nerve. The sciatic nerve leaves the pelvis through the greater sciatic notch and most commonly runs posteriorly below the inferior border of the piriformis.

Pregnant women often complain of back pain, located laterally in the gluteal area and which radiates into the posterior part of the thigh resembling sciatica. However, as the pain does not usually radiate below the knee, and the associated deep tendon reflexes are normal, it cannot be considered as a radicular pathology. Maternal postural imbalance

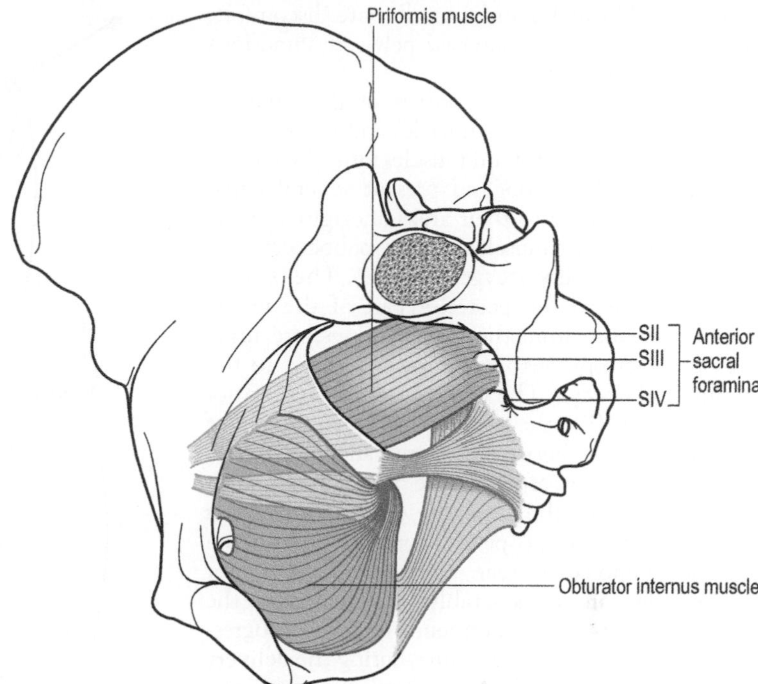

Figure 1.18. *Soft tissues: piriformis and obturator internus muscles.*

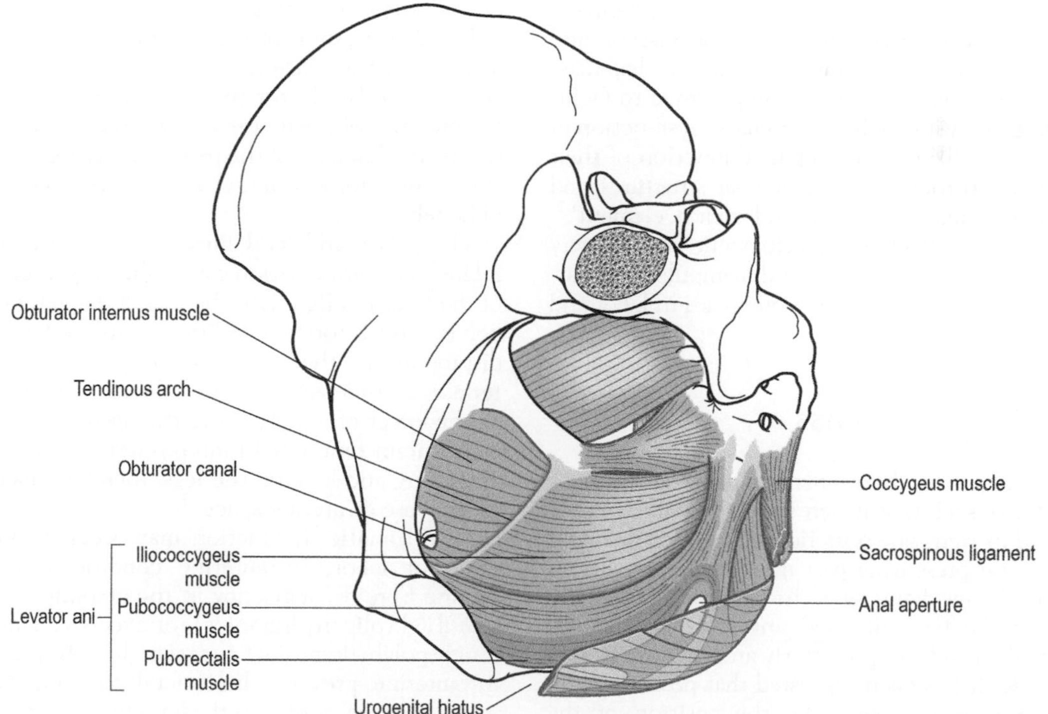

Figure 1.19. *Soft tissues: levator ani and coccygeus muscles.*

should be addressed in order to alleviate discomfort, further knowing that maternal pelvic dysfunctions affect normal parturition.

The pelvic diaphragm consists of the bilateral levator ani and coccygeus muscles and their fasciae (Fig. 1.19). The levator ani muscles form the greater part of the pelvic floor and present several parts, described according to their areas of origin and the relationships of the muscles, i.e. the pubococcygeus, puborectalis and iliococcygeus muscles. The coccygeus muscles form the posterior part of the pelvic diaphragm, arise from the ischial spines, are fused with the sacrospinous ligaments, and insert to the sacrum and coccyx. The central tendinous point of the perineum (i.e. the perineal body) is an area of connective tissue between the anus and the vagina. During parturition, after rupture of the chorioamniotic membranes, the fetal presenting part exerts great pressure on the pelvic floor. The perineum must accommodate or tear. The fibers of the levator ani muscles are considerably stretched and the central portion of the perineum becomes progressively thinner. At the same time, during the delivery process, in the case of a cephalic presentation, the pelvic floor resistance acts as a fulcrum, allowing the fetal head to rotate and extend. In the absence of sufficient rotation, the use of forceps is more likely to be necessary.

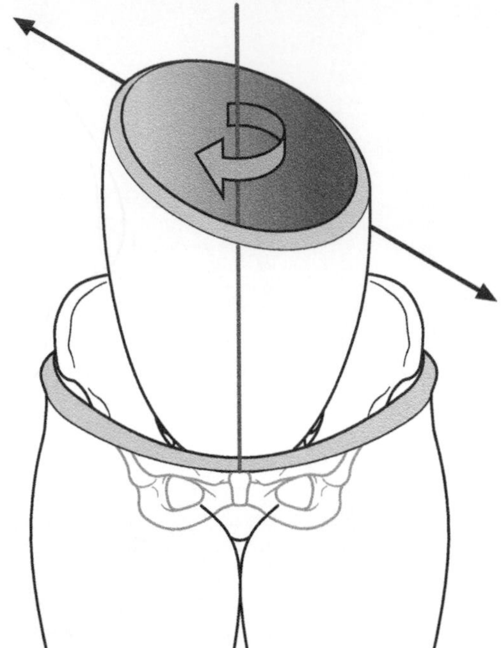

Figure 1.20. *Right rotation of the uterus.*

A functional pelvic floor that should accompany a well-balanced pelvis and intrapelvic viscera, and functional abdominal muscles with a balanced lumbar spine, is of paramount importance to facilitate pregnancy and delivery. Somatic dysfunction of these areas will result in impaired function of their 'skeletal, arthroidal and myofascial structures and related vascular, lymphatic and neural element',[13] and therefore affect the development and delivery of the child. The use of prenatal manipulative treatment of the mother improves outcomes in labor and delivery.[14]

The birth process

Most commonly, the uterus is turned to the right (Fig. 1.20), such that its left side is displaced anteriorly and its right side posteriorly. The long diameter of the fetal presenting part most frequently lies in the left oblique diameter of the pelvic inlet, with the spine of the fetus directed anteriorly and to the maternal left side, or posteriorly and to the maternal right side. It has been suggested that positioning of the uterus is influenced by the position of the descending colon and the sigmoid flexure. Fetal positioning is also thought to be determined by the right-sided location of the maternal liver,[3] but the location of the placenta appears to have no influence.[15] Another factor that affects fetal position is the presence of the iliopsoas muscles that reduce the transverse diameter of the pelvis. In vertex presentations, the iliopsoas muscles direct the fetal head obliquely.

The pelvis and fetal presentation appear to be related. Accommodation causes the largest diameter of the fetus to align with the largest diameter of the pelvis. Under normal conditions, without fetopelvic disproportion, the typical vertex presentation, at term, is considered to be physiologic. It is attributed to the effect of gravity[16] and the need for the fetus to maintain functional limb position by stretching, extending and kicking the legs, therefore maximizing the use of uterine space.[17]

Fetal somatic dysfunction may occur before the onset of labor. Intrauterine conditions such as uterine fibroids, deficiency in the amount of amniotic fluid (oligohydramnios), or excessive amniotic fluid (polyhydramnios) associated with increased intrauterine pressure, limit fetal movements and may, therefore, constrain the fetus in a dysfunctional position. Multiple births may have the same effect, where one fetus applies pressure on the other(s). Intermittent uterine contractions are also source of compression. They increase in force and frequency as gestation advances and augment intrauterine pressure. They also push the fetal head down in the direction of the lower uterine segment and, consequently, the pelvic inlet. The resilience of the fetal tissues usually allows for adaptation to these pressures. When this does not happen, or when the pressure is significant, compression of the fetal head may occur.

Before the onset of labor, the frontoparietal area of the fetal head is particularly vulnerable to compressive forces. The fetus most commonly lies on the maternal left side, i.e. with their back toward the mother's left side. In such cases, the left side of the fetal head is more constrained by the maternal pelvis and lumbar spine than is the right. If the fetus stays in this position for any length of time, the frontoparietal area may remain in contact with part of the bony pelvis, usually the sacral promontory. This can result in the left frontal bone or the left frontoparietal area being compressed by a force that is directed toward the base of the fetal head, with a resultant lower frontal bone and decreased orbital size on that side.

The beginning of labor is defined as the onset of regular, intense, uterine contractions, with dilatation of the cervix. The process of labor is described as three stages:

- the first stage lasts from onset of labor to full dilatation of the cervix
- the second stage ends with the delivery of the child
- the third stage is the time from delivery of the child until the delivery of the placenta.

During these stages, several mechanisms influence the delivery and determine the best route for the fetus to pass through the maternal birth canal.

Accommodation and orientation of the fetal presenting part are two processes that occur during labor to result in normal delivery. Accommodation is the process by which the fetal volume decreases in order to pass through the maternal birth canal. This may occur through changes in the fetal body position or by displacement of fetal body fluids. Orientation is the process by which the fetal presenting part is positioned to best fit the shape of the birth canal.

The increase in frequency and intensity of contractions cause the fetus to move inferiorly and to approach the pelvic inlet. During that time, fetal positional adjustments are constant. It is a dynamic process, with a combination of movements that adapt the fetus to the birth canal. The understanding of these mechanisms of labor, involving a passenger (i.e. the fetus), a passage (i.e. the maternal birth canal) and expulsive forces, is very helpful in appreciating the complexity of somatic dysfunction in the newborn and, therefore, in the future adult.

Molding of the fetal head is another frequently described process of accommodation during labor. Some authors have linked molding depressions with excessive forces applied to the skull through the use of forceps, from digital pressure of the obstetrician's hand, and more commonly from compression of the fetal head on the pubic symphysis or the sacral promontory.[18] As a result of molding during parturition, a displacement of the bones of the calvaria is also commonly described, associated with overlapping of the parietal, frontal and occipital bones at the sutural level. Furthermore, in severe cases, molding has been reported potentially to exert tension on the great cerebral vein to the point of rupture.[2] The classic pattern of overlapping usually described consists of the parietal bones overlapping the frontal and the occipital bones. Of the two parietal bones, the one that receives the greater pressure – always the one lying posteriorly in the pelvis – is said to slide under its counterpart.[19]

Overlapping of the parietal bones at the sagittal suture seems, however, to be less common than usually thought.[20] A locking mechanism in the sutures of the calvaria possibly acts as a protective mechanism for the fetal brain. The dural reciprocal tension membranes may also be part of this locking mechanism. Most often the skull changes shape, demonstrating shortening of the suboccipitobregmatic diameter and a tendency for flattening of the parietal bones.[20] When labor is prolonged, significant stresses can be applied to the dural membranes. Membranous articular strains can result, which, unless treated, persist throughout life, acting as a framework upon which additional dysfunctional mechanisms can arise.

As well as molding, orientational processes occur as mechanisms of labor. These include engagement, descent and expulsion. They occur mainly during the second stage, although engagement may start before the onset of labor, particularly in primigravidae.

ENGAGEMENT

Engagement is defined as the time when the fetal head passes through the pelvic inlet. The biparietal

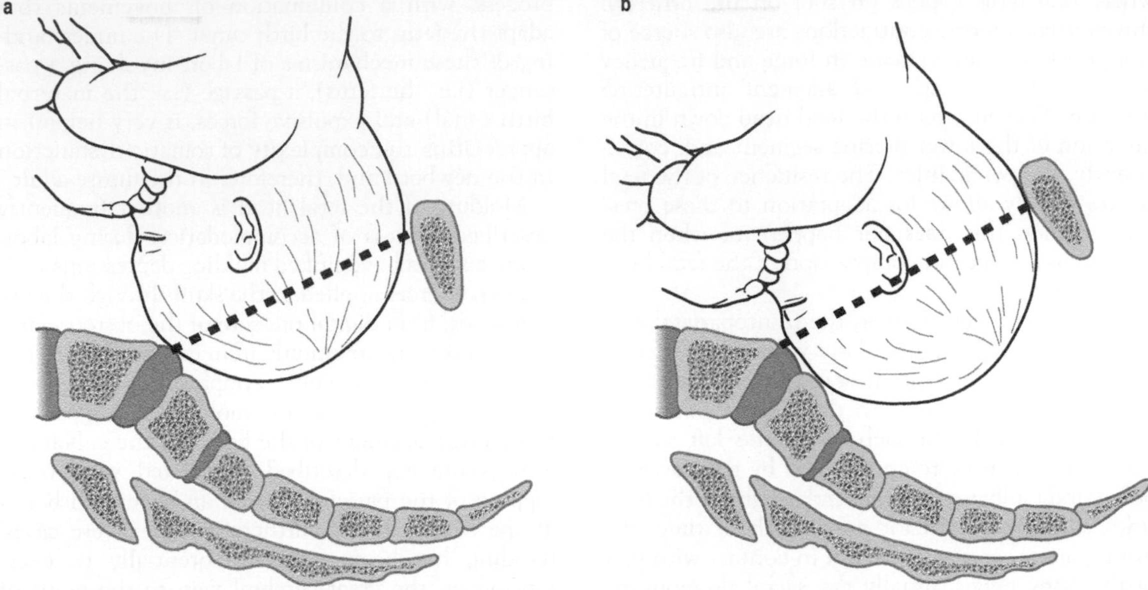

Figure 1.21. *Engagement: (a) head not engaged; (b) head engaged.*

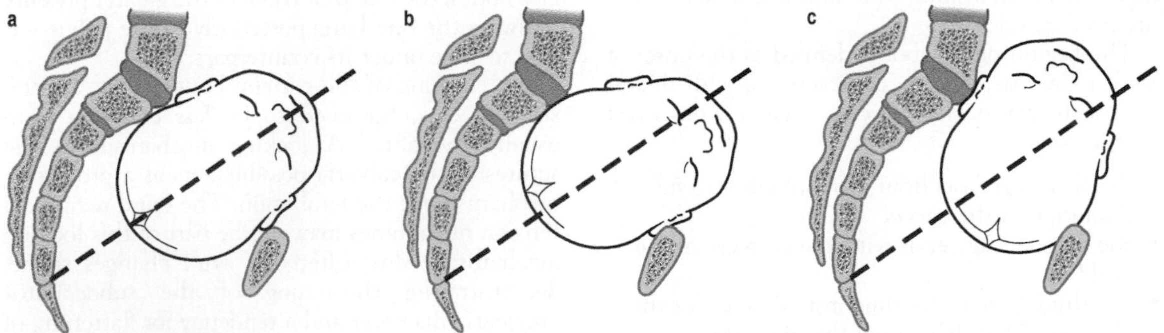

Figure 1.22. *Synclitism and asynclitism: (a) synclitism; (b) anterior asynclitism, fetal head sidebent toward the maternal sacrum; (c) posterior asynclitism, fetal head sidebent toward the maternal pubic symphysis.*

plane, the largest diameter of the normally flexed fetal head, is the reference. The head is engaged when this diameter is below the pelvic inlet (Fig. 1.21). In nulliparous women, engagement usually starts in the last few weeks of pregnancy. It may also occur as late as the beginning of the second stage of labor, as is the case for most multiparous women.

Engagement normally occurs with the fetal sagittal suture aligned in the transverse pelvic diameter, or, more often, in one of the two oblique pelvic diameters. Normal-sized fetuses do not usually orient their heads in the smaller AP diameter. Furthermore, in order to facilitate engagement, the fetal head should be oriented in a direction perpendicular to the plane of the pelvic inlet. This phenomenon is referred to as synclitism (Fig. 1.22a). Consequently, when the head is laterally deflected, asynclitism is present. Asynclitism may be anterior, when the fetal head sidebends toward the maternal sacrum (Fig. 1.22b), the sagittal suture is closer to the sacrum and the anterior parietal bone closer to the pubic symphysis is palpable intravaginally. Posterior asynclitism occurs when the fetal head sidebends toward the maternal pubic symphysis (Fig. 1.22c) and the posterior parietal bone is palpable intravaginally. Although moderate asynclitism is usual, a greater degree of asynclitism may be a cause for a difficult engagement, resulting in fetopelvic disproportion.

Asynclitism also causes a greater amount of pressure to one side of the calvaria, with the resultant potential for cranial dysfunction. A sidebending–rotation of the sphenobasilar synchondrosis (SBS) on the side of the pressure on the parietal bone may result, with an associated sidebending of the craniocervical junction and cervical spine. This pressure may also produce an intraosseous dysfunction of the homolateral temporal bone and associated temporomandibular structures. Under normal circumstances, the fetal head will move from anterior to posterior asynclitism alternatively, like the clapper of a bell, in order to progress toward the direction of the pelvic outlet.

DESCENT

Increased uterine contractions push the fetus inferiorly. Cervical flexion causes the chin of the fetus to be brought into contact with their sternum. This is part of the accommodation process. Consequently, the shortest diameter of the fetal head, the suboccipito-bregmatic diameter, becomes the presenting diameter, and facilitates better passage through the birth canal. Normally internal rotation follows. (*Note*: In this instance, the term internal rotation refers to a rotation of the fetus that occurs inside the pelvic cavity, whereas external rotation refers to a fetal rotation that occurs outside the pelvic cavity. These terms are used in the context of obstetrics and have a different meaning from the one used in the rest of this book.)

After engagement of the fetal head, failure to progress further, or lack of fetal descent, may occur. Either malposition of the fetal head or ineffective uterine contractions is usually responsible. Malposition of the fetal head may arise, for instance, from a brow presentation with resultant increase in the head circumference. In such circumstances, the fetus is compressed against the maternal pelvis in response to the contractions of the uterine fundus putting pressure on the breech. The compressive forces are transmitted along the fetal spine to the cranial base and skull, against the resistance of the maternal pelvis. Some areas are, therefore, placed under stress. The stress may be localized to the anterior part of the fetal calvaria and may produce a vertical strain or frontal bone dysfunction, with compression of the frontoethmoidal suture. A sphenobasilar compression dysfunction may result if the pressure is applied in the direction of the AP diameter of the fetal head. The craniocervical junction and the upper thoracic area may also be placed under stress, resulting in somatic dysfunction and associated parasympathetic and sympathetic hyperactivity, respectively. Normally, in vertex presentation, with an anterior-occiput engagement, the descent that follows is easier and more rapid.

In the process of descent, the fetus will have to turn their head when approaching the pubic symphysis to align the sagittal suture along the AP diameter of the pelvic outlet. This process is called internal rotation. With the progression of the presentation inferiorly, the maternal coccyx is pushed posteriorly. This increases the tension of the pelvic floor and normally results in a greater amount of resistance posteriorly. As such, the levator ani muscles, together with the surrounding tissues, which are shaped like a gutter, act as a fulcrum and a guide for the fetal head. The internal rotation that is essential to achieve delivery may occur at this time, if it has not already happened. The contribution of the muscles of the pelvic floor to this process is significant. First, they provide sufficient support to resist the pressure of the fetal head, and therefore serve as a guide to direct the head anteriorly towards the vulva. Second, the muscles of the pelvic floor must relax to allow the expulsion of the presenting part. A hypotonic pelvic floor does not provide sufficient resistance, nor can it effectively serve as a fulcrum and guide during this stage of the delivery process. Other means, such as the use of forceps, may be necessary to assist the rotation of the head. On the other hand, a hypertonic pelvic floor does not allow the necessary relaxation at the time of expulsion, and episiotomy may be required to avoid perineal tear.

After being guided anteriorly through the mother's true pelvis, the base of the occiput is pushed under the inferior margin of the pubic symphysis (Fig. 1.23). The vulvar outlet is oriented anteriorly and superiorly. As a result, the fetal cervical spine and craniocervical junction must change from an attitude of flexion to an attitude of extension in order for the fetal head to pass through it. Extension of the cervical spine and passage of the head under the pubic symphysis are significant points during delivery, as this is the time when cranial dysfunction may develop. The pubic symphysis acts as a fulcrum for the craniocervical junction that turns around it. A significant amount of this extension takes place at the level of the condyles of the occiput. They have to move forward on the atlantal articular surfaces to provoke extension of the craniocervical junction. In so doing, an extension dysfunction

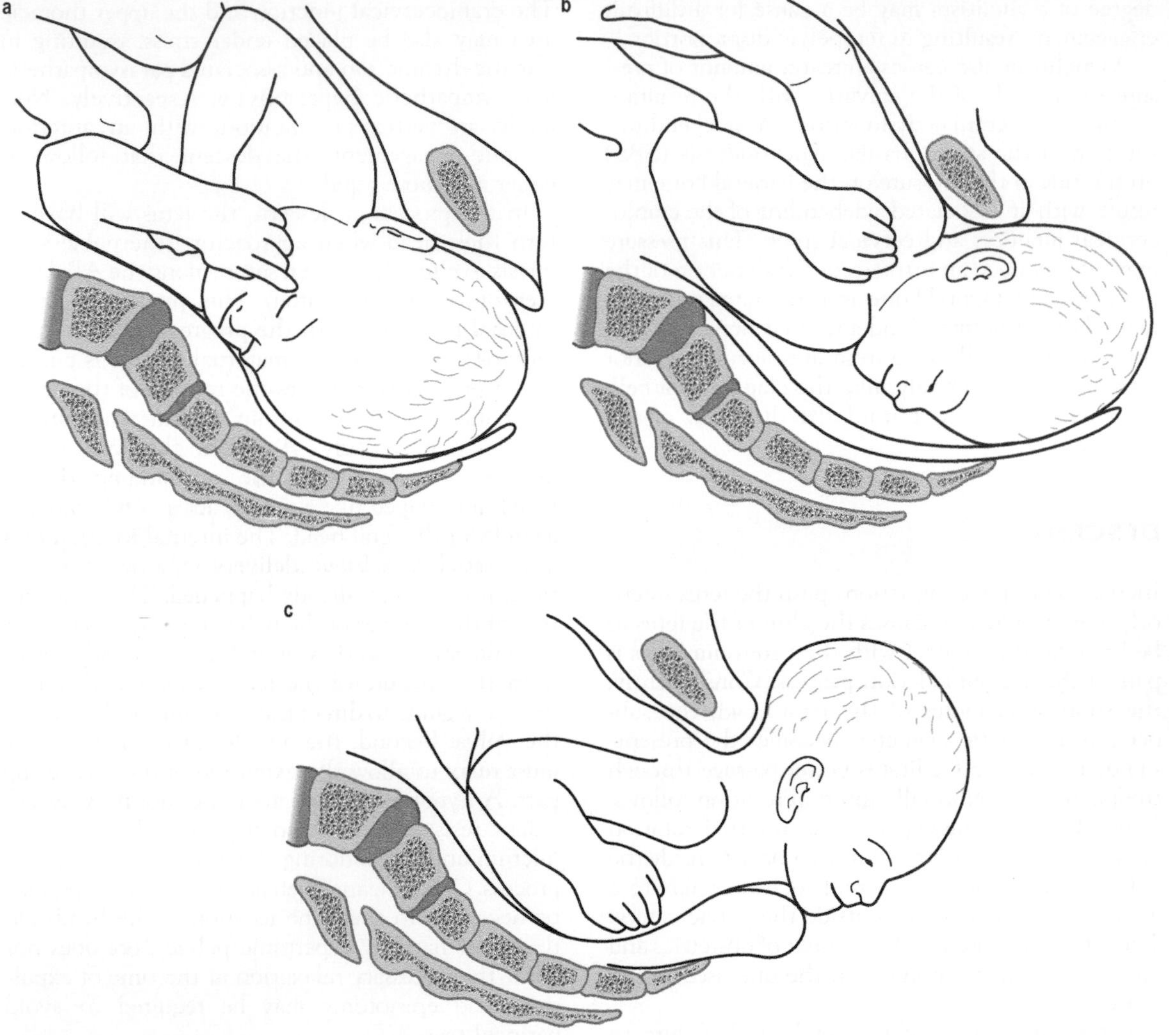

Figure 1.23. *Passage of the head under the pubic symphysis.*

between the occiput and the atlas may develop. The extension may also take place in the synchondroses of the cranial base. The posterior intraoccipital cartilaginous synchondrosis participates in the extension. When the resilience of the tissue is overwhelmed, this can produce an intraosseous dysfunction within the occiput.

Most of the time extension of the head does not occur in the pure sagittal plane, but rather in association with lesser or greater amounts of rotation and sidebending. Consequently, the resultant dysfunctions may be asymmetric, with one occipital condyle being more compressed than the other, or one side of the squamous occiput being more anterior, superior or inferior to the other. This, in turn, may be the foundation for future axial skeletal disorders such as plagiocephaly or scoliosis.

Gradually, and with further extension of the occiput, the head will emerge from the pelvis. The forehead, the nose, the mouth and the chin will appear after sliding along the perineal gutter. This sequence may be another cause of cranial somatic dysfunction, particularly if the maternal coccyx is anteriorly hooked. At this time the forces applied to the forehead and the facial skeleton are directed inferiorly, toward the fetal chin, and may result in vertical strain of the SBS or other dysfunctional patterns involving the frontal bone and/or the facial bones. The areas of the frontoethmoidal and frontonasal sutures, as well as the maxillae, are particularly vulnerable. Once again, these motions, as they occur during the delivery process, and, consequently, any resultant dysfunction, are never perfectly symmetrical.

When the head is delivered occiput anterior, it declines anteriorly, with the newborn's chin close to the maternal anal area. The next phase of the delivery process consists of the restitution of the head to its original rotation. In an LOA presentation, the head rotates to face the right maternal thigh. This restitution results in an external rotation that positions the infant's head in the transverse diameter of the maternal pelvis, and an internal rotation of the fetal trunk. The shoulders usually enter the pelvic inlet in the oblique diameter opposite to the one in which the head entered. Therefore, during delivery, the global motion of the body follows a dynamic spiral. There is a limit to the resilience of the fetal tissues, however, and during the process of producing the external rotation this limit may be exceeded. As a consequence, dysfunction that develops during this period may result in the establishment of a torsional pattern between the pectoral and pelvic girdles. This is a global pattern involving the whole body – fasciae, membranes, muscles and joints included. Interestingly, this pattern is quite frequently encountered with newborn babies.

EXPULSION

Once the shoulders are engaged in the pelvic inlet, the bisacromial diameter must fit the AP diameter of the pelvic outlet. The anterior shoulder is expelled as it passes under the pubic symphysis and then the posterior shoulder is delivered (Fig. 1.24). After the shoulders, the rest of the body follows. Difficulty at the time of delivery of the shoulders can result in myofascial and ligamentous articular strain in the cervical and upper thoracic regions. In severe cases this can result in brachial plexus injury and clavicular fractures.

A child delivered in the LOA presentation may demonstrate a flattening of the area between the brow and the anterior fontanelle, and, typically, an asymmetric vault, with one parietal bone (the one located on the presenting side) being more arched, while the opposite parietal bone is more flattened. Asynclitism further increases the pressure of the infant's head against the pelvic bones. If the right side of the infant's occipital bone is in contact with the maternal pubic symphysis while the left frontal bone is against the sacrum, it will result in occipital flattening on the right and frontal flattening on the left. The reverse – occipital flattening on the left and frontal flattening on the right – would follow the LOP position. At the end of the descent, the head contacts the pelvic floor and turns in such a way as to position the occiput under the pubic symphysis. In the occiput-anterior position, the right side of the occiput, eventually the occipitomastoid area, can be exposed to greater pressure. Later, during expulsion, compressive forces may be applied to both sides of the occipital bone by the pubic symphysis.

In the presence of calvarial molding, the presenting part, which is the lowest, is usually forced out, and is cone shaped (Fig. 1.25). In an LOA presentation, the apex of the cone is commonly the postero-

Figure 1.24. *Expulsion of the shoulders.*

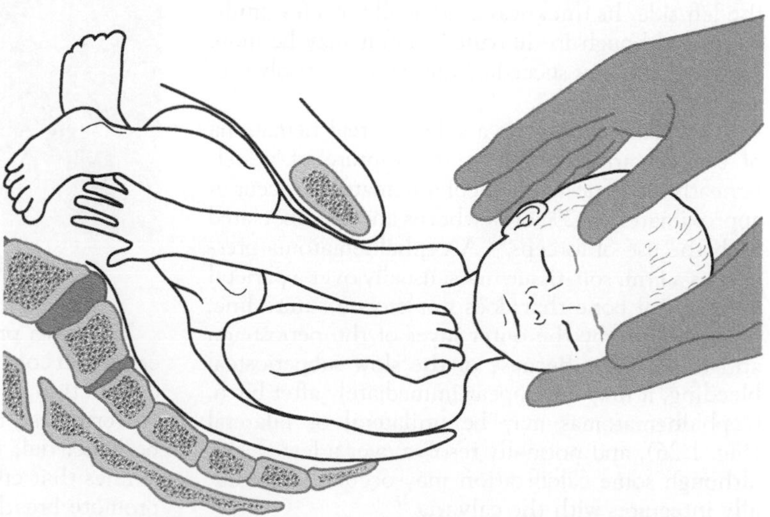

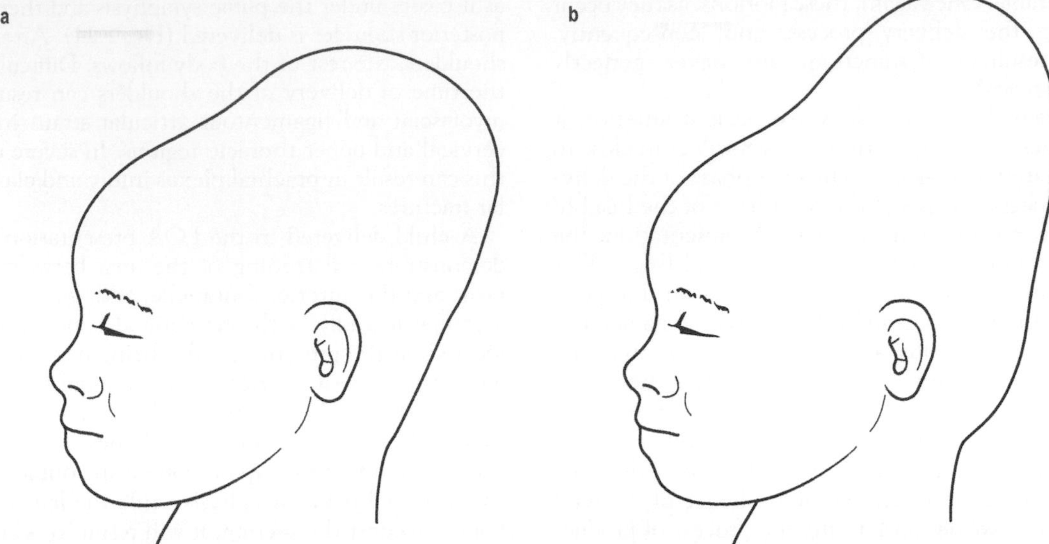

Figure 1.25. *Calvarial molding: (a) occiput-anterior presentation; (b) occiput-posterior presentation.*

superior (or occipital) angle of the right parietal bone, at the lambda. This is frequently the location of caput succedaneum and of cephalhematoma. Caput succedaneum, a serosanguineous fluid collection above the periosteum, results from the changes in the pressure to which the presenting portion of the scalp is subjected. The swelling occurs on the posterior and superior part of the vault. In an LOA presentation, it is on the right side, but may extend across suture lines; in an ROA presentation, it is on the left side. Its thickness is generally of a few millimeters, although in difficult labors it may be more significant. Caput succedaneum typically resolves in a few days.

A cephalhematoma is a subperiosteal hematoma of the calvaria, caused by the rupture of vessels beneath the periosteum. Cephalhematomas occur in approximately 1–2% of newborns and are associated with the use of forceps.[21] A cephalhematoma presents as a firm, soft-tissue mass, usually over a parietal or occipital bone that does not cross a suture line, being limited by the outer layer of the periosteum and the sutures. Because of the slow subperiosteal bleeding, it may not appear immediately after birth. Cephalhematomas may be unilateral or bilateral (Fig. 1.26), and normally resolve over a few weeks, although some calcification may occur that gradually integrates with the calvaria.[21]

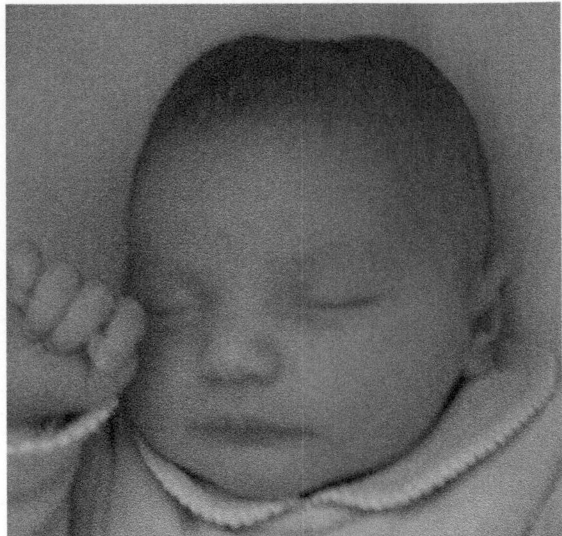

Figure 1.26. *Cephalhematomas.*

The birth process, through normal vaginal delivery, when considered as a potential source for cranial dysfunction, may appear as an undesirable life event. Nevertheless, the stress of being born is thought to be beneficial, through the production of catecholamines that enhance the infant's ability to survive, promote breathing, speed up the metabolic rate at birth and increase blood flow to vital organs.[22] This stressful process also appears to be beneficial to the child's health in assisting the development of their immune system.[23]

DYSTOCIA

Dystocia means difficult childbirth, as compared to eutocia, i.e. normal labor. Dystocia most often results from a combination of fetal and pelvic dynamics. Maternal pelvic structures are of paramount importance, as addressed by Still: 'The first duty of the obstetrician is to carefully examine the bones of the pelvis and spine of the mother, to ascertain if they are normal in shape and position.'[24] During fetal engagement, in order to increase the pelvic inlet diameter, the sacral base should move posteriorly in anatomic extension (craniosacral flexion) while the sacral apex moves anteriorly. During the phase of expulsion, in order to increase the pelvic outlet diameter, the coccyx and apex of the sacrum should move posteriorly and the sacral base anteriorly, i.e. anatomic flexion (craniosacral extension). The need for sacral mobility has always been recognized.[25]

Somatic dysfunction or disproportions in the maternal pelvis may be responsible for dystocia by influencing the fetal position during labor. A dysfunctional pattern of uterine contraction may follow, with the need for increased use of oxytocin, establishing a vicious cycle that ends with the need for the performance of a cesarean section.[26]

Over the years, in order to deliver their babies, women have tried various positions, such as squatting, sitting on birthing chairs or lying down. The dorsal lithotomy position, where the mother is lying on her back with her buttocks at the end of the delivery table, her hips and knees flexed, and her legs or feet supported and strapped into stirrups, is typical. This position may increase the pelvic outlet diameter by 1.5–2 cm, but at the same time the posterior displacement of the sacral base, in anatomic extension (craniosacral flexion), may be restricted by the resistance of the table. Furthermore, this position is less efficient for pushing. Women should be advised to change position during labor as needed and, if possible, to give birth in the position that they find most comfortable. This may facilitate sacral positional release and, therefore, facilitate delivery.

Occiput-posterior presentation

All vertex presentations follow the same principles and mechanics as occiput-anterior presentations. Occiput-posterior presentations, either right occiput-posterior (ROP) or left occiput-posterior (LOP), represent 15% of all presentations.[27] They may be associated with prolonged stages of labor. Internal rotation of the fetal head is greater. The fetal head has to turn 135° in order for the occiput to move from a posterior position, adjacent to one of the maternal sacroiliac joints, to an anterior position near the pubic symphysis.

The position of caput succedaneum, when present, reflects the position of the presentation. In ROP presentations, it is located on the anterosuperior angle of the left parietal bone, but may extend across the coronal suture. In LOP presentations caput succedaneum is to be found on the anterosuperior angle of the right parietal bone, with frequent overlapping of the coronal suture.

In some instances, the head will not turn, leading to a persistent occiput-posterior presentation. However, in 62% of persistent occiput-posterior presentations, sonography at the onset of labor has demonstrated that the initial presentation is an occiput-anterior position followed by a malrotation during labor.[27] Persistent occiput-posterior presentation is associated with induction of labor, use of oxytocin to increase labor and epidural use.[28,29] Additionally, persistent occiput-posterior presentation is related to greater risk of poor neonatal outcome, including birth trauma, when compared to occiput-anterior presentation.[30] With persistent occiput-posterior presentation, operative deliveries are more frequent, and spontaneous vaginal delivery in nulliparas occurs in only 26% of cases.[29]

Breech presentation

Breech presentation at term occurs in about 3% of all deliveries,[31] and prematurity is a risk factor.[3] Term breech presentation is less frequent because of the increased practice of external fetal version at 37 weeks' gestation. External version should be performed in a setting in which the fetus can be monitored and only by physicians familiar with this procedure. In this instance, having skilled osteopathic touch and an appreciation for the use of indirect manipulative techniques can be a significant advantage. External version should never be forced: the umbilical cord may be too short, or it may be coiled around the neck, therefore not allowing fetal version.

Breech presentation is classified according to the location of the fetal sacrum, i.e. left sacroanterior, which is the most frequent, right sacroanterior, right sacroposterior or left sacroposterior. Further, according to the position of the fetal legs, breech presentations may be complete when the legs are flexed (see Fig. 1.9) or incomplete when the legs are extended (see Fig. 1.10). During engagement and descent the principles and mechanics described for vertex presentations apply.

During delivery, when the breech reaches the pubis, the fetal trunk sidebends, followed by the delivery of the hips. This may be the cause of articular or intraosseous somatic dysfunction for the infant, including hip, pelvic bone, and sacrum or lumbar spine dysfunctions. Expulsion of the head in the occiput-anterior position occurs, with the fetal chin, mouth, nose and forehead sliding along the anterior surfaces of the maternal sacrum and coccyx. This can produce facial dysfunction, particularly affecting the maxillae, frontonasal and frontoethmoidal sutures.

The outcomes for breech deliveries are controversial. Vaginal delivery of term infants presenting as breech, when compared to infants delivered by elective cesarean section, demonstrates greater risks of neonatal mortality and morbidity.[32,33] On the other hand, a higher risk of maternal complications has been correlated with cesarean delivery without corresponding improvement in neonatal outcomes.[31]

Face presentation

Face presentations are associated with a hyperextension of the fetal cervical spine. The occiput is positioned contacting the fetal back and the presenting part is the chin (mentum). Four varieties of face presentation exist. The two mentum posterior presentations, with the fetal brow being compacted against the maternal pubic symphysis, and resultant diffi cult labor, require cesarean section. The two mentum anterior presentations may deliver vaginally, but usually with signifi cant molding of the fetal skull. Swelling and edema of the facial tissues are typically present and change the appearance of the face (Fig. 1.27). Cranial somatic dysfunction is common and affects the cervical spine, particularly the occipitoatlantal joint, and the viscerocranium.

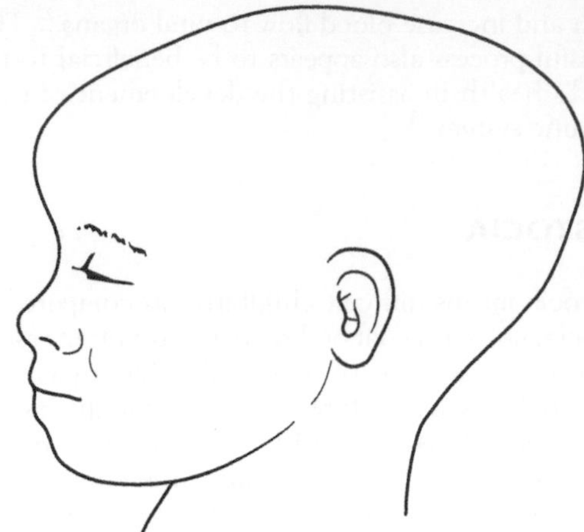

Figure 1.27. *Calvarial molding: face presentation.*

Shoulder dystocia

The incidence of shoulder dystocia varies from 0.2 to 3% of all deliveries.[34,35] Changes in fetal body with increasing birth weight disproportion between the fetal shoulders and the maternal pelvis, significantly greater shoulder-to-head and chest-to-head disproportions and increased bisacromial diameters are commonly described risk factors. During fetal descent, the posterior fetal shoulder may be forced against the maternal sacral promontory. After delivery of the head, the anterior shoulder may be lodged against the maternal pubic bones. Deliveries with associated shoulder dystocia necessitate the use of specifi c maneuvers to release the impacted shoulders: the McRoberts' maneuver reorients the pelvis by pushing the mother's knees to her chest, the Barnum maneuver delivers the posterior shoulder fi rst and other procedures attempt to release the shoulders by maneuvering the fetal trunk.

Delivery with shoulder dystocia can result in significant neonatal morbidity, including asphyxia and trauma. Shoulder dystocia is associated with a second stage of labor greater than 2 hours' duration and an increased need for operative vaginal delivery.[36] In the process of delivery, traction applied to the neonate may introduce significant sidebending, with the potential for obstruction of the venous return from the head. Intracranial hemorrhage and anoxia may result.

Traction applied to the head may also be responsible for brachial plexus injury, most often affecting the right arm in cases of LOA presentations. Greenstick fracture of the clavicle may also occur. The forces responsible for these injuries will also readily result in somatic dysfunction of the upper thoracic area, associated ribs, pectoral girdle and cervicothoracic junction.

Forceps delivery

Forceps deliveries are completed in 5–10% of deliveries.[37] The use of forceps may be an aid to the mother who is exhausted or in whom anesthesia prevents spontaneous delivery. Forceps may also be indicated by fetal conditions, such as bradycardia and malposition.[38,39] Although associated with neonatal complications, including facial nerve palsy, skull fractures and intracranial hemorrhage, the use of forceps is described as a fairly safe procedure in the hands of experienced practitioners.[39,40]

The use of forceps may, however, be a potential source for cranial dysfunctions. Compressive forces that are applied through the forceps blades may be slight or of greater intensity. In delivery of the head, pulling forces are also involved. These pulling forces are rarely directed in a straight line, and membranous dysfunction, reflecting the combination of compression and traction, may result. The forceps blades are usually set up on each side of the head and the areas of contact may demonstrate cranial dysfunction. The frontal bone, the greater wings of the sphenoid, the zygomatic bones and the temporomandibular joints may be involved.

Vacuum extraction

Vacuum extraction is another alternative when instrumentation is needed to assist vaginal delivery. Although various devices are available, most of the time a soft suction cup is applied to the scalp. Negative pressure is raised while the cap is held on the head. Traction is then applied to deliver the head. Vacuum extraction may be indicated to assist in the delivery of an infant when the mother is exhausted or when anesthesia results in the inability to deliver spontaneously. It may also assist in addressing fetal malposition.

Both forceps and vacuum extraction present advantages and disadvantages. Vacuum extraction appears to be less traumatic for the mother, but is associated with a greater incidence of subarachnoid hemorrhage and cephalhematoma than forceps deliveries.[41]

Instrumental vaginal deliveries sometimes result in scalp laceration. The underlying structures, the bones of the calvaria and the cranial membranes may also be subject to stress. Extracting forces most often affect one side, with resultant asymmetry in the pattern of the parietal bones. The cranial membranes are stretched. The falx cerebri and tentorium cerebelli may be placed under significant strain, possibly transmitted to the spinal dura mater, and, through the connection of the spinal dura mater, from the occiput to the sacrum. Dysfunction of the cranial and spinal membranes may follow.

Epidural anesthesia

Lumbar epidural block is used in 80% of vaginal deliveries for relief of pain in labor.[42] An epidural catheter is introduced under local anesthesia at the L2–L3 or L3–L4 interspace. Normally, when correctly applied, epidural anesthesia eases the pain from cervical dilatation without influencing uterine contractions, and later, when delivery is imminent, it produces a perineal anesthesia. However, epidural anesthesia in some instances may slow the labor, with a decrease in abdominal pushing and relaxation of the pelvic floor. It may also predispose to incomplete fetal internal rotation during the descent. Epidural anesthesia has been associated with an increased incidence of occiput-posterior presentation[43] and with the need for the physician to employ more force to deliver the fetus.[42]

REFERENCES

1. Arbuckle BE. The selected writings of Beryl E. Arbuckle, D.O., F.A.C.O.P. Newark OH: American Academy of Osteopathy; 1971:179.
2. Williams PL (ed). Gray's anatomy, 38th edn. Edinburgh: Churchill Livingstone; 1995.
3. Lansac J, Body G. Pratique de l'accouchement. Paris: SIMEP; 1988.
4. Vrahas M, Hern TC, Diangelo D, Kellam J, Tile M. Ligamentous contributions to pelvic stability. Orthopedics 1995;18(3):271–4.
5. Caldwell WE, Moloy HC. Anatomical variations in the female pelvis and their effect in labor with a suggested classification. Am J Obstet Gynecol 1933;26:479–505.
6. Abitbol MM. The shapes of the female pelvis. Contributing factors. J Reprod Med 1996;41(4):242–50.
7. Sporri S, Thoeny HC, Raio L, Lachat R, Vock P, Schneider H. MR imaging pelvimetry: a useful adjunct in the treatment of women at risk for dystocia? AJR Am J Roentgenol 2002;179(1):137–44.
8. Weisl H. The movements of the sacroiliac joint. Acta Anat (Basel) 1955;23(1):80–91.
9. Colachis SC Jr, Worden RE, Bechtol CO, Strohm BR. Movement of the sacroiliac joint in the adult male: a preliminary report. Arch Phys Med Rehabil 1963;44:490–8.
10. Glossary of Osteopathic Terminology. In: Ward RC (ed). Foundations for osteopathic medicine, 2nd edn. Philadelphia: Lippincott, Williams & Wilkins; 2003:1246.
11. Mitchell FL Sr. Structural pelvic function. Academy of Applied Osteopathy (American Academy of Osteopathy). Yearbook 1965;2:186.
12. Kristiansson P, Svardsudd K, von Schoultz B. Serum relaxin, symphyseal pain, and back pain during pregnancy. Am J Obstet Gynecol 1996;175(5):1342–7.
13. Glossary of Osteopathic Terminology. In: Ward RC (ed). Foundations for osteopathic medicine, 2nd edn. Philadelphia: Lippincott, Williams & Wilkins; 2003:1249.
14. King HH, Tettambel MA, Lockwood MD, Johnson KH, Arsenault DA, Quist R. Osteopathic manipulative treatment in prenatal care: a retrospective case control design study. J Am Osteopath Assoc 2003;103(12):577–82.
15. Ververs IA, De Vries JI, van Geijn HP, Hopkins B. Prenatal head position from 12–38 weeks. II. The effects of fetal orientation and placental localization. Early Hum Dev 1994;39(2):93–100.
16. Sekulic SR. Possible explanation of cephalic and noncephalic presentation during pregnancy: a theoretical approach. Med Hypotheses 2000;55(5):429–34.

17. Clarren SK, Smith DW. Congenital deformities. Pediatr Clin North Am 1977;24:665–7.
18. Axton JH, Levy LF. Congenital molding depressions of the skull. Br Med J 1965;5451:1644–7.
19. Magoun HI. Osteopathy in the cranial field, 2nd edn. Kirksville, MO: The Journal Printing Company; 1966:218.
20. Carlan SJ, Wyble L, Lense J, Mastrogiannis DS, Parsons MT. Fetal head molding. Diagnosis by ultrasound and a review of the literature. J Perinatol 1991;11(2):105–11.
21. Glass RB, Fernbach SK, Norton KI, Choi PS, Naidich TP. The infant skull: a vault of information. Radiographics 2004;24(2):507–22.
22. Lagercrantz H, Slotkin TA. The 'stress' of being born. Sci Am 1986;254(4):100–7.
23. Thilaganathan B, Meher-Homji N, Nicolaides KH. Labor: an immunologically beneficial process for the neonate. Am J Obstet Gynecol 1994;171(5):1271–2.
24. Still AT. The philosophy and mechanical principles of osteopathy. Kirksville, MO: Osteopathic Enterprise; 1986:312.
25. Dunn PM. Henrick van Deventer (1651–1724) and the pelvic birth canal. Arch Dis Child Fetal Neonatal Ed 1998;79(2):F157–8.
26. Compton AA. Soft tissue and pelvic dystocia. Clin Obstet Gynecol 1987;30(1):69–76.
27. Gardberg M, Laakkonen E, Salevaara M. Intrapartum sonography and persistent occiput posterior position: a study of 408 deliveries. Obstet Gynecol 1998;91(5 Pt 1):746–9.
28. Fitzpatrick M, McQuillan K, O'Herlihy C. Influence of persistent occiput posterior position on delivery outcome. Obstet Gynecol 2001;98(6):1027–31.
29. Ponkey SE, Cohen AP, Heffner LJ, Lieberman E. Persistent fetal occiput posterior position: obstetric outcomes. Obstet Gynecol 2003;101(5 Pt 1):915–20.
30. Cheng YW, Shaffer BL, Caughey AB. The association between persistent occiput posterior position and neonatal outcomes. Obstet Gynecol 2006;107(4):837–44.
31. Sanchez-Ramos L, Wells TL, Adair CD, Arcelin G, Kaunitz AM, Wells DS. Route of breech delivery and maternal and neonatal outcomes. Int J Gynaecol Obstet 2001;73(1):7–14.
32. Roman J, Bakos O, Cnattingius S. Pregnancy outcomes by mode of delivery among term breech births: Swedish experience 1987–1993. Obstet Gynecol 1998;92(6):945–50.
33. Rietberg CC, Elferink-Stinkens PM, Brand R, van Loon AJ, Van Hemel OJ, Visser GH. Term breech presentation in The Netherlands from 1995 to 1999: mortality and morbidity in relation to the mode of delivery of 33824 infants. BJOG 2003;110(6):604–9.
34. Gherman RB. Shoulder dystocia: prevention and management. Obstet Gynecol Clin North Am 2005;32(2):297–305, x.
35. Ouzounian JG, Gherman RB. Shoulder dystocia: are historic risk factors reliable predictors? Am J Obstet Gynecol 2005;192(6):1933–5; discussion 1935–8.
36. Mehta SH, Bujold E, Blackwell SC, Sorokin Y, Sokol RJ. Is abnormal labor associated with shoulder dystocia in nulliparous women? Am J Obstet Gynecol 2004;190(6):1604–7; discussion 1607–9.
37. Chamberlain G, Steer P. ABC of labour care: operative delivery. BMJ 1999;318(7193):1260–4.
38. Patel RR, Murphy DJ. Forceps delivery in modern obstetric practice. BMJ 2004;328(7451):1302–5.
39. Roshan DF, Petrikovsky B, Sichinava L, Rudick BJ, Rebarber A, Bender SD. Soft forceps. Int J Gynaecol Obstet 2005;88(3):249–52.
40. Gardella C, Taylor M, Benedetti T, Hitti J, Critchlow C. The effect of sequential use of vacuum and forceps for assisted vaginal delivery on neonatal and maternal outcomes. Am J Obstet Gynecol 2001;185(4):896–902.
41. Wen SW, Liu S, Kramer MS, Marcoux S, Ohlsson A, Sauve R, Liston R. Comparison of maternal and infant outcomes between vacuum extraction and forceps deliveries. Am J Epidemiol 2001;153(2):103–7.
42. Poggi SH, Allen RH, Patel C, Deering SH, Pezzullo JC, Shin Y, Spong CY. Effect of epidural anaesthesia on clinician-applied force during vaginal delivery. Am J Obstet Gynecol 2004;191(3):903–6.
43. Sizer AR, Nirmal DM. Occipitoposterior position: associated factors and obstetric outcome in nulliparas. Obstet Gynecol 2000;96(5 Pt 1):749–52.

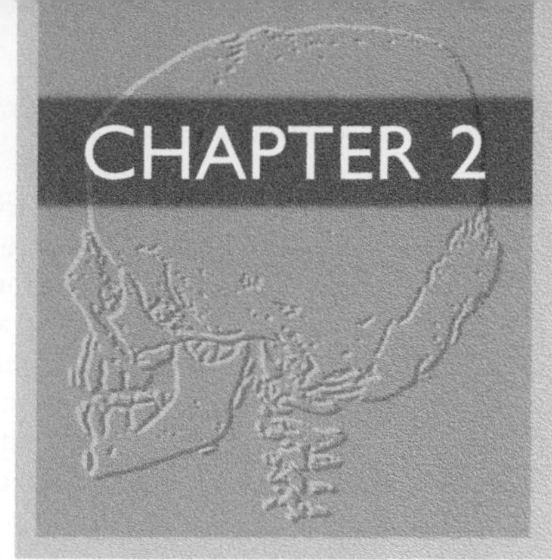

NORMAL GROWTH AND DEVELOPMENT OF THE CHILD

The term growth is usually employed to describe the increase in the size of the total body or one region of the body, while the term development commonly refers to changes in function in a broad sense, comprising musculoskeletal functions as well as any function under the influence of environmental, emotional or social conditions.

The skull consists of two portions: the neurocranium, which surrounds the brain, and the viscerocranium or splanchnocranium, which forms the face. The neurocranium is further divided into the skull base and the cranial vault. Growth of the skull is complex; the various parts that form the skull develop from several origins and demonstrate different functions. Although it is complex, knowledge of this process is important for the understanding and treatment of dysfunction of developmental origin in infants, children and adolescents.

Neurocranium

The human neurocranium develops from the mesenchymal cells that condense around the cerebral vesicles of the developing brain. Although most of the skeleton passes through blastemal and cartilaginous stages before ossification occurs, some parts of the neurocranium do not follow this process and do not pass through chondrification. Thus, the bones of the vault and certain parts of the cranial base develop within a membrane of primitive mesenchymal tissue without prior formation of cartilage. They are referred to as membranous bones. The rest of the bones that constitute the cranial base are derived from the chondrocranium and are referred to as cartilaginous bones.

At the end of the 1st month of gestation, during the blastemal stage of skull development, the mesenchymal cells surrounding the cerebral vesicles increase in number and start to condense. This forms the desmocranium, from which both membranous bones and cartilaginous bones are derived. At this time, the mesenchymal cells, located between the cranial part of the neural tube and the foregut, thicken to constitute the primordium of the basicranium that will go through chondrification.

At the beginning of the 2nd month, the arrangement of the mesenchymal cells is referred to as meninx primitiva, or primary meninx. From this primary meninx, two layers develop that will differentiate into an outer layer, the ectomeninx (pachymeninx), and an inner layer, the endomeninx (leptomeninges). The endomeninx will form the arachnoid and piamater, while the ectomeninx will evolve to become the dura mater and the future cartilaginous and membranous parts of the neurocranium.

At the end of the 2nd month, at about the 7th week, multiple chondrifi cation centers develop in the desmocranium. They organize in masses of chondroid tissue resembling plates. The first cartilaginous plates to appear are located in front of the notochord near its rostral end. They form the parachordal plates and will take part in the development of the basal plate in the area of the dorsum sellae of the sphenoid bone. Chondrification progresses in the occipital region to form the occipital cartilage. This cartilage incorporates the sclerotomes from the occipital somites to form the future basilar portion of the occiput. Because of the incorporation of the sclerotomes, the accessory (CN XI) and hypoglossal (CN XII) nerves, initially extracranial in location, are also incorporated. As this process progresses, the mesenchymal condensation expands on each side, giving rise to the condylar portions of the occiput. They develop surrounding CN XII and initiate the formation of the hypoglossal canal as well as the circumference of the foramen magnum (Fig. 2.1).

It should be remembered that nerves do not traverse bones. Rather, nerves and vascular structures are present before the initiation of skeletal development, and the cartilaginous anlagen develop by surrounding them while establishing close relationships with the connective tissues of their epineurium, or adventitia. There is consequently continuity between the different tissues of the body.

As development continues, the primitive chondrobasicranium extends forward, in the region of the future sella turcica, around the developing pituitary, and forms the polar and hypophyseal cartilages. In concert with the trabecular cartilage, they participate in the formation of the primordium of the body of the sphenoid. Additionally, on each side, the cartilages of the orbitosphenoid and alisphenoid develop. They will later become the lesser wings and the greater wings of the sphenoid bone, respectively.

Chondrifi cation continues to progress forward around the nasal placodes to form the nasal capsules. These will later develop into the ethmoidal labyrinths and nasal conchae. The central part constitutes the nasal septum that remains cartilaginous after birth and plays an important role in facial growth, acting as a 'functional matrix'.[1,2]

At approximately the 5th week the otic capsules develop bilaterally around the auditory vesicles, anlagen of the future semicircular canals and cochlea. They will fuse with the parachordal cartilages to form the future petrous and mastoid portions of the

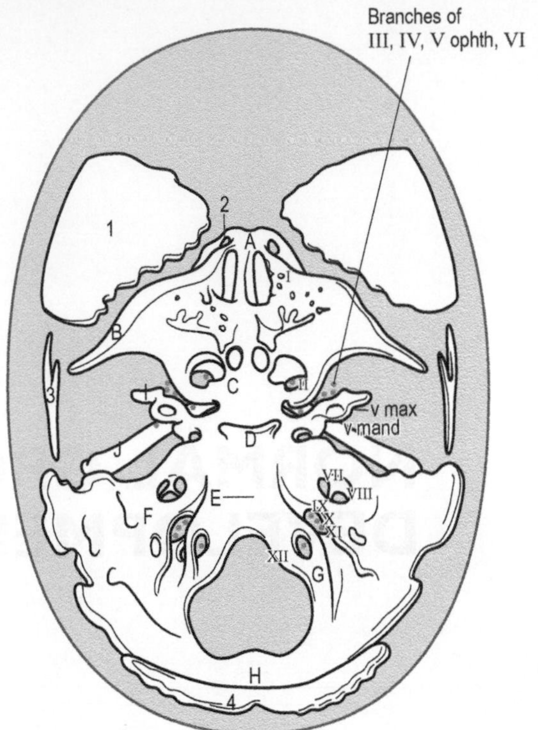

Figure 2.1. *Development of the cranium: superior aspect of the cranium of a human embryo at 40 mm.*

Chondral elements:
- A *Nasal capsule*
- B *Orbitosphenoid*
- C *Presphenoid*
- D *Postsphenoid*
- E *Basiocciput*
- F *Otic capsule*
- G *Exoccipital*
- H *Supraoccipital*
- I *Alisphenoid*
- J *Meckel's mandibular cartilage*
- K *Cartilage of malleus*
- L *Styloid cartilage*
- M *Hyoid cartilage*
- N *Thyroid cartilage*
- O *Cricoid cartilage*
- P *Arytenoid cartilage*

Membranous elements:
- 1 *Frontal bone*
- 2 *Nasal bone*
- 3 *Squama of temporal bone*
- 4 *Squama of occipital bone*
- 5 *Parietal bone*
- 6 *Maxilla*
- 7 *Lacrimal bone*
- 8 *Zygomatic bone*
- 9 *Palatine bone*
- 10 *Vomer*
- 11 *Medial pterygoid plate*
- 12 *Tympanic ring*
- 13 *Mandible*

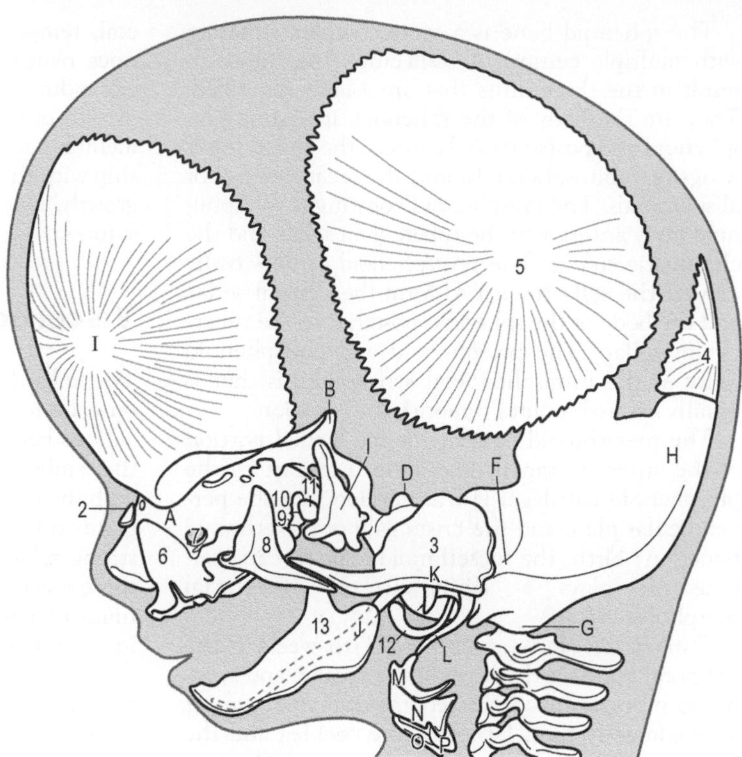

Figure 2.2. *Development of the cranium: lateral aspect of the cranium of a human embryo at 80 mm. (See Figure 2.1 for key to symbols.)*

temporal bone. Thus, they surround the internal jugular vein and the glossopharyngeal (CN IX), vagus (CN X) and accessory (CN XI) nerves, and this hiatus will become the jugular foramen.

At about the 8th week of gestation, the chondrocranium has almost totally replaced the mesenchyme of the desmocranium in the cranial base.[3] It forms a stable foundation that will thereafter develop less rapidly than the calvaria and facial skeleton. The occipital, sphenoid, temporal, frontal and ethmoid bones that form the cranial base (or basicranium) develop through endochondral ossification. However, all these bones, except the ethmoid, also have membranous components that do not go through the stage of chondrification, whereas the ethmoid and inferior nasal conchae develop completely from endochondral ossification.[2] In comparison, the bones of the calvaria form primarily through intramembranous ossification.

Ossification begins in the occipital bone at precisely 12 weeks and 4 days of gestation.[4] It then progresses rostrally in the cranial base, with ossification progressing into the postsphenoid around the sella turcica, in the presphenoid around the area of the chiasmatic sulcus, and lastly to the ethmoid bone. The progression of this pattern of ossification is constant.

Most individual bones of the skull arise from multiple centers of ossification. Some authors have identified up to 110 ossification centers within the embryonic skull.[3] Part of the complexity of this ossification process lies in the multiplicity of terms utilized to describe these centers. These ossification centers develop within the chondrocranium and expand peripherally to meet with their counterparts. Thus, they establish cartilaginous intraosseous relationships between the ossification centers that, depending on the bone being considered, may or may not be totally ossified at birth. The chondrocranium is the foundation within which the centers of ossification of the basicranium develop.

The cartilaginous portion of the occipital bone is derived from five primary centers of ossification that surround the spinal cord to form the foramen magnum. There is one primary center for the anterior basilar portion of the occipital bone or basiocciput, one for each of the paired lateral exoccipital segments, and two for the lower part of the squama. These different cartilaginous portions are not fused at birth.

The sphenoid bone is a more complex structure with multiple centers of ossification that unite to result in the three units that are usually described. They are the body of the sphenoid, including presphenoid and postsphenoid centers, the paired lesser wings or orbitosphenoids, and the greater wings or alisphenoids. The presphenoid constitutes the sphenoid body anterior to the tuberculum sellae and the chiasmatic sulcus. The postsphenoid centers ossify around the sella turcica to form the dorsum sellae and the body of the sphenoid posterior to the tuberculum sellae. The presphenoid and postsphenoid unite at the intrasphenoidal synchondrosis that is usually ossified around 8 months of gestation.

The mesethmoid cartilage is the medial portion of the anterior cranial base, formed in part by the presphenoid cartilage. It will develop into the perpendicular plate and the crista galli of the ethmoid bone.[4] At birth, the mesethmoid remains cartilaginous. It plays a significant part in facial morphogenesis.[5]

Ossification starts around the 17th week in the temporal bones at the level of the squama and zygomatic process, in condensed mesenchyme and, at approximately the 21st week, the cochlea and the lateral semicircular canal attain adult size.[6] They are embedded in the cartilaginous otic capsule, where the centers of ossification of the petromastoid portion appear during the 5th month. The tympanic portion of the temporal bones also develops from the mesenchyme.

Again, the cranial base of the neurocranium develops through an arrangement of endochondral and intramembranous ossification. The occiput, sphenoid and temporal bones demonstrate both types of ossification, whereas the ethmoid and nasal conchae are derived completely from endochondral ossification.[3]

The membranous neurocranium develops into the cranial vault or calvaria. Ossification centers within the desmocranial mesenchyme expand peripherally, separated by membranous tissues that become sutures. When developed, the ossification centers form the bones of the calvaria. They are the frontal bones, the parietals, the squamous portions of the temporal bones and the upper portion of the occipital (supraoccipital) squama. The sutures separating these bones are the sagittal suture between the parietal bones, the metopic suture between the frontal bones, the paired coronal sutures between the two frontal and two parietal bones, the paired lambdoid sutures between the supraoccipital and parietal bones, and the squamous sutures between the parietal, temporal and sphenoid bones. The membranous neurocranium is under the influence of the expanding brain that exerts a significant stimulus for growth of the calvaria during the fetal period. The membranous neurocranium is also in close relationship with the dura that regulates the sites of calvarial growth, much of it occurring on the edges of the sutures.[7]

Viscerocranium

The cells that constitute the viscerocranium demonstrate multiple origins and follow complex interactions between the neural crest cell migration and the embryonic displacement of tissue associated with the neurulation, i.e. the formation of the neural plate and its closure to form the neural tube.[8,9] The strong relationship between the brain, the special sense organs and the development of the viscerocranium remains constant throughout facial development and growth. The neural crests originate in the dorsal aspect of the neural folds (neural tube). They migrate and differentiate into various cell types, including sensory ganglia cells of the cranial nerves – trigeminal (CN V), glossopharyngeal (CN IX) and vagus (CN X) – as well as part of the meninges and part of the skull.

The migrating neural crests will form several prominences that constitute the face. They are the midline frontonasal prominence and two paired structures derived from the first pharyngeal (branchial) arch, the maxillary and mandibular prominences. The frontonasal prominence forms the forehead, the middle of the nose, the philtrum of the upper lip and the primary palate, while the lateral nasal prominence forms the sides of the nose (Figs 2.3–2.6).

After head fold formation, the primitive oral cavity or stomodeum is delimited cranially by the forebrain and caudally by the cardiac prominence. In that area, between the stomodeum and the thorax, the mandibular region and the neck develop from six paired pharyngeal arches. The first pharyngeal arch is quite different from the other arches. It presents, on either side, a ventral part (mandibular prominence) and a dorsal part (maxillary prominence). A cartilaginous portion that is the cartilage of Meckel develops bilaterally in the first arches, from which the malleus and incus are derived, although the latter is subject to debate.[10] In the mesenchyme located in the ventral part of the cartilage, the mandible and maxillae develop from

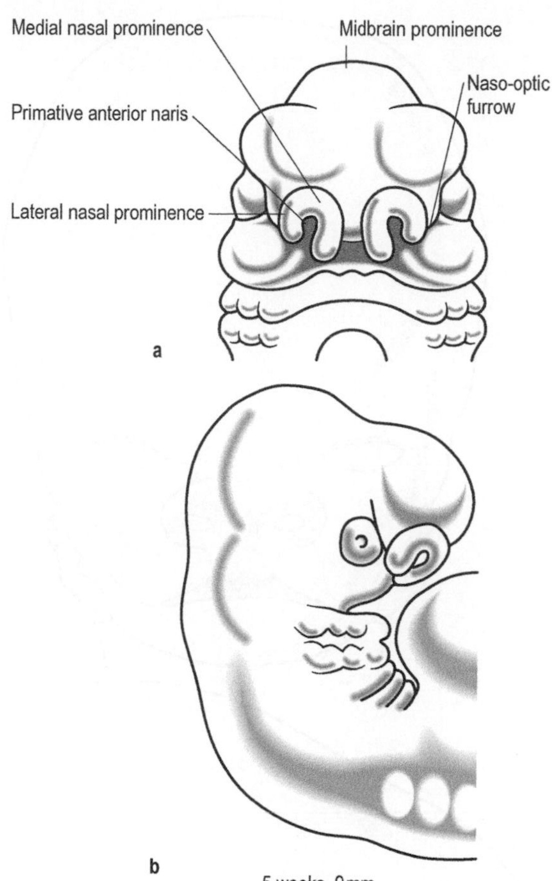

Figure 2.3. *Development of the viscerocranium at 5 weeks: (a) frontal view; (b) lateral view.*

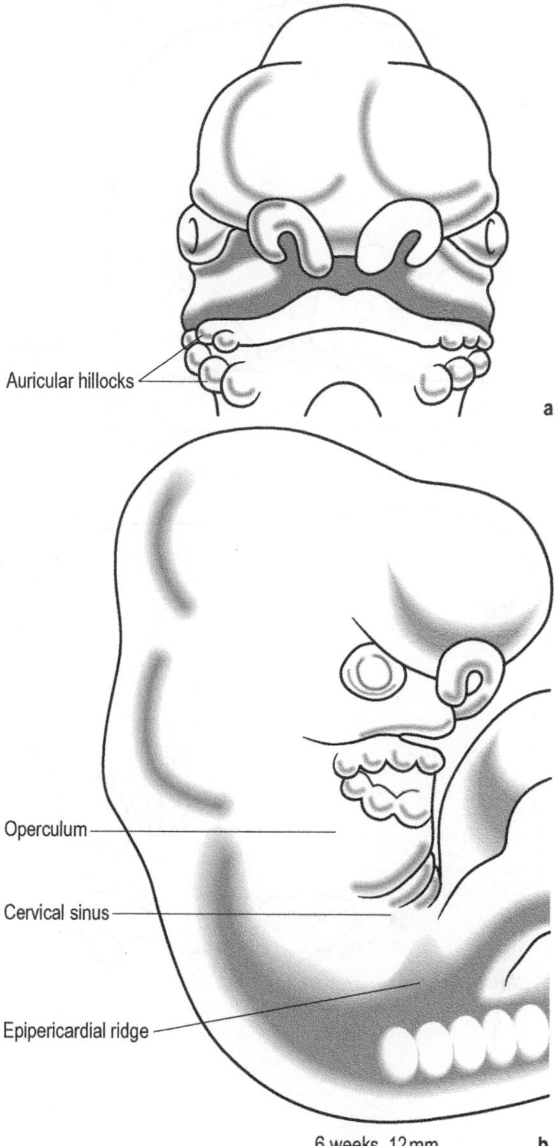

Figure 2.4. *Development of the viscerocranium at 6 weeks: (a) frontal view; (b) lateral view.*

membranous ossification.[9,11] On either side, the zygomatic bones, the squamous portions of the temporal bones, the tympanic ring and the lacrimal and nasal bones will also derive from the mesenchyme of the first arch through membranous ossification. The muscles of mastication also develop from the first arch, whereas the muscles of facial expression come from the second arch. The cartilage of the second arch, or Reichert's cartilage, gives rise to the stapes, the styloid process of the temporal bone, the stylohyoid ligament, the lesser cornu and part of the body of the hyoid bone.

The medial migration of the maxillary prominences and the merging of the two sides form the roof of the oral cavity or primitive palate, and also result in the formation of the philtrum of the upper lip. At about the 6th week of gestation, the secondary palate is derived from the palatine processes or shelves developed from the lateral nasal prominences, which fuse in the midline. Cleft lip or cleft palate arises from failure of the midline fusion. During the formation of the palate, the nasal septum derives from the frontonasal prominence and grows downward to meet the palate.[3]

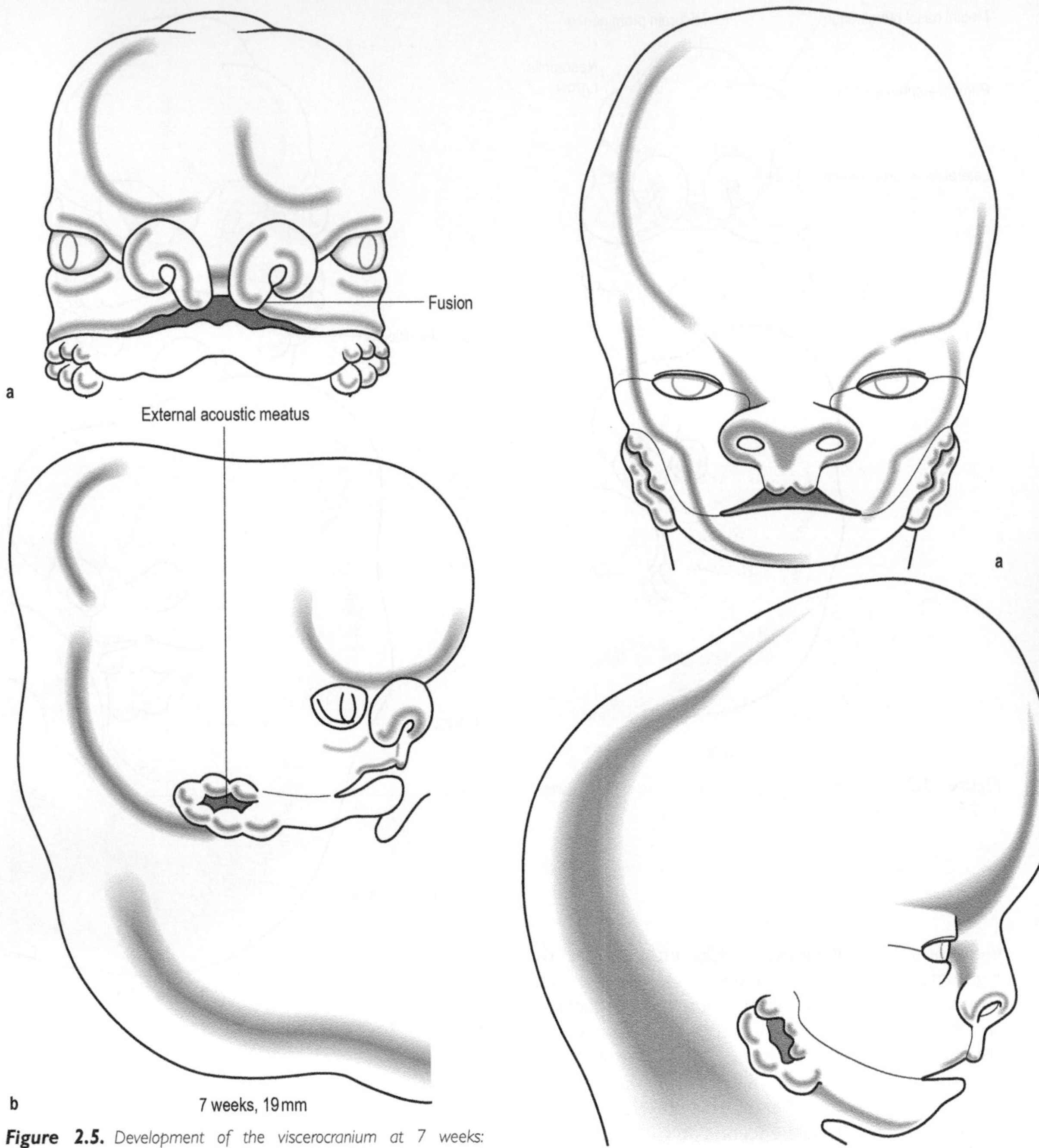

Figure 2.5. *Development of the viscerocranium at 7 weeks: (a) frontal view; (b) lateral view.*

Figure 2.6. *Development of the viscerocranium at 8 weeks: (a) frontal view; (b) lateral view.*

Postnatal development

Normally, the head circumference is 35 cm at birth. It should reach 47 cm at the end of the first year, with a growth of approximately 6 cm in the first 3 months. In comparison, the length at birth is about 50 cm and around 75 cm at the end of the first year; by 4 years of age, the child's height will normally be double their birth length.

At birth, ossification is not yet complete for most of the bones and they still consist of several component parts. Cranial somatic dysfunction may already be present, i.e. an impaired or altered function of the components of the skull and their related myofascial, vascular, lymphatic and neural elements. It may be the result of any cranial constraint during the fetal period or trauma during labor or delivery (see Chapter 4). Any of the bones of the skull may be involved, resulting in interosseous dysfunction. Additionally, dysfunction may be between the different parts of one bone resulting in intraosseous dysfunction.

CRANIAL BASE

The different articulations of the cranial base are named synchondroses. By definition they are cartilaginous joints in which two bones are united by a fibrocartilage. In fact, in these synchondroses, the cartilage is a remnant of the chondrocranium. Thus, bones should not be considered as separated by fibrocartilages, rather they should be considered as parts of a continuum of tissue where the dura and the cartilaginous, membranous and osseous portions of bones are intimately interrelated.

Synchondroses are found in the cranial base. They can be interosseous synchondroses, between two adjacent bones, as well as intraosseous synchondroses, between intraosseous constituents of a single bone. Synchondroses present at birth include:

- the spheno-occipital synchondrosis (sphenobasilar synchondrosis, SBS) between the basisphenoid and the basiocciput
- the petro-occipital synchondrosis between the petrous portion of the temporal bone and the basiocciput
- the sphenopetrosal synchondrosis between the sphenoid and the petrous portion of the temporal bone
- the sphenoethmoidal synchondrosis between the sphenoid body and the ethmoid

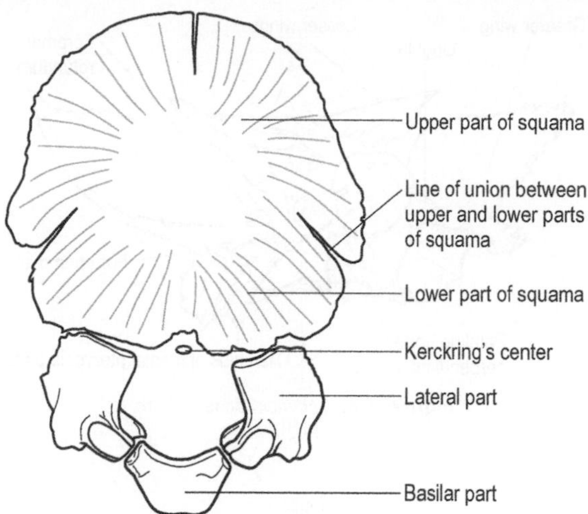

Figure 2.7. *Occipital bone at birth.*

- the intraoccipital posterior and anterior synchondroses, between the exocciput and the squama, and between the basiocciput and the exocciput, respectively.

At birth, the occiput consists of four portions: the basiocciput, two exocciputs and the squama. They represent the development of the five primary occipital cartilaginous centers, i.e. one for the basiocciput, one for either lateral exocciput and two for the portion of the squama located below the highest nuchal line (Fig. 2.7). The occipital squama is completed with a superior part that develops in the membranous cranium. This is of significance because the nuchal line may act as a hinge around which movement may occur between the superior membranous portion of the occipital squama and the inferior cartilaginous portion. During delivery and expulsion of the fetus, the occiput is positioned under the pubic symphysis around which deflexion of the craniocervical junction takes place. The superior and inferior parts of the occipital squama may be stressed with resultant cranial somatic dysfunction. Furthermore, infants with bilateral posterior flattening in non-synostotic plagiocephaly sometimes demonstrate severe flattening that is specifically localized to the area of the membranous squama.

Between 2 and 4 years of age the exocciputs and squama on either side unite, at the posterior intraoccipital synchondroses. The basiocciput and the bilateral exocciputs join between 7 and 10 years of age at the anterior intraoccipital synchondroses.[12] These anterior synchondroses are located within the

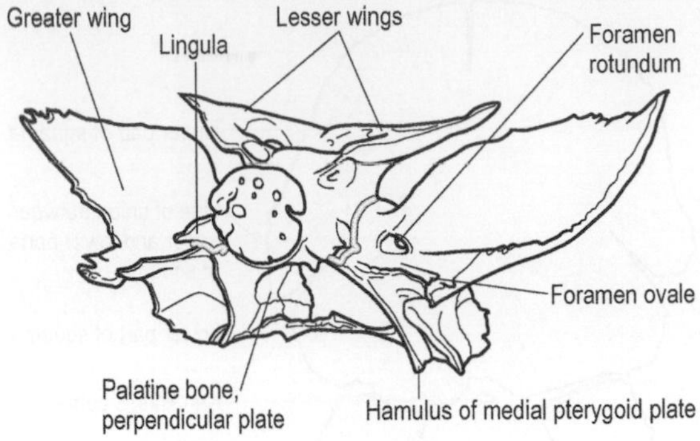

Figure 2.8. *Sphenoid bone at birth.*

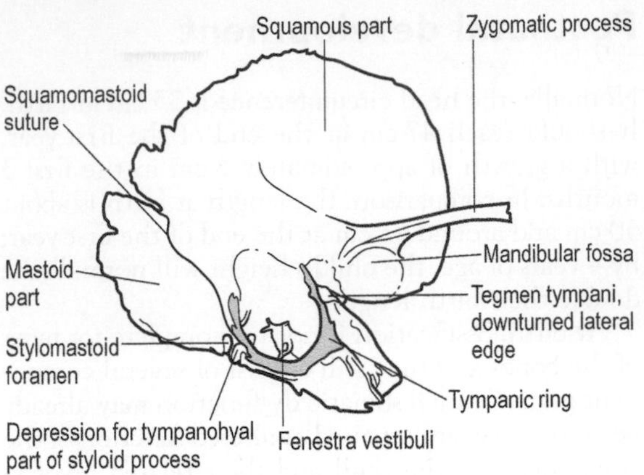

Figure 2.9. *Temporal bone at birth.*

middle of the occipital condyles. The occipital condyles, formed in two parts, are relatively flat at birth and become prominent later during childhood. The flexibility of these occipital synchondroses can result in intraosseous dysfunctions that through any number of possible infantile and childhood traumas can affect the shape of the occipital squama and condyles.

Even though most are in some intermediate stage of closure, nine synchondroses have been identified in the sphenoid at birth.[12] At birth, however, the sphenoid presents essentially as three main parts: a central part that is the body and the lesser wings, and two lateral parts, each consisting of a greater wing and the associated pterygoid process (Fig. 2.8). Most of the fusion between the different parts of the sphenoid occurs after the 1st year of life. The greater wings join the body by surrounding the Vidian nerve forming the pterygoid canal.

Postpartum, the sphenoid undergoes significant changes. The dorsal surface of the sphenoid follows the same pattern of growth as that of the neurocranium to which it is related. Most of this growth occurs in the first 10 years of life. The ventral surface of the sphenoid, however, continues to grow during puberty, as do the facial bones to which it forms the posterior limit.[13] The medial plates of the pterygoid processes form the lateral boundaries of the nasopharynx. Muscular activity significantly contributes to their development. The tensor veli palatine muscles act to stabilize the action of the medial pterygoid muscles that originate mainly from the pterygoid fossa and exert a downward and lateral force, while the lateral pterygoid muscles originate on the lateral surface of the lateral pterygoid plate and exert a lateral force upon it. The actions of these muscles shape and elongate the pterygoid process, and thus its development is dependent on functional orofacial activities such as suckling and later mastication.

At birth the temporal bones each consists of four parts: the squamous, petrous and tympanic portions, and the styloid process (Fig. 2.9). The petrous portion is cartilaginous in origin; the squamous and tympanic portions are membranous in origin. The styloid process is derived from the cartilaginous part of the second pharyngeal arch. The tympanic and squamous portions form the squamotympanic suture, the petrous and squamous portions form the petrosquamosal suture, and the petrous and tympanic portions form the petrotympanic suture.

The squamotympanic suture is closed just before birth.[10] The petrosquamosal suture may ossify after birth, although in some individuals a fissure remains patent up to 19 years of age. Finally, the petrotympanic suture fuses before the end of the first year. The petrosquamosal and petrotympanic sutures contribute to the constitution of the mandibular fossa that forms the roof of the temporomandibular joint (TMJ). At birth, the fossa is quite shallow and lacks its articular tubercle. The shape of the mandibular fossa develops in association with orofacial functions such as suckling, swallowing and later mastication. Dysfunction between the petrous, squamous and tympanic portions can affect the shape of the mandibular fossa and the function of the TMJ.

The anterior third of the mastoid region develops from the squamous portion and the posterior two-thirds from the petrous portion. It is incompletely formed at birth, and the mastoid process develops at the end of the 1st year of life. The traction of the sternocleidomastoid muscle as the child begins to hold their head in an upright position contributes to that development. The mastoid air cells are very small in infancy and do not fully develop until the growth spurt of puberty. Their physiology exerts a significant effect on the equilibration of pressure within the middle ear and because of this they need to be fully developed. Compression with resultant decreased development of these cells, as in plagiocephaly, has been associated with predisposition to develop otitis media.

The ethmoid is derived from the cartilaginous nasal capsule and consists of three portions: the perpendicular plate medially and a labyrinth on either side. At birth the labyrinths are incompletely ossified. The ethmoid center of ossification for the perpendicular plate and crista galli appears during the first year in the upper portion of the cartilaginous nasal septum.[14] The perpendicular plate unites with the labyrinths in the 6th year.[10]

The anteroinferior portion of the nasal septum remains cartilaginous and becomes the septal cartilage, while the posteroinferior part develops into the vomer. The spatial orientation of the vomer changes between birth and adolescence. Through progressive posterior growth its superior border completely covers the inferior sphenoidal rostrum to reach the sphenobasilar synchondrosis.[15]

The growth of the cranial base responds to diverse influences such as the growth of the brain and changes in posture. Brain growth is greatest in the first postnatal year,[16] resulting in changes that produce cranial base flexion at the intrasphenoidal synchondrosis, the sphenoethmoidal synchondrosis and the SBS. Increased chondrogenic activity in the superior part of these synchondroses results in flexion. This chondrogenic activity seems to be most active in the SBS.[17] Growth in the sphenoethmoidal synchondrosis also contributes to facial development and this growth continues as the result of neural expansion up to the age of 8 years, when most of the brain size is achieved.[18] The increase in the length of the anterior cranial base through sphenoethmoidal synchondrosis growth is completed at the same time as that of the sphenofrontal and frontoethmoidal sutures.

The basiocciput and the basisphenoid form the clivus at the SBS. It has been reported that ossification of the SBS begins as early as the age of 8 years.[12] The majority of authors, however, state that the SBS begins fusion shortly after puberty, and that the process lasts to approximately 25 years of age.[10,17,19–21] Consequently, the greatest potential for cranial manipulation to affect the SBS is probably prior to adolescence.

On either side, the petro-occipital synchondroses never ossify, the petrous portions of the temporal bones and the basiocciput being separated throughout life by a cartilaginous remnant of the chondrocranium.[12,20] The occipitomastoid sutures between the occipital squama and the two mastoid parts of the temporal bones demonstrate variable patterns of ossification.[20] These start slowly around 30 years of age, and usually, although incompletely ossified, the occipitomastoid sutures are no longer ossifying after 70 years of age.[22,23] In the anterior part of the cranial base, the sphenofrontal sutures begin ossification around 5 years of age and are fused at about 15 years of age.[12,20]

During the first 2 years of life, the growth of the cranial base is associated with significant changes in the surrounding structures, such as the pharynx, larynx and sensory organs. The cranial base at birth (Fig. 2.10) is slightly arched with the spheno-occipital synchondrosis and basion aligned in the same plane. In the infant, the tongue is located totally within the oral cavity. The larynx is situated in a high position with contact maintained between the epiglottis and the soft palate during both deglutition and respiration.[24] Gradually the larynx descends from this high position in the neck, at the level of C1–C3 during the first 2½ to 3 years of life, to a lower position in the adult, where it is located at the level between the upper borders of C4 and C7.[25] The hyoid bone rests at the level of C1–C2 in newborns and descends to C3–C4 in adults. These changes occur concomitantly with the growth of the cervical spine and traction on the aerodigestive tract. As the larynx descends, the posterior part of the tongue is drawn posteriorly and inferiorly to form part of the superior anterior wall of the pharynx, which becomes the oropharynx. At the same time, the superior constrictor of the pharynx that arises bilaterally from the lower third of the posterior margins of the medial pterygoid plate and its hamulus contributes to the inferior and posterior growth of the pterygoid processes. This pharyngeal differentiation occurs during the first 4 years of life, when functions such as suckling, swallowing and later mastication and speech, all involving the pharyngeal, lingual and orofacial muscles, are significant contributory factors to the normal development of the cranial base. Conversely, dysfunction in the cranial base adversely affects the function of these structures and therefore their development (Figs 2.11, 2.12).

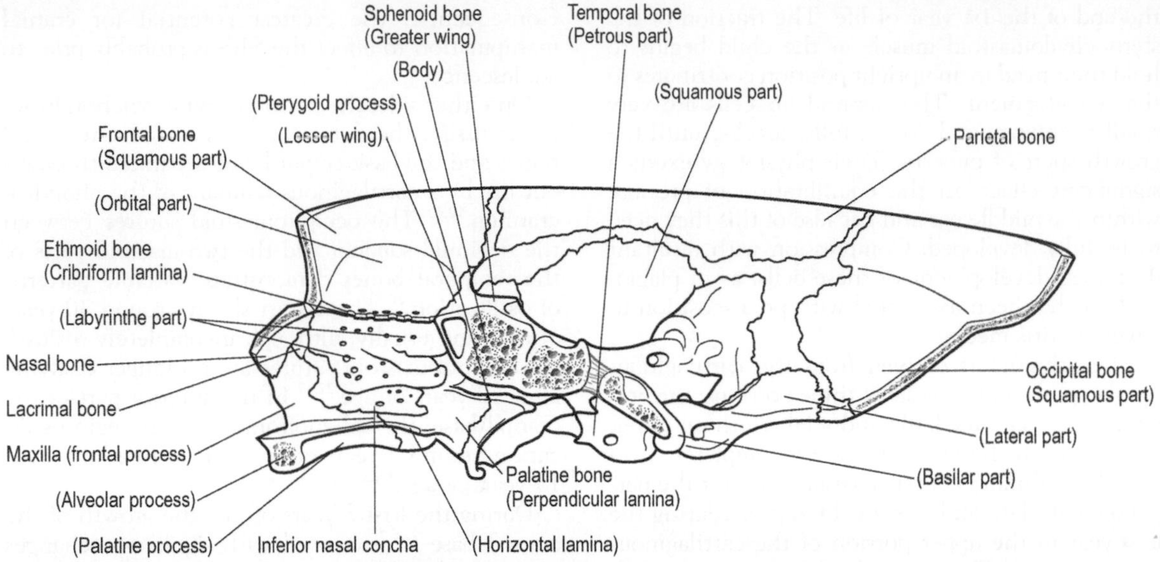

Figure 2.10. *Sagittal section of the cranial base at birth.*

CALVARIA

While the bones of the cranial base are separated by cartilaginous spaces, the synchondroses, the bones of the vault are separated by membranous spaces, the sutures. The fontanelles, unossifi d membranous intervals, are present at the angles of the parietal bones at the junctions between several sutures of the calvarial bones. There are six fontanelles: two are medial and unpaired (the anterior or bregmatic, and posterior or lambdatic) and four are lateral and paired (the sphenoid and mastoid), two on either side. Accessory fontanelles can be present in the sagittal and metopic sutures. The fontanelles are typically closed by the growth of the surrounding bones. Additional centers of ossification may develop within the sutures.

During the growth of the neurocranium, the cranial vault sutures, as long as they remain patent, are, as are the synchondroses, major sites of bone growth. Sutural premature osseous fusion, as in craniosynostosis, prevents further bone formation at the site, resulting in craniofacial dysmorphology.[7] Obliteration of the sutures of the vault of the skull normally begins between the ages of 20 and 40; it is usually first observed on the inner surface of the skull and about 10 years later on the outer surface. Fusion commonly occurs first in the posterior part of the sagittal suture around age 22, then in the coronal and lambdoidal sutures at about age 25. Ossification of these sutures is typically complete between 35 and 47 years of age.[22,23] Sutural fusion may occur over a long period of time that varies from individual to individual. This can, in part, account for the reported variation in age of fusion. Different authors employ various methods of assessment and this may also provide different results. As an extreme example, some authors using radiographic imaging state that the sphenosquamosal suture commences fusion between 2 and 6 years of age,[12,20] whereas others examining dry skulls have identified the age of commencement of fusion at 40 years, with complete fusion rarely occurring.[22,23] Fusion of a suture, however, does not mean that manipulation cannot be employed to affect bony compliance. Again, when using cranial manipulation, the greatest potential for best results is at the youngest possible age.

Morphogenesis of the bones of the calvaria, as of the bones of the cranial base, is the result of both intracranial and extracranial forces. The internal forces exerted by the growing brain are balanced with external muscular forces. These external forces come from muscles that insert on the skull, in particular postural muscles posteriorly and muscles from the aerodigestive tract anteriorly. The dural reciprocal tension membranes modulate muscular influences and maintain balance between the anterior and posterior parts of the skull. Dysfunction, however, in either the dural membranes or the postural or aerodigestive muscles will result in imbalance of cranial growth.

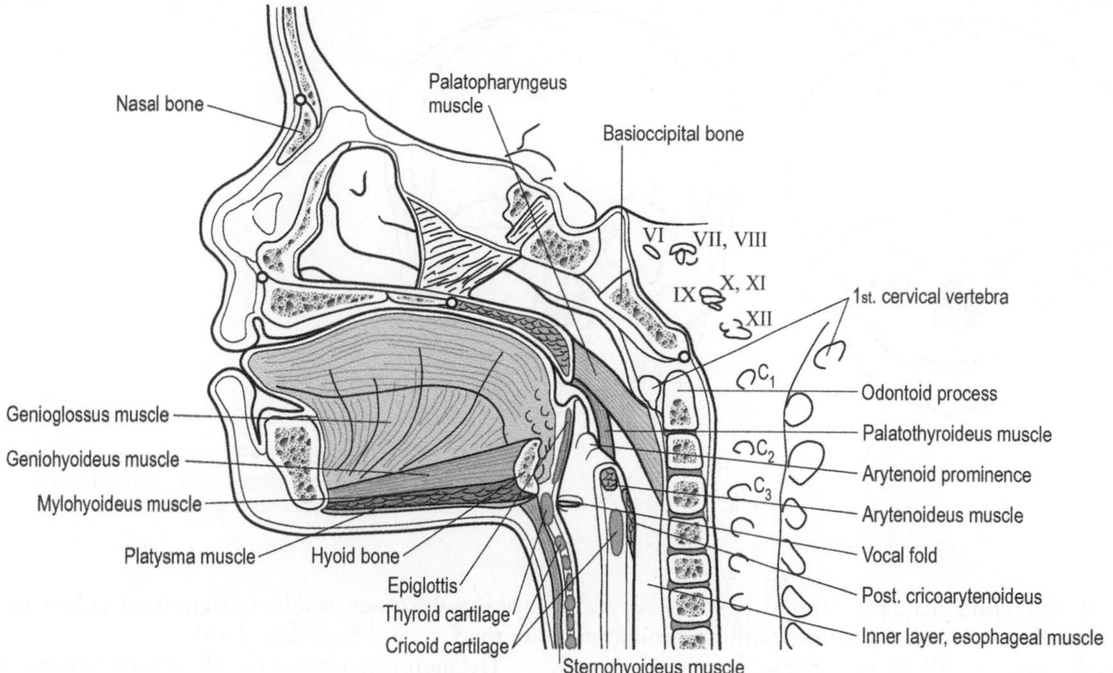

Figure 2.11. *Sagittal section of the oral and pharyngeal regions in the infant. Reproduced with permission from Bosma J. Oral and pharyngeal development and function. J Dent Res 1963;2:375–80.*

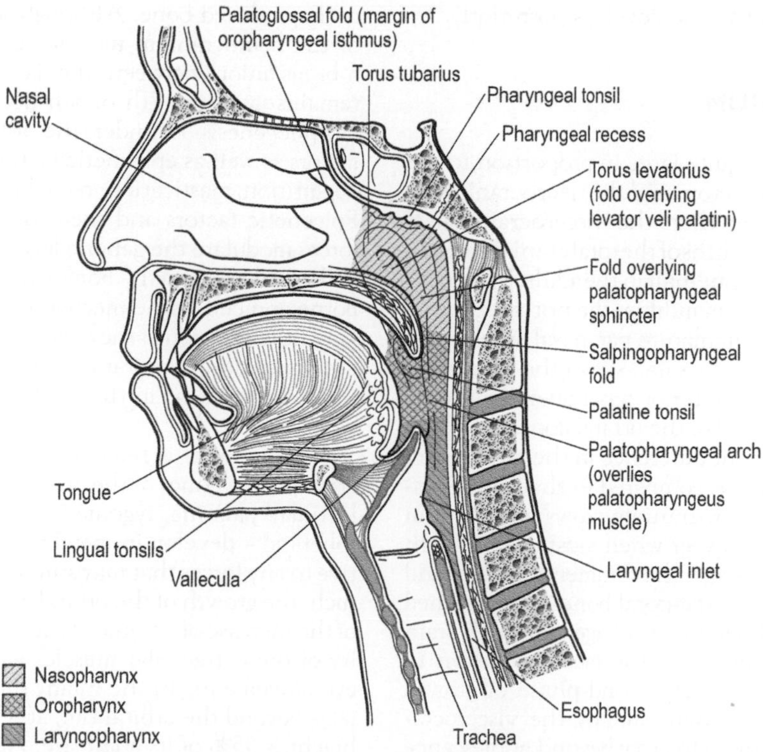

Figure 2.12. *Sagittal section of the oral and pharyngeal regions in the adult: lateral view.*

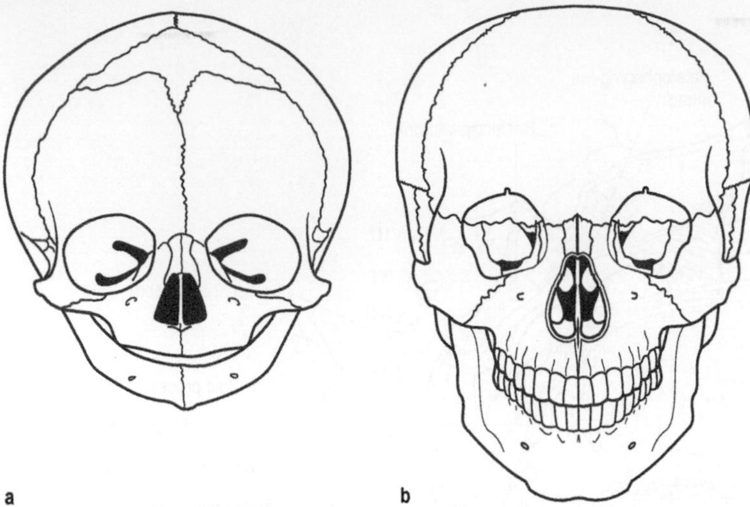

Figure 2.13. *Development of the viscerocranium: difference in the growth rates of the neurocranium and viscerocranium.*

As the child acquires bipedal posture, several cranial characteristics associated with hominization usually appear. While the cranial base undergoes flexion, the cranial vault increases its volume, the frontal and parietal eminences become more prominent and the biparietal diameter increases. At the same time, the frontal bones become more vertical while the occipital squama develops posteriorly.[26]

VISCEROCRANIUM

At birth the skull is quite large in proportion to the other parts of the skeleton, and the neurocranium is, in turn, much larger than the viscerocranium. It equals about seven-eighths of the total cranial volume, as compared to about one-half in the adult. The undeveloped maxillae and mandible, the not yet erupted teeth, as well as the immature paranasal sinuses and nasal cavities explain the small size of the face in the infant. The infantile anterior nasal aperture is only slightly below the level of the orbital floor.

There is a significant difference in the growth rate of the neurocranium as compared to that of the viscerocranium. The neurocranium grows quickly from birth to about the 7th year when most of its growth is completed. At this age, the foramen magnum and petrous portions of the temporal bones have reached their full size. At about 5 years of age, although brain growth is almost complete, the face has grown to only half its adult size.[5] A second phase of growth occurs at puberty involving mainly the viscerocranium that will continue to grow beyond adolescence into adulthood. Eruption of the deciduous and later the permanent teeth, as well as pneumatization of paranasal sinuses, results in significant enlargement of the face and jaws (Fig. 2.13).

The morphogenesis of the viscerocranium extends over a long period of time up until the 3rd decade of life. The bones of the viscerocranium undergo a mechanism of appositional growth as the result of the addition of new layers and resorption of previously produced bone. Although some of the sutures of the neurocranium fuse, in the viscerocranium a fibrous union between the facial bones typically remains until the 7th or 8th decade of life.[7] Facial morphogenesis is under the influence of genetic factors as well as epigenetic factors such as suckling, deglutition, mastication, nasal breathing and speech. Epigenetic factors and their associated mechanical forces modulate the genetic legacy and thereby bone and cartilage growth. Forces transmitted as tissue-borne and cell-borne mechanical strain act to regulate the expression of the genes, and the proliferation, differentiation, maturation and matrix synthesis of the cells, resulting in the totality that is growth and development.[27]

Facial growth is related to orbital and maxillary growth. The bones of the orbital cavity – the frontal, lacrimal, palatine, zygomatic, ethmoid, maxilla and sphenoid – develop in membrane and are very reactive to any forces that may stimulate their growth. As such, the growth of the orbital cavity is the net result of the increase of volume of the eyeball and the activity of the extraocular muscles with their associated eye movements. In the infant the large eyeball projects beyond the orbital rim, at which time the orbit height is 55% of its adult size. At 3 years of age it is 79% and at age 7 about 94%, although facial height is only 80% of its definitive size.[1]

The morphologic changes in the orbit are associated with modification of the optic foramen, which evolves from a foramen into a canal, about 4 mm long, in the 1st year, and from a horizontal position in the infant to a forward inclination of about 15–20° before the 5th year.[28] This change occurs in association with structural changes of the sphenoid wings as well as cranial base growth.

Facial morphogenesis is greatly influenced by the development of the cartilaginous nasal capsules. The multidirectional forces that these capsules exert are thought to have the same effect on the viscerocranium that the growing brain exerts on the neurocranium.[5] The nasal capsules will form the chondroethmoid that is considered to be the facial skeleton in the first 2 years of life. The chondroethmoid further differentiates into a central mesethmoid (with ossification and growth starting in the first year of life and lasting well into the end of adolescence) and two bilateral ectethmoids. All these cartilaginous structures are linked together through the facial aponeurosis and soft tissues. The mesethmoid forms the nasal septum that acts as a 'functional matrix', propulsing and positioning the lower portion of the frontal bones as well as the nasal bones and premaxillae.[1,2,5] Consequently, trauma to the nose, as can often occur during delivery and normal childhood activities, can result in dysfunction that can, in turn, affect the development and growth of the viscerocranium and dentition.

The maxillary complex is moved downward and forward as a result of orbital development and mesethmoid propulsion. On either side, growth occurs in the frontomaxillary, zygomaticomaxillary and pterygomaxillary sutures. At the same time as the maxillary complex moves downward, its transverse length increases. This is the result of growth at the median palatine suture influenced by the pterygoid processes expanding laterally and inferiorly, and the growth in the internasal and frontal sutures. Additionally, increase of the sagittal length of the maxillary complex occurs at the transverse palatine suture between the palatine plates of the maxillae and the horizontal plates of the palatine bones, and also at the posterior border of the palatine bones. Sagittal growth of the maxillae correlates with the developmental expansion of the nasopharynx.[28] The palatal sutures may remain present in young adults.

The development of the paranasal sinuses in the facial bones proceeds at different rates, differing significantly between individuals. The maxillary and sphenoidal sinuses develop first, about the 4th month of gestation. This is followed by frontal and ethmoidal sinus development, in the 6th month.

The paranasal sinuses are quite small at birth. The maxillary sinuses are approximately 7 mm long and 4 mm wide, while the ethmoid cells measure 2–5 mm.[29] The ethmoidal air cells reach mature size at 12–13 years of age. The maxillary sinuses assume their pyramidal shape between 5 and 8 years, reaching full size by age 15. The sphenoidal sinuses become pneumatized at about 5 years.[30] Around the age of 6, when brain growth slows down, the frontal sinuses are developed such that they may be seen on X-ray. Although the inner table of the frontal bone becomes stable, the outer table continues to be pulled forward by nasomaxillary growth, thus increasing the sinusal space. The increase in size of the sinuses has been linked to the mechanical forces of mastication and the actions of growth hormones.[31] Under normal conditions paranasal sinus development continues well into adolescence. Somatic dysfunction of the cranial base, or of the bones of the viscerocranium, may exert untoward effects on the development and growth of the sinuses. Spinal dysfunction and dysfunctional postural mechanics can also impact orofacial functions and consequently the paranasal sinuses.

Similar to the paranasal sinuses, the pharyngotympanic tube (PT) undergoes significant developmental changes in relation to growth of the maxilla, pterygoid process and associated muscles. In the infant it is about half the length of that of the adult and by the age of 7 has attained 97% of its final length. The direction of the PT is horizontal in the newborn whereas in the adult it passes downward, forward and medially from the middle ear.

Psychomotor development

Multiple factors contribute or interfere with infant motor development and therefore multiple theories have been proposed. The theory of progressive maturation of the central nervous system is based on the existence of pre-established patterns regulating the development of the infant, whereas environmental theories stress the various factors modulating the genetic inheritance through diverse influences such as intrauterine or familial environment. A more recent theory proposes the existence at birth of a myriad of neuronal networks capable of modification through cell migration, division and death that can be selected by trial and error, with reinforcement of the most positive experiences.[32]

Development of the musculoskeletal system initiates functional actions during embryonic life and they first appear at the 7th gestational week as simple movement of extremities or extension of the neck.[10]

These simple movements, most often twisting and stretching, can also involve the whole body. They promote normal skin growth and suppleness and contribute to establishing the neurophysiologic organization and development of the musculoskeletal system. Two weeks later, the fetus demonstrates single arm movements that can involve only one side and are the first sign of laterality.[33,34] In the following weeks, jaw movements develop with rhythmical swallowing after 11 weeks and movements of the fetal tongue visible after 14 weeks. When the fetus approximates their hand against the lips they suck their thumbs reflexively.[35] Furthermore, examination by means of ultrasound between 15 weeks and term demonstrates a preference for sucking the right thumb in approximately 90% of fetuses,[36] and this preference is related to postnatal handedness.[37] More complex movement involving a combination of movements of limb, trunk and head are observed between 12 and 16 weeks of gestation, and at about 20 weeks bilateral movement such as bilateral leg extension or arm flexion, with both hands often observed near the face, can be seen. Normally, the occurrence of flexion and stretching during fetal life is greatest at 28–31 weeks, and at 40–41 weeks the movements of the upper half of the trunk and rolling movements are increased.[38] Typically, at birth, an infant has developed a motor behavior sufficiently elaborate for survival, with the capability to suck, swallow and masticate, in association with protective reflexes such as blinking and coughing.

Orofacial activities as well as any other fetal movements such as stretching the limbs or kicking the legs are essential for the development of cortical–motor–neuronal pathways. However, the maturation of the nervous system and motor development may be hampered by environmental factors. Amplitude and velocity of fetal movements can be altered by intrauterine constraints,[39] and maternal viscera such as the liver,[40] rectum or bladder[41] can influence fetal positioning. Usually, the fetus is in a cross-legged posture and in the vertex presentation (left occiput-anterior, LOA) and most frequently lies on the maternal left side, with their back to the left side of the mother and their head against the maternal pelvis.[42] The vertex presentation LOA is also associated with a predilection for fetal head rotation to the right at 38 weeks,[43] as well as neonatal head rotation to the right when placed in a supine position, and a tendency for right-hand utilization in visually guided reaching tasks at 19 weeks.[44] Then again, surrounding factors such as maternal lumbosacral somatic dysfunctions may impede fetal positioning and ability to move. For instance, a maternal left on left sacral torsion affects the left oblique diameter of the pelvic inlet, between the maternal right sacroiliac joint and the opposite iliopubic eminence, with subsequent fetal positioning adjustment and asymmetry. (*Note*: The oblique diameter of the pelvic inlet should not be confused with the sacral oblique axis described in osteopathic mechanics.) Additionally, greater stimulation of the left utricle, the result of fetal positional asymmetry, predisposes to developmental neurologic asymmetry of the ear and labyrinth, and a left-sided otolithic dominance at birth.[41]

Following birth, infant motor activity contributes to the development of muscle tone. The lower and upper extremities flexed at birth demonstrate positioning in extension around 3–5 months of age. Nevertheless, the extremities should reveal rather symmetrical movements. At the same time, the axial musculature progressively builds up, allowing a stable vertical posture of the head and trunk against the force of gravity. Stimulation of the child, however, is necessary and placing infants in the prone position for supervised playtime contributes to the postural development necessary for sitting, standing and walking. The 'Back to Sleep' campaign initiated in 1992 by the American Academy of Pediatrics (AAP) recommend that healthy 'infants be placed down for sleep on either their side or back' to prevent sudden infant death syndrome (SIDS).[45] Nevertheless, the upper trunk, upper extremities and shoulder girdle muscles are less stimulated when an infant is placed in a supine position, and since that sleep campaign, delay in early gross motor milestones have been observed in infants placed to sleep in a supine position, particularly in rolling prone to supine, tripod sitting, creeping, crawling and pulling to stand.[46]

The sleeping posture is also associated with the timing of independent walking, and infants sleeping in a prone position start to walk 1.5 months earlier than those sleeping supine.[47] The AAP guidelines advocate that infants should spend supervised wakeful time in the prone position. A certain amount of stimulation is necessary to encourage the child to explore the environment. In turn, their motor and intellectual abilities will improve. Additionally, the repetition of movements and activities provides sensory feedback through visual, vestibular and somatosensory input necessary for the attainment of posture and gross motor development as well as fine motor abilities. Somatic dysfunction should be sought out and treated as soon as possible to avoid any dysfunctional sensorimotor integration during the early developmental periods in order for the

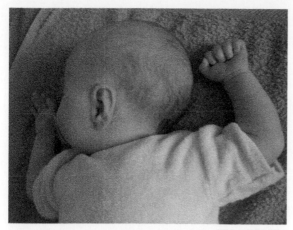

Figure 2.14. *Neonatal head rotation to the right when the infant is placed in a supine position.*

infant to develop the best head and trunk postural control and mechanics. The craniocervical junction, upper thoracic spine and pelvis should be particularly considered. A child should be able to turn their head to both sides and an asymmetry of this motion should be considered as an anomaly. When there is a preference, usually on the right side,[48] this should disappear at approximately 12 weeks of age.[49] An asymmetry in the rotation of the head may predispose to plagiocephaly associated with the development of musculoskeletal dysfunction,[50] scoliosis[51] and psychomotor retardation.[46]

The period around 3 months of age is a time of major neurologic transition where the quality of general movements attains its major developmental predictive value.[52] At that time, the child can typically balance their head and is gradually facing situations where they must control and stabilize their head as well as their body against the force of gravity. Thus, postural adjustments must occur. These result from activation of muscular patterns regulated through visual, vestibular and somatosensory input. Vision is a major contributor to motor development, providing significant feedback to the vestibular and proprioceptive systems, and to the development of cerebellar functions. This is confirmed by the observation of blind children where initial visuomotor coordination (e.g. coordinated eye–head scanning) present in the first weeks of life disappears after several weeks; additionally, these children demonstrate delayed development, particularly in self-initiated postures and locomotion.[53]

Practically, head and trunk stabilization and postural control are involved in every motor activity. Normally, in early infancy, the frequency of activation of the dorsal muscles is higher than for the ventral muscles, and the latencies to onset of activation much shorter for the dorsal trunk and the leg muscles than for the ventral muscles.[54] Additionally, postural synergies develop early in the trunk muscles, where forward sway of the body results in a synergy of the dorsal extensor muscles and backward sway a synergy of the ventral flexors.[55] Before they can sit up independently, typically during the second half-year of postnatal life, children are able to sit with arms propped at 3 or 4 months and unsustained at approximately 5–6 months of age, controlling weight shifts and rotations of the head and trunk, and without any significant postural asymmetry.

Naturally, when the child is able to crawl, at about 9 or 10 months, they are also able to move in and out of the seated position. Most of the time infants crawl on their bellies prior to crawling on hands and knees. This developmental stage requires unencumbered function of the pelvis, limbs and spine. Any delay or absence of crawling may be associated with somatic dysfunction of the hip, innominate bones, sacrum or lumbar spine. For instance, some children stay seated on the floor and move by scooting their bottoms, or they attempt to creep while one leg (always the same one) stays in a semi-extended position without being able to flex alternately with the other side. In this last example a somatic dysfunction of the innominate bone in an anterior rotation (external) pattern is frequently found. Any dysfunction should be addressed since early crawling experience is of paramount importance in the development of sensory system and general motor skills.[56] Thus, early appropriate timing of treatment is important to allow for optimal postural development. It may also have additional cognitive effects, since faster development during the 1st year of life is correlated with an increased chance of attaining higher education in adult life.[57]

Development of gross motor skills occurs concomitantly with fine motor skills, social interaction and development of language. At 3 months when children sit head steady, they should also be able to put their hands together, regard their own hand and begin to imitate speech sounds. At 6 months they sit with no support and can pronounce single syllables. At 9 months when they pull to stand they are able to combine syllables and demonstrate thumb–finger grasp.

When considering development during infancy, 'nature' vs. 'nurture' has always been a matter of debate. There are, however, neurophysiologic indications that postural control may be enhanced through daily training. Through trial and error, the reinforcement of the most positive responses allows the child to find the best connections among the numerous neuronal networks of a genetically predetermined repertoire.[58] Training at an 'opportune time' affects the development of automatic motor patterns involved in postural control and, through multisensory interactions, finetunes the various sensory systems.

Moving to an erect position is an important motor achievement in a child's life. This occurs progressively, starting around 9–10 months of age, with significant body oscillations as a result of postural instability. The spine reacts to this newly upright posture by adapting through the lumbar lordosis and associated protuberance of the abdomen. Children evolve from postural instability to successful balance control through neural maturation, when stability of the head and development of coordination occur, fine-tuned by visual, vestibular and proprioceptive sensory indications. Walking will, in turn, enhance sensory integration.[59] Thus, at 18 months, most children walk without assistance and become more autonomous, with the possibility of getting closer to, or further from, people in their environment. Coordination while walking improves significantly during the first months of walking, with an increase in step length and frequency, and a decrease in the oscillatory movements of the head and trunk. The ability to maintain a static quiet stance equilibrium defines normal motor development. At 18 months, the child can walk fast and walk up stairs with one hand held. At 24 months, they will run and walk up and down stairs alone, while at 36 months, they alternate feet when walking up stairs, are able to jump from a step, walk on toes or hop two or three times. The intricate system of standing stability attains adult levels at age 7–8 years.[60]

Dominance of laterality appears generally between 6 and 12 months of age at the level of the hand as well as at the level of the foot and eye. The child understands words some time between 8 and 10 months of age and may repeat words between 10 and 17 months of age. During their 2nd year of life, word comprehension, production and knowledge of grammar improve tremendously. They start to combine two words between 20 and 24 months. The use of 'I' appears at this time, and they reach more personal consciousness between 30 and 36 months. At approximately 3 years, a child can draw a representation of themselves and knows the different parts of their body.

This dynamic developmental musculoskeletal and cognitive progression, based on feedback from trial-and-error experience, may be impaired by musculoskeletal dysfunction. Functional impairments in early life that interfere with symmetrical head motion, or the ability to sit or crawl, can slow the development of motor functions that are, in turn, necessary for the acquisition of future developmental motor and cognitive milestones. Furthermore, as the child grows older and develops self-awareness, functional impediments can foster feelings of inadequacy. Thus it is imperative that somatic dysfunction, which is reversible and readily amenable to appropriately applied manipulative procedures, be identified and treated at the earliest possible age.

REFERENCES

1. Scott JH. The growth of human face. Proc Roy Soc Med 1954;47(2):91–100.
2. Sperber GH. The cranial base. In: Sperber GH. Craniofacial embryology. Chicago, Year Book Medical; 1976:78–87.
3. Ricciardelli EJ. Embryology and anatomy of the cranial base. Clin Plast Surg 1995;22(3):361–72.
4. Nemzek WR, Brodie HA, Hecht ST, Chong BW, Babcook CJ, Seibert JA. MR, CT, and plain film imaging of the developing skull base in fetal specimens. AJNR Am J Neuroradiol 2000;21(9):1699–706.
5. Couly G. Le mésethmoïde cartilagineux humain. Son rôle morphogénétique sur la face humaine en croissance. Applications. Rev Stomatol Chir Maxillofac 1980;8:135–51.
6. Nemzek WR, Brodie HA, Chong BW et al. Imaging findings of the developing temporal bone in fetal specimens. AJNR Am J Neuroradiol 1996;17(8):1467–77.
7. Opperman LA. Cranial sutures as intramembranous bone growth sites. Dev Dyn 2000;219(4):472–85.
8. Couly GF, Coltey PM, Le Douarin NM. The triple origin of skull in higher vertebrates: a study in quail-chick chimeras. Development 1992;117:409–29.
9. Helms JA, Cordero D, Tapadia MD. New insights into craniofacial morphogenesis. Development 2005;132(5):851–61.
10. Williams PL (ed). Gray's anatomy, 38th edn. Edinburgh: Churchill Livingstone; 1995.
11. Delaire J. Le rôle du condyle dans la croissance de la mâchoire inférieure et dans l'équilibre de la face. Rev Stomatol Chir Maxillofac 1990;91:179–92.
12. Madeline LA, Elster AD. Suture closure in the human chondrocranium: CT assessment. Radiology 1995;196(3):747–56.
13. Nakamura S, Savara BS, Thomas DR. Norms of size and annual increments of the sphenoid bone from four to sixteen years. Angle Orthod 1972;42(1):35–43.
14. Scott JH. The cranial base. Am J Phys Anthropol 1958;16(3):319–48.
15. Takagi Y. Human postnatal growth of vomer in relation to base of cranium. Ann Otol Rhinol Laryngol 1964;73:238–41.
16. Bosma JF (ed). Symposium on development of the basicranium. Bethesda, MD: US Department of Health, Education, and Welfare (DHEW publication (NIH) 76–989); 1976.
17. Melsen B. Time of closure of the spheno-occipital synchondrosis determined on dry skulls. A radiographic craniometric study. Acta Odontol Scand 1969;27(1):73–90.
18. Lieberman DE, Ross CF, Ravosa MJ. The primate cranial base: ontogeny, function, and integration. Am J Phys Anthropol 2000;Suppl 31:117–69.

19. Irwin GL. Roentgen determination of the time of closure of the spheno-occipital synchondrosis. Radiology 1960;75: 450–3.
20. Mann SS, Naidich TP, Towbin RB, Doundoulakis SH. Imaging of postnatal maturation of the skull base. Neuroimaging Clin N Am 2000;10(1):1–21, vii.
21. Okamoto K, Ito J, Tokiguchi S, Furusawa T. High-resolution CT findings in the development of spheno-occipital synchondrosis. Am J Neuroradiol 1996;17(1):117–20.
22. Todd TW, Lyon DW. Endocranial suture closure. Its progress and age relationship. Part I. Adult males and white stock. Am J Phys Anthropol 1924;7:325–84.
23. Todd TW, Lyon DW. Cranial suture closure. Its progress and age relationship. Part II. Ectocranial closure in adult males of white stock. Am J Phys Anthropol 1925;8:23–45.
24. Laitman JT, Heimbuch RC, Crelin ES. Developmental change in a basicranial line and its relationship to the upper respiratory system in living primates. Am J Anat 1978;152: 467–82.
25. Laitman JT, Crelin ES. Developmental change in the upper respiratory system of human infants. Perinatol Neonatol 1980;4:15–22.
26. Delaire J. Essai d'interprétation des principaux mécanismes liant la statique à la morphogenèse céphalique. Actualités Odonto-Stomatologiques 1980;130:189–219.
27. Mao JJ, Nah HD. Growth and development: hereditary and mechanical modulations. Am J Orthod Dentofacial Orthop 2004;125(6):676–89.
28. Moss ML, Greenberg SN. Post-natal growth of the human skull base. Angle Orthod 1955;25:77–84.
29. Gruber DP, Brockmeyer D. Pediatric skull base surgery. 1. Embryology and developmental anatomy. Pediatr Neurosurg 2003;38(1):2–8.
30. American Academy of Pediatrics. Subcommittee on Management of Sinusitis and Committee on Quality Improvement. Clinical practice guideline: management of sinusitis. Pediatrics 2001;108(3):798–808.
31. McLaughlin RB Jr, Rehl RM, Lanza DC. Clinically relevant frontal sinus anatomy and physiology. Otolaryngol Clin North Am 2001;34(1):1–22.
32. Changeux JP. Variation and selection in neural function. Trends Neurosci 1997;20:291–3.
33. Ververs IA, de Vries JI, van Geijn HP, Hopkins B. Prenatal head position from 12–38 weeks. II. The effects of fetal orientation and placental localization. Early Hum Dev 1994; 39(2):93–100.
34. Hepper PG, McCartney GR, Shannon EA. Lateralised behaviour in first trimester human foetuses. Neuropsychologia 1998;36(6):531–4.
35. Gaspard M. Acquisition et exercice de la fonction masticatrice chez l'enfant et l'adolescent. Première partie. Rev Orthop Dento-Faciale 2001;35(3):349–403.
36. Hepper PG, Shahidullah S, White R. Handedness in the human fetus. Neuropsychologia 1991;29:1107–1111.
37. Hepper PG, Wells DL, Lynch C. Prenatal thumb sucking is related to postnatal handedness. Neuropsychologia 2005; 43(3):313–5.
38. Kozuma S, Okai T, Nemoto A et al. Developmental sequence of human fetal body movements in the second half of pregnancy. Am J Perinatol 1997;14(3):165–9.
39. Sival DA, Visser GH, Prechtl HF. Does reduction of amniotic fluid affect fetal movements? Early Hum Dev 1990;23(3):233–46.
40. Lansac J, Body G. Pratique de l'accouchement. Paris: SIMEP; 1988.
41. Previc FH. A general theory concerning the prenatal origins of cerebral lateralization in humans. Psychol Rev 1991;98(3):299–334.
42. Fong BF, Savelsbergh GJ, van Geijn HP, de Vries JI. Does intra-uterine environment influence fetal head-position preference? A comparison between breech and cephalic presentation. Early Hum Dev 2005;81(6):507–17.
43. Ververs IA, de Vries JI, van Geijn HP, Hopkins B. Prenatal head position from 12–38 weeks. I. The effects of fetal orientation and placental localization. Developmental aspects. Early Hum Dev 1994;39:83–91.
44. Goodwin RS, Michel GF. Head orientation position during birth and in infant neonatal period, and hand preference at nineteen weeks. Child Dev 1981;52(3):819–26.
45. AAP Task Force on Infant Positioning and SIDS: positioning and SIDS. Pediatrics 1992;89:1120–6.
46. Davis BE, Moon RY, Sachs HC, Ottolini MC. Effects of sleep position on infant motor development. Pediatrics 1998;102: 1135–40.
47. Widhe T. Foot deformities at birth: a longitudinal prospective study over a 16-year period. J Pediatr Orthop 1997; 17(1):20–4.
48. Vles J, van Zutphen S, Hasaart T, Dassen W, Lodder J. Supine and prone head orientation preference in term infants. Brain Dev 1991;13(2):87–90.
49. Hopkins B, Lems YL, van Wulfften Palthe T, Hoeksma J, Kardaun O, Butterworth G. Development of head position preference during early infancy: a longitudinal study in the daily life situation. Dev Psychobiol 1990;23(1): 39–53.
50. Biggs WS. Diagnosis and management of positional head deformity. Am Fam Physician 2003;67:1953–6.
51. Wynne-Davies R. Infantile idiopathic scoliosis: causative factors, particularly in the first six months of life. J Bone J Surg 1975;57B:138–41.
52. Prechtl HF. General movement assessment as a method of developmental neurology: new paradigms and their consequences. The 1999 Ronnie MacKeith lecture. Dev Med Child Neurol 2001;43(12):836–42.
53. Prechtl HF, Cioni G, Einspieler C, Bos AF, Ferrari F. Role of vision on early motor development: lessons from the blind. Dev Med Child Neurol 2001;43(3):198–201.
54. Hedberg A, Carlberg EB, Forssberg H, Hadders-Algra M. Development of postural adjustments in sitting position during the first half year of life. Dev Med Child Neurol 2005;47(5):312–20.
55. Hadders-Algra M, Brogren E, Forssberg H. Development of postural control – differences between ventral and dorsal muscles? Neurosci Biobehav Rev 1998;22(4):501–6.
56. McEwan MH, Dihoff RE, Brosvic GM. Early infant crawling experience is reflected in later motor skill development. Percept Mot Skills 1991;72(1):75–9.
57. Taanila A, Murray GK, Jokelainen J, Isohanni M, Rantakallio P. Infant developmental milestones: a 31-year follow-up. Dev Med Child Neurol 2005;47(9):581–6.
58. Hadders-Algra M, Brogren E, Forssberg H. Training affects the development of postural adjustments in sitting infants. J Physiol 1996;493(Pt 1):289–98.
59. Bril B, Ledebt A. Head coordination as a means to assist sensory integration in learning to walk. Neurosci Biobehav Rev 1998;22(4):555–63.
60. Steindl R, Kunz K, Schrott-Fischer A, Scholtz AW. Effect of age and sex on maturation of sensory systems and balance control. Dev Med Child Neurol 2006;48(6): 477–82.

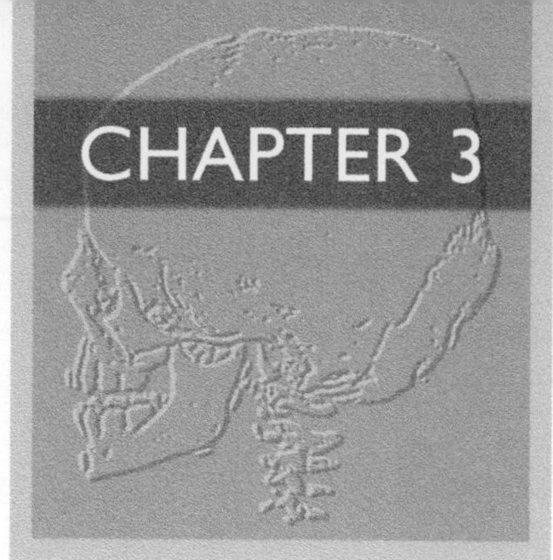

THE CRANIAL CONCEPT

Anatomy of the skull

The skull is divisible into two parts: the neurocranium surrounds and protects the brain and consists of eight bones; the facial skeleton or viscerocranium consists of 13 bones. The mandible is not part of the neurocranium, nor is it part of the viscerocranium. This total of 22 bones, to which may be added the three paired bones of the middle ear, and the midline hyoid bone attached to the base of the skull, results in a total of 29 bones:

- Neurocranium, eight bones:
  - occipital bone
  - two parietal bones
  - frontal bone
  - two temporal bones
  - sphenoid
  - ethmoid
- Facial skeleton, 13 bones:
  - two nasal bones
  - two maxillae
  - two lacrimal bones
  - two zygomatic bones
  - two palatine bones
  - two inferior nasal conchae
  - vomer
- Mandible
- Hyoid bone
- Middle ear, three bones or ossicles:
  - malleus
  - incus
  - stapes.

The neurocranium can be divided into two parts: the vault or calvaria, from a membranous origin, and the base, from a cartilaginous origin. The exterior of the skull may be viewed from above, from behind, from the side, from the front and from below. The interior of the skull may be described in two parts: the vault and the cranial base.

SUPERIOR VIEW OF THE SKULL
(Fig. 3.1)

Four bones form the vault of the skull. In an anterior to posterior direction, they are:

- the frontal bone that articulates with the two parietal bones at the coronal or bregmatic suture
- the two parietal bones that articulate with each other at the sagittal suture and with the occipital bone at the lambdoid suture
- the occipital bone.

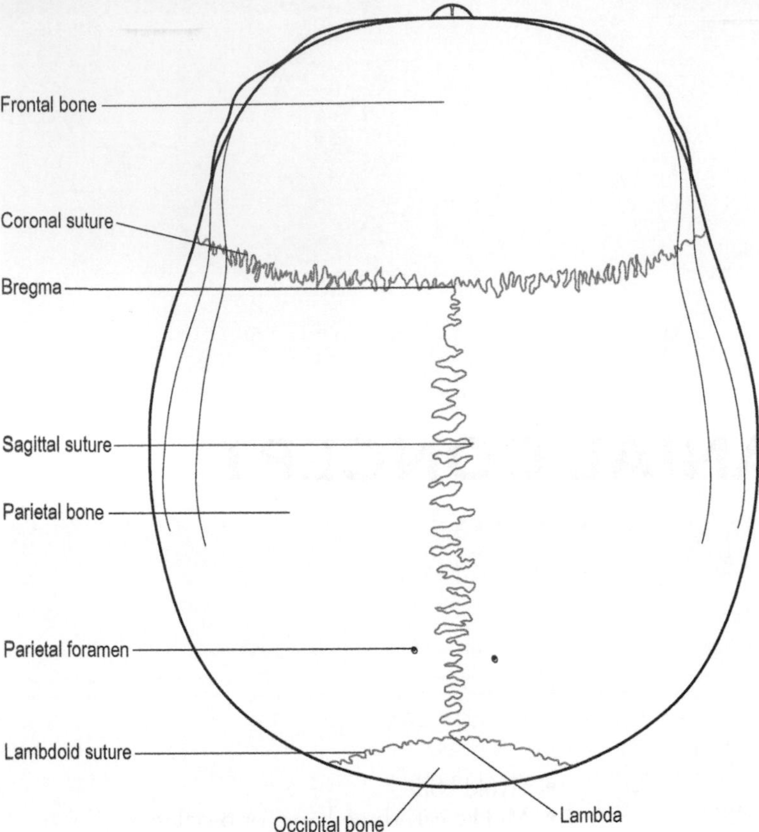

Figure 3.1. *Superior view of the skull.*

The junction of the coronal and sagittal sutures is the bregma; the junction of the lambdoid and sagittal sutures is the lambda. Some sutural (wormian) bones may be present at or near the lambda, such as the 'interparietal' or Inca bone.

POSTERIOR VIEW OF THE SKULL

(Fig. 3.2)

The posterior view includes the occipital bone and the two parietal bones. On each side and below the parietal bones, parts of the temporal bones are visible.

Occipital bone

The squamous part of the occiput is the central structure visible in the posterior view. Slightly convex, it presents the inion, summit of the external occipital protuberance, with two curved lines on each side – the superior and inferior nuchal lines. The occipital bone articulates superiorly with the two parietals at the lambdoid suture. Bilaterally, it articulates with the two mastoid parts of the temporal bones at the occipitomastoid sutures.

LATERAL VIEW OF THE SKULL

(Fig. 3.3)

The lateral view consists of part of the neurocranium, part of the facial skeleton, or viscerocranium, and the mandible. The neurocranium includes the frontal, parietal, temporal, sphenoid, occipital and ethmoid bones; the facial skeleton includes the maxilla, the zygomatic, lacrimal and nasal bones.

Frontal bone

A part of the forehead is visible in the lateral view of the skull. The temporal surface of the frontal bone forms the anterior part of the temporal fossa. The parietal border of the frontal bone articulates with the parietal bone at the coronal suture. Inferiorly,

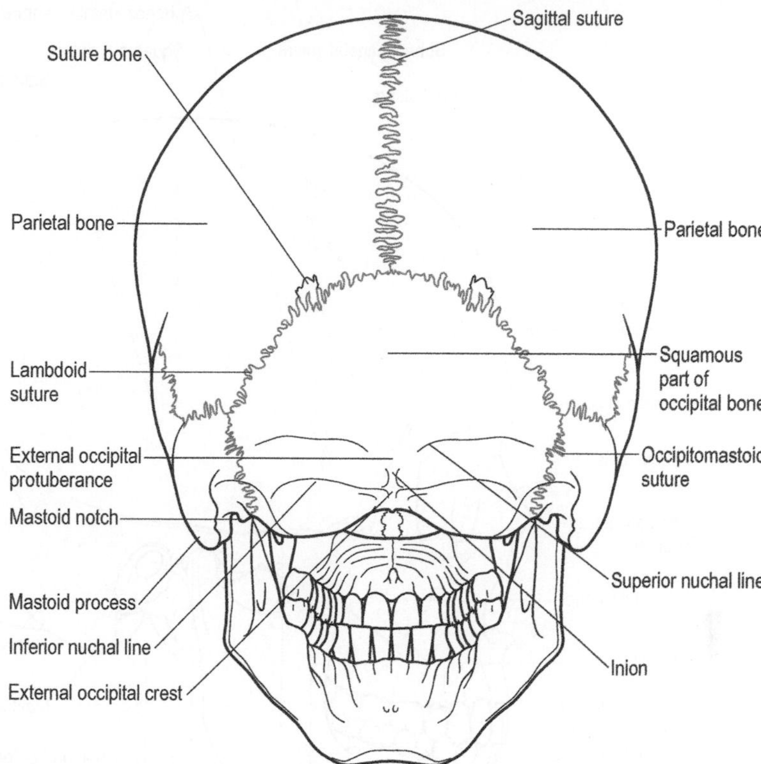

Figure 3.2. *Posterior view of the skull.*

the frontal bone articulates with the greater wing of the sphenoid in an L-shaped articulation.

Parietal bone

The external surface of this bone is completely visible. The frontal border of the parietal articulates with the frontal bone to form half of the coronal suture. The occipital border articulates with the occipital bone to form half of the lambdoid suture. The squamosal or inferior border articulates anteriorly with the greater wing of the sphenoid to form the sphenoparietal suture, in the middle with the squamous part of the temporal bone to form the squamous suture, and posteriorly with the mastoid part of the temporal bone to form the parietomastoid suture.

The parietal bone is somewhat rectangular with four angles: the anterosuperior or frontal angle is at the bregma; the anteroinferior or sphenoidal angle is between the frontal bone and the greater wing of the sphenoid. The point where the greater wing of the sphenoid joins the sphenoidal angle of the parietal is the pterion. At this level, the sphenoparietal suture between the parietal and the apical border of the greater wing of the sphenoid forms the horizontal line of an 'H'. The frontal, parietal, temporal squama and sphenoid meet in this area. The posterosuperior or occipital angle of the parietal is at the lambda. The posteroinferior or mastoid angle articulates with the mastoid part of the temporal bone and the occiput. The point of meeting of the lambdoid, parietomastoid and occipitomastoid sutures is called the asterion.

Temporal bone

The temporal bone is developmentally separable into three parts: the squamous, tympanic and petromastoid. The petromastoid part is frequently divided into a mastoid part and a petrous part for descriptive purposes. All of the parts of the temporal bone are visible in the lateral view, except for the petrous part which is seen in the inferior view.

The squamous part or squama is the anterosuperior part of the temporal bone. It contributes to the lateral wall of the cranium. The superior border is beveled internally and overlaps the parietal to form the squamous suture. The anteroinferior border beveled above internally and below externally

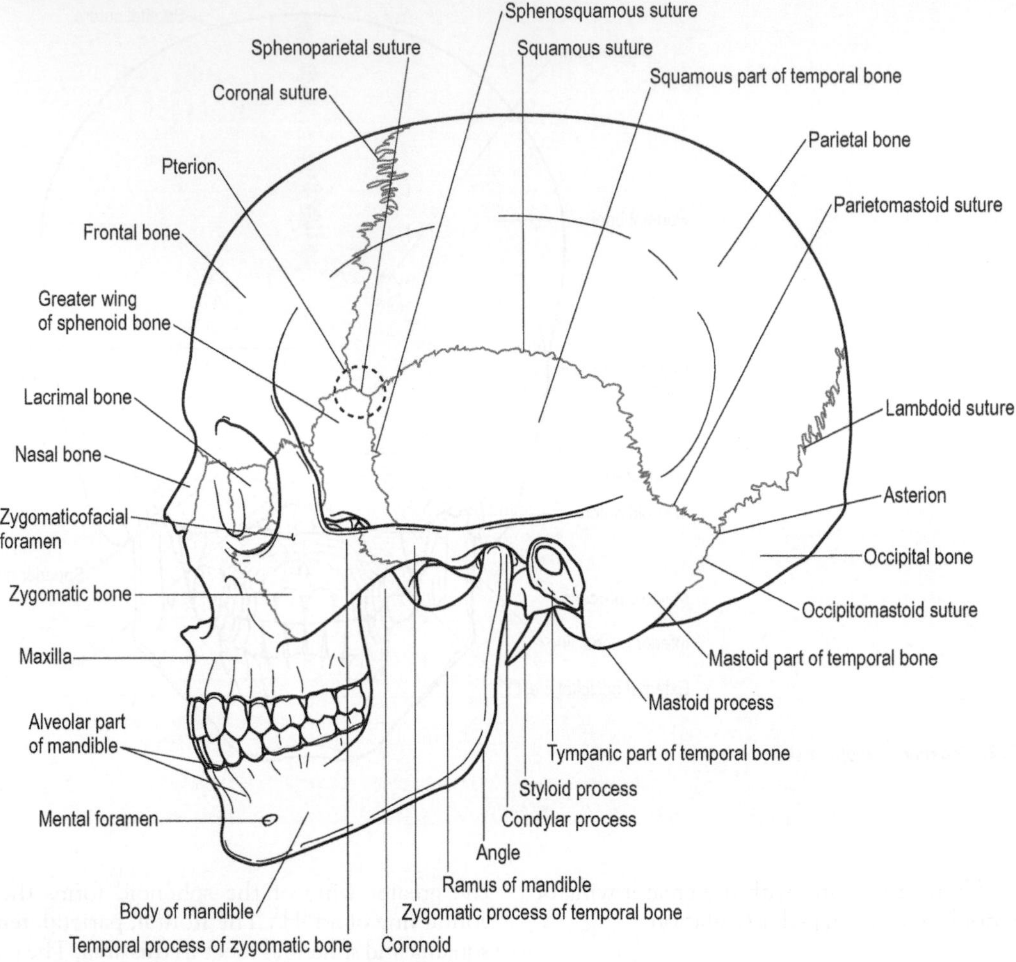

Figure 3.3. *Lateral view of the skull.*

articulates with the greater wing of the sphenoid to form the sphenosquamous suture.

The zygomatic process of the temporal bone consists of two roots, anterior and posterior, surrounding the mandibular fossa. Anteriorly, the zygomatic process articulates with the temporal process of the zygomatic bone to form the zygomaticotemporal suture.

The tympanic part of the temporal bone is located below the posterior zygomatic root and anterior to the mastoid process. It is a curved plate surrounding the external acoustic opening and meatus.

The mastoid part is the posterior part of the temporal bone. It projects downward as the mastoid process that is not fully developed in children until the age of 2 years, and is small in the female. The posterior border of the mastoid part articulates with the occiput to form the occipitomastoid suture. Anterior and medial to the mastoid process, the styloid process descends anteromedially toward the posterior margin of the ramus of the mandible.

Sphenoid

Part of the lateral surface of the sphenoid greater wing is visible anterior to the squama of the temporal bone. This is the temporal surface or upper part of the greater wing. The lower part, not visible on the lateral view, projects downward, medial to the coronoid process of the mandible, and is continuous with the pterygoid process. Only part of the lateral surface of the lateral plate of the pterygoid process is visible in the lateral view.

Occipital bone

Half of the squamous part of the occiput is visible. The deeply serrated lambdoid border extends from the superior to the lateral occipital angles and articulates with the parietal bone to form half of the lambdoid suture. Inferiorly, the mastoid border articulates with the mastoid part of the temporal bone at the occipitomastoid suture.

Ethmoid bone

Part of the lateral surface of the ethmoidal labyrinth is visible in the lateral view. It is the orbital plate of the ethmoid bone that assists in the formation of the medial wall of the orbit. It articulates superiorly with the frontal bone, anteriorly with the lacrimal bone, inferiorly with the maxilla and the palatine bone, and posteriorly with the sphenoid.

Zygomatic bone

The anterolateral surface of the zygomatic bone forms the prominence of the cheek. The zygomatic bone is located anterior to the sphenoid, its posterior border articulating with the greater wing of the sphenoid to form the sphenozygomatic suture. This bone is lateral to the maxilla, to which its anteroinferior border articulates to form the maxillozygomatic suture. It is inferior to the frontal bone with which its frontal process articulates to form the frontozygomatic suture. Laterally, its temporal process articulates with the zygomatic process of the temporal bone to form the zygomaticotemporal suture. The temporal and zygomatic processes together form the zygomatic arch.

Maxilla

The maxilla contributes to the middle part of the viscerocranium. Inferiorly, the alveolar process of the maxilla contains the teeth and forms, with the other side, the upper jaw. Superiorly it forms part of the inferior and medial borders of the orbit. The zygomatic process of the maxilla articulates with the zygomatic bone. The frontal process articulates superiorly with the frontal bone, anteriorly with the nasal bone and posteriorly with the lacrimal bone. Near the posterior border of the lateral surface of the frontal process is a vertical groove that combines with a groove on the lacrimal bone to form the lacrimal fossa.

Lacrimal bone

The smallest of the cranial bones, the lacrimal bone is seen on the medial wall of the orbit. The posterior lacrimal border articulates with the orbital plate of the ethmoid bone, the inferior border with the maxillary orbital surface, the anterior border with the frontal process of the maxilla and the superior border with the frontal bone. The anterior part of the lateral or orbital surface demonstrates a vertical groove that combines with a groove on the maxilla to form the fossa for the lacrimal sac.

Nasal bone

The nasal bone is small and oblong. The superior border articulates with the frontal bone, the lateral border articulates with the frontal process of the maxilla, the medial border joins the opposite nasal bone to form the nasal bridge and the inferior border is continuous with the lateral nasal cartilage.

Mandible

Half of the mandible is seen in the lateral view. One half of the horizontal curved body joins one of the two vertical mandibular rami. The angle of the mandible is the meeting point between the inferior margin of the mandible and the posterior margin of the vertical mandibular ramus. The upper border of the mandibular body is the alveolar part that contains alveoli for the roots of the teeth. The superior part of the ramus extends upward to form, anteriorly, a coronoid process and, posteriorly, a condylar process. The head or condyle of the condylar process articulates with the mandibular fossa of the temporal bone to form the temporomandibular joint. (*Note*: The hyoid bone, a small U-shaped bone, is located in a horizontal plane, under the mandible. The body of the hyoid bone is anterior and forms the base of the U, with the two greater horns forming the two arms of the U. The tip of the greater horn is at the level of the angle of the mandible.)

ANTERIOR VIEW OF THE SKULL

(Fig. 3.4)

The anterior view includes the frontal bone superiorly that forms most of the anterior part of the calvaria. On each side and below the frontal bone, part of the parietal bone and sphenoid are visible. Below the parietal bone, part of the temporal bone is seen. Inferiorly, the facial skeleton is hanging under the frontal bone.

Frontal bone

The frontal bone forms the forehead and the roof of the orbits; the asymmetric frontal eminences are found on each side. The two superciliary arches

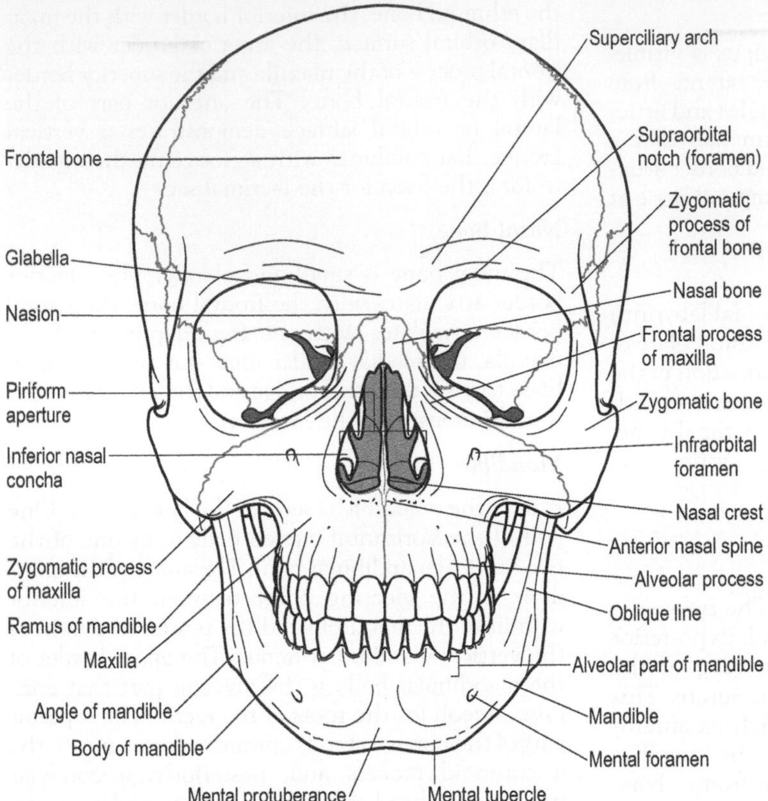

Figure 3.4. *Anterior view of the skull.*

superior to the rim of the orbit are joined by a soft elevation, the glabella. They illustrate the location of the frontal sinuses and are absent in children and small in the female. The orbital rim ends laterally in a zygomatic process that articulates with the frontal process of the zygomatic bone. Medially, between the supraorbital margins, the nasal notch articulates with the nasal bones and laterally with the maxillary frontal processes.

Zygomatic bones

Their convex anterolateral surfaces bilaterally form the prominence of the cheeks. The orbital surface forms the anterolateral part of the orbital floor and part of the lateral orbital wall. The anteroinferior border articulates with the maxilla; the posterior border articulates with the greater wing of the sphenoid.

Nasal bones

The nasal bones are located above the piriform aperture, or anterior opening, of the nasal cavity. Laterally, they articulate with the frontal processes of the maxillae. They articulate medially with each other in the midline and above with the frontal bone. The nasion is the center of the frontonasal suture and the root of the nose.

Maxillae

The maxillae are large bones that occupy the space between the orbit and the upper teeth. They articulate with each other in the midline, below the piriform aperture, and together form the upper jaw. Superiorly, the orbital surface forms most of the orbital floor; the frontal process articulates with the frontal bone. Laterally, the zygomatic process articulates with the zygomatic bone. Inferiorly, the alveolar processes contain the upper teeth.

Piriform aperture

The piriform aperture is limited laterally and inferiorly by the maxillae and above by the nasal bones. A vertical septum divides the nasal cavity in two: its upper part is the perpendicular plate of the ethmoid and its inferior part is the vomer. The inferior border

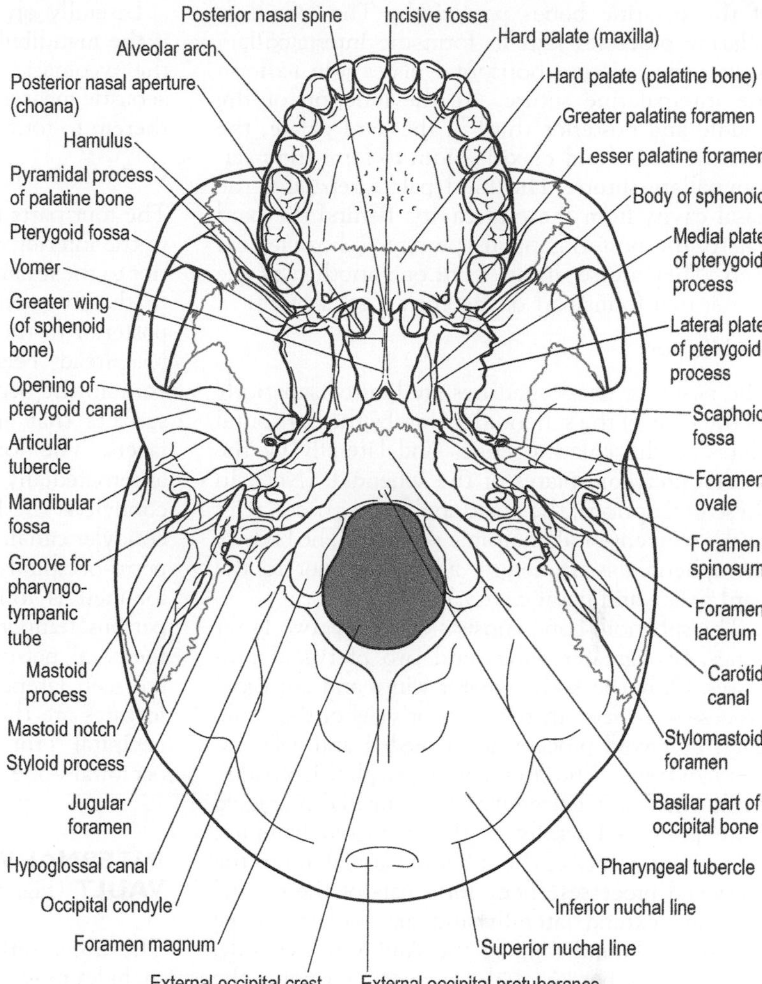

Figure 3.5. *Inferior view of the skull.*

of the vomer articulates with the median maxillary and palatine nasal crests.

Mandible

The mandible forms the lower jaw and represents the lowest bone in the anterior view of the skull. It has a horizontal body convex forward and two rami ascending posteriorly. The symphysis menti is the union of the two halves of the mandible. It is prominent inferiorly as the mental protuberance and on either side as the mental tubercles. The upper part of the body of the mandible is the alveolar part that contains the teeth. A mental foramen is visible below the alveolar part.

INFERIOR VIEW OF THE SKULL
(Fig. 3.5)

The inferior view of the skull is complex. It is usually divided into anterior, middle and posterior parts: the anterior part consists of the hard palate and the alveolar arches, the middle part is located between the hard palate and the foramen magnum, and the posterior part extends to the external occipital protuberance and the superior nuchal lines.

Anterior part

The hard palate consists of the palatine processes of the maxillae anteriorly and of the horizontal plates of the palatine bones posteriorly. The maxillary palatine processes join to form the intermaxillary suture; the palatine horizontal plates join to form the interpalatine suture. At the junction of the middle and posterior third of the hard palate, the palatine bones and maxillae join to form the palatomaxillary suture. The hard palate separates the nasal cavity from the oral cavity. Behind the hard palate, the posterior nasal apertures (choanae) are seen. They are separated from one another by the vomer that forms part of the bony nasal septum.

Middle part

The posterior nasal apertures are limited superiorly by the body of the sphenoid, below by the horizontal plates of the palatine bones and laterally by the medial pterygoid plates of the sphenoid. (*Note*: In these descriptions, the positional terms chosen refer to the conventional anatomic position. The body of the sphenoid is, therefore, always superior to the hard palate and nasal cavity.)

The sphenoid bone consists of a body, two lesser wings, two greater wings and two pterygoid processes. Only the body, greater wings and pterygoid processes are seen in the inferior view of the skull. Each pterygoid process has a medial and a lateral pterygoid plate. The lateral pterygoid plate is broader, while the lower extremity of the medial pterygoid plate projects laterally as the pterygoid hamulus. The greater wings of the sphenoid are lateral to the pterygoid processes. They form part of the cranial base and extend laterally and superiorly to shape part of the lateral walls of the skull. On each side, the posterior border of the greater wing joins the petrous part of the temporal bone to form the sphenopetrosal synchondrosis. The lateral border articulates with the squamous part of the temporal bone to form the sphenosquamous suture.

Behind the sphenoidal body is the basilar part of the occipital bone. It forms the spheno-occipital (or sphenobasilar) synchondrosis (SBS) with the posterior surface of the sphenoidal body, and the petro-occipital (or petrobasilar) suture with the petrous part of the temporal bone.

The petrous parts of the temporal bones are wedge shaped, located lateral and anterior to the basilar part of the occipital bone, and medial and posterior to the greater wings of the sphenoid. Each petrous part contains an opening for the carotid canal and, laterally, with the greater wing of the sphenoid, forms a groove for the cartilaginous part of the auditory tube. This groove runs on, in the petrous part of the temporal bone, as the bony canal of the auditory tube.

Laterally, on each side of the temporal bone, there is the mandibular fossa, below the posterior end of the zygomatic arch and in front of the external acoustic meatus. The head of the mandible is lodged therein to form the temporomandibular joint.

Posterior part

The four parts that constitute the occiput are seen in the inferior view. They are the basilar part, anterior to the foramen magnum, the lateral parts, lateral to the foramen magnum, and the squamous part, posterior to the foramen magnum. The basilar part has already been described above. The lateral parts contain the occipital condyles, which have convex surfaces that articulate with the superior atlantal facets. The long axes of the condyles converge anteromedially. Anterior and superior to each condyle is the hypoglossal canal, and posterior the condylar canal. Laterally, at the posterior end of the petro-occipital suture, on each side, the jugular foramen is formed between the occiput and the petrous temporal bone. The mastoid parts of the temporal petromastoid parts and styloid processes are seen laterally in this view. The most posterior features are the superior nuchal lines and external occipital protuberance visible on the squamous occipital bone.

INTERNAL VIEW OF THE CRANIAL VAULT (Fig. 3.6)

The inner surface of the skullcap is concave and includes most of the frontal and parietal bones, and the upper occipital squama. In front is the coronal suture, along the midline the sagittal suture, and behind the lambdoid suture. Anteriorly, a midline ridge of bone, the frontal crest, marks the attachment of the falx cerebri. It forms a longitudinal groove that continues posteriorly for the superior sagittal sinus. On either side, granular foveolae mark the location of arachnoid granulations.

INTERNAL VIEW OF THE CRANIAL BASE

The internal surface of the cranial base is clearly divided into anterior, middle and posterior fossae.

Anterior fossa (Fig. 3.7)

The anterior cranial fossa is above the nasal cavity and the orbits. The frontal bone forms the front and sides of this fossa. The orbital plates of the frontal

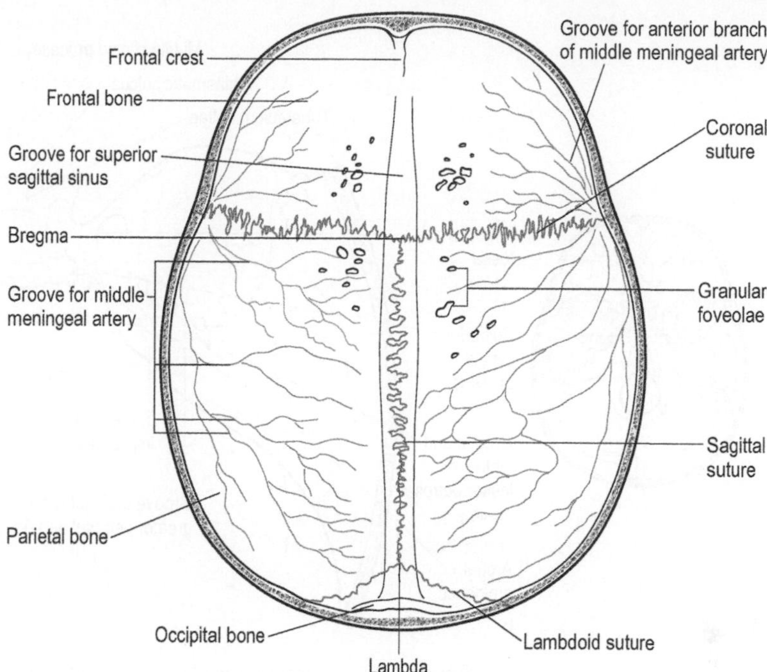

Figure 3.6. *Internal view of the cranial vault.*

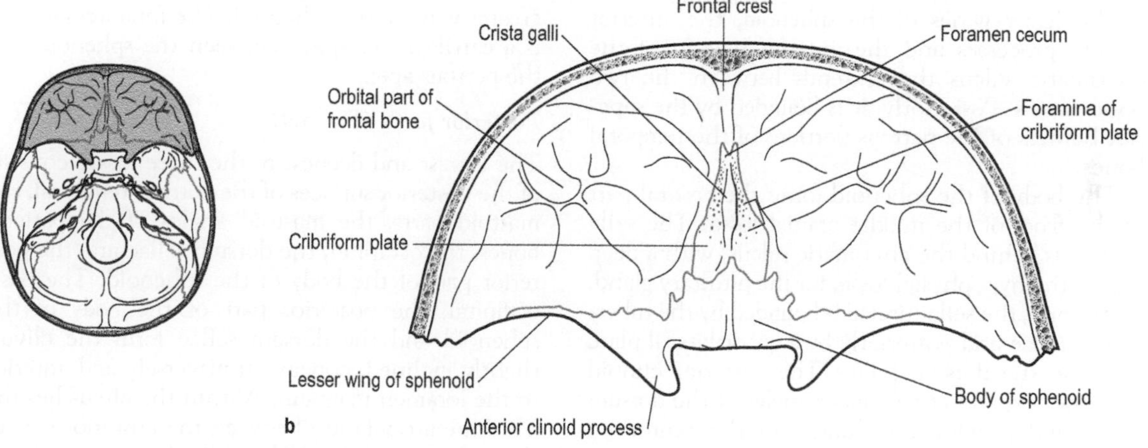

Figure 3.7. *(a,b) Internal view of the cranial base: anterior cranial fossa.*

bone, the cribriform plate of the ethmoid and the anterior part of the body and lesser wings of the sphenoid form the floor of the fossa. The crista galli is a superior projection of the ethmoid, behind the frontal crest, and where the falx cerebri attaches. Medially, each lesser wing joins the sphenoidal body by two roots surrounding the optic canal. The posterior border of the lesser wing projects medially as the anterior clinoid process, where the tentorium cerebelli attaches.

Middle fossa (Fig. 3.8)

The middle fossa is deeper than the anterior fossa. It is bounded in front by the posterior borders

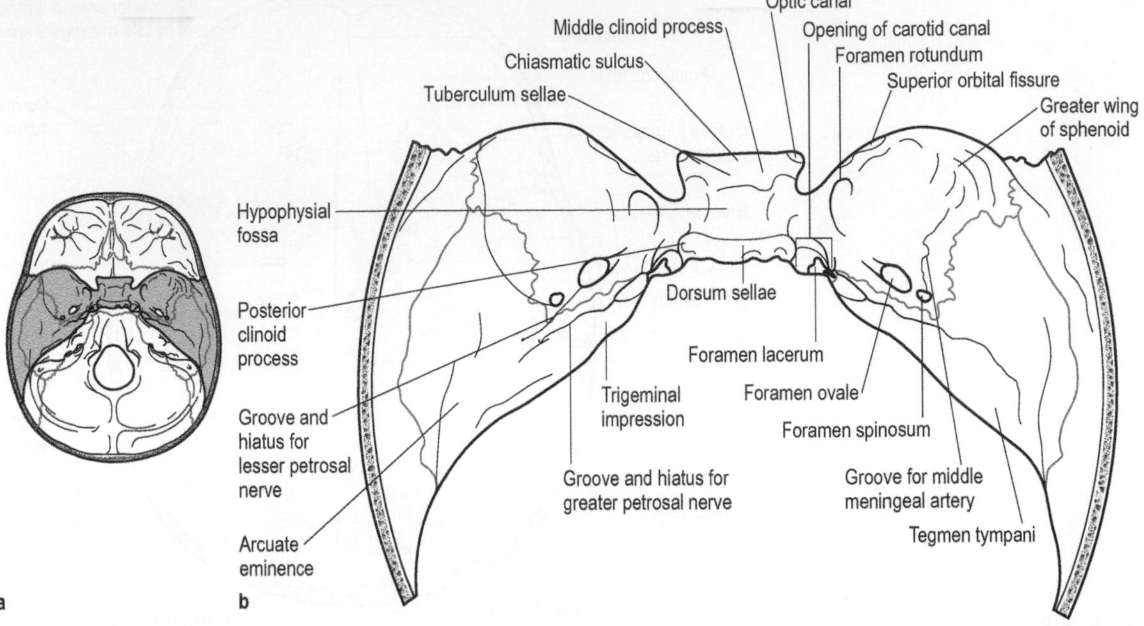

Figure 3.8. *(a,b) Internal view of the cranial base: middle cranial fossa.*

of the lesser wings of the sphenoid, the anterior clinoid processes and the anterior margin of the chiasmatic sulcus that extends between the two optic canals. Posteriorly, it is bounded by the superior borders of the petrous portions of the temporal bones.

The body of the sphenoid forms the central part of the floor of the middle cranial fossa. The sella turcica is behind the chiasmatic sulcus, with a deep recess, the hypophysial fossa, for the pituitary gland. Anteriorly, the sella turcica is bounded by the tuberculum sellae and posteriorly by a quadrilateral plate of bone, the dorsum sellae. The posterior clinoid processes expand at the upper angles of the dorsum sellae and provide attachment to the tentorium cerebelli.

Laterally, on each side, the middle fossa consists of the cerebral surface of the greater wing of the sphenoid, the cerebral surface of the temporal squama and the anterior surface of the petrous temporal bone. The superior orbital fissure, bounded above by the lesser wing of the sphenoid, below by the greater wing and medially by the sphenoidal body, allows communication between the middle fossa and the orbit. The foramina rotundum, ovale and spinosum are located between the roots of the greater wing of the sphenoid. The foramen lacerum is a cartilaginous space between the sphenoid and the petrous apex.

Posterior fossa (Fig. 3.9)

The largest and deepest of the three fossae consists of the posterior surfaces of the petrous temporal, the mastoid parts, the mastoid angles of the parietal bones, the occipital, the dorsum sellae and the posterior part of the body of the sphenoid. The basi-occipital, the posterior part of the body of the sphenoid and the dorsum sellae form the clivus, slightly inclined, concave transversely and anterior to the foramen magnum. Within the clivus lies the SBS, the articulation between the posterior part of the body of the sphenoid and the basi-occipital. On each side, the clivus is joined to the petrous portions of the temporal bones by the petro-occipital (petrobasilar) sutures. The jugular foramina are located posteriorly. The internal acoustic meatus is above the jugular foramina, on the petrous portions of the temporal bones. The inferior occipital fossae are separated by the internal occipital crest, where the falx cerebelli attach. The occipitomastoid and parietomastoid sutures are also located in the posterior fossa.

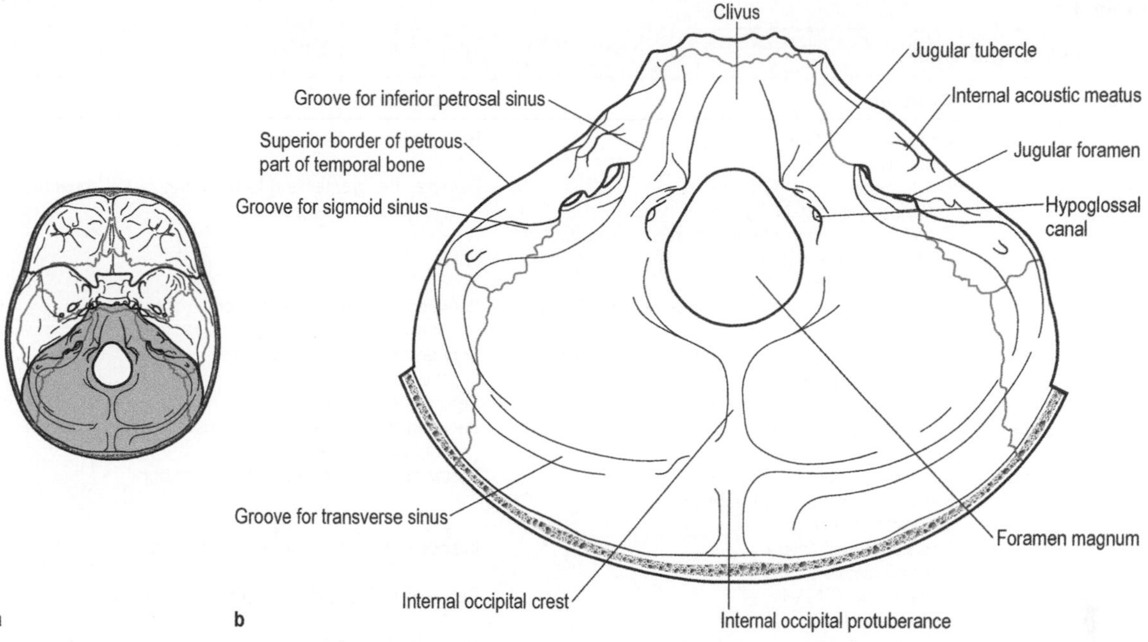

Figure 3.9. *(a,b) Internal view of the cranial base: posterior cranial fossa.*

The content and localization of the foramina of the skull are outlined in Table 3.1.

Dural attachments

'All these parts of bones are held together by the dura mater, "mother dura", functioning as an intraosseous membrane.' —WG SUTHERLAND[1]

In the fetus, a loose mesenchyme surrounds the neural mass. This tissue, referred to as meninx primitiva, or primary meninx, is the source of the different meningeal layers.[2] According to Arbuckle, in the early days of Sutherland's teaching, he was speaking of these layers as the dura mater and the 'dura pater'.[3] This image stresses well the common origin of, and interrelationship between, all of the structures derived from the primary meninx.

Two layers develop from the primary meninx. They differentiate into an outer layer, the ectomeninx (pachymeninx) and an inner layer, the endomeninx (leptomeninges). The arachnoid, subarachnoid space and pia mater originate from the endomeninx, while the ectomeninx will become the dura mater and the future cartilaginous and membranous parts of the neurocranium.

By the end of the 2nd month of gestation (57 days),[2] the developing endomeninx covers a significant portion of the rostral segment of the developing central nervous system – the rhombencephalon, the mesencephalon and part of the prosencephalon – and has developed into the arachnoid mater and the pia mater. By that time, the cerebrospinal fluid (CSF) is being secreted by the choroid plexus, entering and fi lling the developing subarachnoid spaces, where collagenous trabeculae connect the arachnoid and pia mater. The pia mater has closely invested the surface of the brain, encasing the developing circumconvolutions, covering every sulcus, and further extends to the roofs of the ventricles where it participates in the development of the choroid plexus.

From its earliest developmental stages, the meninx primitiva – the mesenchymatous matrix that surrounds the brain – resembles a capsule. While the inner part of the capsule evolves into the endomeninx, the progressive transformation of the outer part of the capsule creates the ectomeninx. At this time the brain expands dramatically, albeit in an eccentric fashion, and the capsule is totally responsive to the expanding spatial demands. Growth of

Table 3.1

Foramina of the skull

Foramen	Content	Localization
Optic canal	Optic nerve (CN II) Ophthalmic artery	Between the roots of the sphenoidal lesser wing
Superior orbital fissure	Oculomotor nerve (CN III) Trochlear nerve (CN IV) Ophthalmic division of the trigeminal nerve (CN VI) Abducent nerve (CN VI) Ophthalmic veins	Between the greater and lesser wings of the sphenoid
Foramen rotundum	Maxillary division of the trigeminal nerve (CN V2) Vein	Between the anterior and middle roots of the sphenoidal greater wing
Foramen ovale	Mandibular division of the trigeminal nerve (CN V3) Lesser petrosal nerve	Between the middle and posterior roots of the sphenoidal greater wing
Foramen spinosum	Middle meningeal artery and vein	Behind the foramen ovale
Foramen lacerum	Greater petrosal nerve	Between the apex of the petrous temporal and the sphenoidal body
Internal acoustic meatus	Facial nerve (CN VII) Vestibulocochlear nerve (CN VIII) Labyrinthine artery	Posterior surface of the petrous temporal
Carotid canal	Internal carotid artery Internal carotid plexus	Inferior surface of the petrous temporal
Stylomastoid foramen	Facial nerve (CN VII) Stylomastoid artery	Between the styloid and mastoid processes
Jugular foramen	Glossopharyngeal nerve (CN IX) Vagus nerve (CN X) Accessory nerve (CN XI) Inferior petrosal sinus Sigmoid sinus	Between the petrous part of the temporal and the basilar part of the occiput
Hypoglossal canal	Hypoglossal nerve (CN XII) Meningeal branch of the ascending pharyngeal artery	Anterior and superior to each occipital condyle
Foramen magnum	End of brainstem Vertebral arteries Spinal roots of the accessory nerve	Behind the basilar part of the occipital bone

the brain and surrounding mesenchyme occurs simultaneously in all three dimensions; biodynamic differentiation, however, causes some areas of the developing brain to grow more rapidly than others. The base of the mesenchymatous capsule, i.e. the anlage (or primordium) of the cranial base, becomes the thickest area of the capsule. This is also the place where the brain expands the least in volume.

During this same period, the cerebral vesicles enlarge and differentiate into the cerebellum and the occipital, temporal and frontal poles of the cerebral hemispheres. Areas of the mesenchymatous capsule between these developing portions of the brain become more dense and thicken as the portions approximate. These areas of thickness are referred to as dural stretches.[4] Five dural stretches are described:

- two orbital stretches between the frontal and the temporal lobes of the developing brain
- two otic stretches between the occipital lobes and cerebellum
- the ethmoidal stretch, in the midline, between the two frontal lobes.

The dural stretches and the dura connecting them are referred to as the dural girdles.[4] The thickened dural stretches act as reinforcement bands. The dura between the stretches offers less resistance and thereby more readily allows for brain growth.

The dural stretches in the vault are partially responsible for the creation of sutures that develop along the lines of stretch, whereas, between the dural stretches, membranous plates form centrally within each of the less resistant areas of the capsule as they are pulled in response to brain growth. These membranous plates will provide the location for the future centers of ossification of the bones of the skull. As these plates ossify, the dura contributes to the formation of periosteum, while the areas between the membranous plates, along the lines of dural stretch, will eventually become the sutures. Throughout life, the patency of the sutures is under the influence of chemical signaling mechanisms from the dura,[5] and dural fibers remain present within the sutures, even though varying degrees of sutural ossification may occur.

In the base of the cranium, the dural stretches and girdles exert similar influences. In response to the biodynamic forces of growth, the dural stretches respond less than the adjacent areas. This causes areas of the dural precursor to fold upon themselves and the dural stretches to form the innermost edges of the tentorum cerebelli and falx cerebelli and cerebri. Within the cranial base anlage, the chondrification of the five dural stretches occurs as a result of the associated traction and forms the otic alae, orbital alae and crista galli. These structures evolve to form the ridges of the petrous portions of the temporal bones, the lesser wings of the sphenoid and the ethmoidal crista galli, respectively.

This developmental relationship between the brain and the dura is very intimate. As the brain grows, the dural girdles develop, with continuity between all of the layers and areas of the cranial dura. Anteriorly and inferiorly, at the level of the anlage of the cranial base, the dural stretches are centrally joined to form the diaphragma sellae at the location of the future sella turcica of the sphenoid bone. They are also continuous caudally with the spinal dura.

The ossification of the skull develops within the initial mesenchymatous capsule surrounding the brain. This explains the close relationship between the dura and the osseous skull. Both the dura mater and the cartilaginous and membranous parts of the neurocranium are derived from the ectomeninx. In the base, the desmocranium is formed within the ectomeninx at about 4 weeks of gestation. By 8 weeks, through chondro-ossification, the desmocranium is replaced with cartilage and ossification begins at precisely 12 weeks and 4 days of gestation, initially within the chondrocranium, to form part of the occipital bone.[6] At this time, the inner part of the chondrocranium – the dura – differentiates into two layers: the inner (or meningeal) layer and the outer (or endosteal) layer.

In the vault, the bones are not preformed in cartilage, but develop from direct ossification within the mesenchyme. At this level, an intimate relationship also exists between the bones of the vault and the dura. The adhesion of the dura to the bones of the skull is strongest in the region of the sutures and the cranial base, and around the foramen magnum, where the endosteal layer is continuous with the spinal dura. This linkage is of paramount importance in cranial osteopathy. The connection of the spinal dura mater from the occiput at the foramen magnum to the pelvis is referred to as the core link.[7]

As previously stated, dural fibers remain present within the sutures throughout life and therefore the endosteal layer of the dura is continuous with the pericranium. In the same fashion, the endosteal layer is continuous with the pericranium through the cranial foramina and with the orbital periosteum through the superior orbital fissure. Because the osseous skull is organized around the pre-existent nervous and vascular structures, the skull should not be considered as having holes and fissures to allow passage for these structures. Instead, it should be remembered that, as nerves grow, they carry with them a protective tubular sheath of the meningeal layer of the dura. When the osseous skull develops around these nerves, foramina result, with some residual adherence between the foramina and the protective dural sheath. Outside the skull, the dural fibers will eventually fuse with the epineurium.

The dura mater consists of a dense fibrous network, with fibers arranged in fascicles, or stress fibers. Composed not only of collagen, it also contains a certain amount of elastic fibers. It is richly innervated essentially by the three divisions of the trigeminal nerve, except for the dura of the posterior cranial fossa that is innervated by the first three cervical spinal nerves.

Although for descriptive purposes the dura is divided in two layers – the meningeal and the endosteal – these two layers, except at the level where the venous sinuses have developed, are intimately united. Additionally, as described above, growth in the different portions of the brain causes areas of the inner (meningeal) layer of the dura to fold upon themselves to form the tentorium cerebelli and falx cerebelli and cerebri. Therefore, these folds also appear to have two layers. These three sickle-shaped folds come together in the area of the straight sinus. This area is referred to as the Sutherland Fulcrum[8] and constitutes a suspended area of reciprocal tension between the three folds.

FALX CEREBRI

The falx cerebri is crescent shaped, and descends vertically in the sagittal fissure between the cerebral hemispheres (Fig. 3.10). Its upper margin is curved, congruent with the internal convexity of the cranial

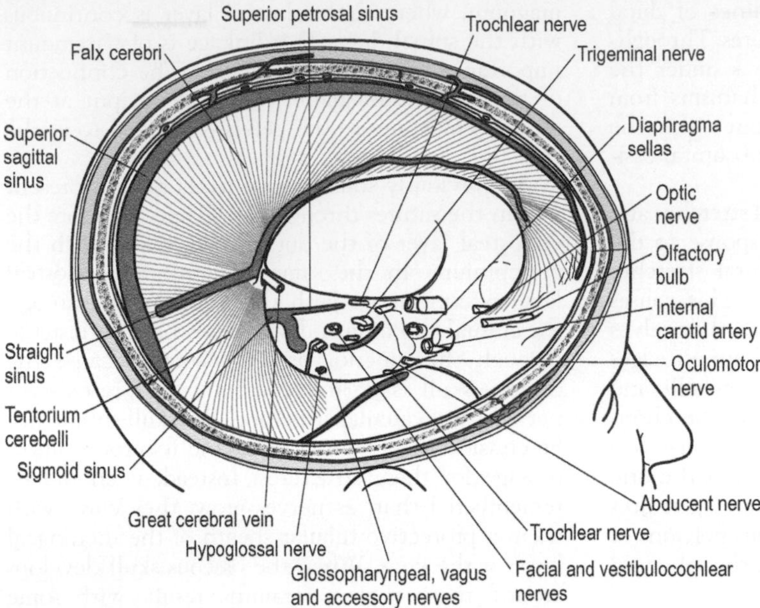

Figure 3.10. *Cerebral dura mater.*

vault. It extends from the frontal crest to the internal occipital protuberance and is affixed to the inner surface of the skull on each side of the midline. There, the two layers of the falx participate in the formation of the walls of the superior sagittal sinus. The inferior border of the falx cerebri is concave and can be divided into three portions:

- anteriorly, it is attached to the crista galli of the ethmoid
- behind, its free portion lies above the corpus callosum, where it contains the inferior sagittal sinus
- posteriorly, it broadens and connects, at the Sutherland Fulcrum, to the summit of the tentorium cerebelli. The straight sinus is located along this line, between the dural layers; it receives the inferior sagittal sinus and the vein of Galen.

The falx cerebri is a link between the anterior and posterior parts of the skull. It is also a strong connection between the neurocranium and the viscerocranium through its attachment to the crista galli. Thus, when the viscerocranium is dysfunctional, it may well be associated with, or secondary to, neurocranial dysfunction, and this relationship between the anterior and posterior skull and the face, through the falx, should be considered. In addition, the occipital bone acts as an interface between the posterior exocranial forces of the myofascial structures attached to it and the anterior intracranial forces that are transmitted posteriorly through the falx cerebri. Consequently, imbalances between the anterior cranium and posterior myofascial structures can result in dysfunctional stresses refl eted in the external shape of the occipital bone or of the viscerocranium. Postural balance, particularly the upper thoracic and cervical spine, is undoubtedly related to the mechanics of the skull and viscerocranium. The falx cerebri is, thus, an important component of this balanced relationship.

TENTORIUM CEREBELLI

The tentorium cerebelli is recognizable by the 8th week of gestation, and by 3 months of gestation its left and right sides are united around the straight sinus.[9] Classically described as a tent, as its name implies, the tentorium cerebelli covers the superior surface of the cerebellum and supports the occipital lobes of the cerebral hemispheres (Fig. 3.11). Its anterior margin, referred to as the lesser circumference, is free and concave. It surrounds a large oval opening, the tentorial incisure, where the midbrain is located. The outer convex border of the tentorium cerebelli is referred to as the great circumference. It

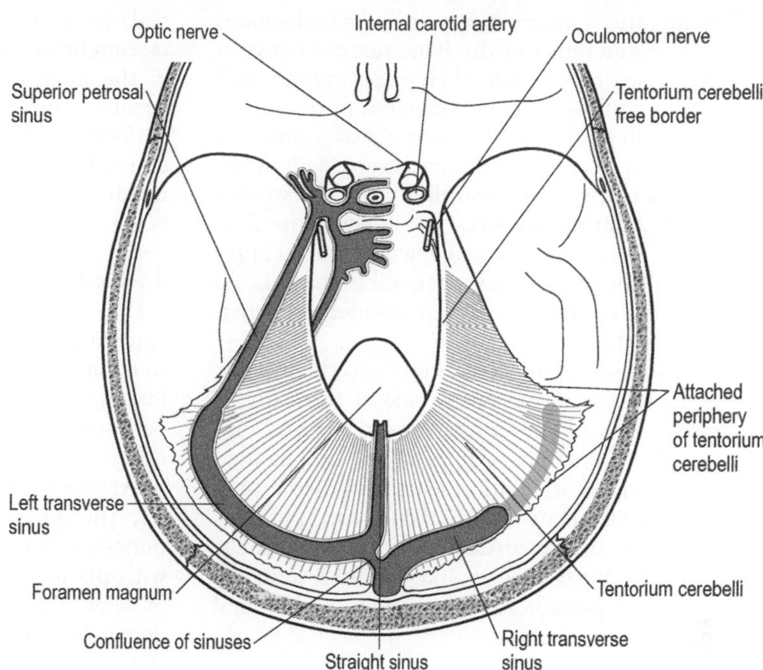

Figure 3.11. *Superior aspect of the tentorium cerebelli.*

is attached at the back to the transverse ridges of the inner surface of the occipital bone, where it encloses the transverse sinuses. On both sides it is attached across the parietomastoid sutures, the upper layer attached to the posterior–inferior angles of the parietal bones and the lower layer to the mastoid. Laterally, the two layers of the tentorium are attached to the superior ridges of the petrous portions of the temporal bones, where the superior petrosal sinuses are located. Next to the apex of the petrous part of the temporal bone, the lower layer of the tentorium forms the trigeminal cave that protects the root and the ganglion of the trigeminal nerve. Both circumferences of the tentorium meet at the apex of the petrous part of the temporal bone, crossing one another in such a way that the free borders of the lesser circumference continue forward to be fixed to the anterior clinoid processes of the body of the sphenoid, and the attached borders to be fixed to the posterior clinoid processes. The posterior border of the falx cerebri meets with the midline of the tentorium cerebelli's upper surface at the Sutherland Fulcrum. The straight sinus is enclosed within this junction.

The tentorium cerebelli is in close relationship with cranial nerves III, IV, V_1 and VI. It may, consequently, become a site for entrapment of these nerves and should be considered when diagnosing trigeminal and ocular dysfunctions.[10] The trigeminal cave may be a site of entrapment for the trigeminal ganglion. Other potential vulnerable locations include the anterior portion of the tentorium cerebelli, where it forms part of the roof of the cavernous sinus. The fi bers located between the lesser and greater circumferences of the tentorium cerebelli are twisted, and change from an oblique direction to a more horizontal one. The oculomotor (CN III) and trochlear (CN IV) nerves pierce the dura at this level as they pass through the cavernous sinus before entering the superior orbital fi ssure. The abducent nerve (CN VI), after bending sharply over the superior border of the petrous portion of the temporal bone, passes under the petrosphenoidal ligament to join cranial nerves III and IV in the cavernous sinus. The petrosphenoidal ligament – a fibrous band that joins the apex of the petrous temporal and the lateral margin of the dorsum sellae – is considered to be a site of entrapment for CN VI.[10]

The external occipital protuberance, or inion, is a palpable landmark that can be used to locate the level of attachment of the tentorium cerebelli. It is located at almost the same level as the internal occipital protuberance where the major venous sinuses enclosed in the dura – the transverse sinuses, straight sinus and superior sagittal sinus – meet. Above the tentorium cerebelli the occipital squama is of membranous origin; below, it is of cartilaginous origin. The difference in the bony texture between these two parts may be felt when palpating the skull of a newborn. This area of attachment of the tentorium cerebelli to the occiput may act as a hinge in the production of occipital intraosseous dysfunctions, particularly those resulting from the stresses encountered during delivery. The upper, more flexible part of the occipital squama may be forced anteriorly, resulting in posterior occipital flattening. As such, balancing of the dura can be effective when treating this dysfunction.

The tentorium is attached laterally to the interior of the neurocranium on either side of the parietomastoid sutures. Here it encloses the transverse sinus at the point where it becomes the sigmoid sinus. Molding in association with the possibility of parietal displacement during labor can put this venous sinus under stress. Cranial hemorrhage following the birth process and impaired drainage have been reported in association with dural dysfunction.[11]

FALX CEREBELLI

The falx cerebelli is a small triangular fold of dura mater, located underneath the falx cerebri. It is attached posteriorly to the lower portion of the vertical crest of the occipital bone where it contains the occipital sinus, and sometimes splits into two smaller folds that disappear laterally on either side of the foramen magnum. Superiorly, it is attached to the posterior portion of the tentorium cerebelli, while its anterior edge is free and located between the two cerebellar hemispheres.

DIAPHRAGMA SELLAE

The diaphragma sellae is a small rounded horizontal fold of dura that covers the hypophysial fossa, in the sella turcica, of the sphenoid bone. There is an opening in the center of the diaphragma that allows the infundibulum and blood vessels to connect the hypophysis (pituitary gland) to the base of the brain.

SPINAL DURA

The cranial dura mater is adherent close to the margin of the foramen magnum. The outer (endosteal) layer ends at this level, turning into the periosteum lining the vertebral canal. The prolongation of the meningeal layer of the cranial dura mater becomes the spinal dura mater, separated from the periosteum of the vertebral canal by the extradural or epidural space. It is attached via the posterior longitudinal ligament to the posterior surfaces of the bodies of vertebrae C2 and C3.

All along the spine, at the level of each intervertebral foramen, the spinal dura mater (Fig. 3.12) extends as a tubular sheath to surround the emerging spinal nerves, and fuses with the epineurium at the level of, or after, the intervertebral foramina.[12] The dural sheath may be adherent to the periosteum, particularly around the C5–C6 spinal nerves.[13]

At the middle one-third[14] or inferior border of S2,[2] the spinal dura mater fuses with the filum terminale, a thin connective tissue filament invested with pia mater that prolongs the conus medullaris, or apex, of the spinal cord. The filum terminale descends in the middle of the spinal nerves that form the cauda equina, and blends, at the level of S2, with the dura. It then descends to the back of the first coccygeal segment where it fuses with the periosteum. It is referred to as the central ligament of the medulla spinalis because of its assistance in preserving the position of the medulla spinalis during movements of the spine. In the newborn, the apex of the conus medullaris is situated at the level of the upper margin of L3, lower than in the adult, where it is located between L1 and L2.

It is important to recognize that these individually named and described structures are, in fact, one continuous structure. Most commonly, the tentorium cerebelli is pictured as a rather horizontal septum, while the falx cerebri is thought to be an anteroposterior link. It should be remembered that the tentorial dura is reflected on each side to cover the temporal bones and the occipital squama posteriorly, whereas the falx continues on each side of the sagittal suture to cover the parietal bones and to meet with the tentorium cerebelli laterally. Anteriorly, at the level of the cavernous sinus, fibers from the tentorium cerebelli are continuous with the upper layer of the diaphragma sellae. Inside the sella turcica the fibers of the dura are intimately blended with the capsule of the hyphophysis. Posteriorly, the dural duplications form a unit in continuation with the spinal dura.

This continuous structure forms the reciprocal tension membranes, an important component of the cranial concept. It unites the different areas of the skull (the cranial bowl) to the pelvis (the pelvic

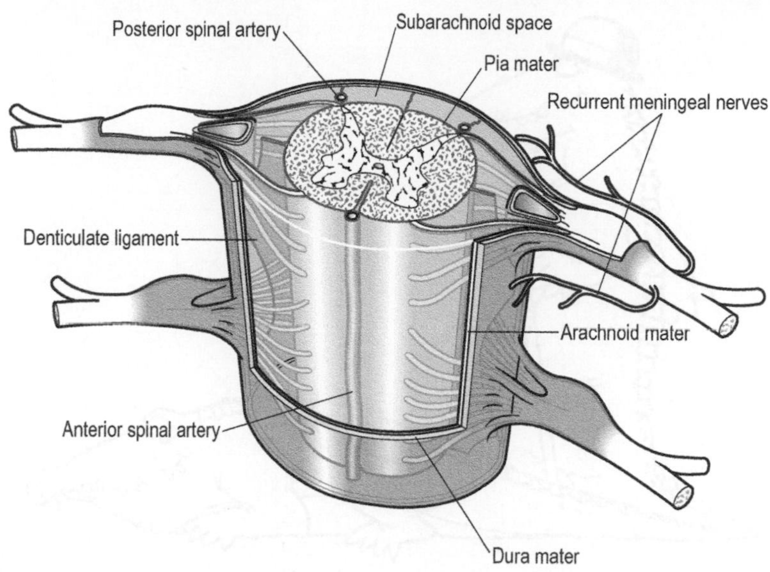

Figure 3.12. *Spinal dura mater.*

bowl), creating the core link. Membranous strain dysfunctions can exist intraspinally as well as intracranially, and may be established prenatally as well as postpartum. Understanding this is of particular importance when diagnosing and treating infants because their bone structure is not completely organized, and any dysfunctional pattern in the membranes may serve as a template for bone growth in the future, resulting in dysfunctional patterns in the structure of the skeleton. A failure to recognize dural dysfunctional mechanics can result in inability to effectively treat somatic dysfunction affecting other areas of the body.

Motion in the cranial concept

PHYLOGENETIC EVOLUTION OF THE SKULL

Comparative anatomic and anthropometric studies between non-human primates and modern humans are of value for not only understanding the evolution of the skull, but also for fostering an appreciation of the development of cranial dysfunctions over time. During the evolutionary process from early primates to anthropoids, and finally to *Homo sapiens*, significant changes in the shape of the cranial base seem to have been extremely important.[15] One of the signifi cant differences between humans and other primates is an increased flexion of the cranial base along the midline for humans. The basicranium (base of the neurocranium; cranial base) includes parts of the occipital bone, most of the sphenoid, the ethmoid and the petrous portions of the temporal bones. These cranial elements develop from the chondrocranium and are sites where early growth and development occur. The basicranium provides support for the brain and contains numerous foramina that allow the passage of important vascular and nervous structures in and out of the brain case. It can also be considered as an interface between the other craniofacial units, the vault of the neurocranium and the viscerocranium. It is logical to assume that interaction occurs between these different constituents – for instance, that the morphogenesis of the base of the skull impacts that of the face and, inversely, that the function and dysfunction of the viscerocranium impacts the basicranium. The different issues affecting behavior also affect structure. In the course of the evolution of the skull, the activities of non-human primates and humans, as determined by the environment, should also be considered.

If a creature with a purely horizontal body structure (e.g. a crocodile) were to shift from the horizontal to an upright vertical position, their eyes would fi nd themselves directed toward the sky. In order for the crocodile to look straight ahead and maintain the eyes in a forward-facing orientation, forward flexion of the head would be necessary. First,

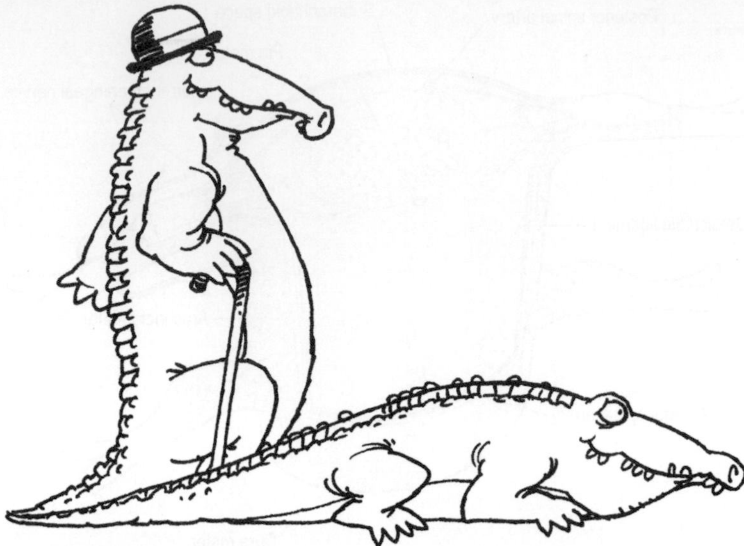

Figure 3.13. *Forward flexion of the cranial base is part of the adaptation to orthograde posture.*

the cervical vertebrae and the occipitoatlantal junction would be flexed. Next, to further orient the position of the eyes, flexion of the synchondroses of the skull base would be necessary. This adaptation to orthograde or bipedal posture is the most common reason proposed to explain the flexion of the base of the skull in humans. Cranial base flexion, or angulation of the basicranium, is one of the most significant characteristics of phylogenetic evolution of the skull, with humans demonstrating more cranial base flexion than other primates[16] (Fig. 3.13).

Another significant difference between humans and other primates is brain growth, considered to be one of the significant factors responsible for changes in the shape of the cranial base. The human brain is far from maturity at birth. It is about 25% of its adult size at birth, reaching 50% of its adult size by the end of the 1st year and about 95% at 10 years.[17] In comparison, chimpanzees achieve 80% of the adult brain size by the end of the 1st year of life.

In terms of evolution, encephalization – the growth in size of the human brain – is another characteristic that explains the differences in basicranial morphology between humans and other primates. Throughout human evolution, the volume of the brain case has tended to increase in size progressively. Cranial volume is about 500 ml in *Australopithecus afarentis*, 700 ml in *Homo habilis*, 1000 ml in *Homo erectus*, 1230 ml in *Homo sapiens* and 1400 ml in *Homo sapiens sapiens*.[18] Human brain growth acts as an expansive force, stimulating the development of the osseous skull. The synchondroses of the cranial base consist of cartilaginous bone growth plates where the anteroposterior length of the base increases. Another effective way to enlarge the volume of the skull, so as to accommodate a bigger brain, is to augment the angulation of the base, consequently creating a flexion of the base. The development of the human cranial base begins prenatally and continues after birth. Flexion is well established before 2 years of age, although brain growth is not yet complete. On the other hand, the non-human primate demonstrates a flexion of the cranial base before birth and an extension after birth.

The cranial base angle is the angulation between the clivus (dorsum sellae of the sphenoid and basiocciptal bone) and the planum sphenoideum (plane of the superior surface of the sphenoid). It opens downward and forward, and measures about 120° in humans and 140° in anthropoids (Fig. 3.14).

The changes in the cranial base that result in flexion (angulation) occur at the level of three synchondroses:

- the intrasphenoidal synchondrosis, between the pre- and the postsphenoid
- the sphenoethmoidal synchondrosis, between the anterior aspect of the sphenoid and the posterior part of the ethmoid
- the spheno-occipital (or sphenobasilar) synchondrosis (SBS), between the basilar process of the occipital bone and the body of the sphenoid.

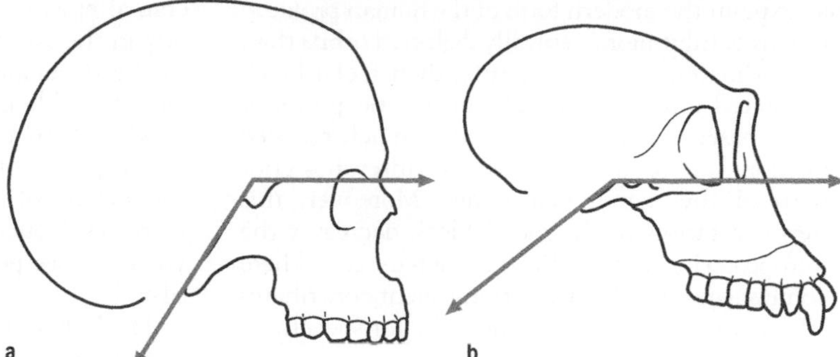

Figure 3.14. *The cranial base angle opens downward and forward and measures about 120° in humans (a) and 140° in anthropoids (b).*

These synchondroses act like hinges, where increased chondrogenic activity in the superior part of the synchondrosis produces flexion and increased chondrogenic activity in the inferior part of the synchondrosis produces extension. In primates, the SBS seems to be the most active.[19] The intrasphenoidal synchondrosis participates in cranial flexion during the prenatal period and in most instances is completely ossified at birth. The sphenoethmoidal synchondrosis continues to be an active site of cranial base growth during neural expansion up to the age of 6–8 years, when most of the brain size is achieved. The sphenoethmoidal synchondrosis also plays a key role in facial development as an interface between the sphenoid and the ethmoid.

Brain growth stimulates sutural osteoblastic deposition and the periosteal remodeling that are the basic phenomena involved in growth of the bony parts of the skull. Simultaneously, osteoclastic resorption occurs at different sites, altering bone deposition. This modulation results in apparent differences in the growth of the multiple parts of the cranial base. The same process occurs between different parts of one bone, giving the impression that the bone is growing at different rates. This phenomenon occurs between the four parts of the occiput. In humans, the basioccipital (anterior) part displays less growth than the other parts of the occiput; the squamous (posterior) part grows more. This difference in growth between the two parts explains why the position of the foramen magnum seems to be more anterior in humans than in non-human primates. The increase of the occipital squama seems to push the foramen magnum forward. A posterior ('positive') rotation of the occiput, i.e. clockwise when looking at the skull from the left side, is described to illustrate the increase in the development of the squamous portion.[20] This modification of the shape of the occipital squama is the result of both the intracranial forces generated by the growing brain and the extracranial forces generated by the muscles that insert on the squama and that contract to maintain the head in a vertical position.

There is, however, a limit to the degree of flexion of the cranial base that can occur without interfering with the function of, and interrelationships between, the basicranium and the viscerocranium, the pharynx and the larynx, and modifications to allow for brain expansion are, therefore, necessary. Concomitant with basicranial base flexion and the development of the squama of the occiput, the size of the temporal bones increases and the petrous portions adjust their orientation. They move downward and laterally, with a greater displacement at their posterior part that increases the posterior width of the skull.[21] Enlargement of the brain, therefore, evolves in a fashion parallel with the augmentation of the skull volume. Complex interactions also occur in other components of the skull, such as lateral expansion of the squamous portions of the temporal bones,[22] increased vertical orientation of the frontal bone and increased biparietal diameter. The dimensions in the three cardinal planes are modified in the modern human skull to diminish the cranial length relative to the endocranial volume, resulting in a more spherical skull and an increased cranial 'globularity'.[23]

The sphenoid occupies a predominant position, centrally located within the skull base. It connects the basicranium and the bones of the viscerocranium. Composed of multiple foramina and fissures that contain numerous vessels and nerves, the sphenoid articulates with many facial bones located in front of it. Additionally, the length of its body influences the degree of facial projection in relation to the anterior cranial fossa. The human sphenoid demonstrates a decrease in its anteroposterior dimension that diminishes the projection of the face and may explain the modern form of the human profile.[24] Humans exhibit more ventrally deflected orbits than other primates.[22] Concomitantly, their facial block has rotated anteriorly in relation to the posterior cranial base; it is associated with a much-reduced dentition and a decrease of the anteroposterior length of the mandibular ramus. Moreover, this anterior rotation of the facial block decreases the anteroposterior length of the nasopharynx.[25] There is some suggestion that this arrangement contributes to the cranial structure that provides for speech.[24]

ONTOGENETIC DEVELOPMENT

Ontogenetic development of the cranial base follows the same sequential pattern as phylogenesis and comparative anatomy described above. At birth, the cranial base forms a slightly arched line with the spheno-occipital synchondrosis and the basion, the most anterior point of the foramen magnum being in the same plane. The larynx is located at a high position in the neck, close to the hyoid bone, and the tongue is contained totally within the oral cavity (Fig. 2.11).[26]

The basilar fl exion initiated during the fetal period continues after birth until the adolescent period.[15] Again, the different synchondroses of the cranial base are involved in producing this basilar fl exion. These are also sites of growth, and the spheno-occipital synchondrosis is one of the most active, contributing to lengthening of the clivus. The sphenoethmoidal synchondrosis between the presphenoid and cribriform plate contributes to the elongation of the anterior part of the cranial base. Growth appears to stop between 6 and 8 years, and this synchondrosis fuses between puberty and adulthood.[15]

In the posterior part of the skull, as the child attempts to lift their head when in the prone position, the squamous portion of the occiput develops because of the pull exerted by the posterior musculature. Later, when crawling and standing, this muscular action is maintained for more prolong periods of time, continuing to shape the occiput.

In the anterior part of the skull, the myofascial components also contribute to the development of the bony structures to which they are attached. Functions of the viscerocranium, such as suckling, swallowing, chewing and speech, are involved. The pharyngeal and palatal muscles particularly affect the pterygoid processes in deglutition, when they pull the pterygoid hamuli in a downward and lateral direction. This contributes to the fl exion of the cranial base, causing the sphenoid to rotate anteriorly in the sagittal plane. Glutition also contributes to the development of the pterygoid hamuli that almost double in size between childhood and adulthood.[27] With age, as the pterygoid hamuli move laterally and inferiorly, the hard palate widens and the height of the posterior nares, the choanae, increases. Concomitantly, the superior border of the vomer grows posteriorly to reach the level of the SBS.[28]

The human brain enlarges rapidly during the first years of life and stimulates the growth of the neurocranium that has considerably increased in size by the age of 2–3 years. This is the age when flexion of the cranial base has almost reached completion. It is also the time when the upper airway structures have changed position.[26] The hyoid bone and larynx are lower. The tongue that was totally contained in the oral cavity at birth moves down in such a way that its posterior part defines the upper anterior wall of the pharynx. A space is created under the concavity of the exocranial base, i.e. the nasopharynx, its vault being formed by the spheno-occipital synchondrosis. This new supralaryngeal airspace, combined with the low position of the larynx and mobility of the tongue, allows for the production of the sounds necessary for speech. Concomitantly with the descent of the tongue and larynx, the pharyngeal constrictor muscles change their orientation to become more vertically oblique. The superior constrictor of the pharynx is, in part, inserted into the cranial base, on the medial pterygoid plate of the sphenoid and on the median pharyngeal raphe that is projected onto the pharyngeal tubercle of the basilar part of the occiput. There is a relationship between the development of these structures and their orientation relative to the basiocciput, and it is suggested that they may contribute to the flexion of the cranial base.[26]

The cranial base, therefore, is under multiple influences. Strong postural muscles posteriorly assist the actions of the anterior myofascial structures to increase the flexion of the cranial base. The meninges, also called reciprocal tension membranes (the falx cerebri, tentorium cerebelli and falx cerebelli), play important roles by counteracting these external muscular forces. The balanced membranous tension applied to the inner surfaces of the skull effectively counters the forces exerted by the external muscles. Skull ridges, processes and crests on the external surfaces, as well as on the internal surfaces, provide evidence of these tractions.

Facial features – the external projection of the viscerocranium – are among the dominant characteristics that identify an individual. Both the human profile and the position of the mandible have been correlated with the basicranial shape.[29] The different ocular, nasal, oral and pharyngeal components that are incorporated within the viscerocranium and under the influence of the cranial base also exert an influence on the human profile. Posture of the cervical spine also contributes to shape the craniofacial morphology. Forward bending of the head is associated with an increase in anterior facial height; backward bending is associated with a decrease.[30,31] Therefore, human activities, part of the epigenetic influences, particularly those that occur early in life, are extremely important in determining structure, function and dysfunction in the developing individual.

Multifactorial influences during phylogeny that result in hominization produce a flexion of the cranial base. This basic flexion pattern is repeated during ontogeny. It demonstrates the interdependence of the different parts of the skull – basicranium, vault and viscerocranium. It also demonstrates the interdependence of the skull with the rest of the body. This same pattern of flexion of the cranial base, coupled with lateral expansion of the squamous portions of the temporal bones and the biparietal diameter increase, is described during cranial movements of the inspiratory phase of the primary respiratory mechanism (PRM).

PATTERNS OF MOTION

The following description of bony movement in the craniosacral mechanism is a simple mechanical model based on principles originally described by Sutherland.[32] The purpose of this presentation is to describe the hypothetical basis for a modality that has been demonstrated to be effective through years of clinical application on countless patients.

Throughout the entire body it is possible to palpate a rhythmic micro movement, the PRM of Sutherland. The PRM is a cyclic phenomenon divided into two phases termed cranial inspiration and cranial expiration. In the inspiratory phase, the midline unpaired structures of the skull and pelvis move in the direction of the fetal curve, termed craniosacral flexion, and the paired structures externally rotate. In the reciprocal expiratory phase, the midline structures move in the direction of craniosacral extension and the paired structures internally rotate. It is important to note here that, in some instances, the craniosacral flexion and extension movements described later in the chapter differ from, and should not be confused with, anatomic flexion and extension. The discussion of bony movements that follows is a description of motion of the respective structures in the absence of somatic dysfunction. Dysfunctional mechanics, the precursor to somatic dysfunction, will be discussed later.

The spine and the thoracic cage, together with the structures of the upper and lower limbs, demonstrate a biphasic motion in association with the inspiratory and expiratory phases of the PRM. The individual vertebral segments demonstrate craniosacral flexion and extension. The global motion of the spine, in synchrony with the PRM, demonstrates a decrease of the normal anteroposterior curves in association with the inspiratory phase and an increase of the anteroposterior curves in association with the expiratory phase. The sternum, as an unpaired structure, demonstrates a motion of flexion in association with the inspiratory phase and a motion of extension in association with the expiratory phase. As would be anticipated, the paired structures – ribs, pectoral girdle, upper and lower limbs – demonstrate external rotation in association with the inspiratory phase and internal rotation with the expiratory phase. These movements are of importance in the whole body approach and particularly when considering appendicular problems in infants and children.

The PRM, palpated as the cranial rhythmic impulse (CRI) by a trained examiner, consists of a cyclic movement having a rate described as 4–14 cycles per minute.[33,34] It is separate from pulmonary respiration and the cardiovascular pulse. It has been demonstrated to be associated with the low frequency Traube–Hering–Mayer oscillation, a manifestation of sympathetic tone within the autonomic nervous system that has 'been measured in association with blood pressure, heart rate, cardiac contractility, pulmonary blood flow, cerebral blood flow and movement of the cerebrospinal fluid, and peripheral blood flow including venous volume and thermal regulation. This whole-body phenomenon, which exhibits a rate typically slightly less than and independent of respiration, bears a striking resemblance to the PRM'.[35] In the peacefully resting individual, pulmonary respiration commonly becomes entrained with the rhythm of the PRM.

Movement of the unpaired structures in craniosacral flexion–extension

The unpaired structures are the sacrum and coccyx, the vertebral segments of the spine, the hyoid bone, the sternum, the occipital bone, the sphenoid, the ethmoid and the vomer. The following discussion describes the movement of the unpaired midline structures, flexion during the cranial inspiratory phase of the PRM and extension during the cranial expiratory phase. Flexion occurs about a transverse axis in the sagittal plane; extension occurs opposite to flexion.

Sacrum and coccyx

The axis of motion for craniosacral flexion–extension of the sacrum is a hypothetical horizontal transverse axis that has been described as passing through the tip of the spinous process of the second sacral segment.[36] The exact location of this axis is open to debate. During craniosacral flexion, the sacral base moves posteriorly and the sacral apex anteriorly; during craniosacral extension, the sacral base moves anteriorly and the sacral apex posteriorly. The sacral segments remain unfused in infants and prepubescent children, and, as such, the normally posterior convex sacral curve decreases during craniosacral flexion and increases during craniosacral extension. The coccygeal bones follow the movement of the sacrum in craniosacral flexion and extension (Fig. 3.15).

Vertebrae

The vertebrae behave both segmentally and as a group. The axis of motion for craniosacral flexion–extension of the vertebrae is a horizontal transverse axis. During craniosacral flexion, the spine demonstrates a decrease of the normal AP curves in association with the inspiratory phase of the PRM (Fig. 3.16a). Therefore, the cervical lordosis decreases as each cervical segment, including the occiput on the atlas, forward bends relative to the segment below. The thoracic kyphosis decreases as each thoracic segment backward bends relative to the segment below. The lumbar lordosis decreases as each lumbar segment, including L5 on the sacral base, forward bends relative to the segment below.

Conversely, during craniosacral extension, the spine demonstrates an increase of the normal AP curves in association with the expiratory phase of the PRM (Fig. 3.16b). Therefore, the cervical lordosis increases as each cervical segment, including the occiput on the atlas, backward bends relative to the segment below. The thoracic kyphosis increases as each thoracic segment forward bends relative to the segment below. The lumbar lordosis increases as each lumbar segment, including L5 on the sacral base, backward bends relative to the segment below.

Hyoid

The hyoid bone is suspended by the stylohyoid ligament from the tips of the styloid processes of the temporal bones and is, therefore, influenced by temporal bone motion. During craniosacral flexion, the hyoid bone demonstrates a movement where the body, or central part, moves inferiorly and posteriorly, and the greater cornua moves superiorly and anteriorly. During craniosacral extension, the body moves superiorly and anteriorly, and the greater cornua moves inferiorly and posteriorly. These motions are normally concurrent with the movements of the mandible and cervical spine.

Sternum

During craniosacral flexion, the entire sternum moves anteriorly and the sternal angle of Louis increases; during craniosacral extension, the sternum moves posteriorly and the sternial angle decreases.

Occiput

The axis of motion for craniosacral flexion–extension of the occiput is a horizontal transverse axis located above the foramen magnum, at the level

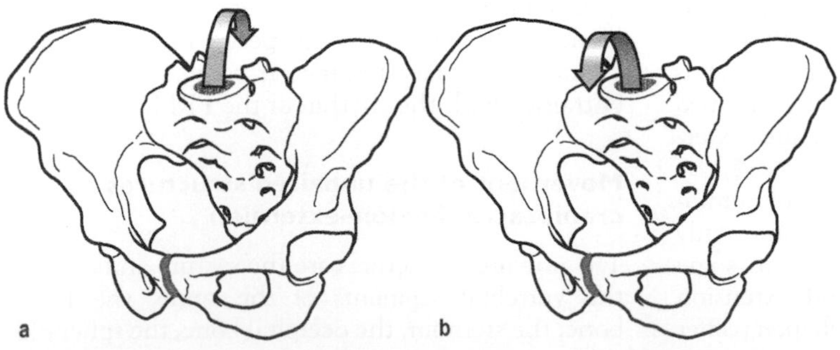

Figure 3.15. *Movement of the sacrum: (a) craniosacral flexion; (b) craniosacral extension.*

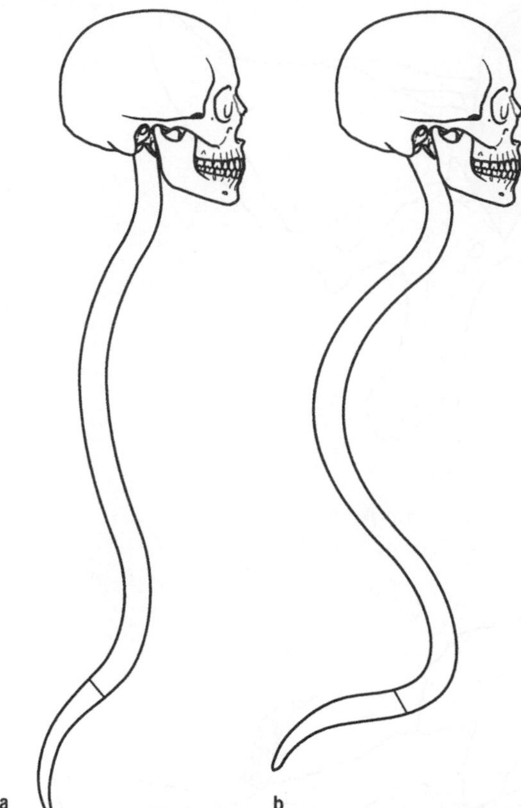

Figure 3.16. *Movement of the vertebrae. (a) Craniosacral flexion: decrease of the normal AP curves of the spine. (b) Craniosacral extension: increase of the normal AP curves of the spine.*

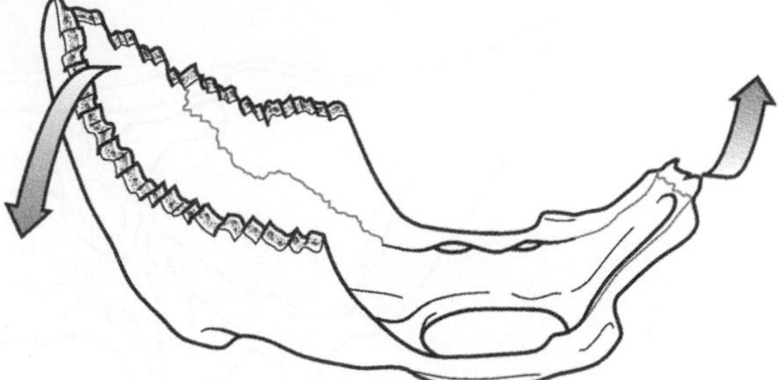

Figure 3.17. *Movement of the occiput in cranial flexion.*

of the jugular processes. During craniosacral flexion, the anterior articular surface of the occipital basilar portion moves anteriorly and superiorly, the lambda moves posteriorly and inferiorly, and the lateral angles move posteriorly and laterally (Fig. 3.17). During craniosacral extension, the anterior articular surface of the occipital basilar portion moves posteriorly and inferiorly, the lambda moves anteriorly and superiorly, and the lateral angles move anteriorly and internally (see 'Remarks', p. 66).

Sphenoid

One cannot completely understand the subtleties of sphenoid motion and its relationship to the rest of the skull without recognizing that this bone consists of three distinct parts at birth. The body and lesser wings form the central part, while the two lateral parts, one on each side of the body, are each created by the combination of the greater wing and pterygoid process. Ossification of the synchondroses between these three parts is usually completed between the 1st and 2nd year of life. The junctional zones between the parts, however, retain a certain degree of flexibility throughout life. Because of this, the body of the sphenoid will be considered as an unpaired structure, and both greater wing–pterygoid units considered as paired structures as discussed below (see 'Movement of the paired structures', p. 71).

The axis of motion for cranial flexion–extension of the body of the sphenoid, the central part, is a horizontal transverse axis located anterior and inferior to the sella turcica. During cranial flexion, the anterior portion of the body moves inferiorly and the dorsum sellae moves superiorly, causing the superior aspect of the body of the sphenoid to rotate anteriorly in the sagittal plane (Figs 3.18, 3.19). During cranial extension, the anterior portion of the body moves superiorly and the dorsum sellae moves inferiorly, causing the superior aspect of the body of the sphenoid to rotate posteriorly in the sagittal plane (Fig. 3.20).

Ethmoid

Similar to the sphenoid, the ethmoid consists of a medial part, the perpendicular plate, which behaves as an unpaired structure, and two paired parts, the lateral labyrinths, which will be discussed below (see 'Movement of the paired structures', p. 71).

The axis of motion for cranial flexion–extension of the medial part of the ethmoid is a horizontal transverse axis, perpendicular to the ethmoidal perpendicular plate. During cranial flexion, the anterior portion of the perpendicular plate moves superiorly, and the crista galli, the point of anterior insertion of the falx cerebri, moves superiorly and posteriorly (Fig. 3.21). The posterior border of the cribriform plate moves inferiorly, accompanying the anterior portion of the body of the sphenoid. During cranial extension, the anterior portion of the perpendicular

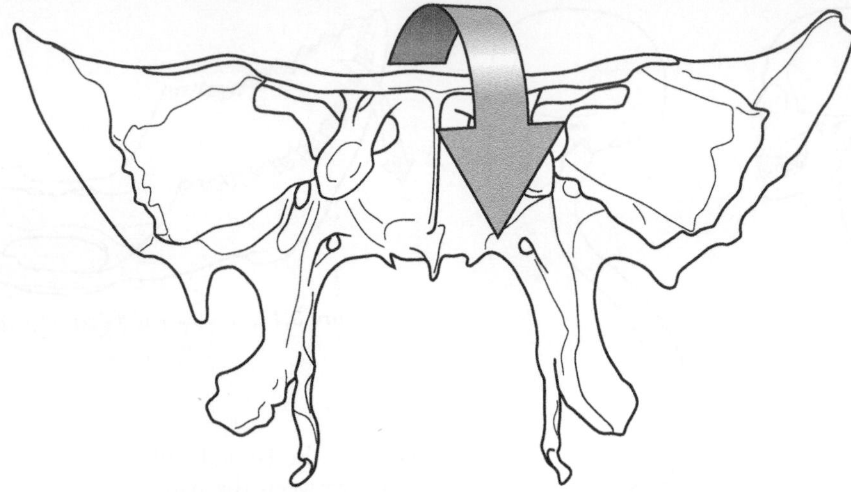

Figure 3.18. *Movement of the sphenoid in cranial flexion.*

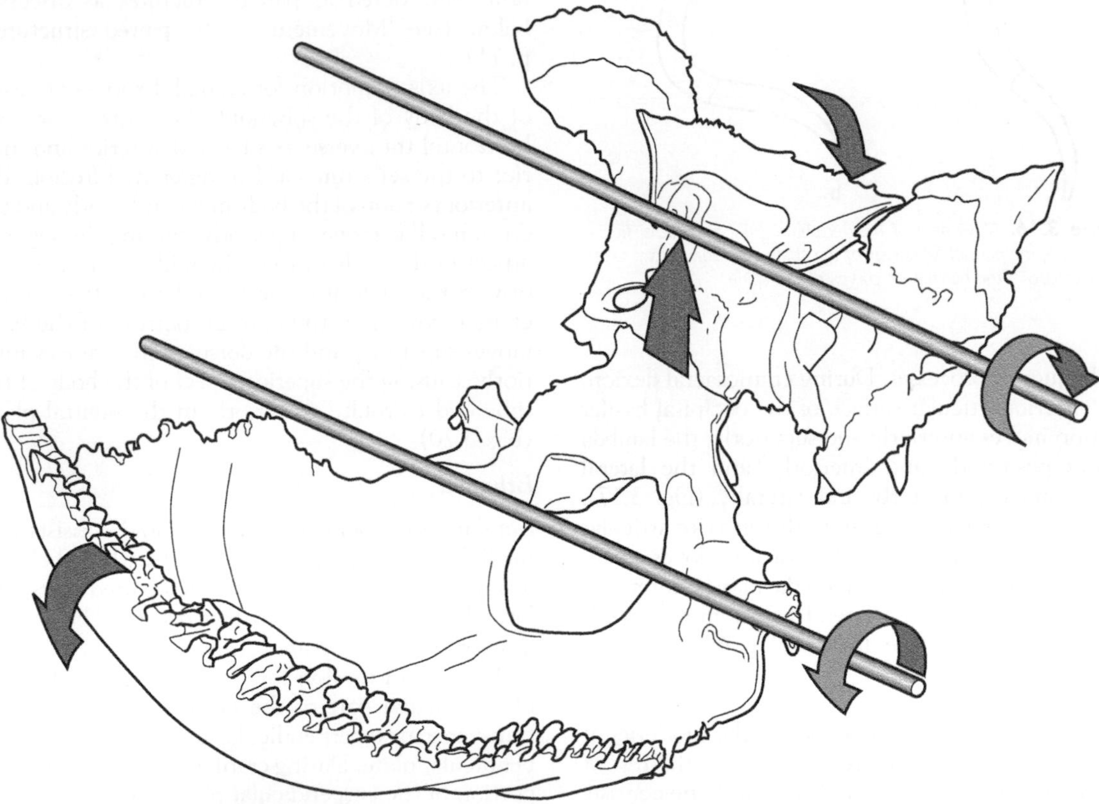

Figure 3.19. *Movement of the sphenobasilar synchondrosis in cranial flexion.*

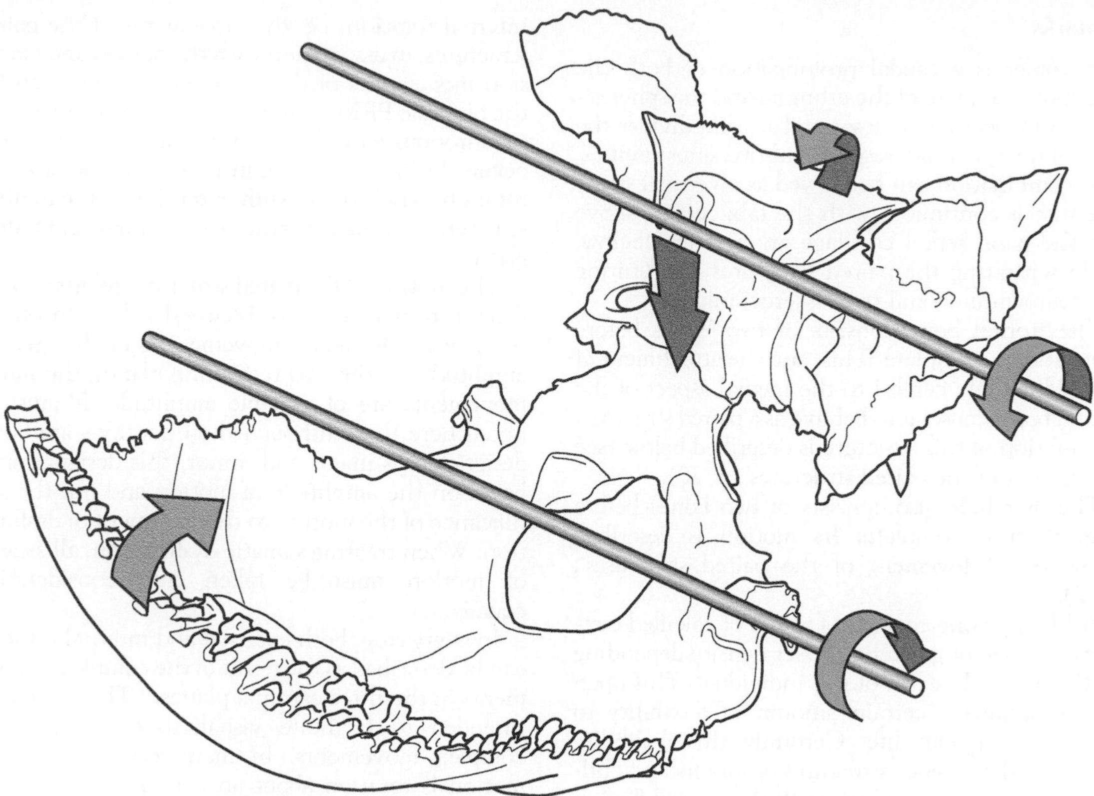

Figure 3.20. *Movement of the sphenobasilar synchondrosis in cranial extension.*

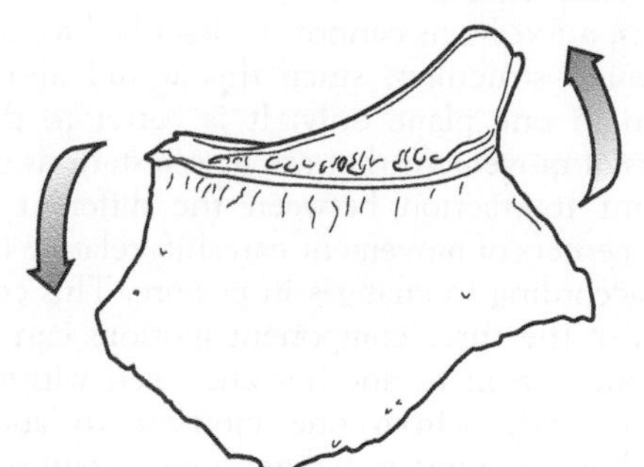

Figure 3.21. *Movement of the ethmoid in cranial flexion.*

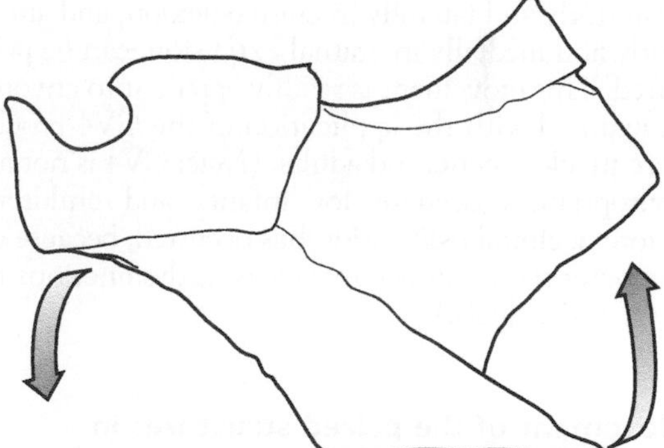

Figure 3.22. *Movement of the vomer in cranial flexion.*

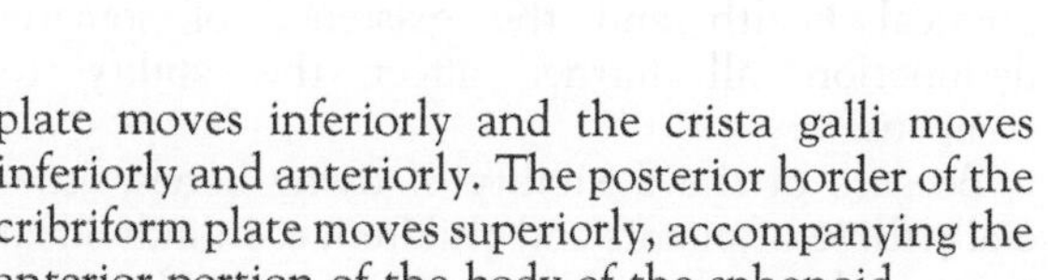

plate moves inferiorly and the crista galli moves inferiorly and anteriorly. The posterior border of the cribriform plate moves superiorly, accompanying the anterior portion of the body of the sphenoid.

Vomer

The axis of motion for cranial flexion–extension of the vomer is a horizontal transverse axis, perpendicular to the vomer. During cranial fl exion, the anterior portion of the vomer moves superiorly and the posterior portion moves inferiorly (Fig. 3.22); during cranial extension, the anterior portion of the vomer moves inferiorly and the posterior portion moves superiorly.

Remarks

The vomer is a caudal prolongation of both the perpendicular plate of the ethmoid and the sphenoidal sagittal septum. The sagittal septum divides the body of the sphenoid, resulting in two sinus cavities. This combination can be viewed as a vertical structure that is continuous with the falx cerebri above and the nasal septal cartilage anterior and below, while separating the paired structures and uniting the neurocranium and the viscerocranium.

The frontal bone consists of two bones before ossification is complete. This, and the attachment of the midline falx cerebri to the medial aspect of the frontal bone, causes it to behave as a paired structure. The motion of this structure is described below (see 'Movement of the paired structures', p. 70).

The mandible also consists of two bones before ossification is complete. Its motion is described below (see 'Movement of the paired structures', p. 72).

All living bone consists of a web of calcified connecting tissue of greater or lesser density depending on the age and health of the individual. This open matrix permits a certain amount of flexibility to remain throughout life. Certainly this flexibility applies to the osseous structures of infants and children. For this reason, along with the cranial flexion and extension movements described above, there is a palpable lateral expansion and contraction of the unpaired bones. This is particularly appreciable in the lateral angles of the occipitut, where movement posteriorly and laterally in cranial flexion, and anteriorly and medially in cranial extension, can be palpated. This movement is readily apparent to anyone acquainted with the application of the CV4 procedure in adolescents and adults. (*Note*: CV4 is not an appropriate procedure for infants and children, before occipital ossification has occurred, because of the potential to induce intraosseous dysfunctions in these individuals.)

Movement of the paired structures in craniosacral flexion–extension

The paired structures are the pelvic bones, the lower limbs, the upper limbs, the ribs, the temporal bones, the parietal bones, the two halves of the frontal bone, the lateral parts of the sphenoid consisting of the greater wings and pterygoid processes, the ethmoidal lateral parts, the zygomae, the maxillae, the two halves of the mandible, the palatine bones, the lacrimal bones, the nasal bones and the conchae. The following discussion describes external and internal rotation, i.e. the movements of the paired structures, in association with the flexion and extension movements of the midlines structures, during the biphasic PRM. External rotation, the movement synchronous with flexion of the midline structures, occurs during the cranial inspiratory phase; internal rotation, synchronous with extension of the midline structures, occurs during the cranial expiratory phase.

The motion of the paired structures relative to the three cardinal planes is discussed below. In one of the planes, the major movement is of the greatest amplitude; in the two remaining planes, the minor movements are of variable amplitude. It must be noted here that, although these motions are being designated as major and minor, this designation is based on the amplitude of motion and not the significance of the motion to the treatment of dysfunction. When treating somatic dysfunction, all aspects of motion must be taken into consideration equally.

In every case, both external and internal rotation can be described as the result of the combined movements in the three cardinal planes.[37] This is a model intended to facilitate visualization of otherwise complex movements. In many cases, the actual motion is rotation about an axis that is not fixed, but is shifting in three-dimensional space. Additionally, anatomic asymmetries result in variations of motion when comparing one structure with its paired counterpart.

Thus, a fixed axis cannot be described for any of the paired structures, since this would allow for motion in one plane only. It is better to discuss centers of movement that are manifestations of the resultant interaction between the different axes. These centers of movement can shift relative to the bone according to changes in posture. This combination of the three component motions can differ from one person to another and even within the same individual from one moment to another, depending on gravitational and muscle pull stresses and the individual's ability to compensate. Age, nutritional status, degree of fatigue, mental status, physical health and the existence of somatic dysfunction all further affect the ability to compensate.

Because of the flexibility of living bones, especially those of infants and children, each individual point within a bone does not move to the same degree or even in the same direction. Zones of variable resistance are palpable according to the trabeculae that result from stress forces. The different parts of a structure do not receive the same influences.

The description of movement is, therefore, relative; it is a model allowing visualization of the system and incorporates a language convention to facilitate communication between osteopathic practitioners.

Overview

During cranial flexion–external rotation, the whole skull widens through the influence of the outward movement of the external rotation of the paired bones (Fig. 3.23a). The back of the skull widens more than the front. The vault of the skull descends, with the posterior portion descending more than the anterior portion. The parietal, orbital and palatine vaults all demonstrate similar movements. Thus, during global cranial flexion–external rotation, the transverse dimension of the skull increases and the vertical dimension decreases. Conversely, during cranial extension–internal rotation, the transverse dimension of the skull decreases and the vertical dimension increases (Fig. 3.23b).

Similarly, at the level of the pelvis, the same association occurs. During craniosacral flexion–external rotation, the pelvic transverse diameter broadens and its vertical dimension decreases; during craniosacral extension–internal rotation, the pelvic transverse diameter narrows and the vertical dimension increases.

Pelvic bones

During craniosacral external rotation, each pelvic bone exhibits complex motion that can be described in the context of the three cardinal planes. In the sagittal plane, they demonstrate anterior rotation, wherein the anterior superior iliac spine (ASIS) moves inferiorly, the pubic tubercle moves inferiorly, the posterior superior iliac spine (PSIS) moves superiorly and the ischial tuberosity moves posteriorly and superiorly. These are the major components of external rotation.

The minor components of pelvic bone external rotation occur in the frontal and horizontal planes. In the frontal plane, the pelvic bone demonstrates abduction of the iliac crest and adduction of the ischial tuberosity. The ASIS and the PSIS both move laterally. In the horizontal plane, the entire pelvic bone moves laterally but to a greater degree at the PSIS than at the ASIS.

The resultant complex motion of pelvic bone external rotation consists of the combination of the three components. This manifests as a net downward movement of the ASIS and a net upward and lateral movement of the PSIS (Fig. 3.24).

Conversely, during craniosacral internal rotation, each pelvic bone exhibits complex motion in the opposite direction to that described above in the context of the three cardinal planes. The major component is again in the sagittal plane and the minor components in the frontal and horizontal

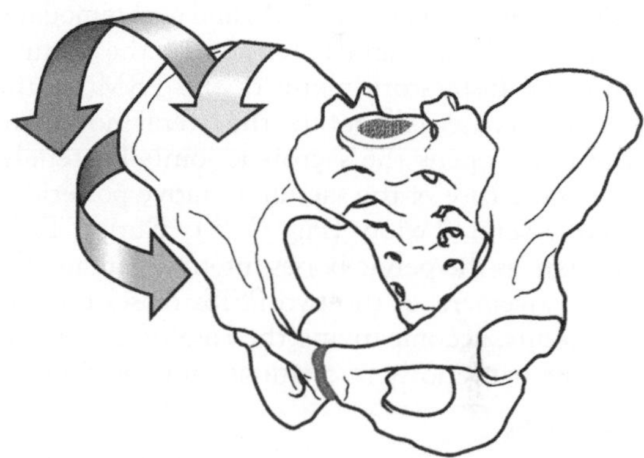

Figure 3.24. *Movement of the pelvic bones in external rotation.*

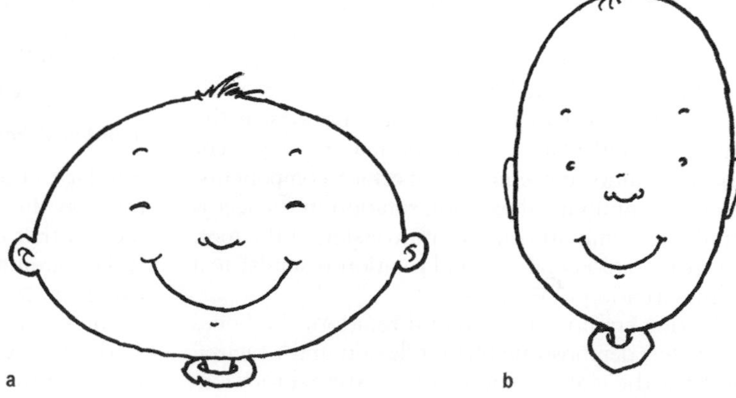

Figure 3.23. *Overview. (a) During cranial flexion–external rotation, the transverse dimension of the skull increases and the vertical dimension decreases. (b) During cranial extension–internal rotation, the transverse dimension of the skull decreases and the vertical dimension increases.*

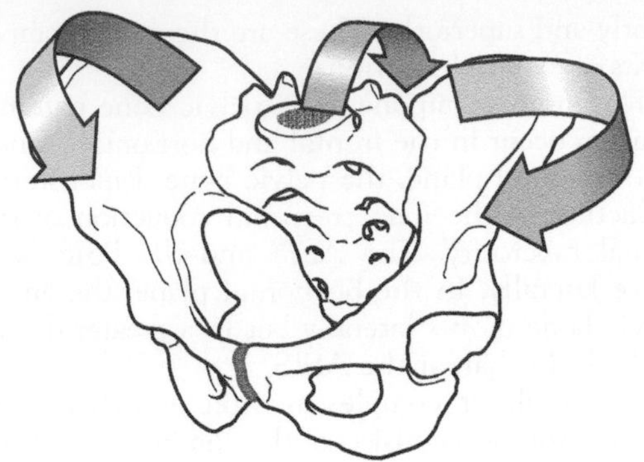

Figure 3.25. *Movement of the pelvis in craniosacral flexion and external rotation.*

planes. The resultant complex motion of pelvic bone internal rotation consists of the combination of the three components and manifests as a net upward movement of the ASIS and a net downward and medial movement of the PSIS.

The biphasic motion of the two PSISs is synchronous with the action of the PRM and accommodates craniosacral flexion and extension of the sacrum. During the inspiratory phase of the PRM, as the pelvic bones externally rotate, the lateral movement of the PSISs opens the sacroiliac joints bilaterally, allowing the base of the sacrum to move posteriorly in craniosacral flexion (Fig. 3.25). During PRM expiration, as the pelvic bones internally rotate, the medial movement of the two PSISs closes the sacroiliac joints, accompanying the base of the sacrum as it moves anteriorly in craniosacral extension.

Lower limbs

All the bones of the lower limbs individually demonstrate biphasic external and internal rotation in synchrony with the PRM. The movements of the long bones are relatively simple in that, as would be anticipated, they demonstrate external rotation with craniosacral flexion and internal rotation with craniosacral extension, around their long axes.

The motion of the bones of the feet is more intricate and consists of the combined motions in the three cardinal planes, with one major component and two minor but equally important components. As such, craniosacral external rotation in the feet is similar to a miniaturization of inversion of the foot, whereas craniosacral internal rotation is similar to a miniaturization of eversion.

During craniosacral external rotation, the bones of the feet demonstrate plantar flexion in the sagittal plane as the major component of external rotation. The minor components of external rotation occur in the frontal and horizontal planes and consist of supination and adduction, respectively.

During craniosacral internal rotation, the bones of the feet demonstrate dorsiflexion in the sagittal plane as the major component of internal rotation. The minor components of internal rotation occur in the frontal and horizontal planes and consist of pronation and abduction, respectively.

Upper limbs

Synchronous with the PRM, the individual bones of the upper limbs demonstrate external and internal rotation. The movements of the long bones, as would be anticipated, are relatively uncomplicated. With craniosacral flexion, they demonstrate external rotation around their long axis and with craniosacral extension, internal rotation.

The motions of the bones of the hand are more elaborate. They each consist of the combined motions in the three cardinal planes, with a major component and two minor but equally important components.

During craniosacral external rotation, the bones of the hand demonstrate extension in the sagittal plane as the major component of external rotation. The minor components of external rotation occur in the frontal and horizontal planes and consist of abduction and supination, respectively.

During craniosacral internal rotation, the bones of the hand demonstrate flexion in the sagittal plane as the major component of internal rotation. The minor components of internal rotation occur in the frontal and horizontal planes and consist of adduction and pronation, respectively.

Ribs

Synchronous with the PRM, each rib exhibits biphasic external and internal rotation. As such, craniosacral external rotation of the ribs is similar to a miniaturization of the movement of respiratory inhalation. Conversely, craniosacral internal rotation is similar to a miniaturization of the rib movement during respiratory exhalation.

Temporal bones

Similar to the pelvic bones, during cranial external rotation the temporal bones demonstrate intricate motion that can be described in the context of the three cardinal planes. In the sagittal plane, they exhibit anterior rotation, wherein the superior edge of the squamous portion moves anteriorly and inferiorly, the zygomatic process moves inferiorly, and the tip of the mastoid process moves posteriorly and

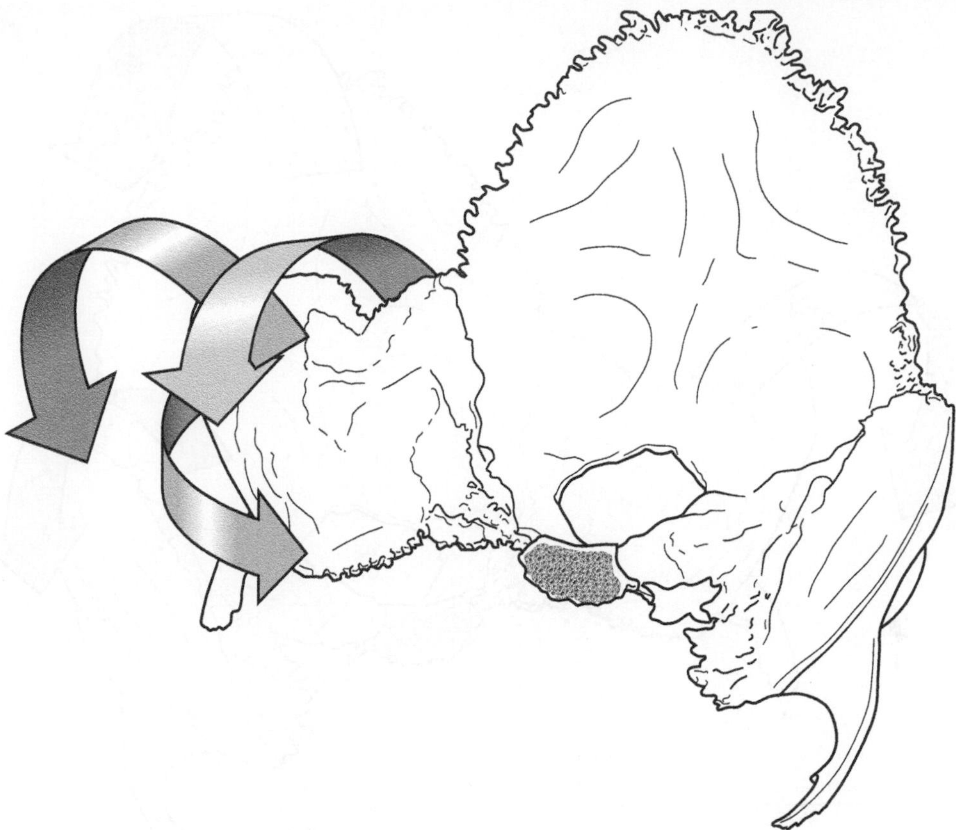

Figure 3.26. *Movement of the temporal bones in external rotation.*

superiorly. This movement in the sagittal plane is the major component of external rotation.

The minor components of temporal bone external rotation occur in the frontal and horizontal planes. In the frontal plane, the temporal bone demonstrates abduction of the superior edge of the squamous portion and adduction of the tip of the mastoid process. In the horizontal plane, the whole temporal bone moves laterally but to a greater degree at the posterior portion than at the anterior portion. The resultant complex motion of temporal bone external rotation consists of the combination of the three components, where the superior edge of the squamous portion moves anteriorly, laterally and inferiorly, and the tip of the mastoid process moves posteriorly, medially and superiorly (Fig. 3.26).

Conversely, during cranial internal rotation, the temporal bones exhibit complex motion in the three cardinal planes, opposite to the directions of those described above. The major component is again in the sagittal plane and the minor components in the frontal and horizontal planes. The resultant complex motion of temporal bone internal rotation consists of the combination of the three components, where the superior edge of the squamous portion moves posteriorly, medially and superiorly, and the tip of the mastoid process moves anteriorly, laterally and inferiorly.

The biphasic motion of the temporal bones is synchronous with the action of the PRM and accommodates cranial flexion and cranial extension of the occiput. During the inspiratory phase of the PRM, as the temporal bones externally rotate, the lateral movement of the posterior portion of the temporal bones opens the occipitomastoid and petro-occipital sutures bilaterally, allowing the squamous portion of the occiput to move posteriorly and inferiorly in cranial flexion (Fig. 3.27). During PRM expiration, as the temporal bones internally rotate, the medial movement of their posterior portions closes the occipitomastoid sutures and petrobasilar joints, accompanying the squamous portion of the

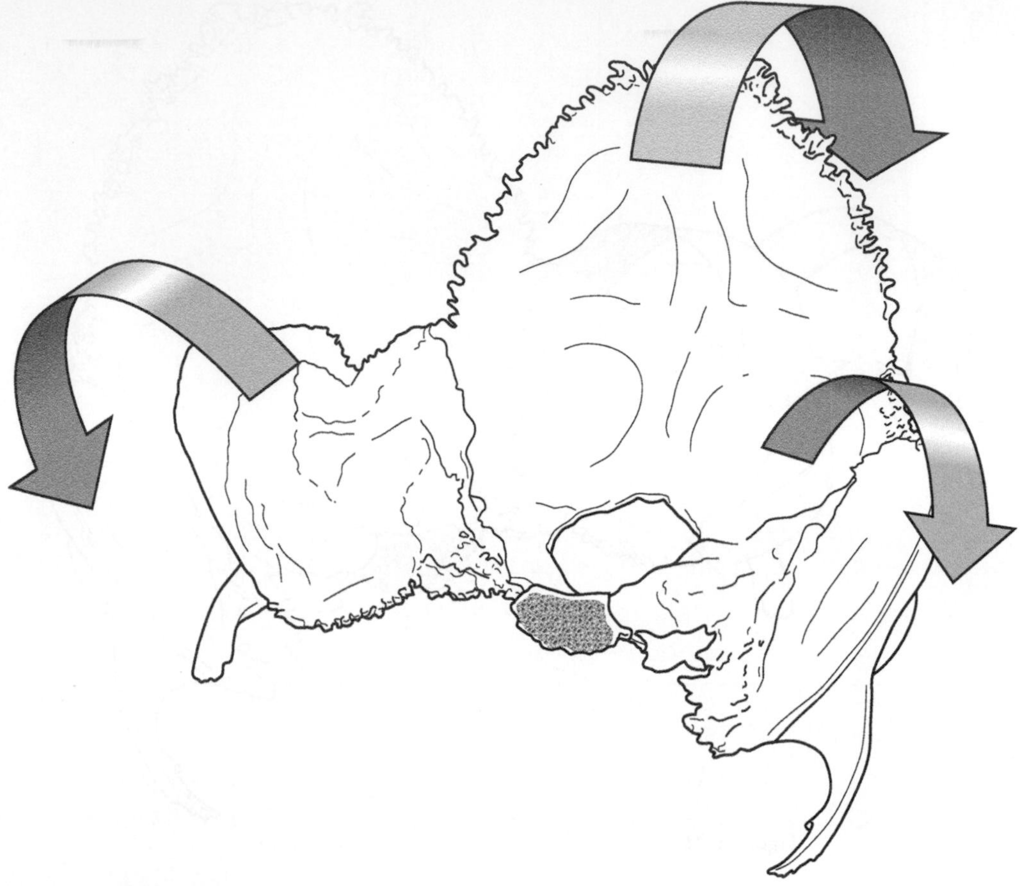

Figure 3.27. *Movement of the occiput and temporal bones in cranial flexion and external rotation.*

occiput as it moves anteriorly and superiorly in cranial extension.

Parietal bones

During cranial external rotation, the parietal bones demonstrate elaborate motion that can be described relative to the three cardinal planes. The major motion occurs in the horizontal plane. The entire parietal bone follows the squamous portion of the temporal bone as it moves laterally. The medial and lateral borders of the parietal bone are, thus, displaced laterally to a greater degree at its posterior portion than at its anterior portion. In the frontal plane, the entire parietal bone moves inferiorly but to a greater degree at its medial border than at its lateral border. The parietals behave as if they were hinged at the sagittal suture, thus accommodating the widening of the skull. In the sagittal plane, the medial border at the sagittal suture moves posteriorly along with the falx cerebri and the squamous portion of the occiput.

Conversely, during cranial internal rotation, the major motion in the horizontal plane consists of the entire parietal bone being displaced medially, with greater displacement at its posterior portion than at its anterior portion. In the frontal plane, the entire parietal bone moves superiorly but to a greater degree at its medial border than at its lateral border. This motion of the parietals accommodates the narrowing of the skull. In the sagittal plane, the medial border at the sagittal suture moves anteriorly along with the falx cerebri and the squamous portion of the occiput.

The two halves of the frontal bone

The two halves of the frontal bone move in a fashion that can be described relative to the three cardinal planes. In external rotation, in the horizontal plane, the metopic suture moves posteriorly in response to the tension of the falx cerebri. The zygomatic processes at the lateral aspects of the frontal bone move anteriorly and laterally and the ethmoidal notch widens. The frontal eminences become less prominent. In the sagittal plane, traction from the falx cerebri causes the metopic suture to move posteriorly and slightly superiorly, the bregma moves posteriorly and inferiorly, and the posterior edges of the orbital plates and the back of the ethmoidal notch move slightly inferiorly.

In internal rotation, the metopic suture moves anteriorly in the horizontal plane and the zygomatic processes at the lateral aspects of the frontal bone move posteriorly and medially. This causes the frontal eminences to become more prominent and the ethmoidal notch to narrow. In the sagittal plane, the metopic suture moves anteriorly and slightly inferiorly, and the bregma moves anteriorly and superiorly. The posterior edges of the orbital plates and the back of the ethmoidal notch move slightly superiorly.

Remarks

The frontosphenoidal articulation and the zygomatic process of the frontal bone are signifi cant hinge-like zones between the sphenoid, whose simplifi ed movement is rotation on a transverse axis, and the frontal bone, whose movement about a similar axis is rotation in the opposite direction. This is an important therapeutic consideration. The inferior angles of the frontal bone are set on the greater wings of the sphenoid. Thus, the greater wings of the sphenoid are restrained by the frontal bone and do not move inferiorly as much as the body.

The lateral parts of the sphenoid consisting of the greater wings and pterygoid processes

The lateral surfaces of the greater wings of the sphenoid can be considered as anterior continuations of the squamous portion of the temporal bones. The sphenoid is often compared to a bird. The pterygoid processes represent the bird's legs and the greater wings represent the bird's wings that are unfolding as it takes off in flight.

During cranial external rotation, the lateral parts of the sphenoid, the greater wings and the pterygoid processes demonstrate complex motion that can be described relative to the three cardinal planes. In the sagittal plane, the greater wings and pterygoid processes rotate anteriorly following the body of the sphenoid, but are restrained by the frontal bone. Thus, they are held in a superior position relative to the inferior movement of cranial flexion of the body of the sphenoid. In the frontal plane, the greater wing portions of the lateral parts move laterally with the squamous portion of the temporal bones and the pterygoid processes move laterally with the palatine bones. In the horizontal plane, the external surfaces of the greater wings move anteriorly and laterally, thus 'fi lling' the temporal fossae. Bilaterally, the angles between the orbital and temporal surfaces of the greater wings increase. During palpation, the superior portion of the temporal surface of the greater wings gives the feeling of lateral movement as the body of the sphenoid moves anteriorly. During cranial external rotation, the tips of the pterygoid processes move posteriorly, laterally and inferiorly.

With cranial internal rotation in the sagittal plane, the greater wings and pterygoid processes rotate posteriorly following the body of the sphenoid, but to a lesser extent because of the influence of the frontal bone. In the frontal plane, the greater wing portions of the lateral parts move medially with the temporal bones and the pterygoid processes move medially with the palatine bones. In the horizontal plane, the external surfaces of the greater wings move posteriorly and medially, enhancing the temporal fossae. The angles between the orbital and temporal surfaces of the greater wings decrease bilaterally. During palpation, the superior portion of the temporal surface of the greater wings gives the feeling of medial movement as the body of the sphenoid moves posteriorly. During cranial internal rotation, the tips of the pterygoid processes move anteriorly, medially and superiorly.

Ethmoidal labyrinths

The ethmoidal labyrinths hang beneath the edges of the frontal ethmoidal notch and articulate inferiorly with the maxillae; thus, they are influenced by both. During cranial external rotation, the ethmoidal labyrinths demonstrate motion in the three cardinal planes. In the sagittal plane, they rotate posteriorly, following the perpendicular plate of the ethmoid. The anterior portions of the ethmoidal labyrinths move superiorly, as does the crista galli, and the posterior portions move inferiorly. In the frontal plane, the ethmoidal labyrinths move apart, similar to the edges of the frontal ethmoidal notch and the maxillae, thus participating in the general widening of the skull. The widening of the ethmoidal labyrinths is greatest in their inferior portions. In the horizontal plane, the ethmoidal labyrinths rotate such that the lateral portions move anteriorly and the medial portions move posteriorly. The latero-posterior portions have the greatest displacement.

During cranial internal rotation in the sagittal plane, the ethmoidal labyrinths rotate anteriorly. The anterior portions of the ethmoidal labyrinths move inferiorly and the posterior portions move superiorly. In the frontal plane, they move together, as do the edges of the frontal ethmoidal notch and the maxillae, thus participating in the general narrowing of the skull. The movement is greatest in their inferior portions. In the horizontal plane, the ethmoidal labyrinths rotate such that the lateral portions move posteriorly and the medial portions move anteriorly. The lateroposterior portions have the greatest displacement.

Zygomatic bones

The zygomatic bones are key structures that balance forces between the sphenoid, the temporal bones and the maxillae. During cranial external rotation, the zygomatic bones demonstrate motion in the three cardinal planes. In the sagittal plane, they rotate in such a manner that their orbital edges move anteriorly and inferiorly, the inferior edges move posteriorly and superiorly, and the cheekbones that are the inferior part of the lateral surface become less prominent. In the frontal plane, the zygomatic bones contribute to the general widening of the skull and orbits. Their superior edges move laterally and the inferior edges move medially. In the horizontal plane, the entire zygomatic bone moves laterally, with the medial portion moving to a greater degree than the lateral portion.

With cranial internal rotation in the sagittal plane, the zygomatic bones rotate such that their orbital edges move posteriorly and superiorly, the inferior edges move anteriorly and inferiorly, and the cheekbones become more prominent. In the frontal plane, they participate in the general narrowing of the skull and orbits. Their superior edges move medially and the inferior edges move laterally. In the horizontal plane, the entire zygomatic bone moves medially and, again, the medial portion moves to a greater degree than the lateral portion.

Maxillae

The maxillae are very important components of the viscerocranium. During cranial external rotation, the maxillae exhibit motion in the three cardinal planes. In the sagittal plane, they rotate such that their anterior portions move superiorly, the posterior portions move inferiorly and the palate descends. In the frontal plane, they move such that the lateral portions move laterally and superiorly, the medial portions move laterally and inferiorly and the palate flattens. The movement is greater at the inferior portion of the maxillae; the teeth are, consequently, everted. In the horizontal plane, they rotate such that their lateral portions move anteriorly, the medial portions move posteriorly with the lateroposterior portions having the greatest movement. The palate, therefore, widens (note the similarity to the parietals; the vault demonstrates the same displacement as the palate). Additionally, the lateral surfaces of the frontal processes move toward the frontal plane.

With cranial internal rotation in the sagittal plane, the maxillae rotate in such a way that their anterior portions move inferiorly, the posterior portions move superiorly and the palate becomes more arched. In the frontal plane, the lateral portions move medially and inferiorly, and the medial portions more medially and superiorly. Again, the movement is greater at the inferior portion of the maxillae and the teeth are, consequently, inverted. In the horizontal plane, the maxillae rotate such that their lateral portions move posteriorly, the medial portions move anteriorly with the lateroposterior portions having the greatest movement. Consequently, the palate narrows and the lateral surfaces of the frontal processes move toward the sagittal plane.

The two halves of the mandible

The two halves of the mandible are joined at the symphysis menti. They are influenced from above by the temporal bones and the upper part of the viscerocranium. From below they are influenced by diverse structures, including the tongue, the hyoid bone and associated muscles, and the myofascial elements of the cervicothoracic area. In cranial external rotation, following the mandibular fossae of the temporal bones, the body of the mandible moves posteriorly and the chin recedes.

With cranial internal rotation, the mandibular fossae of the temporal bones and the body of the mandible move anteriorly. As a result, the chin becomes more prominent.

Palatine bones

The palatine bones are located posterior to the maxillae and anterior to the sphenoid. Their horizontal plates unite to form the posterior portion of the hard palate. The palatine bones follow the movement of the maxillae in cranial external and internal rotation. During cranial external rotation, they exhibit motion in the three cardinal planes. In the sagittal plane, they rotate such that the two palatine bones move inferiorly, but the posterior portions move to a greater degree than the anterior portions. In the frontal plane, they move like the maxillae, the lateral portions moving laterally and superiorly and the medial portions laterally and inferiorly. This movement is greater for the inferior portion of the palatine bones. In the horizontal plane, they again rotate like the maxillae, the lateral portions moving anteriorly and the medial portions moving posteriorly. Consequently, the posterior portion of the palate widens.

With cranial internal rotation in the sagittal plane, the palatine bones rotate such that the two bones move superiorly, but the posterior portions move to a greater degree than the anterior portions. In the frontal plane, the lateral portions move medially and inferiorly while the medial portions move medially and superiorly, with greater movement of the inferior portion of the palatine bones. In the horizontal plane, the lateral portions move posteriorly and the medial portions move anteriorly. Consequently, the posterior portion of the palate narrows.

Lacrimal bones

The lacrimal bones are small and delicate. They follow the movement of the lateral surfaces of the ethmoidal labyrinths in cranial external and internal rotation. During cranial external rotation, they demonstrate motion in the three cardinal planes. In the sagittal plane, they rotate such that their anterior borders move superiorly and the posterior borders move inferiorly. In the frontal plane, the inferior lacrimal border moves laterally and superiorly, and the superior border moves laterally and inferiorly, the lateral displacement being greater for the inferior border than for the superior border. In the horizontal plane, the anterior borders move posteriorly and the posterior borders move anteriorly, with the greatest displacement at the posterior borders.

With cranial internal rotation in the sagittal plane, the lacrimal bones rotate such that their anterior borders move inferiorly and the posterior borders move superiorly. In the frontal plane, the inferior lacrimal border moves medially and inferiorly, and the superior border moves medially and superiorly, the lateral displacement being greatest for the inferior border. In the horizontal plane, the anterior borders move anteriorly and the posterior borders move posteriorly, with the greatest displacement at the posterior borders.

Nasal bones

The nasal bones are located anterior to the frontal processes of the maxillae, which lie immediately anterior to the lacrimal bones. Consequently, the nasal bones demonstrate motion in the three cardinal planes that is similar to that of the maxillary frontal processes and lacrimal bones, as described above. Although small, these bones contribute significantly to the functional mechanics of the nasal passages in infants and children.

Inferior nasal conchae

The inferior nasal conchae each articulates laterally with the nasal surface of the homolateral maxillary bone and superiorly with the ethmoid uncinate process and the descending process of the lacrimal bone. Their motion in the three cardinal planes follows most closely that of the maxillary bones, as described above.

Other physiologic movements

Cranial flexion–extension and the associated external and internal rotations are perceived as a succession of micro movements that repeat rhythmically and are palpable throughout the body unless impaired by dysfunctional mechanics. This movement is palpable throughout life. Both endogenous and exogenous factors can affect the unencumbered motion pattern of the PRM described above. For example, sidebending the head while fixing the eyes on an object, and while keeping the gaze horizontal, causes the estraocular muscles to hold the sphenoid, preventing it from completely following the occiput. The point of balance between the sphenoid and the occiput is located at the level of the SBS that is consequently placed in compensatory torsion. Because this is a response to position, and is not fixed, it is not dysfunctional. Thus, a functionally balanced individual should be capable of bilaterally and symmetrically assuming such compensatory mechanical patterns while maintaining the biphasic rhythm of the PRM. Therefore, in addition to cranial flexion–extension and external and internal rotations, variable movement patterns can be identified. It must be stressed that, in the absence of dysfunction, the biphasic rhythm of the PRM remains present when palpating these other movement patterns. The movement patterns to be considered here include those of the sacrum and pelvis, the spine and the skull.

Sacrum and pelvis

The other physiologic movements that the sacral vertebrae demonstrate are sidebending and rotation: sidebending occurs around a horizontal anteroposterior axis; rotation occurs around a vertical axis. Although the sacral segments are not totally fused during infancy and early childhood, in the absence of dysfunction the sacrum sidebends and rotates as a single unit. Coupled sidebending and rotation of the sacrum results in sacral torsion, as if occurring around an oblique axis.[38] Sidebending of the spine above determines the side of the oblique axis (e.g. sidebending right engages the right oblique axis).

Sacral torsion is named for the side toward which sacral vertebral rotation occurs. Sacral rotation to the left is named a left torsion. In the absence of dysfunction, the pelvic bones follow the motion of the sacrum. Therefore, with a left sacral torsion, the left pelvic bone demonstrates internal rotation, where posterior movement is the major displacement, and the right pelvic bone exhibits external rotation, where anterior movement is the major displacement.

Spine

The other physiologic movements that the spinal vertebrae demonstrate are sidebending and rotation similar to those described by Fryette.[39] Sidebending occurs around a horizontal anteroposterior axis and is named for the side of the resultant concavity. The transverse process on the side of the concavity is approximated to the transverse process below, whereas on the side of the convexity they are separated. The spinous process is inclined toward the side of the concavity.

Rotation occurs around a vertical axis and is named for the direction toward which the anterior aspect of the vertebral body has rotated. The transverse process on the side of the rotation is posterior, whereas on the other side it is anterior. The tip of the spinous process is deviated toward the side opposite to which rotation has occurred.

These movements are most often encountered coupled and can occur in the same direction or in opposite directions. (*Note*: These mechanical patterns are not dysfunctional.) When an individual is in a sidebent and rotated position, the biphasic PRM will still be palpated, reflecting the position taken by the subject. Therefore, what will be felt is not a pure flexion–extension, but a biphasic motion, including a combination of flexion–extension and the positional sidebending–rotation to one side. In the absence of underlying somatic dysfunction, this palpated asymmetry will revert to a pure flexion–extension when the individual reverts to the symmetric anatomic position (see Chapter 5, 'Physical examination', p. 106).

Skull

During one's entire life, the skull retains a certain amount of flexibility, allowing for the movements of flexion–extension and compensating adjustments. This capacity for micro movement decreases with age, and, as such, is rather prominent in infants and children relative to adults and geriatrics. The other physiologic movements encountered involve the spheno-occipital synchondrosis which demonstrates torsion and sidebending–rotation. These motions occur as part of physiologic activities (e.g. chewing) and as an accommodation to spinal movement below. Although these motions are traditionally described as occurring at the spheno-occipital synchondrosis, the rest of the skull must also accommodate. In order to understand these motions, it must be remembered that living bones are compliant and demonstrate a capacity for adjustment to stresses placed upon them. As such, with torsion and sidebending–rotation, movements occur not only at the level of the SBS but also throughout the skull, with sutural and intraosseous manifestations.

Torsion

Torsion of the SBS occurs as a movement around a single anteroposterior axis. This axis lies along a line joining the nasion and opisthion. During torsion, the sphenoid and the occiput rotate in opposite directions around this axis. Thus, as the body of the sphenoid rotates on the axis, one side will be higher than the other. The greater wing of the sphenoid on that side is displaced superiorly, whereas the greater wing on the other side is displaced inferiorly. At the same time, the occiput rotates, moving inferiorly on the higher side of the sphenoid and superiorly on the opposite side (Fig. 3.28).

Torsion is named for the side on which the greater wing of the sphenoid moves superiorly. For instance, during a right torsion, the right lateral part of the body of the sphenoid and the right greater wing move superiorly, while the right lateral part of the occiput moves inferiorly. In the absence of cranial somatic dysfunction, this movement exists symmetrically, with the motions of torsion left and torsion right demonstrating the same quantity and quality.

Associated movements of the paired bones accompany a movement of torsion, with a tendency toward external rotation on the side for which the torsion is named, and internal rotation on the other side. With a right torsion, the right temporal bone will follow the occiput in its inferior displacement and tend to externally rotate. The right temporal bone, however, also articulates anteriorly with the right greater wing of the sphenoid, which moves superiorly during right torsion. Therefore, the pattern of the right temporal bone, in this instance, is not purely that of external rotation – there is some

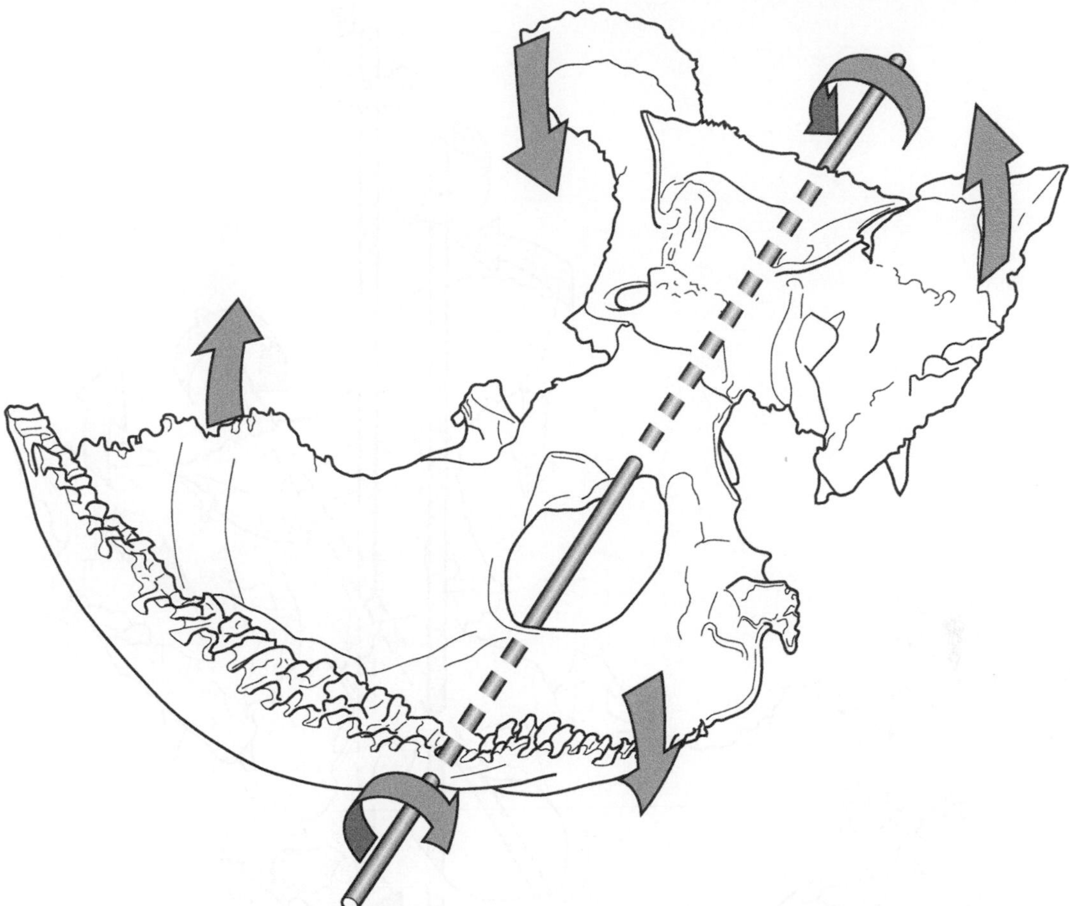

Figure 3.28. *Movement of the sphenobasilar synchondrosis in right torsion.*

modulation in the pattern. Modulation occurs mainly at the level of the membranous squamous portion of the temporal bone. This squamous intraosseous torsion is most likely to occur in the flexible skulls of infants and children.

Sidebending–rotation

Sidebending–rotation of the SBS occurs as a complex movement that consists of two components involving three distinct axes of motion. The occiput and the sphenoid rotate in the same direction around an anteroposterior axis. This axis lies along a line joining the nasion and opisthion. As the body of the sphenoid rotates on the axis, one side will be higher than the other. The greater wing of the sphenoid on that side is displaced superiorly and the greater wing on the other side is displaced inferiorly. Concomitantly, the occiput rotates with the sphenoid, moving superiorly on the higher side of the sphenoid and inferiorly on the opposite side.

Simultaneous with the above motion, the occiput and sphenoid move in opposite directions around two vertical axes, one for each bone, one through the center of the body of the sphenoid, the other through the foramen magnum. The greater wing of the sphenoid and the occiput on one side move apart, the greater wing moving anteriorly and the occiput on the same side moving posteriorly. On the other side, the greater wing and the occiput move together. This produces sidebending between the sphenoid and occiput at the SBS and results in a convexity on one side and a concavity on the other (Fig. 3.29).

Sidebending–rotation is named for the side where the greater wing and occiput move inferiorly. For instance, during a left sidebending–rotation, the left

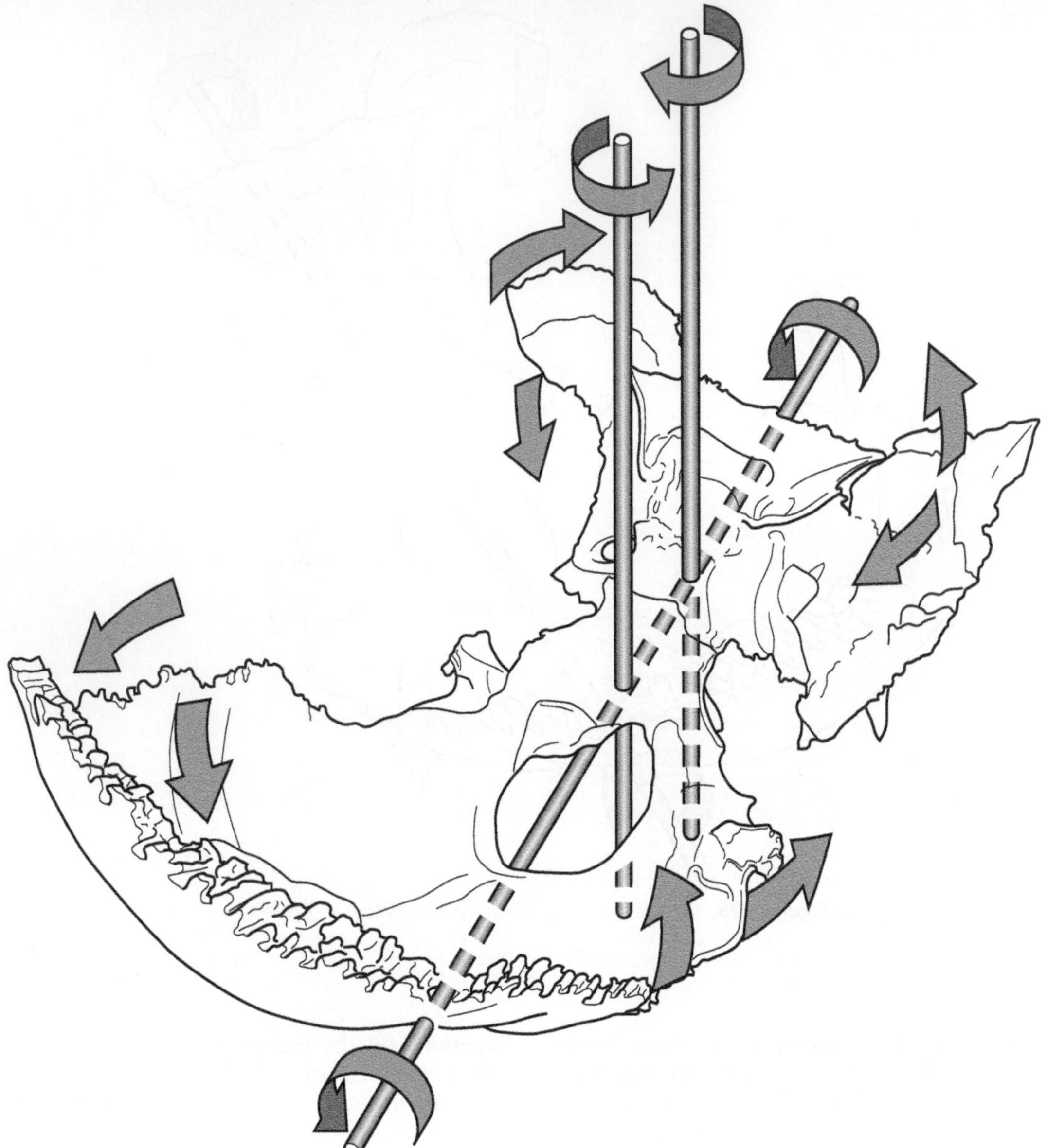

Figure 3.29. *Movement of the sphenobasilar synchondrosis in left sidebending–rotation.*

lateral part of the body of the sphenoid and the left greater wing move inferiorly and anteriorly, while the left lateral part of the occiput moves inferiorly and posteriorly. In the absence of cranial somatic dysfunction, this movement exists symmetrically, with the motions of left sidebending–rotation and right sidebending–rotation demonstrating the same quantity and quality.

Associated movements of the paired bones accompany the movement of sidebending–rotation. On the side for which the sidebending–rotation is named, where the greater wing moves inferiorly, bones influenced by the sphenoid tend to demonstrate internal rotation. On that same side there is a tendency toward external rotation of the temporal bone that follows the occiput. The temporal bone also articulates anteriorly with the greater wing of the sphenoid that itself moves inferiorly and anteriorly during sidebending–rotation. Two influences are present affecting the temporal bone, one pulling anteriorly and one pulling posteriorly. The temporal bone is in the middle, and although it follows the occiput, its anterior squamous portion will also be affected by the sphenoid; however, if the posterior influence is greater than the anterior influence, the sphenoid will be affected by the temporal. A compromise must occur, either at the level of the greater wing of the sphenoid or at the level of the squamous part of the temporal bone. Therefore, the pattern of the temporal bone, in this case, is not purely that of external rotation. Once again, remember that to fully appreciate the pattern of sidebending–rotation, the modulation of the associated paired bones must be understood. This modulation, which is highly probable in the flexible skulls of infants and children, occurs essentially at the level of the membranous portions of the bones, such as the squamous part of the temporal bone or the greater wing of the sphenoid.

Remarks

The motion of torsion and sidebending may be compared to spinal mechanics. The SBS can be considered as a modified intervertebral joint, whose orientation when compared to the rest of the spine, relative to the anatomic position, has shifted. Although the orientation of the spinal intervertebral discs is predominantly in the horizontal plane, because of the flexion of the craniocervical junction that occurs to accommodate the bipedal posture of human beings, the orientation of the plane of the SBS is obliquely oriented inferiorly and anteriorly.

Torsion, therefore, can be compared to simple vertebral rotation, where the displacement of the body of the sphenoid can be compared to the displacement of the vertebral body and the displacement of the greater wings to that of the transverse processes. Sidebending–rotation, as coupled movements, differs from spinal mechanics because the sphenoid and occiput are rotating together in the same direction. The sidebending component is, however, quite similar to sidebending mechanics in the spine below. Since the majority of individuals are acquainted with spinal mechanics, and have experienced diagnosing and treating spinal somatic dysfunctions in particular with indirect procedures, the recognition of the similarities between SBS and vertebral motions may make the diagnosis and treatment of the SBS less intimidating. Obviously the amplitude of motion in the cranial mechanism is significantly smaller than that of the spine.

In cranial osteopathy, whichever physiologic movement is under consideration, it must be recognized that the entire cranium will be involved through the influence of the intracranial membranes. The external layer of the dura mater is contiguous with the inner cranial periosteum, thereby functionally uniting all of the cranial bones. The falx cerebri plays a significant role in linking the frontal and ethmoid bones in the anterior portion of the skull with the occiput in the posterior portion of the skull. Because of these reciprocal tension membranes, torsion and sidebending–rotation mechanics unite the sphenoid and all the bones located in the anterior portion of the cranium with the occiput and its associated structures. Additionally, this link continues through dural fibers into the vertebral canal, functionally uniting the skull with the spine and sacrum. This is part of the core link and these principles of functional unity must be continuously borne in mind when diagnosing and treating somatic dysfunction in any area of the body. Cranial osteopathy is not, as its name seems to imply, limited to the head.

REFERENCES

1. Sutherland WG. Teachings in the science of osteopathy. Fort Worth, TX: Sutherland Cranial Teaching Foundation Inc.; 1991: 107.
2. Williams PL (ed). Gray's anatomy, 38th edn. Edinburgh: Churchill Livingstone; 1995.
3. Arbuckle BE. The selected writings of Beryl E. Arbuckle, D.O., F.A.C.O.P. Newark, OH: American Academy of Osteopathy; 1971:67.
4. Bosma JF (ed). Symposium on development of the basicranium. Bethesda, MD: US Department of Health, Education, and Welfare (DHEW publication (NIH) 76–989); 1976.
5. Opperman LA, Passarelli RW, Morgan EP, Reintjes M, Ogle RC. Cranial sutures require tissue interactions with the dura mater to resist obliteration in vitro. J Bone Mineral Res 1995;10(12):1978–87.
6. Nemzek WR, Brodie HA, Hecht ST, Chong BW, Babcook CJ, Seibert JA. MR, CT, and plain film imaging of the developing skull base in fetal specimens. AJNR Am J Neuroradiol 2000;21(9):1699–706.
7. Glossary of Osteopathic Terminology. In: Ward RC (ed). Foundations for osteopathic medicine, 2nd edn. Philadelphia: Lippincott, Williams & Wilkins; 2003:1232.
8. Sutherland WG. Teachings in the science of osteopathy. Fort Worth, TX: Sutherland Cranial Teaching Foundation; 1991: 45.
9. Klintworth GK. The ontogeny and growth of the human tentorium cerebelli. Anat Rec 1967;158(4):433–41.
10. Magoun HI Sr. Entrapment neuropathy of the central nervous system. II. Cranial nerves I–IV, VI–VIII, XII. J Am Osteopath Assoc 1968;67(7):779–87.
11. Arbuckle BE. The selected writings of Beryl E. Arbuckle, D.O., F.A.C.O.P. Newark, OH: American Academy of Osteopathy; 1971:135.

12. Wiltse LL. Anatomy of the extradural compartments of the lumbar spinal canal. Peridural membrane and circumneural sheath. Radiol Clin North Am 2000;38(6):1177–206.
13. Sunderland S. Mechanisms of cervical nerve root avulsion in injuries of the neck and shoulder. J Neurosurg 1974;41(6):705–14.
14. Macdonald A, Chatrath P, Spector T, Ellis H. Level of termination of the spinal cord and the dural sac: a magnetic resonance study. Clin Anat 1999;12(3):149–52.
15. Lieberman DE, Ross CF, Ravosa MJ. The primate cranial base: ontogeny, function, and integration. Am J Phys Anthropol 2000;Suppl 31:117–69.
16. Scott JH. The cranial base. Am J Phys Anthropol 1958;16(3):319–48.
17. Coqueugniot H, Hublin JJ, Veillon F, Houet F, Jacob T. Early brain growth in Homo erectus and implications for cognitive ability. Nature 2004;431(7006):299–302.
18. Kamina P. Précis d'anatomie clinique. Paris: Maloine; 2002.
19. Melsen B. Time of closure of the spheno-occipital synchondrosis determined on dry skulls. A radiographic craniometric study. Acta Odontol Scand 1969;27(1):73–90.
20. Delattre A, Fenart R. Le développement du crâne du gorille et du chimpanzé comparé au développement du crâne humain. Bull Mem Soc Anthropol Paris 1956;6:159–73.
21. Delattre A, Fenart R. La torsion du rocher des primates et de l'homme. J Sci Med Lille 1961;79:304–7.
22. Ross C, Henneberg M. Basicranial flexion, relative brain size, and facial kyphosis in Homo sapiens and some fossil hominids. Am J Phys Anthropol 1995;98(4):575–93.
23. Lieberman DE, McBratney BM, Krovitz G. The evolution and development of cranial form in Homo sapiens. Proc Natl Acad Sci USA 2002;99(3):1134–9.
24. Lieberman DE. Sphenoid shortening and the evolution of modern human cranial shape. Nature 1998;393(6681):158–62.
25. McCarthy RC, Lieberman DE. Posterior maxillary (PM) plane and anterior cranial architecture in primates. Anat Rec 2001;264(3):247–60.
26. Laitman JT, Heimbuch RC, Crelin ES. Developmental change in a basicranial line and its relationship to the upper respiratory system in living primates. Am J Anat 1978;152:467–82.
27. Krmpotic-Nemanic J, Vinter I, Marusic A. Relations of the pterygoid hamulus and hard palate in children and adults: anatomical implications for the function of the soft palate. Ann Anat 2006;188(1):69–74.
28. Takagi Y. Human postnatal growth of vomer in relation to base of cranium. Ann Otol Rhinol Laryngol 1964;73:238–41.
29. Moss ML, Greenberg SN. Post-natal growth of the human skull base. Angle Orthod 1955;25:77–84.
30. Solow B, Tallgreen A. Head posture and craniofacial morphology. Am J Phys Anthropol 1976;44:417–36.
31. Solow B, Siersbaek-Nielsen S. Growth changes in head posture related to craniofacial development. Am J Orthod 1986;89:132–40.
32. Sutherland WG. The cranial bowl. Mankato, MN: Free Press; 1939. Reprinted: Indianapolis, IN: American Academy of Osteopathy; 1986.
33. Becker RE. The stillness of life. In: Brooks RE (ed). Portland, OR: Stillness Press; 2000:122.
34. Nelson KE, Sergueef N, Glonek T. Recording the rate of the cranial rhythmic impulse. J Am Osteopath Assoc 2006; 106(6):337–41.
35. Nelson KE, Sergueef N, Lipinski CL, Chapman A, Glonek T. The cranial rhythmic impulse related to the Traube–Hering–Mayer oscillation: comparing laser-Doppler flowmetry and palpation. J Am Osteopath Assoc 2001;101(3):163–73.
36. Magoun HI. Osteopathy in the cranial field. Kirksville, MO: The Journal Printing Company; 1951:19.
37. Sergueef N. L'odyssée de l'iliaque. Paris: Spek; 1985.
38. Mitchell FL Sr. Structural pelvic function. Academy of Applied Osteopathy (American Academy of Osteopathy). Yearbook 1965;2:186.
39. Fryette HH. Principles of osteopathic technic. Carmel, CA: Academy of Applied Osteopathy (American Academy of Osteopathy, Indianapolis, IN); 1954.

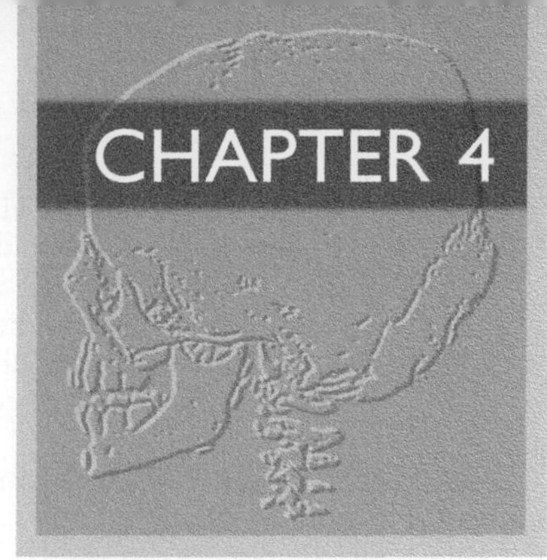

DYSFUNCTIONS

Definition of dysfunction

'In describing spinal lesions, I prefer the term ligamentous articular strains; for lesions in the cranium, membranous articular strains. The spinal lesions include the ligaments as well as the joints. The cranial lesion includes the intracranial membranes as well as the articulation.' —WG SUTHERLAND[1]

Every living creature has to be able to adjust to the environment. Health can be defined as the ability to receive different stresses and to answer favorably, with an appropriate dynamic response, at whatever level of reference (articular, myofascial, vascular, cellular, etc.).

Life is movement. The term movement applies to a broad range of dynamic conditions. These can involve muscles, fasciae, bones, viscera, fluids and a wide variety of phenomena, often referred to as bioenergetic, that link body, mind and spirit.

Dysfunction is the loss of these dynamics. The osteopathic practitioner appreciates this as a variation from the movement perceived in a healthy state. This is manifest in the body as somatic dysfunction that is defined as: 'Impaired or altered function of related components of the somatic (body framework) system: skeletal, arthrodial and myofascial structures and related vascular, lymphatic and neural elements.'[2]

Somatic dysfunction can be further classified according to the tissues that are involved, such as osseous, articular, ligamentous, membranous, fascial, muscular, visceral and vascular. It can be classified according to etiology as physiologic, following normal range of motion; traumatic, as a result of exogenous forces; and reflex, as a neurologically mediated response to conditions elsewhere in the body. It can also be classified according to the movement involved in the dysfunctional pattern such as flexion, extension, rotation, sidebending, external rotation, internal rotation and torsion. It may be classified as primary or secondary, depending on whether it exists independently or is compensatory for adjacent or distant dysfunction(s). Finally, it can be classified according to duration, as acute immediately following the cause of the dysfunction, subacute, or chronic as present for more than 3 months.

In practice, somatic dysfunction, when encountered, may be identified using several of these classifications. For instance, immediately after an athletic injury, a teenager may present with a primary, acute, traumatic, externally rotated talus with subtalar articular dysfunction. If not treated, this same individual may present months later with a secondary, chronic, sacral torsion with myofascial dysfunction. Therefore, caution should be exercised not to become overly focused on one aspect of dysfunction, such as myofascial tension, ligamentous articular strain or membranous articular strain, and thereby lose appreciation of the complexity of somatic dysfunction.

Somatic dysfunction may be considered in the context of four dimensions, the three cardinal planes and time. All components of the body must move freely, each in its individually complex spatial pattern. Understanding dysfunction in this context may be simplified by defining it in terms of the three cardinal planes. During the physical examination, however, we assess the movement of a structure in the three cardinal planes in the context of its relationship in time with the biphasic primary respiratory mechanism (PRM).[3]

When describing dysfunction relative to the three cardinal planes, one component usually presents with greater amplitude. This is the major movement; the two other components, of variable amplitude, in the two remaining planes are the minor movements. It should be recognized that, even though these motions are being identified as major and minor, this classification is an indication of the amplitude of motion and not necessarily its significance to the treatment of the dysfunction. When treating somatic dysfunction, all the aspects of motion must be taken equally into consideration. Often the solution to effective treatment lies in the recognition of the contribution of a minor movement.

These descriptive mechanical patterns of dysfunction are basic templates for diagnosis and treatment. It should be stressed that children's bones are not totally ossified, often consisting of several parts demonstrating motion, and dysfunctional patterns between these different parts, as well as potentially dysfunctional patterns of compliance within any given part. Therefore, dysfunction of any bone (e.g. occiput, temporal bone or sacrum) cannot always be simply described relative to the three planes because of the potential for an intraosseous dysfunction.

The factor of time that is manifest as movement during the inspiration and expiration of the PRM is a fourth consideration. The motion in healthy individuals consists of the two cranial respiratory components. Dysfunction, however, presents a restriction of one of these two phases. Therefore, a dysfunction can be described as an inspiratory or expiratory dysfunction.

Dysfunction is named according to the direction of the freest motion. Consider the movement of a midline structure. In the absence of somatic dysfunction, it demonstrates equilibrium between craniosacral flexion and craniosacral extension, with a central point of balance between the two. If the structure can move freely in only one direction – for example, toward craniosacral flexion with restriction of movement toward craniosacral extension – then, by convention, the dysfunction is named for the direction of the freest movement, in this case craniosacral flexion. Furthermore, the biphasic PRM will not be present, as in a non-dysfunctional individual, but will be more prominent in one phase, i.e. the phase of the dysfunction, in this case inspiration.

Somatic dysfunction is often associated with physical discomfort. Neurologically, this discomfort is typically a manifestation of nociception. Afferent nociceptive activity from the area of the dysfunction impacts the central nervous system. This results in a state of irritability, referred to as facilitation, at the anatomic level of the central nervous system supplied by the activated nociceptive neurons. This irritability is the source of the neurologic, viscerosomatic, somatovisceral, somatosomatic and viscerovisceral reflex manifestations of somatic dysfunction. In a more complicated ascending pathway, the spinal segmental facilitation of somatic dysfunction can manifest somato-emotionally, resulting in the irritability that often affects infants and children.[4,5]

Craniosacral dysfunctions can affect:

- membranous structures and thus vascular and nervous elements associated with them
- osseous structures: dysfunction can modify bony shape and bony interrelationships
- articular structures: dysfunction within a joint produces a state of unbalanced strain and interferes with normal movement
- low pressure fluid dynamics: dysfunction with consequent motion impairment interferes with venous and lymphatic flow with resultant passive congestion and decreased tissue perfusion
- neurovascular physiology, thus potentially affecting all areas of the body
- viscera.

Patterns of dysfunction

PHYSIOLOGIC DYSFUNCTIONS

A physiologic dysfunction is a restriction of mobility within the limits of normal range of movement. For example, the right temporal bone is dysfunctional in external rotation when it moves freely in external rotation but cannot move into internal rotation. Physiologic dysfunction may result from any trauma that stresses a structure but does not exceed the physiologic range of motion of that structure. Such trauma can occur prenatally, during the birth process or at any time during the individual's life.

Physiologic dysfunctions of the sphenobasilar synchondrosis

The physiologic dysfunctions of the sphenobasilar synchondrosis (SBS) include cranial flexion, cranial extension, torsion left and right, and sidebending–rotation left and right. These dysfunctions, however, cannot exist alone without affecting other parts of the skull and body.

Cranial flexion and cranial extension dysfunctions

A cranial flexion dysfunction is present when the SBS moves freely into cranial flexion but cannot move into cranial extension. Consequently, the entire skull can be in a state of cranial flexion–external rotation (see Chapter 3). The PRM is facilitated in the inspiratory phase. A cranial extension dysfunction is present when the SBS moves freely into cranial extension but cannot move into cranial flexion. Consequently, the entire skull can be in a state of extension–internal rotation. The PRM is facilitated in the expiratory phase.

Cranial flexion and cranial extension dysfunctions of the SBS may affect thoracoabdominal diaphragmatic excursion. A flexion dysfunction of the SBS may result in limitation of the end of the expiratory phase of pulmonary respiration, whereas a cranial extension dysfunction can similarly limit the inspiratory phase of pulmonary respiration. Likewise, cranial flexion and cranial extension of the SBS may affect spinal and appendicular mechanics. The spine, being a midline structure, demonstrates decreased cervical, thoracic and lumbar anteroposterior curvatures with SBS flexion and increased curvatures with SBS extension. The paired extremities demonstrate external rotation with SBS flexion and internal rotation with SBS extension. Consequently, a child presenting with increased lumbar lordosis and genu valgum is demonstrating a craniosacral extension, internal rotation pattern that may be related to SBS extension dysfunction.

Pure cranial flexion and cranial extension dysfunctional patterns are not commonly encountered because of the tendency for somatic dysfunction to manifest asymmetries. It is more common to find either a cranial flexion or cranial extension pattern in association with one of the bilaterally asymmetric dysfunctions described below.

Torsional dysfunctions

A torsional dysfunction is present when the motion of the SBS occurs freely in one direction only in its torsion on its AP axis. Torsion normally occurs equally to the right and to the left. Indicating the side on which the greater wing of the sphenoid is elevated identifies torsional dysfunction. Therefore, when torsion occurs in only one direction, for example, toward the right, with restriction of torsion in the opposite direction, in this case the left, the patient has a right torsional dysfunction.

Associated movements of the paired bones accompany a torsional dysfunction, with a tendency toward external rotation on the side for which the torsion is named, and internal rotation on the other side. With a right torsional dysfunction, the right half of the skull on the side of the elevated greater wing of the sphenoid is in relative external rotation. The right temporal fossa is higher than the left temporal fossa. The right orbit is wider and the right eyeball more prominent than the left. The right naris and right nasal passage are more open. The right half of the palate is wider and lower and the upper molars on the right are everted. The right temporal bone follows the occipital bone in its inferior displacement and tends to externally rotate, carrying the ear with it, thus causing the right ear to stick out.

With a right torsional dysfunction, the pectoral and pelvic girdles and upper and lower extremities will tend toward external rotation on the right. Consequently, the right pelvic bone will tend to be externally rotated and the right knee and foot will lie in a preferentially varus position; however, on the left side of the skull and body, structures will tend to be internally rotated. The opposite findings are anticipated in response to a left torsional dysfunction.

Sidebending–rotation dysfunctions

A sidebending–rotation dysfunction is present when the occiput and the sphenoid both rotate in the same direction around an anteroposterior axis while simultaneously sidebending by moving in opposite directions around two vertical axes. Sidebending–rotation normally occurs equally to both sides. A sidebending–rotation dysfunction is named by indicating the side where the greater wing of the sphenoid and the occiput move inferiorly. Therefore, when a sidebending–rotation pattern occurs in only one direction, for example toward the right, with restriction of the opposite sidebending–rotation pattern, in this case the left, the patient has a right sidebending–rotation dysfunction. In such a right sidebending–rotation dysfunction, the occiput and the sphenoid are lower on the right and the SBS is sidebent, so that the resultant convexity is on the right. Thus, the right greater wing of the sphenoid moves anteriorly and the occiput moves posteriorly on the right. (*Note*: The opposite combination, however, can occasionally occur wherein the sphenoid and occiput are atypically inferior on the side of the sidebending–rotation concavity of the SBS.[3])

Associated movements of the paired bones accompany a sidebending–rotation dysfunction. On the side for which the sidebending–rotation is named, in the above example the right side, there is a tendency toward external rotation of the temporal bone influenced by the occiput. Similarly, as the greater wing moves inferiorly on the right, bones influenced by the sphenoid tend to demonstrate internal rotation. In the front of the skull, on the side of the sidebending–rotation to the right, the skull and face seem to be vertically shortened, the right half of the frontal bone is lower and more anterior, the orbital cavity is smaller and the eyeball less prominent. Posteriorly, the right occipital squama is lower, the right mastoid process is displaced medially and inferiorly. External rotation of the right temporal bone causes the mandibular fossa on the right to be displaced posteriorly, whereas internal rotation of the left temporal bone, in association with a right sidebending–rotation, causes the mandibular fossa on the left to be displaced anteriorly. Consequently, the chin is displaced to the right. On the left side of the skull, with a right sidebending–rotation dysfunction, structures tend to be externally rotated in the front of the skull and internally rotated posteriorly. The opposite findings will be anticipated in response to a left sidebending–rotation dysfunction.

Note: The whole skull, including the membranes, is involved in the patterns of flexion, extension and torsion or sidebending–rotation. This is what is felt when globally palpating the skull. With infants, before ossification has occurred, however, articular motion of the SBS is present. Therefore, mental visualization of the structure and function of the SBS is important for precision of diagnosis and treatment.

Other physiologic dysfunctions of the skull

Aside from the SBS, cranial somatic dysfunction can involve any bone of the skull. Unpaired structures become dysfunctional in cranial flexion or extension. Paired structures become dysfunctional in external or internal rotation.

In a fashion similar to those mechanics described for the SBS, a cranial flexion dysfunction of any unpaired structure is present when the structure moves freely into cranial flexion but cannot move into cranial extension with the PRM facilitated in the inspiratory phase. A cranial extension dysfunction is present when motion is freer in cranial extension, restricted in cranial flexion and the PRM facilitated in the expiratory phase.

External and internal rotation dysfunctions can occur unilaterally or bilaterally, and may involve any of the paired bones of the skull. An external rotation dysfunction is present when a structure moves freely into external rotation during cranial flexion and does not move into internal rotation during cranial extension. The PRM is facilitated in the inspiratory phase. Conversely, in an internal rotation dysfunction, the structure moves into internal rotation during cranial extension, is restricted in external rotation during cranial flexion and the PRM is facilitated in the expiratory phase.

Physiologic dysfunctions of other areas of the body

Any area of the body can demonstrate dysfunctional mechanics similar to those of the cranium and face. A physiologic dysfunction of these areas is a restriction of mobility within the limits of the normal range of movement and consists of restriction of the patterns of motion described in Chapter 3. They include flexion, extension, rotation left and right, and sidebending left and right for the midline bones, and external and internal rotation for the paired bones. These dysfunctions do not exist alone; they affect and are affected by the mechanics in other parts of the body.

Physiologic dysfunctions of the sacrum and pelvic bones

A craniosacral flexion dysfunction of the sacrum is present when the sacrum moves freely into craniosacral flexion but cannot move into craniosacral extension. Consequently, the entire pelvis may be in a state of craniosacral flexion–external rotation. Because of the core link – the connection of the spinal dura mater from the occiput, at the foramen magnum, to the sacrum – the PRM is facilitated in the inspiratory phase. A craniosacral extension dysfunction of the sacrum is present when the sacrum moves freely into craniosacral extension but cannot move into craniosacral flexion. Consequently, the entire pelvis may be in a state of craniosacral extension–internal rotation and the PRM will be facilitated in the expiratory phase.

Craniosacral flexion and craniosacral extension dysfunctions of the sacrum may affect the spine above, and particularly through the influence of the lumbar spine and diaphragmatic crura, thoracoabdominal diaphragmatic excursion. Craniosacral flexion dysfunctions of the sacrum are associated with decreased lumbar anteroposterior curvature and limitation of the end of the expiratory phase of pulmonary respiration, whereas craniosacral extension dysfunctions of the sacrum are associated with increased lumbar anteroposterior curvature and limitation of the end of the inspiratory phase of pulmonary respiration. Craniosacral flexion and craniosacral extension of the sacrum may also affect the paired lower extremities that demonstrate external rotation with craniosacral flexion and internal rotation with craniosacral extension.

Torsional dysfunctions of the sacrum manifest as coupled sidebending and rotation. These dysfunctions characteristically present as a combination of sacral sidebending and rotation in opposite directions. In newborn infants the whole pelvis typically follows the pattern of the sacral torsion. Thus, a left sacral torsion dysfunction occurs when the sacrum moves freely into coupled left rotation and right sidebending but cannot move into right rotation and left sidebending. In this instance, the right pelvic bone accompanies the left torsion with external rotation, wherein the major component of the movement is anterior rotation, and the left pelvic bone demonstrates internal rotation with a major component of posterior rotation. In an accommodative pattern to a right sacral torsion, the sacrum moves freely into coupled right rotation and left sidebending, and does not move into left rotation and right sidebending, whereas the left pelvic bone moves into external rotation with significant anterior rotation and the right pelvic bone demonstrates internal rotation with significant posterior rotation.

These patterns of pelvic accommodation are extremely common and, unless treated, persist throughout life, acting as a foundation upon which additional dysfunctional mechanics occur. The existence of this underlying asymmetry can create confusion when diagnosing iliosacral and sacroiliac somatic dysfunction encountered in later life.

Iliosacral dysfunctional mechanics – the impact of the lower extremity on the relationship between the pelvic bone and the sacrum – are commonly encountered later in infancy and childhood. In this instance, although the pelvis may demonstrate a pattern of accommodation, the dysfunctional pelvic bone exhibits an overlying pattern that is inconsistent with sacral mechanics. Iliosacral dysfunctional mechanics occur as pelvic bone external rotation or internal rotation dysfunctions. In external rotation dysfunction, the pelvic bone can move into external rotation but cannot move into internal rotation. In internal rotation dysfunction, the pelvic bone can move into internal rotation but is restricted in external rotation.

The motion of the PRM is manifested in the pattern of iliosacral dysfunctional mechanics. On the side of an external rotation dysfunction of the pelvic bone, the inspiratory phase of the PRM is unencumbered and the expiratory phase is restricted. On the side of an internal rotation dysfunction, the expiratory phase is unencumbered and the inspiratory phase is restricted.

Physiologic dysfunctions of the vertebral segments

A craniosacral flexion dysfunction of a vertebral segment is present when the segment moves freely during craniosacral flexion but does not move during craniosacral extension. In this case, the PRM is facilitated in the inspiratory phase. A craniosacral extension dysfunction is present when the vertebral segment moves during craniosacral extension, does not move during craniosacral flexion and the PRM is facilitated in the expiratory phase.

Dysfunctions of the vertebrae manifest as coupled sidebending and rotation that can occur in the same direction or in opposite directions. As with all other dysfunctions discussed, vertebral somatic dysfunction is named for the direction of freedom of motion. In infants, group spinal mechanics, demonstrating coupled sidebending and rotation in opposite directions, are most often found in association with dysfunctions of the cranial base, the occiput and atlas, or the sacrum and pelvis.

Although the biphasic PRM will be palpable, it will be modified by the vertebral dysfunction. Therefore, it will not demonstrate pure inspiratory or expiratory phases as seen during craniosacral flexion–extension, but rather a motion pattern that includes the dysfunctional combination of flexion–extension and sidebending–rotation, with greater freedom of movement in the direction of the dysfunctional combination. The inspiratory phase of the PRM is associated with a decrease of the spinal AP curves, whereas the expiratory phase is associated with an increase of the AP curves. Therefore, if the dysfunction of the vertebral segment results in a decrease of the spinal AP curve at that vertebral level, the inspiratory phase of the PRM will be unrestricted and the expiratory phase will be restricted. When the dysfunction of the vertebral segment results in an increase of the spinal AP curve, the expiratory phase will be unrestricted and the inspiratory phase will be restricted.

Physiologic dysfunctions of the limbs

In an external rotation dysfunction of any component of the upper or lower extremities, that component moves freely into external rotation during craniosacral flexion; during craniosacral extension, however, it does not move into internal rotation. In this case, the PRM is facilitated in the inspiratory phase. Conversely, in an internal rotation dysfunction, the component moves into internal rotation during craniosacral extension, is restricted in external rotation during craniosacral flexion and the PRM is facilitated in the expiratory phase.

NON PHYSIOLOGIC DYSFUNCTIONS

A non physiologic dysfunction is commonly associated with a total loss of mobility following any trauma. This results when a given structure is displaced beyond its normal and physiologic range of movement. (*Note*: Traumatic forces that move a structure within its normal and physiologic range of motion produce a physiologic dysfunction.)

Cranial non physiologic dysfunctions

Non physiologic dysfunction can affect any area of the skull. The following are among the most commonly encountered cranial non physiologic dysfunctions.

Compression of the sphenobasilar synchondrosis

Compression of the SBS can be the result of a difficult birth or any trauma compressing the skull, and thus the SBS, along its anteroposterior axis (Fig. 4.1). External constraints, such as headbands, can also produce compression. Following a traumatic compression, the SBS loses all mobility and the PRM is dampened, demonstrating less amplitude and power.

Strains of the sphenobasilar synchondrosis

Strains result from forces that shift the articular surfaces of the SBS between the basilar portion of the occiput and the body of the sphenoid. They occur in the plane of the articular surfaces of the SBS that, in the anatomic position, declines anteriorly and inferiorly. Thus, the anterior articular surface of the basilar portion of the occiput faces anteriorly and superiorly, whereas the posterior articular surface of the body of the sphenoid faces posteriorly and inferiorly. Strains occur either vertically with superior or inferior displacement, or laterally with left or right displacement. They are named for the direction of displacement of the posterior articular surface of the sphenoidal body and occur before ossification of the SBS is complete.

Vertical strain follows an upward or downward force, applied either anterior or posterior to the SBS, resulting in a vertical shift between the occiput and the sphenoid. A superior vertical strain (Fig. 4.2) is present when the posterior articular surface of the sphenoidal body is elevated and the anterior articular surface of the basiocciput is low. Conversely, an inferior vertical strain is present when the posterior sphenoidal body is low and the anterior articular surface of the basiocciput is elevated.

Lateral strain follows a lateral force applied anterior or posterior to the SBS, resulting in a lateral shift between the occiput and the sphenoid. A right lateral strain (Fig. 4.3) is present when the posterior articular surface of the sphenoidal body is shifted to the right and the anterior articular surface of the basiocciput is shifted to the left. Conversely, in a left lateral strain, the posterior sphenoidal body is shifted to the left and the anterior articular surface of the basiocciput is shifted to the right. In either case, when viewed from above, the resultant lateral shift between the sphenoid and occiput at the SBS produces a parallelogram-shaped deformity of the skull (Fig. 4.10).

When strain dysfunctions result from significant traumatic forces, the motion restriction at the SBS is proportionate to the causative forces. Minor SBS strains can be compensatory for other imbalances or can follow a minor physical stress. SBS strains may be encountered in conjunction with other dysfunctional patterns such as torsion and sidebending–rotation of the SBS. As such, the combination of a lateral strain and a torsion or sidebending–rotation will result in the palpatory sensation of shifting of the sphenoid in association with an elevation of the greater wing of the sphenoid on one side. In these cases the displacement of the SBS results in the sensation of freedom of motion in the direction of the strain with some restriction in the opposite direction. Such strain dysfunctions may be considered as minor movements within other complex

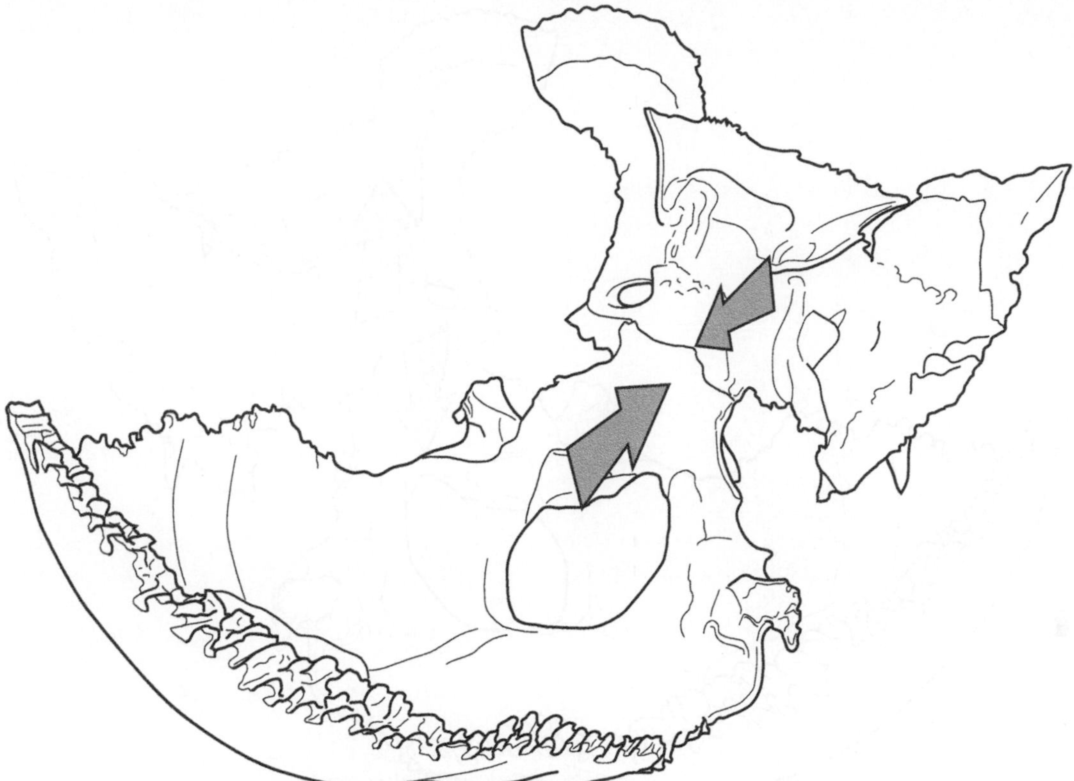

Figure 4.1. *Dysfunction of the sphenobasilar synchondrosis: compression.*

patterns of SBS dysfunction, but still are of great significance in diagnosis and treatment.

Note: Cranial dysfunctions are membranous articular dysfunctions. Membranous imbalance is combined with alteration of motion, as dictated by the articular anatomy, in the production of the dysfunction. In infants and children the membranous component is dominant; however, articular anatomy still dictates available patterns of motion. As such, focusing on membranous influences as opposed to articular influences, or vice-versa, is naive. As Sutherland said: 'The cranial lesion includes the intracranial membranes as well as the articulation.'[1]

Other non physiologic cranial dysfunctions

By definition, the forces that produce a traumatic dysfunction do not respect range of movement. Thus, after any significant trauma, cranial non physiologic dysfunctions affecting any area of the skull can result. Dysfunctions of the articular relationships of the zygomatic bone and the frontosphenoidal articulations are very common with facial trauma.

Non physiologic dysfunctions of other areas of the body

Non physiologic dysfunction can also affect any other area of the body. The following are among the most commonly encountered non physiologic dysfunctions.

Dysfunctions of the cranial base

Dysfunctions of the cranial base, although involving the cranium, are classified here under the heading of other areas of the body because of the involvement of the cervical spine. These dysfunctions can be the result of any trauma where the base of the skull is impacted on the upper cervical spine, such as a significant blow to the head or an abrupt fall onto the buttocks. The motion between the occiput, the atlas and one or both of the temporal bones becomes locked. The palpatory sensation of the PRM in the region of the cervico-occipital junction is dampened, demonstrating decreased amplitude and power.

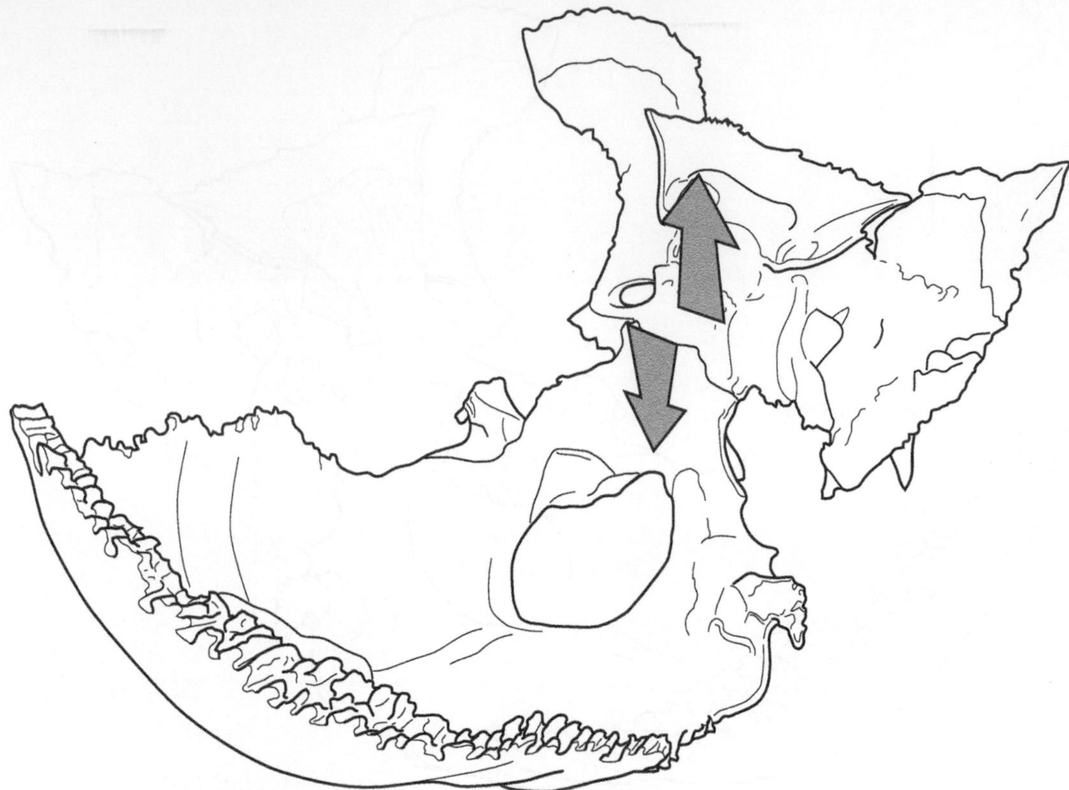

Figure 4.2. *Dysfunction of the sphenobasilar synchondrosis: superior vertical strain.*

Traumatic dysfunctions of the sacrum and pelvic bones

Dysfunction of the sacrum and pelvic bones can be the result of any trauma where the pelvis is impacted. This can be the result of an abrupt fall onto the buttocks, bilateral or unilateral traumatic forces applied to the lower extremities or even a significant blow to the top of the head. The motion between the sacrum and one, or both, of the pelvic bones is consequently restricted. The palpatory sensation of the PRM in the region of the pelvis is decreased in amplitude and power. This can, in turn, affect the cranial mechanism through the core link and the total body through the interrelationship between the PRM and the autonomic nervous system (ANS).

INTRAOSSEOUS DYSFUNCTIONS

All living bone consists of a web of calcified connective tissue of greater or lesser density depending on the age and health of the individual. In the absence of somatic dysfunction, this open matrix permits a certain amount of flexibility to remain throughout life. The bones of infants and children frequently consist of multiple centers of growth joined by flexible cartilaginous or membranous tissues that remain particularly subject to dysfunction until ossification occurs.

An intraosseous dysfunction, therefore, can result in the loss of the normal flexibility of the fibrous components of the matrix of bone tissue and/or of the cartilaginous or membranous unossified areas. Skeletal ossification is not complete until some time between the ages of 20 and 30 years and, in principle, an intraosseous dysfunction can be produced in any structure that is not completely ossified. This type of dysfunction occurs most often during intrauterine life or at the time of delivery when the skull is particularly vulnerable. Traumas experienced during childhood can also produce these dysfunctions, which can occur in any bone, resulting in a modification of shape and, thus, function. Intraosseous dysfunction should be differentiated from

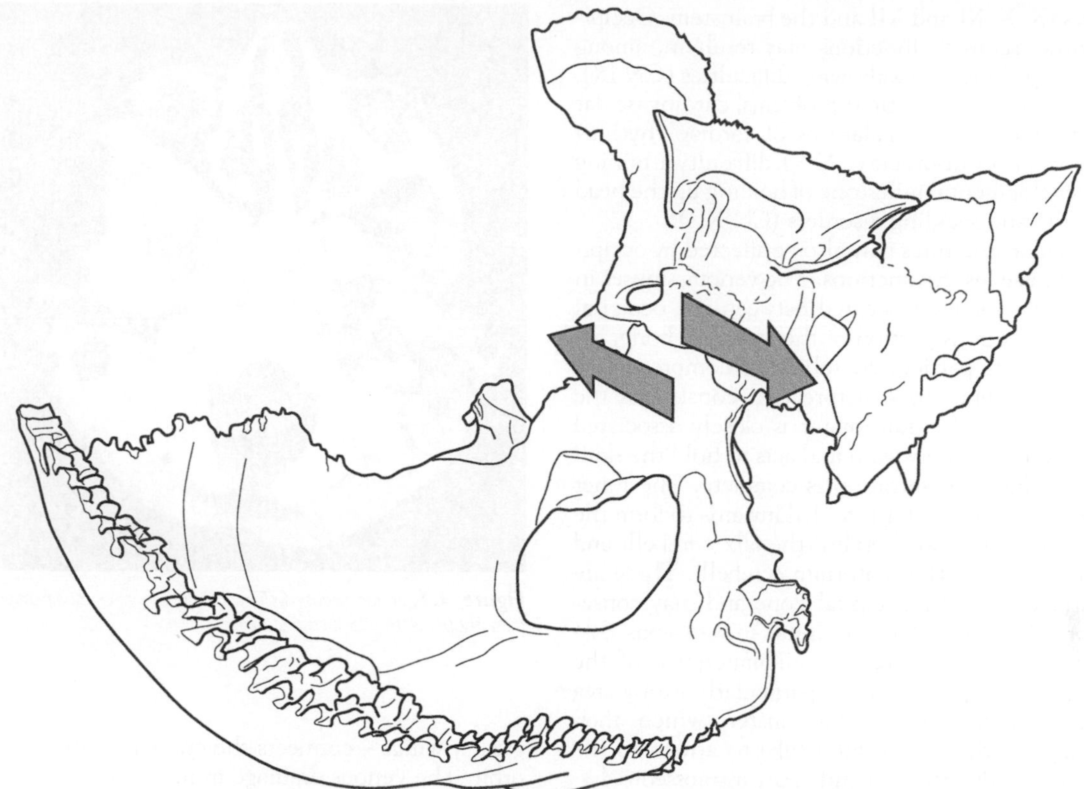

Figure 4.3. *Dysfunction of the sphenobasilar synchondrosis: right lateral strain.*

interosseous dysfunction: intraosseous dysfunction occurs within the structure of a single bone; interosseous dysfunction occurs between adjacent bones.

Cranial intraosseous dysfunctions

Intraosseous dysfunctions of the occipital bone

At birth, the occipital bone consists of four main parts: the basilar part, two lateral parts and, most posteriorly, the squamous part. The ossifi ation between the squamous part and the lateral parts is complete by 2–3 years of age and between the lateral parts and the basilar part by 7–9 years of age. The occipital condyles are situated on the junction between the lateral and basilar parts. As such, the anterior portion of each condyle is derived from the basilar part and the posterior portion from the lateral part. Their fusion also results in the formation of the hypoglossal canal.

Intraosseous dysfunctions of the occipital bone result from compressive or shearing forces affecting the junctions between the different parts and/or the osseous matrix of any individual part. These can produce modifi cations of the circumference of the foramen magnum, the shape of the condylar parts and the outline of the occipital squama. The deformity of the occipital bone encountered in non-synostotic plagiocephaly is a readily apparent example of intraosseous dysfunction, where asymmetric compressive forces result in gross asymmetry of the left and right halves of the occipital squama and the intraoccipital synchondroses.[6] Because of the structural changes in the occiput and consequent modifi cations of high spinal mechanics, this may be an etiologic factor in the development of infantile scoliosis. The often-stated association between intraosseous dysfunction and infantile scoliosis[7,8] is further upheld by the association between non-synostotic plagiocephaly and scoliosis.[9]

In addition to the accommodative impact of occipital intraosseous dysfunctions on the spine below, they are of particular consequence because of the relationship of the occiput with associated structures. Associated nervous structures include cranial nerves IX, X, XI and XII and the brainstem. Occipital intraosseous dysfunctions may result in, among other impediments, swallowing difficulties (CN IX), functional gastrointestinal problems, cardiovascular dysfunction (e.g. irregularities of cardiac rhythm) and respiratory disorders (CN X), difficulty attaining the developmental milestone of holding up the head (CN XI) and suckling disorders (CN XII).

Vascular structures may also be affected by occipital intraosseous dysfunctions. The venous sinuses in the jugular foramen, located between the occipital bone and petrous portion of the temporal bone, are thought to be particularly subject to compression.

The membranous structure that constitutes the outer layer of the dura mater is closely associated with the inner periosteum and acts to hold the skull together before ossification is complete. The inner layer of the dura mater is folded inwards to form the four septa – the falx cerebri, the falx cerebelli and the two parts of the tentorium cerebelli. These are all attached to the occipital bone and may consequently be affected by occipital intraosseous dysfunctions. Furthermore, the circumference of the foramen magnum provides a particularly strong area of attachment for the dura mater, which then descends as the spinal dural tube to attach to the sacrum, forming the core link. Any intraosseous dysfunction of the occipital bone can affect distant areas through the core link. The intraosseous occipital dysfunctions are among the most frequently reported of cranial intraosseous dysfunctions (Fig. 4.4).

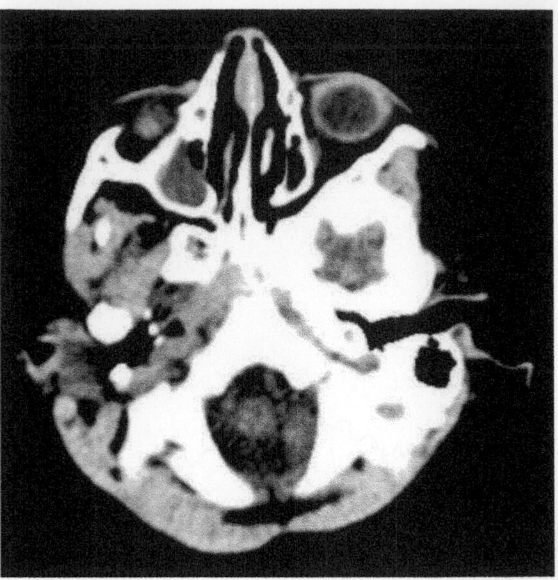

Figure 4.4. *Intraosseous dysfunctions result in a modification of bony shape. Note SBS lateral strain.*

Intraosseous dysfunctions of the sphenoid

The sphenoid develops from multiple centers of ossification. At birth, up to 12 synchondroses have been identified within the sphenoid. Because of the various stages of ossification of these synchondroses, the sphenoid is commonly described as consisting of three parts: the body and lesser wings form the central part; the two lateral parts, one on each side of the body, are created by the combination of the greater wing and pterygoid process. Additionally, the sphenoidal body consists of a presphenoidal part and a postsphenoidal part that are typically fused by 8 months of gestation. The remaining synchondroses between the central and lateral parts are usually fused between 1 and 2 years of age.

The sphenoid exerts an important influence on the orbital region. Six of the seven extraocular muscles originate on the sphenoid. Among them the four recti are attached posteriorly to a common annular tendon near the optic canal. The superior orbital fissure – the space between the lesser and greater wings – connects the cranial cavity and the orbit. The venous drainage from the region, and all the nerves that supply the contents of the orbit, except the optic nerve, pass through the superior orbital fissure As such, intraosseous dysfunction of the sphenoid may impact a myriad of ocular functions.

The greater wings and pterygoid processes unite bilaterally with the body of the sphenoid in the basisphenoidal–alisphenoidal synchondrosis to form the two pterygoid canals. Each canal transmits the Vidian nerve – the nerve of the pterygoid canal – from the foramen lacerum to the pterygopalatine ganglion. This nerve includes both the parasympathetic and the sympathetic roots of the pterygopalatine ganglion. Branches from this ganglion are distributed to the orbital region, the lacrimal gland, the mouth, and the nasal and pharyngeal areas. Therefore, intraosseous dysfunction between the body and greater wing of the sphenoid can result in functional complaints referable to the eyes, nose, mouth and pharynx. These synchondroses are usually fused between 1 and 2 years of age.

The cavernous sinus lies on either side of the body of the sphenoid, above the basisphenoidal–alisphenoidal synchondrosis. This venous network surrounds the internal carotid artery and cranial nerves III, IV, V_1 and VI. Therefore, intraosseous dysfunction of the sphenoid at this level can functionally affect venous drainage of the orbit, the carotid artery and its surrounding sympathetic plexus, and the cranial nerves listed above.

The pterygoid process – a component of the lateral part of the sphenoid – serves as the origin of the pterygoid muscles and, through fascial connections, influences the oropharyngeal muscles. Consequently, an intraosseous dysfunction involving the basisphenoidal–alisphenoidal synchondrosis will affect oropharyngeal muscular function. Dysfunction of the above muscles can, alternatively, result in intraosseous dysfunction of this area of the sphenoid.

Intraosseous dysfunctions of the temporal bone

The temporal bones develop as the union of the squamous, petromastoid, tympanic and styloid parts. The tympanic ring unites with the squama just before birth; consequently, it is not a commonly identified area of intraosseous dysfunction. The petrosquamosal suture between the petromastoid and squamous parts is not united until the end of the 1st year of life, making this area and the relationship between these two parts of the temporal bone subject to the development of intraosseous dysfunction. Because the petromastoid part of the temporal bones contains the organ of hearing in the cochlea, and that of balance in the vestibule and the semicircular canals, an intraosseous dysfunction here may be the cause of disturbance of the sensory receptors for hearing and balance.

The posterior part of the temporal bone is cartilaginous in origin; the anterior part is membranous. The posterior cartilaginous part follows the occiput, while the anterior membranous part can be influenced by the greater wing of the sphenoid. In patterns of cranial motion such as torsion, as the greater wing is displaced superiorly on the side of the torsion and the occiput is displaced inferiorly, the anterior and posterior parts of the temporal bone are exposed to opposing forces. Depending on the severity of the torsional forces and the resilience of the petrosquamosal suture, there is potential for the development of an intraosseous dysfunction.

Intraosseous dysfunction may also occur as a result of exogenous forces that asymmetrically affect the development of the temporal bone. The mastoid processes develop bilaterally from the petromastoid parts in response to traction from the sternocleidomastoid muscles. Asymmetric muscular tension will result in asymmetry of the mastoid processes. A chronic asymmetric resting position, as can be responsible for the development of non-synostotic plagiocephaly, will asymmetrically affect the growth of the temporal bones.

Between birth and adulthood a significant number of changes occur at the level of the cranial base. The pattern of flexion of the cranial base is coupled with lateral expansion of the squamous portions of the temporal bones and external rotation of the petromastoid portions. This will amend the position of major structures linked to the temporal bones. Although the ossicles have reached adult size by the middle of gestation, the internal and external auditory canals and the vestibular aqueduct continue to grow after birth.[10] The pharyngotympanic tube (PT), at birth, is more horizontal than in adults.[11] It demonstrates an inclination of 10° from the horizontal plane, reaching about 45° in the adult. Intraosseous dysfunction of the temporal bone complex can result in functional compromise of the PT and tympanic cavity of the temporal bone. In children with secretory otitis, the bony portion of the PT, the vertical portion of the tensor veli palatini and the mastoid air cell system are demonstrably smaller than in normal children.[12]

The petrous parts of the temporal bones are anatomically and functionally linked to one another through the tentorium cerebelli and, as such, dysfunction of one will affect the other. This dysfunctional relationship can, in turn, affect the global balance of the cranium.

Intraosseous dysfunctions of the vault

The parietal bones present the greatest potential for accommodation during the birth process. Consequently, they are often subject to intraosseous dysfunctions. These dysfunctions present as deformations induced by cranial molding and sometimes in association with certain conditions such as extradural hematoma and periosteal edema, and certain procedures such as the use of forceps and vacuum extraction.

The longitudinal venous sinus lies between the two parietal bones, beneath the sagittal suture, in the duplication of dura mater that forms the falx cerebri. Unilateral parietal intraosseous dysfunction will result in asymmetric stresses between the two parietal bones and associated dura. It has been proposed that these stresses on the dura can affect venous blood flow through the sagittal sinus.[13]

Intraosseous dysfunctions of the frontal bones

Intraosseous dysfunctions of the frontal bones are commonly encountered because they are often the first structures to contact the maternal pelvis in vertex presentation. As a result of asynclitism, greater pressure is often applied to one side of the frontal region. The use of forceps during delivery is another potential source of asymmetric forces applied to the frontal bone. These influences result in asymmetry of the frontal bones that can impact the shape of the forehead, the orbit and the eye. A fibrocartilagenous loop is located near the medial end of the supraorbital margin of the frontal bone. It serves as a trochlea for the superior oblique muscle on its way from the body of the sphenoid to the sclera of the eye. Any frontal intraosseous dysfunction may affect the position of the trochlea and consequently the function of the superior oblique muscle. Imbalances in the visual axis may follow. The nasolacrimal duct, through the relationship between the superior border of the lacrimal bone and the frontal bone, is another area where function may be potentially affected by frontal intraosseous dysfunction.

As the frontal bones have an intimate relationship with many of the bones of the viscerocranium, frontal intraosseous dysfunction must be taken into consideration when problem solving dysfunction in the face. The function of the upper respiratory tract may be impacted. Because the ethmoid is suspended from the ethmoidal notch between the frontal bones, any frontal intraosseous dysfunction will affect the frontoethmoidal and frontonasal sutures. Nasal breathing will be impaired on the side of the dysfunction. As the role of the ethmoid and nasal cartilage is important in facial growth, frontal intraosseous dysfunction has the potential to influence facial growth.

As part of the facial complex articulating with the frontal bone, the maxillae may also be affected by frontal bone intraosseous dysfunction. The frontomaxillary sutures are important sites of maxillary development. Children with this dysfunctional relationship commonly demonstrate underdeveloped maxillae.

Intraosseous dysfunctions of the maxillae

The maxillae consist of two parts: a premaxilla (also referred to as os incisivum) and a maxilla. The suture between the two is sometimes observable postnatally, anterior on the palate, joining the two incisive canals on each side. Intraosseous dysfunctions of the maxillae may occur in utero secondary to any direct pressure placed on the face, during delivery secondary to facial pressure against the maternal sacrum in vertex occiput-anterior presentations, postpartum secondary to thumb sucking or exaggerated use of a pacifier, or following facial trauma.

During infancy the maxillae are not fully developed and thus their potential for growth is major. Consequently, intraosseous dysfunctions of the maxillae have the potential to exert significant impact that can only be increased as the dysfunctional bones grow. The consequences of such dysfunction include orofacial problems (e.g. malocclusion) and impaired nasal breathing.

Intraosseous dysfunctions of other areas of the body

Any bone that consists of different parts separated by cartilage before ossification may be subject to the development of intraosseous dysfunction when the cartilaginous junction is placed under stress before ossification. Such dysfunctions may also result in the loss of the normal flexibility of the fibrous components of the affected bone.

Intraosseous dysfunctions of the pelvic bones and sacrum

At birth the sacrum consists of five unfused vertebral segments and the innominates, each of three portions: the ischium, the pubis and the ilium. These different portions are separated by cartilage that is subject to stress when the child is young. Breech deliveries or abrupt falls on the buttocks may be the origin of intraosseous pelvic dysfunctions.

Pelvic intraosseous dysfunctions can affect the craniosacral mechanism, posture and, through the sympathetic and parasympathetic systems, the autonomic nervous balance.[14]

Intraosseous dysfunctions of the sternum and ribs

The sternal body consists of four sternebrae that unite between puberty and 25 years of age.[15] Any trauma prior to ossification may be responsible for intraosseous dysfunction. Intraosseous sternal dysfunctions may also result from postural as well as myofascial imbalances, such as protracted scapular girdles, occipitocervical and associated cervical fasciae dysfunctions. Pectus excavatum and pectus carinatum are the two more often described sternal intraosseous dysfunctions. Pectus excavatum is associated with imbalance of the diaphragm or other internal myofascial structures. It may also result from direct trauma to the sternum, with a dysfunction at the junction between two sternebrae, and appears most of the time as a depression.

Rib ossification follows a pattern similar to that of the sternum. Trauma and postural adaptations are responsible for intraosseous dysfunctions of the ribs. This is well illustrated in scoliosis, where ribs can change shape to accommodate vertebral dysfunctions.

MEMBRANOUS DYSFUNCTIONS

The dural membranes consist of a dense fibrous network arranged in fascicles, or stress bands. The cranial bones develop in close relationship with the dura mater. Balance and imbalance of forces within the dural web directly influence their development. Later in life, after complete ossification of the cranial bones, the dural web still connects and exerts influence on the different parts of the craniosacral mechanism. Alternatively, the dural web may be affected by somatic dysfunction, anywhere within the mechanism. This is a global system, wherein every component is interdependent with every other component and, as such, membranous dysfunctions impact the PRM.

During the latter weeks of pregnancy, the fetus is subjected to stresses from uterine contractions. If the fetal head is engaged in a vertex presentation, forces transmitted through the fetal spine impact the base of the skull. This can, in turn, compress the skull with resultant membranous strain.

During labor, the forces affecting the fetus from uterine contractions are increased significantly and are opposed by the resistance of the maternal pelvis against the fetal head. Even in the easiest delivery, stresses applied to the fetal head can result in dural membranous strains, shears and compression. These dysfunctional membranous patterns provide a template for future membranous dysfunctions and, because of the intimate relationship between the dural membranes and the cranial bones, the pattern is created for articular dysfunctions as the skull, spine and pelvis mature.

Intracranial circulation can be impaired by membranous dysfunctions because of the relationship between the dura and the venous sinuses. Additionally, dural membranous dysfunctions can result in entrapment syndromes of the cranial nerves.

Because of the intimate relationship between the dura and the cranial bones, membranous strain patterns mirror, and are accompanied by, osseous dysfunctional patterns. Therefore, they are named the same as the articular pattern that will develop as a result of the membranous strain.

COMPENSATORY DYSFUNCTIONS

Somatic dysfunction anywhere results in altered tension and imbalances that will affect areas of the body distant from the site of the primary dysfunction. The individual is forced to respond to these imbalances and the response often results in functional compromise. These compensatory dysfunctions manifest as imbalances in soft tissue tensions. They typically allow movement in all directions with, however, qualitative changes in the available motion. This compensation is a demonstration of osteopathic holism, the interdependency of all parts of the body.

A dysfunctional pattern in the skull will result in compensatory responses throughout the membranous and fascial structures of the body. Thus, a child with a dominant flexion–external rotation craniosacral pattern will be apt to assume a postural pattern of flexion and external rotation. The associated sacral flexion will be combined with a decrease of the lumbar lordosis. The legs and feet may be externally rotated, demonstrating genu varum and pes cavus. An asymmetric craniosacral pattern (e.g. torsion) that is associated with external rotation on one side of the skull and internal rotation on the other side will likely show an asymmetric postural pattern.

In similar fashion, a dysfunctional pattern in the pelvis may result in membranous and fascial compensatory responses throughout the body. It is easy to see how pelvic dysfunction can affect the lower extremities; however, it can also affect more distant areas, with compensatory mechanisms manifesting as far away as the skull.

Etiologies of dysfunction

FETAL PERIOD

To understand somatic dysfunction one must understand the difference between deformation and malformation. Deformation occurs when shape or configuration of otherwise normally developed structures is affected in fetal life as the result of mechanical factors.[16] Osteopathic procedures may be employed to improve such deformations, and the earlier the treatment is initiated, the better the potential for positive outcome. Errors in morphogenesis that can occur during the first 2 months of embryonic fetal life cause fetal malformation and are not within the scope of this chapter.

The effect of mechanical factors acting on the fetus during intrauterine life, as a source of fetal deformities, has been described since Hippocrates.[16] Mechanical pressure may be applied directly on the fetus as a result of an abnormal constriction in the intrauterine environment. This may result from increased intrauterine pressure, as in oligohydramnios. It may be caused by physical constraint, as can occur in the presence of a unicornuate uterus, uterine fibroids or multiple births, when one fetus applies pressure on the other(s). Mechanical pressure may also result from extrauterine constraints placed on the fetus, such as pressure from neighboring abdominal organs or increased tonus of the abdominal muscles, as encountered in athletic mothers, particularly primipara. Additionally, maternal sacral and lumbar somatic dysfunctions may influence fetal positioning and interfere with fetal ability to move and consequently with development. Anterior displacement of the maternal sacral base in craniosacral extension may constrain the fetal head. Every part of the fetal body may be affected by mechanical pressure, the feet being the most commonly deformed in an exaggerated talipes equinovarus or calcaneovalgus position. External tibial torsion is also frequently associated with deformities of the knees, resulting in bowing of the legs. Congenital dislocation of the hip, acetabular dysplasia, congenital torticollis, congenital scoliosis and plagiocephaly are also often described as the result of uterine constraint.[16–20] Congenital knee recurvatum, overlapping toes, deformations of the thorax and upper limbs or asymmetric mandible may also occur, but less commonly.

Normally the fetus should be able to move, to stretch their limbs and to kick their legs. These movements are critical for development of the musculoskeletal system. Most mothers notice fetal movements – quickening – from about 4 months of gestation. Abnormal constriction in the intrauterine environment, as described above, may impair these movements. Oligohydramnios, a diminution of the amount of amniotic fluid, found in association with maternal hypertension, may also result in lack of fetal movement and is associated with fetal deformation.[16,18] Fetal ability to change position is of paramount importance, as the fetus may suffer as a result of the pressure from the walls of the uterus due to a prolonged static position.

The usual fetal position is a cross-legged posture. In the vertex presentation (left occiput anterior or LOA) the fetus most commonly lies on the maternal left side, with the fetal back to the left side of the mother (Fig. 4.5).[21] This fetal positioning is thought to be determined by the right-sided location of the maternal liver[22] and the position of the maternal rectum and bladder.[23] Consequently, when the fetus is in the LOA position, the uterus of the pregnant woman becomes oriented in a right torsion, the anterior surface of the uterus facing the right maternal side and the posterior surface facing the left maternal side. More space is available on the maternal left side for the fetal trunk and head. Therefore, the left side of the fetal trunk is compressed back against the maternal spine, while the fetal head is against the maternal pelvis. This may explain the greater frequency of left-sided deformities, such as hip dysplasia, that occurs twice as often on the left side as on the right,[16,17,24] the left hip being compressed against the maternal lumbar spine. Similarly, prolonged adduction of the left leg may result in varus deformities of the left knee or left tibial torsions.[18]

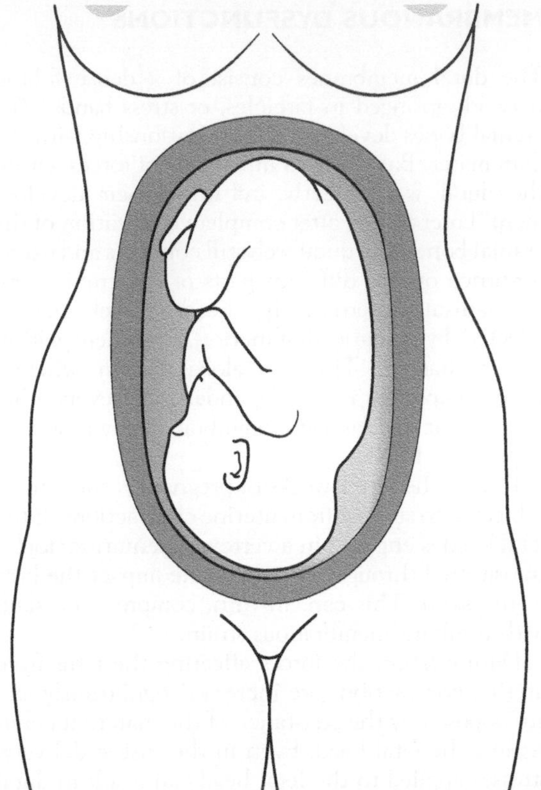

Figure 4.5. *Typical fetal position: head bent forward on the sternum, forearms crossed on the chest, lower limbs flexed.*

Fetal position varies from one fetus to another. However, consideration of the mechanical forces acting on the fetus that limit their ability to change position allows one to understand some of the dysfunctions present at birth, such as limitation of hip abduction or muscle imbalances, with adductor, or abductor, muscle hypertonicity. Mechanical factors play a significant role in fetal and neonatal histogenesis of bone, and any constraint applied to the fetal skeleton may be responsible for congenital deformities or may impair growth in the future.[25]

Multiple authors have described fetal malposition and its consequences. It is referred to as the 'molded baby',[24] 'molded baby syndrome',[26] 'compression baby',[27] 'wind-swept baby',[16] 'packaging defect'[28] or 'faulty fetal packing'.[29] At birth, in such cases, the newborn demonstrates a position that reflects their fetal position. When placed in this fetal position, the newborn is relaxed and enjoys 'the position of comfort'.[30] Several deformities are commonly associated with this positional syndrome, including, most often, plagiocephaly, torticollis, scoliosis and pelvic obliquity. Correlations are observed between these deformities, supporting their mechanical origin. With infantile scoliosis, the pelvis is usually higher on the side of the concavity of the lumbar spinal lateral curve with the hip adducted, demonstrating restricted abduction on the side of the lumbar convexity.[26] When plagiocephaly is present, forehead flattening is reported to be on the side of the restricted hip abduction,[24] always on the side of hip dislocation and convexity of the scoliotic thoracic curve,[19] and also on the side of the sternocleidomastoid muscle mass with congenital torticollis.[17]

Any part of the neurocranium and viscerocranium may also be deformed from fetal malposition or from the 'molded baby syndrome'. Amniotic bands – fibrous bands within the walls of the amniotic sac – may entrap fetal parts in utero and apply untoward pressures on the vault or the face, resulting in hypoplasias and clefting.[29] Positioning of the fetal hand, arm, shoulder or foot can compress part of the head and deform the nose, mandible or frontal region. Furthermore, in the last trimester of pregnancy, some antenatal skull molding occurs when the fetal head is compressed by repetitive Braxton Hicks contractions.[31] Coils of umbilical cord around the fetal neck may also be present, applying mechanical stress to the cranial base and cervical spine.

Deformities are about 10 times more frequent with breech presentations than with vertex presentations.[16] In the breech presentation position, the pelvis and lower limbs are under stress, especially if the fetal legs stay extended, without the potential for the movement of kicking and therefore difficulty converting to a vertex presentation. In this case, genu recurvatum is frequent. Additionally, the head, which is located in the uterine fundus, may be molded into an oblong and contracted shape.[18]

Besides the influence of asymmetry of the maternal environment, early fetal positional asymmetries may also be involved. The fact that in a vertex LOA presentation the fetus lies on the left maternal side has been linked to a left-sided otolithic dominance theory. During the linear acceleration of normal maternal locomotion, the hair cells of the fetal utricles are stimulated with an inertial force directed toward the left fetal side, located posteriorly in the maternal pelvis. This results in greater stimulation of the left utricle.[23] Consequently, because of the fetal positional asymmetry, asymmetric neurologic development of the ears and labyrinths may occur, with a left-sided otolithic dominance present at birth. This may contribute to the noticeable preference of the newborn for a right-sided head position when placed in supine.[32] Breech fetuses that have more liberty to move their head demonstrate less distinct vestibular lateralization.[21]

BIRTH PROCESS

The fetal freedom to move and position themselves impacts the presentation at birth. In about 97% of deliveries, the fetus delivers in the vertex presentation.[33] Maternal environment – the uterus, lumbopelvic soft tissues, bony pelvis and lumbar spine – exerts a significant impact on the fetal presentation and delivery process. Maternal somatic dysfunction, such as sacral and thoracolumbar somatic dysfunction, may affect the normal parasympathetic and sympathetic control of myometrial contractility, respectively. In addition, prolonged periods of uterine contraction during the delivery process increase the mechanical forces applied to the infant as they pass through the birth canal. Compression of the fetal spine may occur, particularly at the level of the occipitocervical and cervicothoracic junctions, with resultant somatic dysfunction.

During pregnancy, ligamentous relaxation of the maternal symphysis pubis and sacroiliac joints occurs due to hormonal changes. Therefore, the available motions of the sacroiliac joints and pubic symphysis are increased. When the fetal head enters the maternal pelvic inlet, it most commonly does so with its anteroposterior orientation in one of the two maternal pelvic oblique diameters. In a vertex LOA presentation, this orientation is along the left oblique pelvic diameter, between the right sacroiliac joints and the opposite iliopubic eminence. Maternal sacral torsional dysfunction decreases the oblique diameter, making orientation of the fetal head in that diameter, and consequently the birth process, more difficult. A prominent maternal sacral base or any fetopelvic disproportion may have the same effect. The fetal head must accommodate the shape

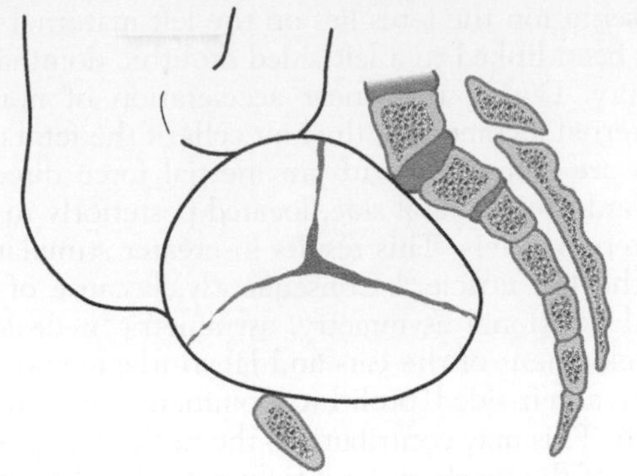

Figure 4.6. *During labor compressive forces result in skull molding.*

of the pelvic inlet and may encounter resistance from the bony pelvis. In a vertex LOA presentation, the left frontal bone is compressed against the sacrum, while the right side of the occipital bone is against the maternal pubic symphysis. The fetal position at the pelvic inlet will impact the final route of delivery.

During an impaired fetal descent, the fetus is still subject to compressive forces and skull molding occurs (Fig. 4.6). Depending on the direction of compressive forces, as well as the position of the fetal head, different molding patterns result. Any joint may be impacted, resulting in cranial compression somatic dysfunction. Any individual cranial bone may be compressed, demonstrating, in turn, intraosseous dysfunction. Any suture may be compacted, with resultant cranial somatic dysfunction. However, because of the fibrous tissue between the two parietal bones, occurrence of overlapping at the level of the sagittal suture is infrequent.[31] Rather, the two parietal bones flatten, losing their convex shape, while the superior portion of the squama of the occipital bone frequently moves forward, locking between the two parietals. This can happen bilaterally or unilaterally, and will result in cranial somatic dysfunction of the lambdoid suture or intraosseous dysfunction of the occipital bone. The line of attachment of the tentorium cerebelli on the inner surface of the occiput separates the inferior portion of the occipital squama of cartilaginous origin from the upper portion that is membranous in origin. This line acts as a hinge in occipital molding. Globally, molding of the head tends to change the shape of the skull, most commonly resulting in a decrease of the suboccipitobregmatic diameter.[31] This anteroposterior decrease may affect the SBS, with resultant cranial somatic dysfunction of SBS compression. Neonates, examined 24–72 hours after delivery, demonstrate posterior or lateral cranial flattening in 13.1% of cases and unusual head shapes in 11.5%.[34]

The dura mater plays an important role in protecting the contents of the skull, as well as in maintaining cohesion between the different bones of the cranium during molding. Dural membranous strains occur frequently as a result of the delivery process. Special dural fibers are organized in strengthening bands and arranged according to the stress patterns that are likely to occur during molding.[35] Nevertheless, dural overstretching may occur, resulting in tearing, particularly at the level of the junction between the tentorium cerebelli and the falx cerebri.[35] When this occurs, the vein of Galen that enters the straight sinus is stretched and the flow of blood is impeded or obstructed. The vein or some of its tributaries may rupture, with subsequent cerebral hemorrhage.[35]

Subarachnoid hemorrhage is the most common intracranial injury identified after birth.[36] Intracranial hemorrhage is reported to occur more often when children are delivered by forceps, vacuum extraction or cesarean section during labor. In the last case, however, abnormal labor is suggested to be the causative factor, since intracranial hemorrhage is encountered less in children delivered by programmed cesarean section.[37]

During descent of the fetal head, asynclitism results in asymmetric sidebending forces on the skull. Soon after, or concomitantly with this sidebending, the head rotates, possibly in response to the resistance of the maternal pelvis. This combination can produce a sidebending–rotation dysfunction of the SBS. Additionally, extension of the cervical spine occurs during the passage of the head under the maternal pubic symphysis and during delivery. The extension takes place at the level of the condyles of the occiput and in the synchondroses of the cranial base. Any exaggerated stress applied to the cranial base may affect the associated structures. The hypoglossal canals situated bilaterally in the anterior intraoccipital synchondroses, between the basiocciput and the bilateral exocciputs, enclose the hypoglossal nerves that supply motor innervation to the tongue. Tissue congestion linked to difficult delivery impacts the hypoglossal nerves and tongue motor function, with resultant suckling difficulties. The glossopharyngeal, vagus and accessory nerves located in the jugular foramina may also be affected, with a consequential wide range of symptoms including dysautonomia, colic and regurgitation, as well as muscular imbalances associated with torticollis and plagiocephaly. Quite frequently, the

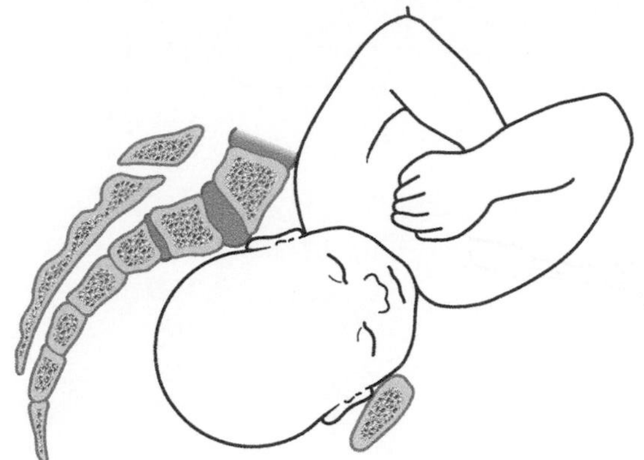

Figure 4.7. *During labor the skull, craniocervical junction and cervical spine are stressed.*

synchondroses of the cranial base are compacted, most often unilaterally.

Birth injuries occur in 3% of all live-born infants, with traumas to the head and neck in 9.56 per 1000 births.[36] Common birth traumas include cephalohematomas, clavicular fractures, facial nerve injury, brachial plexus injury and fracture of the appendicular long bones. Phrenic nerve injury, laryngeal nerve injury or skull fractures occur less frequently. Additionally, male gender is a risk factor for greater fetal distress during labor, with a resultant higher incidence of operative delivery.[38,39] The male fetus demonstrates an increased metabolic rate that might augment his vulnerability.[38] Being a male fetus has also been observed to be a risk factor for a prolonged second stage of labor, which can be associated with the use of epidural anesthesia, labor induction and oxytocin, as well as macrosomia and nulliparity.[40]

Among the common birth traumas, cephalohematoma is caused by subperiosteal rupture of vessels and is considered to be the result of friction during the birth process.[36] Cephalohematomas occur in approximately 1–2% of newborns and are associated with the use of forceps.[29] Clavicular fracture is more common with shoulder dystocia and macrosomia, and may be associated with vacuum-assisted deliveries. Normally, after delivery of the head and its restitution to the original rotation, the anterior shoulder passes under the pubic symphysis and then the posterior shoulder is delivered. When resistance to the delivery of the shoulders occurs, traction through the neck might be necessary, with resultant risk for the production of somatic dysfunction of the upper thoracic spine, the first and second ribs, the cervical spine, clavicle and all of the myofascial components of the thoracic outlet. The joints between the occipital condyles and the upper articular surfaces of the atlas, and those between the atlas and the axis, are particularly stressed, with the possibility of resultant somatic dysfunction in this area; this is a risk factor for congenital torticollis and plagiocephaly.[41] In more severe cases this traction can result in clavicular fractures and brachial plexus injuries. Brachial plexus trauma is usually produced by lateral traction with resultant sidebending of the neck, stretching the brachial plexus. Injury of the fifth and sixth cervical nerves – Erb's paralysis – represents most of postpartum brachial plexus paralysis.[36] Less commonly encountered, Klumpke's paralysis results from injury of the fifth, sixth and seventh cervical nerves.

In addition to the dysfunction and injuries of the neurocranium and trunk, injuries of the face may occur. During the birth process, the viscerocranium is very commonly under stress. With the descent of the fetal head in an LOA presentation, the forehead and nose slide along the perineal gutter before delivery of the head. This may produce somatic dysfunction of the face between the frontal and nasal bones, the ethmoid and the maxillae that may be the origin of noisy breathing and recurrent rhinitis. The nose is more vulnerable than any other structure of the face during delivery; consequently, nasal deformities are frequently encountered. Compression of the nasal tip during delivery is common and may be associated with mucosal edema. Normally, the perpendicular plate of the ethmoid, the vomer and the septal cartilage are aligned to form the midline nasal septum. Nasal septal asymmetry is found in about 1% of newborns,[42] with spontaneous labor causing more septal deviations than cesarean section.[43] In severe cases, nasal dislocation of the cartilaginous septum from the vomerine groove may need special procedural care requiring reduction with a septal elevator within a few days postpartum.

The first breath of the child should be full and unencumbered. In the case of nasal obstruction, the thoracoabdominal diaphragm is required to exert greater inspiratory force, in turn inducing somatic dysfunction of this muscle. Additionally, somatic dysfunction of the cranial diaphragm, the tentorium cerebelli and of any bone to which the cranial diaphragm is attached will also impair the thoracoabdominal diaphragmatic function. Dysfunction of the temporal bone, to which the tentorium cerebelli is firmly attached, can impact the cranial diaphragm and is of particular significance in its association with thoracoabdominal diaphragmatic dysfunction.

Breech presentation is more stressful for the infant's lumbar and pelvic areas. Intraosseous

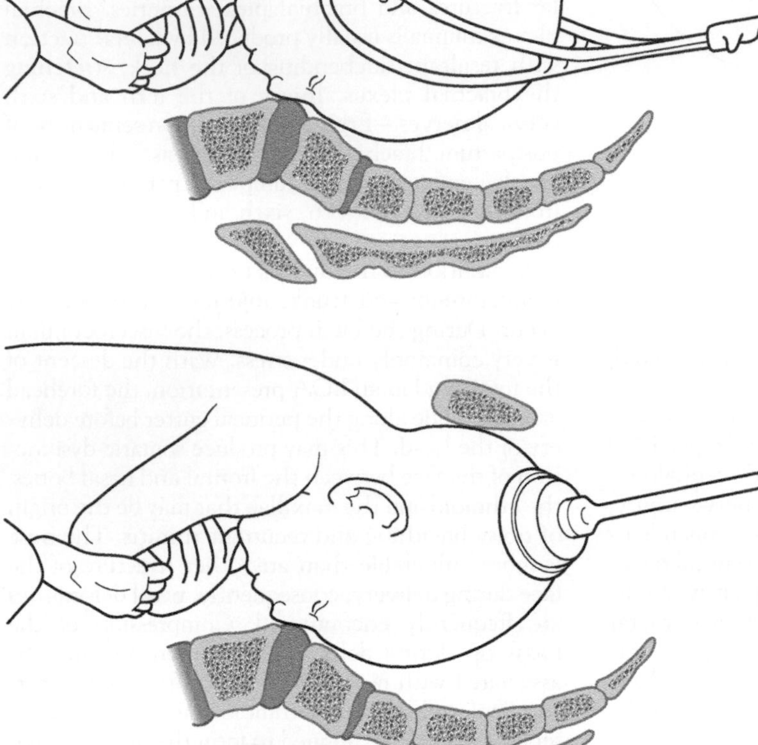

Figure 4.8. *Most often the forceps blades are positioned on the lateral parts of the skull.*

Figure 4.9. *Vacuum extraction consists of a suction cup applied to the scalp.*

dysfunction of the pelvic bones and of the sacrum may occur. The lumbar spine is usually sidebent, with possible resultant lumbosacral somatic dysfunction. After delivery of the breech and trunk, the head may be difficult to deliver, being less compressible than the rest of the body. Therefore, infants born with a breech presentation may also demonstrate cranial somatic dysfunction. During breech deliveries the viscerocranium is usually compressed against the maternal sacrum with the potential for dysfunctions in the viscerocranium affecting the development of the face.

Forceps delivery applies compressive forces and traction combined with rotation. Different patterns of dysfunction may follow, according to the placement of the forceps blades. Most often, they are positioned at the lateral parts of the skull, in the area of the pterion (Fig. 4.8). Thus, the frontal bone may be compressed, with resultant intraosseous dysfunction and the possibility of a prominent metopic suture. The forceps blades may be positioned lower at the level of the temporal bones, applying pressure on the stylomastoid foramen or on the temporal bone at the level of the vertical segment of the facial canal, both risk factors for facial nerve injury. The occipitomastoid area may also be compressed, affecting the jugular foramen. The forceps blades are sometimes placed on the areas of the temporomandibular joints, potentially causing intraosseous dysfunction of the mandible and temporal bone, and the possibility of future temporomandibular joint disorders.

Vacuum extraction (Fig. 4.9) produces local cephalohematoma at the site where the suction cup is applied to the scalp, as well as dural strain dysfunctions when the falx cerebri and tentorium cerebelli are overstretched. These strain patterns may also involve the tubular sheath of the spinal dura mater, linking the cranial somatic dysfunction to a somatic dysfunction of the pelvis.

Vacuum extraction and forceps have been associated with the occurrence of plagiocephaly.[41] The placement of these devices can result in asymmetric forces being applied to the skull, and the traction employed during delivery can impact not only the cranium, but also the cervical spine. Horizontal strain dysfunctions of the SBS and rotational dysfunction of the occiput on the atlas have been shown to be significantly related to the presence of nonsynostotic plagiocephaly.[41]

Onset of labor before 37 weeks of gestation defines preterm labor and any infant born before that time is premature. Most of the time, the preterm newborn is small with a weight less than 2.5 kg. Immaturity of the central nervous system may be responsible for several disorders such as apneic spells or inadequate coordination of sucking and swallowing. Preterm birth can affect many neurologic functions ranging from mild cognitive impairments[44] to more severe neurologic handicaps such as mental retardation or cerebral palsy. Children born preterm may also demonstrate a higher incidence of cranial deformation, with a typical dolichocephalic head shape. The cranial base synchondroses of the premature infant are vulnerable to the normal physical stress of the birth process. In particular, the intrasphenoidal synchondrosis, between the presphenoid and the postsphenoid that fuses at about 8 months of gestation, is at risk in proportion to the degree of prematurity. The fragility of these infants necessitates that they be approached with the utmost delicacy.

CHILDHOOD AND ADOLESCENCE

After birth, the sleeping position is a significant factor affecting the infant's cranial shape as well as the shape of other parts of the body. The young skeleton may be deformed by constant pressure due to having the child in the same position. This is particularly true with preterm neonates where side-to-side flattening of the skull is frequent when lying on one side of the head. Prone sleeping may affect the frontal bone, the mandible and temporomandibular joint, thus affecting occlusion later in life. Alternatively, when the infant sleeps supine, the pressure of the mattress on the infant's head contributes to modifying the shape of the occipital bone[45] and posterior flattening of the skull occurs when a supine sleeping position is maintained. Sleeping supine has been commonly proposed as a cause of posterior plagiocephaly.[34,46] This is supported by the fact that the incidence of posterior plagiocephaly has increased since it was recommended that infants sleep in a supine position to prevent sudden infant death syndrome (SIDS). The young infant demonstrates a significant decrease in swallowing frequency and respiratory rate when sleeping in the prone position, which is, therefore, a risk factor for SIDS.[47] The 'Back to Sleep' campaign started in 1992 by the American Academy of Pediatrics recommended that healthy 'infants be placed down for sleep on either their side or back'.[48] Obviously this recommendation does not apply to certain cases such as preterm neonates or infants with gastroesophageal reflux or obstructive sleep apnea.

Posterior plagiocephaly may be the flattening of the occipital area in the midline or on one side, depending if the infant maintains the head in a central position or turned to one side. The fetal asymmetric position is proposed as a contributing factor to the preference of the newborn for a right-sided head position when placed in supine.[32] Additionally, during a difficult delivery, a dysfunction of the occipitocervical junction may occur, resulting in the inclination to maintain the head turned on one side. Because of this preference, pressure from the weight of the infant's head on the mattress is asymmetric and a plagiocephaly follows. The compressive forces flatten the occipitoparietal area on the side toward which the head is chronically rotated and the opposite side develops markedly. Significant correlation has been identified between rotational dysfunction of the occiput on the atlas and the side of posterior plagiocephaly.[41] Anteriorly, the skull demonstrates frontal bossing on the same side as the occipital flattening with a frontal flattening on the opposite side. When the head is seen from above, it has a 'parallelogram' shape (Fig. 4.10). This has been shown to be correlated with lateral strain dysfunctions of the SBS.[41] Conversely, significant cranial asymmetry present at birth because of fetal molding may prevent the infant from turning the head with equal facility in both directions, thus reinforcing their asymmetry.

When applied over a prolonged time or during a critical period of growth, asymmetric pressures from the mattress can also create asymmetries on the growing spine. A preference to turn towards their right side when in a supine position is proposed to explain the association between plagiocephaly and scoliosis. The immature thorax follows the same pattern of deformation as the skull. When an infant

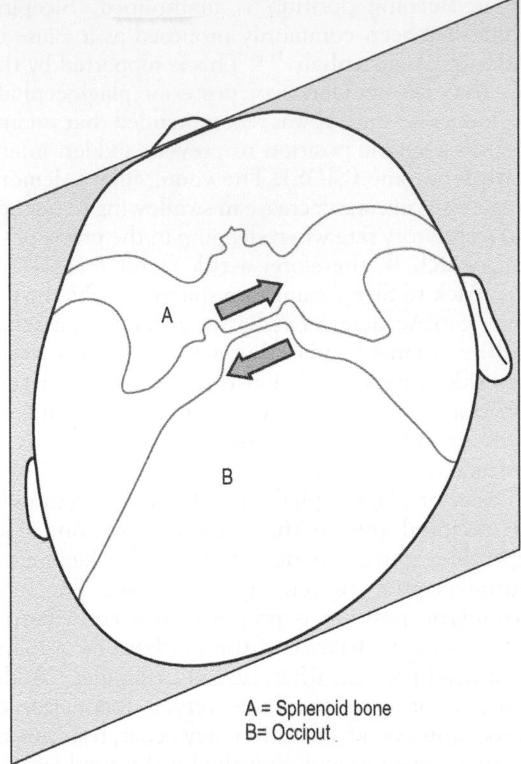

Figure 4.10. *Posterior plagiocephaly: the head seen from above has a 'parallelogram' shape. A lateral strain dysfunction is associated with plagiocephaly. A, Sphenoid bone; B, occiput.*

demonstrates a chronic rotation of the head, the back of the head will flatten on the side of the rotation, permitting growth of the skull on the opposite side. When the infant prefers to turn towards the right side when in a supine position, pressure from the weight of the infant's thorax on the mattress is applied on the right hemithorax; the left hemithorax, under the influence of gravity, has a propensity to expand freely backwards with a left rotation of the thoracic vertebrae.[49]

Additionally, the supine sleeping position of the infant appears to play a strong role in the formation of the sacral curvature. At birth, the sacrum consists of five sacral vertebrae. The ossification of the sacral bodies has begun. Although the union of the vertebral arches with the bodies appears in the lower sacral segments in the 2nd year, it does not occur in the upper segments before the 5th or 6th year.

In humans, as in tailed animals, the sacral curvature seems to be minimal at birth and its formation appears to be strongly influenced through positioning of the child.[50] In the supine position, the inferior segments of the sacrum and coccyx that are under pressure are pushed anteriorly, creating a sacral curvature that will increase through childhood. Constant asymmetry in supine positioning may, therefore, influence the shape of the pelvis. The sleeping position of the infant, with a preference to lie on one side – the 'side-lying syndrome' – has also been proposed as a contributing factor to congenital dislocation of the hip.[51]

The bilateral symmetry of human anatomy is ideally related to bilateral functional symmetry. Neural mechanisms responsible for keeping a midline position of the head, while present at birth, are not functional until later because of a lack of muscular strength of the neck.[52] An infant should turn the head with equal facility in both directions by 12 weeks of age.[53] However, symmetry of cervical motion may be impaired in the presence of cranial or cervical somatic dysfunction. Spinal or pelvic somatic dysfunction may also influence the infant's posture. This may follow a difficult delivery, but may also result from aggressive handling or bad positioning of the child, such as in a car seat where the cervical spine is particularly sensitive to exaggerated sidebending and rotation maintained for a long time when traveling. In every instance, it should be stressed that constant asymmetric positioning of infants and children should be avoided, and that when a particular position is not accepted by the child, a somatic dysfunction may be present that should be treated.

Various methods of carrying the infant are common causes of infantile somatic dysfunctions. The procedure of holding the infant kangaroo style, by suspending the baby against the caregiver's chest in a hammock-type piece of cloth for prolonged periods of time, can be particularly stressful to the upper cervical area. Carrying the child in such a way that they straddle one side of the pelvis is quite common among caregivers in order to free the arm on the other side. This position often fosters existent infantile asymmetries and when maintained for a long time can reinforce pelvic torsion or any other spinal or cranial asymmetry.

Early stimulation in daily activities such as feeding must also be bilateral. Normal breastfeeding is spontaneously done on both sides. In a similar fashion, alternating right- and left-sided bottle feeding is crucial for infants in order to develop bilateral orofacial reflexes and avoid a pattern of asymmetric cervical rotation. Breastfeeding and bottle feeding involve different muscular patterns. Breastfeeding engages significant effort and the increased muscular activity stimulates growth of the bones to which the muscles are attached. Furthermore, maternal milk odor brings out more frequent sucking from the infant with higher milk expression pressure than does formula or water.[54] However, breastfeeding may be impaired when somatic dysfunctions of the cranial base affect the hypoglossal nerve or the relationships between the structures to which the maxillofacial muscles as well as the muscles of the tongue are attached. Ankyloglossia – a tight lingual frenulum – may also be the cause of ineffective latch. Under these circumstances parents often resort to bottle feeding. When difficulties persist, the common solution is to supply a nipple with a larger opening or of softer consistency for successful nursing. This, in turn, reduces the amount of muscular effort required and the variety of muscular activity associated with breastfeeding, hampering a well-balanced maxillofacial development. Breastfeeding appears to have a protective outcome on the occurrence of posterior cross-bite in deciduous dentition.[55]

If the need to suck is not satisfied during habitual feeding, then a non-nutritive sucking habit develops, usually in the form of thumb sucking or pacifiers or dummies. It is suggested that this habit is linked to forms of malocclusion of infancy such as open bite and posterior cross-bite.[55] Non-nutritive sucking seems to be a greater risk factor for development of a dysfunctional occlusion than the type of feeding in the first months of life. However, when non-nutritive sucking activity is associated with bottle feeding, the risk of posterior cross-bite is more than double.[55] During infancy, the premaxillae can easily be influenced through non-nutritive sucking and pushed forward. Sucking a pacifier is commonly associated with malocclusion, followed by the practice of sucking fingers.[56] Until the age of 2–3 years, the risk of developing a dysfunctional occlusion may be reduced proportionally to the time the child will use the pacifier, and under these circumstances the dental arches should be regularly evaluated.[57] At the age of 4 years a significant correlation exists between malocclusion and sucking habits,[58,59] with posterior cross-bite and increased amount of overjet that seems to persist further than the end of the practice of the non-nutritive sucking habit.[60]

Facial development follows genetically determined sequences that are, in turn, influenced by environmental factors. Fetal molding is among the first of these sequences, followed by the impact of delivery on the infant's viscerocranium. Their influence with possible somatic dysfunction can be observed by the trained osteopathic practitioner as early as the first days of life. The orofacial functions of sucking, swallowing, mastication, respiration and speech are environmental factors of paramount importance in the development of the facial skeleton. These functions also contribute to the development of a good posture as they may be influenced by dysfunctional postural balance. Adequate nose breathing plays a significant part in the development of the maxillae. Alternatively, mouth breathing is associated with an inferoposterior displacement of the hyoid bone, an anteroinferior positioning of the tongue[61,62] and an anterior mandibular rotation.[63] Unencumbered tongue mobility and mastication are necessary in order for oral praxis skills to develop in infants. Direct trauma to the face may also disrupt this balance. At birth, the maxillae consist of two parts: the maxilla and premaxilla. The closing of the suture separating them occurs between 6–7 years[64] and 12 years of age.[65] Falls, in particular on the upper teeth, may cause maxillae prognathism that involves a posterior rotation of the premaxillae.

Impact on the mandible may produce somatic dysfunction of the temporomandibular joint, responsible for dysfunctional mastication and occlusal patterns. Among the environmental factors, modern diets and food processing are shown to influence facial growth. A child needs to exert some muscular effort. Chewing softer food contributes to decreased stimulation of periosteal growth with resultant smaller faces.[66,67]

The programming effect of genetics on skeletal growth is also influenced by environmental and cultural factors. Extreme cultural examples include the practice of head or foot deformation. The acquisition of developmental milestones is influenced by cultural norms and expectations. The normal daily physical activity of the infant or child increases bone mineralization and growth. Excessive or premature activity, therefore, may contribute to the creation of dysfunctions. As such, the shape of the pelvis is influenced by the time of attainment of the bipedal ambulation, 14 months of age being the average. When it is achieved earlier, the pelvis tends to develop a platypelloid shape; when achieved later, it develops an anthropoid shape.[68] Additionally, arduous physical activity during adolescence contributes to the development of an android pelvis in females. These issues can exert a significant effect on an individual's obstetrical future.

Spinopelvic balance in the sagittal and frontal planes reflects the influence of the entire spine, globally, regionally and segmentally, as well as that of the postural balance in the lower limbs. Children who demonstrate a slight dysfunctional pattern of

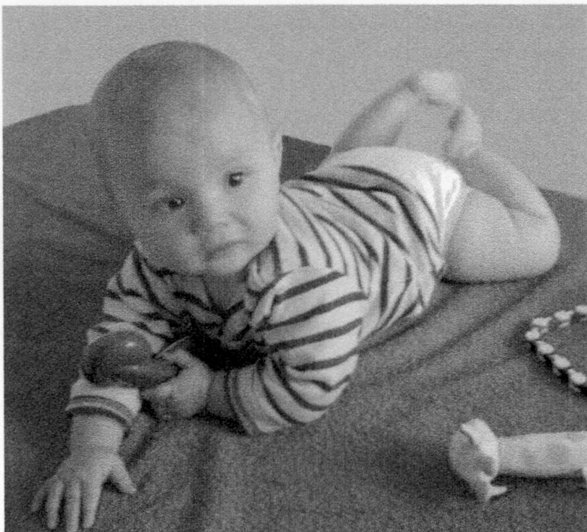

Figure 4.11. *Children who crawl stimulate the postural tone of the paravertebral musculature prior to assuming the gravitational stress of bipedal weight bearing.*

cervical rotation may balance their posture with thoracic or lumbopelvic compensatory patterns. These patterns tend to be greater if the child is encouraged to stand up early in life. Alternatively, children who crawl stimulate the postural tone of the paravertebral musculature prior to assuming the gravitational stress of bipedal weight bearing (Fig. 4.11). Pelvic dysfunction can, in turn, discourage a child from crawling.

Intraosseous dysfunctions of the pelvic bone or sacrum may occur following trauma such as torsional injury of the lower extremity or an abrupt fall on the buttocks during the first years of life. In these cases the child may often present with a limp or hip pain.

Additionally, lower extremity dysfunction impacts the relationship between the pelvic bones and the sacrum. Laterally shifting weight-bearing forces to one leg, as the infant progresses through the developmental milestones and begins to stand, chronically apply asymmetric stress to the pelvis and structures above.

Postural dysfunction may also develop in accommodation to dysfunctional mechanics from above. Minor head traumas are not uncommon during childhood. In the first years of life such traumas can result in intraosseous as well as interosseous dysfunctions. Cranial somatic dysfunction can, in turn, produce global body accommodative postural changes as well as visual, equilibrial, orofacial, cognitive, behavioral and focal pain complaints.

Asymmetric activities, such as tennis or practice of the violin, result in asymmetric postural accommodation. Similarly, asymmetric carrying of a heavy object (e.g. a book bag) or postural accommodation to chronic ergonomically stressful postures (e.g. when studying) can result in or aggravate preexistent somatic dysfunctions. Postural habits (e.g. slumping) may be interpreted as shyness or lack of motivation to stand erect when they may, in fact, be accommodative postures resulting from somatic dysfunction.

As the child ages and enters adolescence, the dysfunctional mechanics encountered begin to approximate those encountered in the adult population. The dysfunction often manifests as the result of trauma, most commonly involving articular strains and sprains of the extremities. The individual's existent underlying functional pattern, however, often predisposes one area to injury over another. As such, when the adolescent presents with repeated injury of the same location, such an underlying predisposing pattern should be sought out and treated.

Although the incidence of adolescent somatic dysfunction approximates that of the adult population, adolescents present less frequently than adults with spinal musculoskeletal complaints. As such, when an adolescent complains of axial musculoskeletal pain, the area of complaint should be thoroughly evaluated for underlying organic pathology or viscerosomatic reflex etiology. The most common viscerosomatic reflex complaints encountered in adolescence originate from the gastrointestinal tract and, in girls, from the pelvic organs. Nociceptive input to the spinal cord from visceral dysfunction or pathology results in spinal segmental irritability (facilitation) and a segmentally related somatic response (viscerosomatic). The associated somatic dysfunction can, in turn, create a feedback loop that maintains or aggravates the visceral condition (somatovisceral) (see Box 7.1.1, Viscerosomatic reflexes).

An untreated dysfunction in a child or adolescent may predispose the individual to disturbance of the physiology of anatomically related viscera, either by direct mechanical effect or through somatovisceral reflex mechanisms. For instance, a somatic dysfunction of the sacrum may affect the position of the uterus through the uterosacral ligament that plays a part in the positioning of the uterus. An upper lumbar somatic dysfunction can affect the sympathetic ANS, thereby affecting normal physiology of the uterus, possibly resulting in dysmenorrhea.

Thorough examination of the back is imperative, even in the absence of pain, because idiopathic scoliosis, which typically has its onset in adolescence, rarely presents with a pain complaint. It is recommended that a skilled osteopathic practitioner preventatively examine the back and posture of children and adolescents once a year.

The growth and functional development of the individual occurs slowly and dysfunction can become apparent at any time. Beginning as mesenchyme, the skeleton evolves through either membranous or cartilaginous phases to become organized in its final articulated osseous structures. Dysfunctions may, therefore, be membranous intraosseous, cartilaginous intraosseous or articular interosseous. These dysfunctions will, in turn, involve all surrounding tissues maintaining the dysfunctional situation and result in a myriad of clinical presentations.

REFERENCES

1. Sutherland WG. Teachings in the science of osteopathy. Fort Worth, TX: Sutherland Cranial Teaching Foundation; 1991: 119.
2. Glossary of Osteopathic Terminology. In: Ward RC (ed). Foundations for osteopathic medicine, 2nd edn. Philadelphia: Lippincott, Williams and Wilkins; 2003:1249.
3. Sergueef N. Le B.A.BA du crânien. Paris: Spek; 1986.
4. Korr IM. The neural basis of the osteopathic lesion. J Am Osteopath Assoc 1947;47:191–8.
5. Korr IM. IV. Clinical signifi cance of the facilitated state. J Am Osteopath Assoc 1955;54(5):277–82.
6. Magoun HI. Osteopathy in the cranial field. Kirksville, MO: The Journal Printing Company; 1951:199.
7. Arbuckle BE. The selected writings of Beryl E. Arbuckle, D.O., F.A.C.O.P. Newark OH: American Academy of Osteopathy; 1971:195.
8. Magoun HI Sr. Idiopathic adolescent spinal scoliosis: a reasonable etiology (1975). In: Peterson B (ed). Postural balance and imbalance. Indianapolis, IN: American Academy of Osteopathy; 1983:94–100.
9. Wynne-Davies R. Infantile idiopathic scoliosis: causative factors, particularly in the first six months of life. J Bone Joint Surg 1975;57B:138–41.
10. Nemzek WR, Brodie HA, Chong BW et al. Imaging findings of the developing temporal bone in fetal specimens. AJNR Am J Neuroradiol 1996;17(8):1467–77.
11. Bluestone CD. Pathogenesis of otitis media: role of the Eustachian tube. Pediatr Infect Dis J 1996;15(4):281–91.
12. Kemaloglu YK, Goksu N, Ozbilen S, Akyildiz N. Otitis media with effusion and craniofacial analysis – II: 'Mastoid–middle ear–Eustachian tube system' in children with secretory otitis media. Int J Pediatr Otorhinolaryngol 1995;32:69–76.
13. Arbuckle BE. The selected writings of Beryl E. Arbuckle, D.O., F.A.C.O.P. Newark OH: American Academy of Osteopathy; 1971.
14. Sergueef N. L'odyssée de l'iliaque. Paris: Spek; 1985.
15. Williams PL (ed). Gray's anatomy, 38th edn. Edinburgh: Churchill Livingstone; 1995.
16. Dunn PM. Congenital postural deformities. Br Med Bull 1976;32(1):71–6.
17. Watson GH. Relationship between side of plagiocephaly, dislocation of hip, scoliosis, bat ears and sternomastoid tumors. Arch Dis Child 1971;46:203–10.
18. Clarren SK, Smith DW. Congenital deformities. Pediatr Clin North Am 1977;24:665–77.
19. Hooper G. Congenital dislocation of the hip in infantile idiopathic scoliosis. J Bone Joint Surg 1980;62B(4):447–9.
20. Dunn PM. Sir Denis Browne (1892–1967) and congenital deformities of mechanical origin. Arch Dis Child Fetal Neonatal Ed 2005;90(1):F88–91.
21. Fong BF, Savelsbergh GJ, van Geijn HP, de Vries JI. Does intra-uterine environment influence fetal head-position preference? A comparison between breech and cephalic presentation. Early Hum Dev 2005;81(6):507–17.
22. Lansac J, Body G. Pratique de l'accouchement. Paris: SIMEP; 1988.
23. Previc FH. A general theory concerning the prenatal origins of cerebral lateralization in humans. Psychol Rev 1991;98(3): 299–334.
24. Good C, Walker G. The hip in the moulded baby syndrome. J Bone Joint Surg 1984;66B(4):491–2.
25. Shefelbine SJ, Carter DR. Mechanobiological predictions of growth front morphology in developmental hip dysplasia. J Orthop Res 2004;22(2):346–52.
26. Lloyd-Roberts GC, Pilcher MF. Structural idiopathic scoliosis in infancy: a study of the natural history of 100 patients. J Bone Joint Surg 1965;47B:520–3.
27. Browne D. Congenital postural scoliosis. Br Med J 1965;5461: 565–6.
28. Scherl SA. Common lower extremity problems in children. Pediatr Rev 2004;25(2):52–62.
29. Glass RB, Fernbach SK, Norton KI, Choi PS, Naidich TP. The infant skull: a vault of information. Radiographics 2004; 24(2):507–22.
30. Chapple CC, Davidson DT. A study of the relationship between fetal position and certain congenital deformities. J Pediatr 1941;18:483–93.
31. Carlan SJ, Wyble L, Lense J, Mastrogiannis DS, Parsons MT. Fetal head molding. Diagnosis by ultrasound and a review of the literature. J Perinatol 1991;11(2):105–11.
32. Goodwin RS, Michel GF. Head orientation position during birth and in infant neonatal period, and hand preference at nineteen weeks. Child Dev 1981;52(3):819–26.
33. Stitely ML, Gherman RB. Labor with abnormal presentation and position. Obstet Gynecol Clin North Am 2005;32(2): 165–79.
34. Peitsch WK, Keefer CH, Labrie RA, Mulliken JB. Incidence of cranial asymmetry in healthy newborns. Pediatrics 2002;110(6):e72.
35. Holland E. Cranial stress in the foetus during labour and on the effects of excessive stress on intracranial contents. J Obstet Gynaecol Br Emp 1922;29:549–71.
36. Hughes CA, Harley EH, Milmoe G, Bala R, Martorella A. Birth trauma in the head and neck. Arch Otolaryngol Head Neck Surg 1999;125(2):193–9.
37. Towner D, Castro MA, Eby-Wilkens E, Gilbert WM. Effect of mode of delivery in nulliparous women on neonatal intracranial injury. N Engl J Med 1999;341(23):1709–14.
38. Bekedam DJ, Engelsbel S, Mol BW, Buitendijk SE, Van Der Pal-De Bruin KM. Male predominance in fetal distress during labor. Am J Obstet Gynecol 2002;187(6):1605–7.
39. Eogan MA, Geary MP, O'Connell MP, Keane DP. Effect of fetal sex on labour and delivery: retrospective review. BMJ 2003;326(7381):137.
40. Myles TD, Santolaya J. Maternal and neonatal outcomes in patients with a prolonged second stage of labor. Obstet Gynecol 2003;102(1):52–8.
41. Sergueef N, Nelson KE, Glonek T. Palpatory diagnosis of plagiocephaly. Complement Ther Clin Pract 2006;12(2):101–10.

42. Olnes SQ, Schwartz RH, Bahadori RS. Consultation with the specialist: diagnosis and management of the newborn and young infant who have nasal obstruction. Pediatr Rev 2000;21(12):416–20.
43. Spiewak P, Kawalski H. Nose deformation as a result of birth injury. Acta Chir Plast 1995;37(3):78–82.
44. Stewart AL, Rifkin L, Amess PN et al. Brain structure and neurocognitive and behavioural function in adolescents who were born very preterm. Lancet 1999;353(9165): 1653–7.
45. Moss ML. The pathogenesis of artificial cranial deformation. Am J Phys Anthropol 1958;16:269–86.
46. Kane AA, Mitchell LE, Craven KP, Marsh JL. Observations on a recent increase in plagiocephaly without synostosis. Pediatrics 1996;97(6 Part 1):877–85.
47. Jeffery HE, Megevand A, Page H. Why the prone position is a risk factor for sudden infant death syndrome. Pediatrics 1999;104(2 Pt 1):263–9.
48. AAP Task Force on Infant Positioning and SIDS. Positioning and SIDS. Pediatrics 1992;89:1120–6.
49. McMaster MJ. Infantile idiopathic scoliosis: can it be prevented? J Bone Joint Surg 1983;65B(5):612–7.
50. Abitbol MM. Sacral curvature and supine posture. Am J Phys Anthropol 1989;80(3):379–89.
51. Wynne-Davies R. Acetabular dysplasia and familial joint laxity: two etiological factors in congenital dislocation of the hip. A review of 589 patients and their families. J Bone Joint Surg 1970;52B(4):704–16.
52. Ronnqvist L, Hopkins B. Head position preference in the human newborn: a new look. Child Dev 1998;69:13–23.
53. Hopkins B, Lems YL, van Wulfften Palthe T, Hoeksma J, Kardaun O, Butterworth G. Development of head position preference during early infancy: a longitudinal study in the daily life situation. Dev Psychobiol 1990;23:39–53.
54. Mizuno K, Ueda A. Antenatal olfactory learning influences infant feeding. Early Hum Dev 2004;76(2):83–90.
55. Viggiano D, Fasano D, Monaco G, Strohmenger L. Breast feeding, bottle feeding, and non-nutritive sucking; effects on occlusion in deciduous dentition. Arch Dis Child 2004;89(12):1121–3.
56. Tomita NE, Bijella VT, Franco LJ. Relação entre hábitos bucais e má oclusão em pré-escolares. Rev Saude Publica 2000;34(3):299–303.
57. Larsson E. Sucking, chewing, and feeding habits and the development of crossbite: a longitudinal study of girls from birth to 3 years of age. Angle Orthod 2001;71(2):116–9.
58. Moore MB, McDonald JP. A cephalometric evaluation of patients presenting with persistent digit sucking habits. Br J Orthod 1997;24(1):17–23.
59. Katz CR, Rosenblatt A, Gondim PP. Nonnutritive sucking habits in Brazilian children: effects on deciduous dentition and relationship with facial morphology. Am J Orthod Dentofacial Orthop 2004;126(1):53–7.
60. Warren JJ, Bishara SE. Duration of nutritive and nonnutritive sucking behaviors and their effects on the dental arches in the primary dentition. Am J Orthod Dentofacial Orthop 2002;121(4):347–56.
61. Behlfelt K, Linder-Aronson S, Neander P. Posture of the head, the hyoid bone, and the tongue in children with and without enlarged tonsils. Eur J Orthod 1990;12(4):458–67.
62. Finkelstein Y, Wexler D, Berger G, Nachmany A, Shapiro-Feinberg M, Ophir D. Anatomical basis of sleep-related breathing abnormalities in children with nasal obstruction. Arch Otolaryngol Head Neck Surg 2000;126(5):593–600.
63. Principato JJ. Upper airway obstruction and craniofacial morphology. Otolaryngol Head Neck Surg 1991;104(6): 881–90.
64. Delaire J, Chateau JP. Comment le septum influence-t-il la croissance prémaxillaire et maxillaire. Déductions en chirurgie des fentes labio-maxillaires. Rev Stomat 1977;78: 241–54.
65. Rouvière H. Anatomie humaine, descriptive et topographique, 9th edn. Paris: Masson; 1962.
66. Beecher RM, Corruccini RS. Effects of dietary consistency on craniofacial and occlusal development in the rat. Angle Orthod 1981;51(1):61–9.
67. Lieberman DE, Krovitz GE, Yates FW, Devlin M, St Claire M. Effects of food processing on masticatory strain and craniofacial growth in a retrognathic face. J Hum Evol 2004;46(6):655–77.
68. Abitbol MM. The shapes of the female pelvis. Contributing factors. J Reprod Med 1996;41(4):242–50.

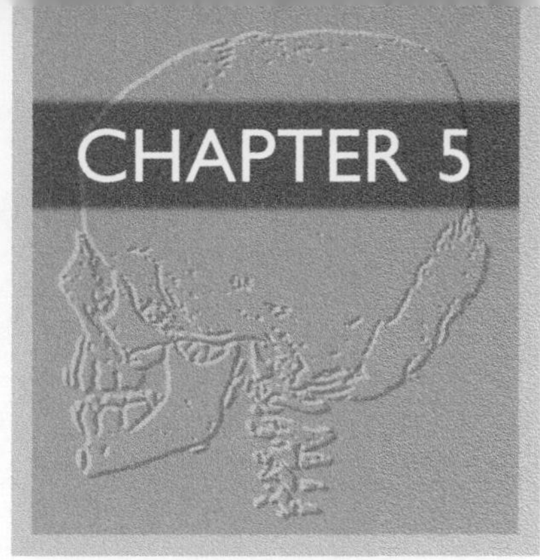

EXAMINATION OF THE PATIENT

The description of the standard procedures to completely assess the newborn and children is beyond the scope of this chapter; rather, we will describe what is distinctively of interest in an osteopathic approach to the diagnosis and treatment of somatic dysfunction in infants and children. This examination is intended to supplement and not to replace the remainder of the complete pediatric physical examination.

The sequence described below, i.e. history followed by physical examination, is a model that provides the necessary information to reach a definitive diagnosis of somatic dysfunction. In actual practice, with infants and young children, this sequence is artificial and should be dictated by the requirements of the individual patient. It is necessary, before anything else, to establish a trusting relationship, particularly with the youngest of infants. This requires that the practitioner interact empathically with the child. It is often useful to present the infant or child with a toy or other object of interest to establish contact.

The physician–patient relationship between adults is often directed by the physician. When treating infants and young children, this relationship is most effective if the physician allows the patient to direct the interaction, in essence applying the principles of indirect technique to the physician–patient relationship. The osteopathic practitioner is well equipped to understand this approach. Not only does the analogy with indirect technique apply, it can also be taken further because it is dynamic: each patient is unique and dictates the direction that the interaction must assume in order to be effective.

Additionally, under these circumstances, the physician–patient relationship is of necessity triangular, involving the child, the physician and the caregiver. With very young infants, the mother–child bond is normally so intense that the establishment of trust between the infant and the physician must include the participation of the mother (Fig. 5.1).

History

The history for the infant or child begins, as with all other patients, with the chief complaint and its history. The complete medical history should then be obtained. The following areas of information within the history are of particular interest to the osteopathic practitioner. The information to be obtained and its relationship to neonatal and childhood somatic dysfunction is best understood in the context of the delivery process. It is therefore appropriate when obtaining the history for a child of any

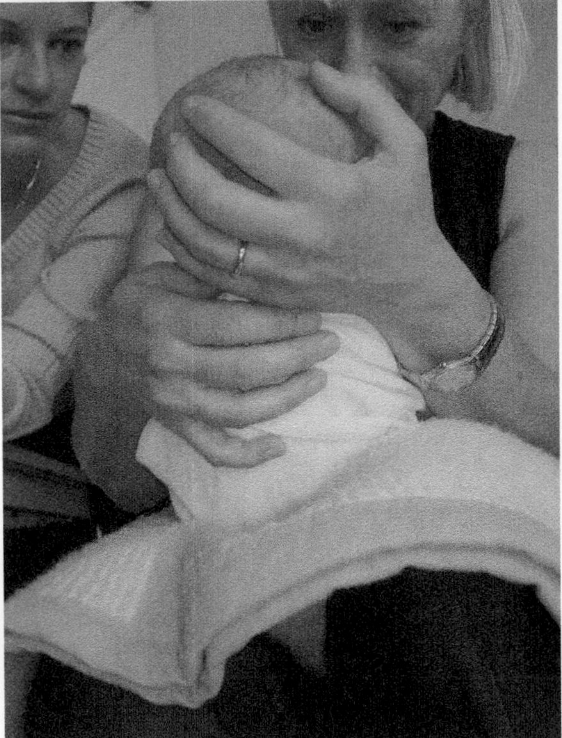

Figure 5.1. *With very young infants the physician–patient relationship must include the participation of the mother.*

age to begin with a history of the pregnancy and their delivery.

MATERNAL INFORMATION AND HISTORY OF THE PREGNANCY

- Age at time of delivery
- Parity
- Obstetrical history including complications of previous deliveries, time elapsed since previous delivery, previous maximal birth weight
- Multiple birth, post-term or prematurity, polyhydramnios or oligohydramnios
- Musculoskeletal history including back pain and pelvic pain during the pregnancy
- Psychological history – how emotionally stressful was the pregnancy?
- When were fetal movements first felt and how active were those movements?
- If a vertex presentation, when did the fetus assume the position?
- When, for any presentation, did the presenting part engage the pelvic inlet?
- In the third trimester, did the fetus press significantly on any particular area – pelvic region, inferior costal border, thoracoabdominal diaphragm?
- Were there Braxton Hicks (false labor) contractions?

BIRTH PROCESS

- Spontaneous or induced? If induced, reason for induction
- Need for oxytocic augmentation of uterine contractions
- Use and type of analgesia or anesthesia
- Type of presentation at delivery: vertex, breech, transverse lie or face
- Presence of a nuchal umbilical cord
- Length and difficulty of labor
- Complication during delivery, cephalopelvic disproportion
- Need for instrumentation, forceps, vacuum extraction or cesarean section
- Episiotomy.

NEONATAL INFORMATION

- Sex
- Birth weight
- Birth length
- Head circumference
- Apgar score
- Need for intubation
- Neonatal paralysis, commonly involving brachial plexus or facial nerve (CN VII)
- Ecchymosis, caput succedaneum, cephalhematoma
- Subconjunctival hemorrhage
- Cranial molding
- Fracture of the clavicle or skull
- Hip dysplasia.

POSTPARTUM HISTORY: INFANTS AND CHILDREN

- Suckling: should be normal from the time of birth
- Feeding method: breast or bottle? If breastfed, until what age?
- Feeding and digestive problems
- Use of pacifier, design (flat, round) and material (silicon, latex) of the teat

- Thumb sucking or finger(s) sucking? Specifically identify digit(s) sucked, of which hand, and the direction placed into the mouth. Does the infant habitually place any other object in their mouth?
- Respiration: should be nasal from the time of birth
- Regurgitation
- Irritability
- Quality of sleep, preferred position and positions refused. 'Nightmares?'
- Play activities, preferred position and positions refused
- Freedom of movement of the extremities. Does the child move all extremities in all directions? Is there difficulty with specific passive movements, as when placing an arm into a sleeve?
- Is there articular noise ('popping' joint) with movement? Commonly hips, shoulders; rarely neck
- Are there motor tics or repetitive behaviors, such as ear pulling? Head banging? Habitual rocking: anteroposterior (AP) or side-to-side?
- Age of onset of teething
- Cross-bites, functional interferences
- Bruxism
- Type of deglutition: infantile or mature?
- Age of attainment of major milestones: rolling to supine, rolling to prone, sitting tripod, sitting unsupported, creeping, crawling, pulling to stand and walking
- Clumsiness
- Age of attainment of social, adaptive and cognitive milestones
- Age of development of language skills
- Diseases of childhood
- Attention deficit or hyperactive disorder
- Academic achievement.

HISTORY: ADOLESCENTS

The information described above relative to infants and children should also be obtained for adolescent patients. These patients are often seen with musculoskeletal or facial developmental complaints and, as such, the following additional information should be sought.

Musculoskeletal complaint

- Duration of complaint and progression of the problem: did it begin at birth, before or after walking, or just recently?
- Family history of limb asymmetries or deformities, and postural abnormalities
- Was a specific trauma involved? Of particular interest would be abrupt falls on the buttocks and blows to the head, as well as details regarding the traumatic force, its direction, its site of impact and its consequences
- Quality, intensity, location and aggravating factors of associated pain, if present
- Side of dominant hand
- Associated postural habits, such as sitting in an asymmetrical position and athletic activities
- Physical fatigability.

Central nervous system and cranial nerve-associated complaints

- Psychological fatigability
- Impaired memory
- Nausea, digestive problems
- Visual disorders
- Olfactory disorders.

Facial developmental complaint

- Infantile oral parafunctional and nutritive sucking habits, as listed above
- History of nasal obstruction, unilateral or bilateral
- Is there a preferred side for mastication?
- Nail biting, chewing on pencils
- Sleeping position
- Associated activities involving the mouth, such as playing a trumpet or flute.

Physical examination

'Therefore, first instruct his fingers how to feel, how to think, how to see, and then let him touch.' —WG SUTHERLAND[1]

The physical examination consists of three components: observation, palpation for structure and palpation for function. Observation – the visual evaluation of the patient – is very important and, when mastered, can provide much of the information necessary to make a diagnosis. By beginning with observation, the necessary time for the child to develop a relationship of trust with the osteopathic practitioner is provided. Palpation may follow, but, in actuality, once a connection is established with the child, these two areas of assessment may be performed almost simultaneously and should be carried out as dictated by the child.

Evaluation by touch may be divided into the tactile appreciation of structure and the tactile appreciation of function. The appreciation of function may be further subdivided into screening tests that are used in the standard medical musculoskeletal examination and the tests of listening that are based on the assessment of the primary respiratory mechanism (PRM) and which are more specifically related to cranial osteopathy. Observation, palpation for structure and palpation for function will be described successively in this section: first for infants, then for children and finally for adolescents. The principles of the treatment that is applicable for all three age groups will be covered in the next chapter, p. 137.

OBSERVATION

Observation may be static (i.e. observation of structure) or dynamic (i.e. observation of function). Static observation requires a thorough knowledge of anatomy, thereby allowing one to observe the different landmarks within the area of consideration, looking for differences between normal configuration and position, and for asymmetries. At this time, it is appropriate to observe physical signs such as respiration, cutaneous features including pallor, hyperemia, lesions, scars and hair distribution.

Dynamic observation is the study of the ease and quantity of both gross and minor movements in the area being examined. It requires functional knowledge of the possible motion that can occur in the area being observed. When observing the patient, it is important to note how the individual moves and verbalizes. Are these activities performed symmetrically and with full available amplitude of motion, or asymmetrically with stiffness or discoordination?

When interpreting these static and dynamic observations, it may be helpful to consider that when you look at a tree, you can see how that tree is being (or has been) blown by the wind and that your observation provides information as to the strength as well as the direction of the wind. Such information about external forces lies within any structure and is available by observing the shape of the structure and how it moves.

PALPATION FOR STRUCTURE

Palpation for structure requires physical contact. It necessitates respect for the patient's willingness to be touched as well as the need for warm, clean hands. First, palpate the skin and note its characteristics. Is it soft, smooth or rough; oily, moist or dry? Note the skin temperature. Using light touch, palpate through the skin to appreciate the feel of the subcutaneous tissues. In young children, the quality of tissue feel differs from that of older individuals. It is normally more flexible and softer because of the open matrix of the connective tissues. Consequently, the fascia is not as dense, offering a less rigid feel.

Palpate deeper in order to palpate the muscles. Palpate for texture, tone, volume and shape. Palpate for areas of tissue inconsistency that might be indicative of hematoma or soft tissue masses. More pressure applied through the layers of tissue will bring your focus of attention to the bones and their articular relationships. By applying graduated pressure it is possible to determine the palpatory differences between skin, connective tissue, muscles, bones and joints. It is also possible through discerning static palpation to identify shape, size and position in space of the area under consideration. It is further possible to compare the area being examined with the normal feel for that area and the age group of the individual patient, as well as, in the case of paired structures, to the same structure on the other side.

In dysfunction, the modification of the parameters that are studied – shape, position and tissue texture – is present. Tactile appreciation of these qualities of the tissues being examined allows for the assessment of normal vs. abnormal, and gives the examiner an idea of the degree of health vs. disease.

PALPATION FOR FUNCTION

The findings obtained by observation and palpation for structure may be further elucidated by palpating for function. Osteopathic diagnosis is ultimately based on the recognition of motion and the restriction thereof. Appreciation of the degree of available motion runs as a continuum from the grossest movement of large joints to the subtlest inherent motility of all living tissue.

Palpation for function consists of the use of gross motion testing and tests of listening. Gross motion testing is employed for the evaluation of the availability, amplitude and ease of motion between adjacent anatomic structures. This can include an appreciation of soft tissue tension and articular mobility. The tests of listening are employed to assess the quality and quantity of available motion and the potency of the PRM in the area being examined. Somatic dysfunction that can manifest as anatomic motion restriction is always accompanied by impediment of the PRM.

In practice, it is far more appropriate to apply the tests of listening before palpating the grosser range of motion. This is because, when performing the physical examination, it is always desirable to begin with the least aggressive procedures and progress to the more aggressive procedures, because the findings from a less aggressive procedure may be influenced by the performance of a more aggressive procedure. In fact, with practice, recognizing the subtle motion changes identified with tests of listening all but eliminates the need for grosser motion testing.

Applying tests of listening to the area to be examined should begin the examination. Visualization of motion may be employed in association with the tests of listening. If listening does not provide sufficient information, or the examiner is uncertain as to the feel observed, it is then appropriate to follow up with more dynamic motion testing. Gross motion testing may be employed if necessary to confirm the findings obtained by listening and visualization.

It is important, here, for the reader to realize that the terms listening and visualization are employed figuratively. Listening refers to the most passive form of no intrusive palpation for function. When visualization is employed in association with this palpation, the examiner pictures the anatomy of the area being palpated in their mind's eye. These terms are used repeatedly in this context throughout this text and should not be confused with the sensations obtained with the ears and eyes.

To test a movement is to compare the response of an anatomic structure to motion, in opposite directions, as illustrated by flexion vs. extension or rotation right vs. rotation left. It is imperative when performing this or any other motion testing that, following the assessment, the body area under consideration is allowed to return to the neutral position before proceeding to the next evaluation. Thus, assess any given motion and specifically return to the neutral position before attempting to assess the opposing motion. The quality of motion observed while returning to the neutral position is often as important as that of the original motion. If a component of motion is dysfunctional, the dysfunction may manifest as a limitation of that movement, with ease of return to neutral, whereas movement in the opposing direction will be free, with resistance of return to neutral.

The hand placement for diagnostic palpation is the same as the hand placement for treatment. For hand placement for all of the following diagnostic procedures, the reader is referred to the descriptions of treatment in Chapter 6.

Tests of listening

Tests of listening provide the examiner with information not only about available motion, but also about the potency of the PRM. Where gross motion testing actively induces the range of motion, test of listening passively observes. The area being examined is observed in the context of the PRM and how the area moves in association with the PRM. All of the information – quality, asymmetry, restriction of motion and tissue texture change – may be evaluated by listening to the inherent motility within the area being examined.

The PRM is referred to as the cranial rhythmic impulse (CRI) when palpated on the head. This rhythm is, however, palpable throughout the body. As such, every structure within the body manifests biphasic motion concomitant with the inspiratory and expiratory phases of the PRM. In the presence of somatic dysfunction, the symmetry and potency of this biphasic function is impaired.

The first contact in the test of listening should be the lightest possible touch, allowing the examiner to observe the PRM by palpating the inherent motility without disturbing it. The sensation of the PRM may be compared to that of the motion of the thoracic cage during quiet respiration. The tissues seem to expand during the inspiratory phase of the PRM and contract during the expiratory phase. The amplitude of this motion is about as great as the amplitude observed when palpating a peripheral arterial pulse, but the frequency is roughly one-tenth that of the pulse. This low frequency, when unaffected by somatic dysfunction, results in the perception of a very slow expansion during the inspiratory phase and an equally slow return during the expiratory phase. As such, the examiner must learn to concentrate in a relaxed manner in order to perceive the PRM.

The rate of the rhythm of the PRM varies between 4 and 14 cycles per minute, with the majority of reported rates, observed by palpation, tending toward the lower half of this range.[2] This frequency – although distinctly separate from, and usually slower than, the rate of pulmonary respiration – occasionally coincides with, and may be entrained with, breathing.[3]

Once the rhythm has been observed and appreciated, the manifest action of the PRM in a given structure is determined by gently increasing the amount of palpatory contact until the inherent motion of the specific structure is palpated. The practitioner should mentally visualize the different anatomic layers until the level of the structure being examined is reached. This must be accomplished while still applying the lightest touch whereby the inherent motion is appreciated. The utilization of proprioceptive awareness from the examiner's flexor pollicis longus and flexor digitorum profundus muscles provides the information being sought.

In cases where the palpable motion is difficult to perceive, it can be useful to mentally visualize the normal motion – cranial flexion, cranial extension, external rotation and internal rotation – of the structure being evaluated as described in Chapter 3. When employing visualization, the examiner mentally focuses on, and compares the availability of, the different opposing motions. Visualization is accomplished by mentally picturing the movement to be evaluated without actively inducing motion. This visualization will cause the transmission of subtle palpatory awareness of the examiner's hands. The direction of unencumbered motion of the PRM will be more readily appreciable, whereas the dysfunctional direction will not.

The appreciation of dysfunctional patterns within the PRM, the rate and potency in any given structure, or between structures, requires quiet listening. Time and patience are often necessary to obtain the desired information. This conscious touching, not just mechanical touching, lends itself particularly well to the examination of infants and children. They are as aware, or more aware, of the palpatory interaction between themselves and the examiner. The direction opposite to that of the dysfunction is the direction of discomfort, whereas the direction of ease is soothing to them. They will respond accordingly and immediately, and, as such, infants and small children are the best teachers of this form of palpatory diagnosis.

During tests of listening the osteopathic practitioner appreciates – 'listens' to – the inherent forces of the tissues. Having employed these tests diagnostically, treatment can follow seamlessly through the manipulation of these inherent forces. The hand placement for tests of listening is consequently the same as the hand placement for treatment and the reader is referred further to the descriptions of treatment in Chapter 6.

Gross motion testing

Gross motion testing consists of the evaluation of the passive range of motion between two adjacent anatomic structures. It is commonly described in terms of anatomic motion: anatomic flexion, anatomic extension, sidebending left, sidebending right, rotation left, rotation right, abduction, adduction, external rotation and internal rotation. These motions are coupled in opposite directions, as flexion and extension or abduction and adduction. There is a neutral point of functional balance between each of the coupled motions and they are limited by physiologic and anatomic barriers. Somatic dysfunction between two adjacent anatomic structures is manifest as the presence of a dysfunctional barrier, limiting motion in one direction between the existent physiologic barriers. As such, in the presence of somatic dysfunction, a limitation of motion in one direction, as well as a new point of balance, the dysfunctional neutral, will be appreciated when motion is evaluated.

Gross motion testing in terms of osteopathic diagnosis should not be confused with gross motion testing as employed in orthopedic diagnosis. Although the ranges of motion evaluated are similar, the forces employed to induce the motion must be very gentle, particularly with infants and children. Dysfunctional mechanics are typically found to be limiting the minor motions between two adjacent anatomic structures, such as abduction and adduction between the ulna and humerus. Because of skeletal immaturity and the high degree of elastin in young connective tissue, the end feel of dysfunctional barriers in infants and children is less distinct than that encountered in adults. For these reasons, gross motion testing must be employed using the lightest possible touch that still provides the perception of motion and barrier. The experienced examiner will soon find that the subtle forces which should be used in gross motion testing, when employed in the gentlest possible manner, point one to the subtle touch employed in tests of listening described above.

PHYSICAL EXAMINATION OF THE INFANT

Observe spontaneous movement and posture as the infant lies on the treatment table in the supine and prone positions. Look for significant positional asymmetries. Look for alignment of the head with the torso and for apparent generalized hypo- or hypertonicity (Fig. 5.2). Newborn infants normally demonstrate flexed elbows and hands, as well as slight flexion and external rotation of the thighs. In the

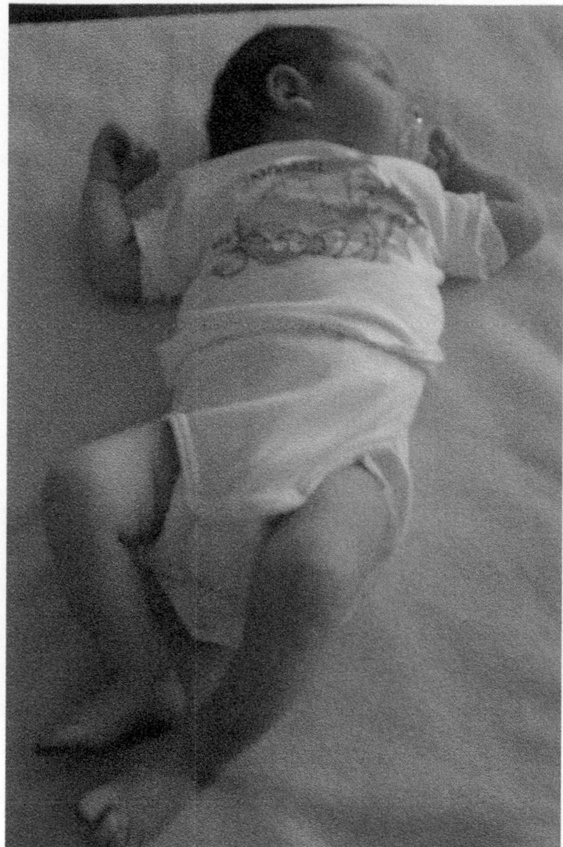

Figure 5.2. *Observe spontaneous movement and posture, alignment of the head with the torso and apparent generalized hypo- or hypertonicity.*

prone position, observe the ability to lift the head according to the age of the child. These observations and the ones that follow may identify the need to do a more thorough neurologic or orthopedic examination and are not intended to replace such examinations.

Look for a global pattern of the body. A twisted or spiral pattern between the pelvis and the head is very common. Carefully observe the different parts of the body to see if they all fit the whole body pattern. Generally, the head will be sidebent and rotated in opposite directions, the cervical and lumbar spine will be sidebent to the same side as that of the head and the pelvis will be rotated in the opposite direction of the head. The observed findings may be confirmed with tests of listening with one hand placed beneath the sacrum and the other beneath the occiput.

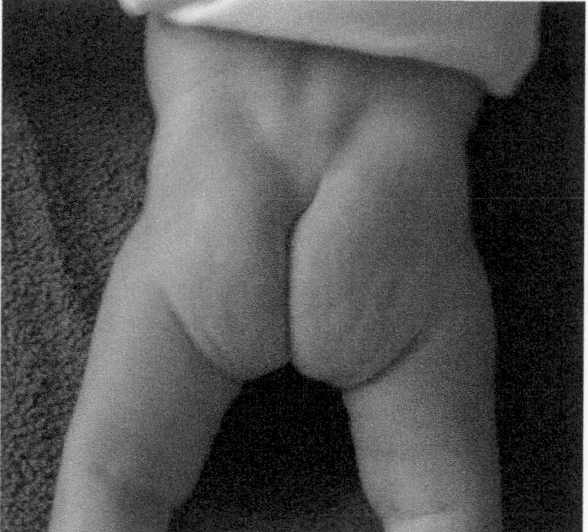

Figure 5.3. *Asymmetry of the gluteal cleft is frequently seen in association with sacropelvic somatic dysfunction.*

Observation and palpation of the pelvic girdle and lower limbs

With the infant in the supine position, observe the pelvic girdle and the lower limbs for spontaneous positions and asymmetries. Normally, a newborn demonstrates slight flexion and external rotation of the hips, a remnant of the fetal position. Look for any differences in the creases of the thighs and any asymmetry in the volume of the thighs. Look for any apparent difference in the length of the lower limb that may be an indication of congenital dysplasia. In the prone position, observe for symmetry of the gluteal musculature as it relates to the sacrum and lower extremities (Fig. 5.3).

Look for a global pelvic torsion, including both pelvic bones, in which one is externally rotated and the other internally rotated. In this case, on the side of the externally rotated pelvic bone, the thigh will be more extended; on the other side, the thigh will be more flexed. This relationship may be observed both when the child is lying still and when they are actively moving their lower extremities. Next note if these observations are consistent with the global body pattern. If they are, then the treatment should be directed at a total body approach with attention simultaneously to the pelvic and cranial areas. If the pelvic mechanics are not consistent with the global body pattern, then treatment should be directed at the dysfunctional pelvic mechanics in an attempt to bring them into functional balance.

The dysfunctional pattern may involve only one side, where one thigh might be more extended in association with a unilateral anteriorly rotated pelvic bone, or flexed with a unilateral posteriorly rotated pelvic bone while the other thigh moves freely in both directions. These observations may reflect a dysfunctional hip or dysfunction between the pelvic bone and the sacrum on that side.

Palpate the pelvic bones, comparing size and shape. Compare the symmetry of the anatomic landmarks: anterosuperior iliac spines, iliac crests and greater trochanters. Assess the range of motion of the hips: flexion, extension, abduction, adduction, and internal and external rotation. Normally, with the pelvis resting flat on the examination table, when the hips are flexed 90°, abduction should be between 70 and 85° and should not be painful to the infant. If abduction is less than 60° there is a restriction of movement that may be associated with shortening of the adductor muscles or with a pelvic dysfunction. The clinical picture of an infant demonstrating a restricted abduction of one hip and a restricted adduction of the other is a sign of instability of the hip joints. Proceed to tests of listening for the pelvis. Pay attention to any crepitation in the pelvis as the child moves as an indication of dysfunction of the pelvic bones. Significant restriction of gross motion, or pain with examination, is an indication for a more complete orthopedic examination.

Observe the legs and feet and compare both sides. Look for asymmetric creases or skin folds. Observe any asymmetric torsional pattern of the limb that may be global or local as is the case with tibiofemoral torsion or intraosseous tibial and femoral torsions. Assess the knees for asymmetry. Because of the fetal position associated with the common left occiput-anterior (LOA) vertex presentation, the left knee is more likely to demonstrate a tendency for varus deformity. Tests of listening for the knee should be employed. If necessary, further assess knee motion – flexion, extension, abduction, adduction and tibiofemoral rotation.

Observe the feet for positional anomalies such as over lapping toes. Look for calcaneovalgus where the foot may appear flat and dorsiflexed. Palpate the feet for configuration of anatomic structures and quality of soft tissue texture, specifically looking for myospasticity. Tests of listening may be applied at this time. Gross motion testing may be used to assess passive inversion and eversion of the feet. The lateral border of the baby's feet may be tickled to assess active abduction. Although most babies demonstrate a small degree of metatarsus adductus, the lateral border of the foot should be relatively straight. A convex lateral border may reflect a significant metatarsus adductus. If a pattern of inversion is associated with a metatarsus adductus, it is a metatarsus varus. In this case it is common to find genu varum and a torsional pattern of the entire limb as a remnant of the fetal position. In these circumstances, treatment should be directed at the entire limb, including the pelvic bone on that side.

Observation and palpation of the thoracoabdominal area

With the infant in the supine position, look for the presence of asymmetry, with attention to the umbilicus. Palpate the abdomen, looking for distension and areas of abdominal tension. Observe the configuration of the inferior border and anterior aspect of the thoracic cage, including the sternal area. Look for sternal depression, usually affecting the lower sternum (Fig. 5.4), or sternal protrusion, usually affecting the upper sternum. Observe resting pulmonary respiratory motion; infants usually demonstrate a pattern of abdominal respiration. Note the frequency and amplitude of the respiratory movements. This motion of the thoracic cage should be symmetrical. Inspiration and expiration should be

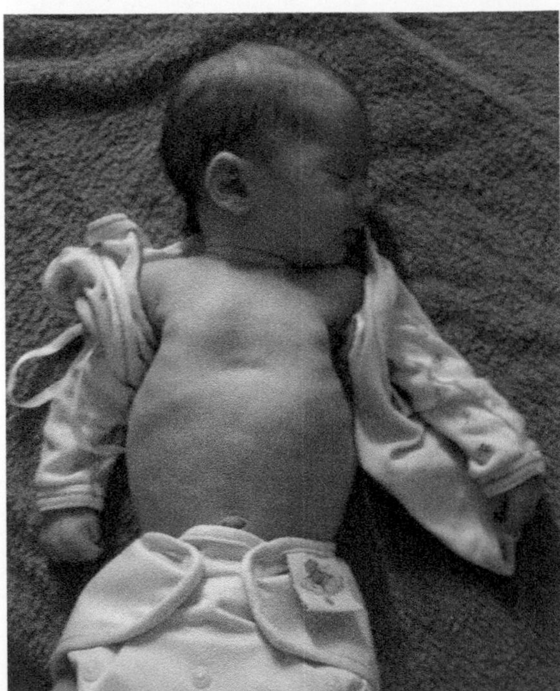

Figure 5.4. *Sternal depression (pectus excavatum).*

unencumbered and should be equal. Apply the principles of the tests of listening to the sternum, ribs and diaphragm.

With the infant either prone or seated, observe the configuration of the spine. In the seated position, observe the normal infantile kyphosis of the lumbar and thoracic spine. Observe the paravertebral musculature for asymmetry. Palpate the muscles to evaluate tone. With the child on their side, palpate the shape and alignment of the spinous processes of the vertebrae. The presence of a sidebent spinal curvature should be evaluated for infantile scoliosis. The dysfunction responsible may be intraosseous, interosseous or membranous. It may be identified in the spine at the level of the curve or at the craniocervical junction, with resultant compensatory spinal curvature below. Dysfunctional intracranial or intravertebral membranous strain should be sought out. Proceed to the tests of listening in any area that appears dysfunctional.

Observation and palpation of the pectoral girdle and upper limbs

Look at the position and symmetry of the pectoral girdle and upper extremities. Compare the position and shape of the clavicles and take note of the anterior axillary folds, looking for asymmetric creasing. Observe the muscular tone, size and mobility of both arms. Even the youngest infant will extend their fingers and open their hands from time to time. Asymmetric inability to perform this action may be consistent with brachial plexus injury, fracture of the clavicle or sequelae of a mild paresis that can present as decreased mobility of the fingers, wrist and arm. In the most common form of brachial plexus injury with damage to the C5 and C6 spinal nerves, the infant will hold their upper extremity in adduction, with the shoulder internally rotated; however, the grasp will still be present. When there is damage to C7, C8 and T1, the muscles of the forearm and hand are involved, with a paralysis of the hand and wrist.

Palpate the superior thoracic cage and shoulder region, with attention to the clavicles. Tissue texture abnormality and crepitus along the clavicle is indicative of clavicular fracture. Bilaterally palpate the arms for increased or decreased muscular tone or contraction.

Using tests of listening, assess the motion between the sternum and clavicle, and clavicle and acromion, as well as that of the shoulder, ulnohumeral, proximal and distal radioulnar articulations, wrist and hand. Somatic dysfunction is uncomfortable but not necessarily painful. Traumatic disruption of tissue, as with clavicular fracture, is quite painful; the infant's response to the examination informs the attentive examiner to the presence of conditions that should not be directly palpated or manipulated. Osteopathic manipulation is the definitive treatment for somatic dysfunction and although it may be appropriate to manipulate areas of compensatory somatic dysfunctions, in the presence of a clavicular fracture it is not appropriate to manipulate the fracture.

Proceed, with respect, to gross motion testing. The shoulders are evaluated in abduction, adduction, flexion, extension, internal and external rotation; the elbows in extension, flexion, abduction and adduction; the forearms in supination and pronation; the wrists in flexion, extension, abduction, adduction and circumduction, and the fingers in flexion and extension.

Observation and palpation of the cervical and upper thoracic area

With the infant in a supine position, observe the spontaneous position of the head. Note the presence of cervical sidebending and cervical rotation. If sidebending or rotation, or both, are present, decide if this is the result of isolated cervical mechanics or part of a global body pattern. When head rotation occurs to the opposite side of the sidebending, the causative dysfunction is often found at the level of the craniocervical junction. When the position of the head is rotated to the same side that it is sidebent, the causative dysfunction is often in the upper thoracic spine. In many cases when upper thoracic dysfunction is present, a coexistent pattern of asymmetry in the motion of the upper extremities corresponds to the causative spinal dysfunction. With right thoracic rotation, the child will present with the left upper extremity extended and internally rotated, and the right upper extremity flexed and externally rotated. In this case, sucking one finger of the right hand is easier and will, in turn, reinforce the causative dysfunctional pattern of the rotational position of the head.

Observe the tone of the cervical musculature and the carriage of the child's head. If the child appears to have difficulty lifting their head, the cause may be craniocervical somatic dysfunction. If it is observed that the child tends to throw their head backward, particularly when being cradled in the arms of the caregiver, the causative dysfunction is often a pattern of extension that may be located at the craniocervical junction, in the upper thoracic spine or occasionally at the level of the sacrum. If the causative dysfunction is found in the upper thoracic spine, both arms will be abducted and externally rotated.

Palpate the cervical region for tissue texture change. A child who has had a difficult birth will often demonstrate edematous tissue texture findings in the suboccipital region, with palpable suboccipital lymph nodes. Bilaterally palpate the sternocleidomastoid (SCM), scalenes, trapezius, semispinalis capitis and splenius capitis muscles, noting tension of the muscle fibers. Look for a hematoma or mass within the SCM; if found, determine its size and location. Remember that an SCM mass is often found in association with torticollis and consequently with an increased risk for the development of non-synostotic plagiocephaly and infantile scoliosis.

With the child, if possible, in the supine position, palpate the vertebrae of the cervical and upper thoracic regions. Palpate the spinous processes, noting their shape and alignment. Assess the first ribs.

Once the region has been screened, the tests of listening may be employed in order to identify membranous, myofascial, ligamentous and interosseous somatic dysfunction. Proceed to gross motion testing and assess active and passive ranges of motion. Because of the risk of torticollis, rotation and sidebending should be carefully evaluated. The normal range of rotation is at least 90° bilaterally. Unimpaired sidebending should bilaterally allow the ear to touch the shoulder on the same side. Following indirect principles, treat upper thoracic and cervical somatic dysfunctions.

Observation and palpation of the cranial vault

Visually observe the shape of the head, usually a refl etion of the presentation during the birth process. Vertex presentations tend to be narrower and more vertical, as compared to the child delivered by programmed cesarean section, who will tend to demonstrate a more symmetric round head. Note the asymmetry of the head. When viewed from above in the presence of plagiocephaly, the infant's head is seen to have the typical 'parallelogram' shape. Observe the shape and symmetry of the ears.

Observe the general appearance of the scalp. Note the presence of cradle cap or more severe atopy. Note also any increased perspiration. Such conditions may be encountered in association with cranial dysfunction. Observe the hair pattern and look for bald spots indicative of chronic positioning where the scalp is rubbed most often by the bed. This can result from chronic asymmetric sleep posture and may be caused by rotational dysfunction of the upper thoracic or upper cervical regions, cranial dysfunction, often sphenobasilar synchondrosis (SBS) horizontal strain, or a combination of these patterns.

The growth of the head, as measured by its greatest circumference (typically 35 cm at birth for a full-term infant), is regularly monitored to appreciate the growth of the brain and the absence of sutural pathology of the skull, such as premature closure. However, caution should be exercised in cases of craniosynostosis, where the circumference may be increasing as the child ages because of distorted cranial shape associated with synostosis of the suture.[4] As such, relying on the circumferential measurements without visually observing the skull is poor practice.

Observe for swelling and/or ecchymosis of the scalp (caput succedaneum). Caput succedaneum – a poorly demarcated soft tissue swelling that crosses suture lines – is an accumulation of blood or serum superficial to the periosteum that results from compressive forces during delivery. It is associated with cranial membranous dysfunctions, and although the soft tissue swelling usually resolves within days postpartum, the membranous dysfunctional pattern can persist. Following prolonged labor, a more severe condition, cephalhematoma – a subperiosteal bleed that does not cross suture lines – may be present (Fig. 1.26). It is readily palpable with clearly delineated edges and may be unilateral or bilateral. It appears on the third or fourth day postpartum and resolves in 4–8 weeks. It is a more serious condition than caput succedaneum because it can result in calcified scar formation. The area of the hematoma may be associated with an intraosseous dysfunction, but should not be directly manipulated until the hematoma has resolved.

Gently touch the vault of the child's head to evaluate tissue texture abnormality and increased tenderness. Areas that have been under physical stress, such as the points of contact of forceps blades or a nuchal cord, or areas associated with cranial somatic dysfunction, can be highly sensitive. The lightest touch during assessment is consequently imperative. The increased tenderness is usually proportional to the compressive forces that were responsible for the dysfunction.

Assess cranial contour and symmetry. Look for deformation, bossing or flattened areas. The bones of the vault are easily accessible for palpation and should be thoroughly evaluated. Deformation can occur as the result of external compressive forces applied in utero as, for example, in multiple gestation when one fetus rests upon the other, or when the fetal head is compacted by the bony maternal pelvis, or in instances of breech presentation by the lower maternal ribs. A step-like relationship between the frontal bones and the parietals may be observed. It may be produced by vertical strain of the SBS as the result of pressure exerted on the uppermost part of the frontal bones.

Bossing may be encountered following vacuum extraction delivery, most often involving one parietal bone. It should be borne in mind that, although the stress of delivery results in the bossing deformation, the dysfunctional pattern also involves membranous strain dysfunction of the dura that through the core link might be transmitted down to the sacrum and pelvis. Contralateral bossing may develop in compensation for plagiocephaly. In these cases the bossing is addressed by treating the plagiocephaly.

Flattening may occur in the occipital, parietal and frontal areas. It may be bilateral or unilateral. The appearance of an area of flattening provides clues as to its etiology. The flattening of the upper part of the occipital squama may result from direct compression of this area by the maternal pelvis in the last weeks of pregnancy or during delivery. When the deformation is associated with a pattern of lateral strain of the SBS and/or rotational dysfunctions of the occipitocervical, cervical or upper thoracic spinal regions, the flattening may extend to include the complete side of the head. Flattening of the right occipital area is usually associated with occipital bossing on the left, whereas in the anterior part of the skull, the reverse occurs with flattening of the left frontal bone and bossing on the right. In this instance, a right lateral strain of the SBS may be present in association with spinal somatic dysfunction that maintains right rotation of the head.

Palpate the fontanelles. Their size can be monitored to evaluate the progressive ossification of the calvaria. The posterior and sphenoid fontanelles are normally obliterated by the age of 6 months, whereas the anterior and mastoid fontanelles are closed in the 2nd year. The anterior fontanelle is diamond shaped. Its size differs from child to child and may be proportionate to the degree of cranial compression experienced in utero or during the birth process. Its palpation provides an estimate of dural tension and intracranial pressure. The triangular posterior fontanelle is smaller and may be closed at birth. Early fontanelle closure can be associated with premature sutural synostosis, while failure to close may be indicative of increased intracranial pressure and other conditions including hypothyroidism or genetic trisomy.[5]

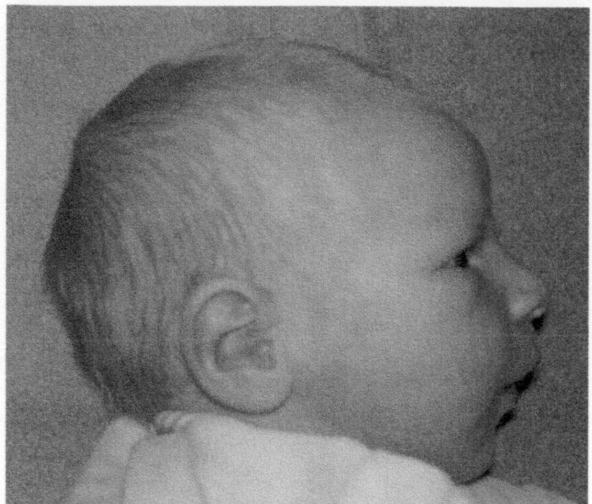

Figure 5.5. *Sutural overlapping in a 2-week-old infant.*

Assess the sutures for quality of tissue texture, inherent motility and for overlapping of adjacent cranial bones. Appreciation of the PRM at the level of the suture may be performed by placing two fingers of one hand in such a fashion that one finger lies on either side of the suture. Sutures that have been compressed are less resilient. The greatest loss of sutural flexibility is palpable in sutural synostosis. Sutural overlapping (Fig. 5.5) can occur anywhere in the vault but is more common in the coronal and lambdoid sutures and is less often encountered in the sagittal, squamous and sphenosquamous sutures. Sutural separation is a sign of rising intracranial pressure and a widened squamous suture is considered a sign of hydrocephalus.[6]

It should be remembered that the fibers of the dura contribute significantly to the sutural anatomy. As such, any dysfunctional suture is inevitably associated with membranous strain dysfunction of the dura.

The inherent motility and the global motion of the bones of the vault, as well as dysfunctional patterns involving individual bones and sutures, may be further evaluated with the tests of listening. These procedures also lend themselves to the assessment of the membranous components of the cranial mechanism.

Although the temporal bone belongs to both the vault and the cranial base, the squamous portion that belongs to the vault may be visually observed

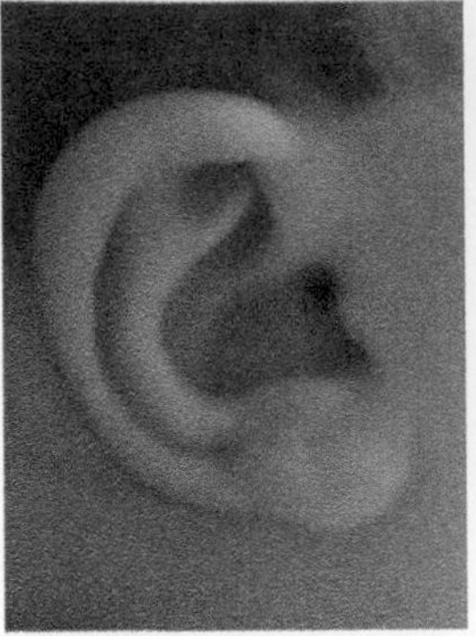
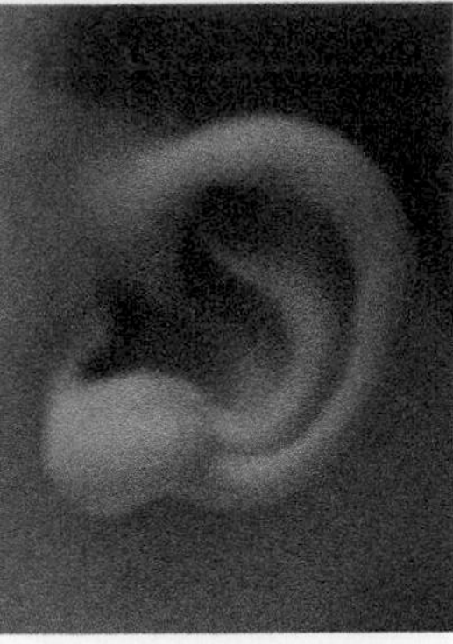

Figures 5.6(left)–5.7(right). *Asymmetry of the position, size and configuration of the ears.*

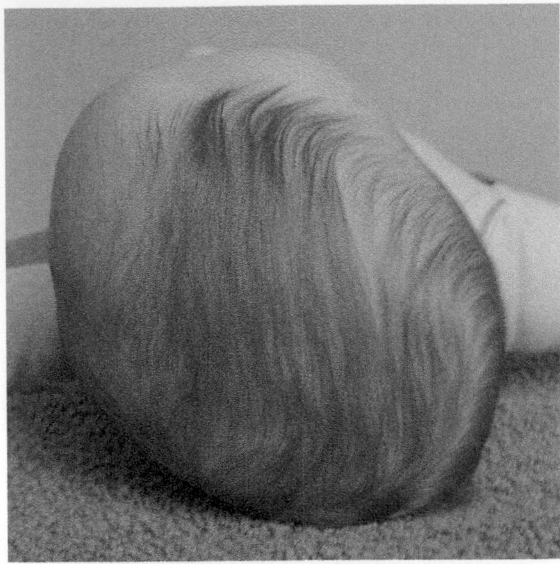

Figure 5.8. *In non-synostotic plagiocephaly, the ear on the side of the occipital flattening is displaced anteriorly.*

through its effect on the ears. Note the position, size and configuration of the ears (Figs 5.6, 5.7). Compare the size of the helix bilaterally; one ear may appear to be smaller. Although differences in folding and creasing of the auricle may be found in association with congenital conditions, this observation is often the result of chronic compression of the smaller ear. This can occur in utero or as the consequence of habitual sleep posture. This observation should lead the examiner to look for possible ipsilateral intraosseous temporal bone dysfunction as well as dysfunctional mechanics that maintain the chronic asymmetric sleep posture.

One ear may be displaced anteriorly or posteriorly. In non-synostotic plagiocephaly, the ear on the side of the occipital flattening is displaced anteriorly compared to the contralateral ear (Fig. 5.8). If the ear is observed to be displaced posteriorly on the fl attened side, additional diagnostic evaluation is indicated because such ear displacement can be the result of synostotic plagiocephaly.[7] It must be noted, however, that this sign is not an exclusive indicator in that synostotic plagiocephaly has also been reported to present with anterior ear position on the flattened side.[8,9] This indicates the importance of palpatory assessment of sutural compliance and, when necessary, diagnostic imaging in such cases.

Wide variations in the position of the auricle are found even in normal neonates.[10] It is of value for the osteopathic practitioner to observe the external ear because it mirrors the temporal bone. The ear may be flared out, usually in association with ipsilateral temporal bone external rotation (Fig. 5.9), or pinned against the side of the head in association with temporal bone internal rotation. Additionally, observing the relative positions of upper and lower

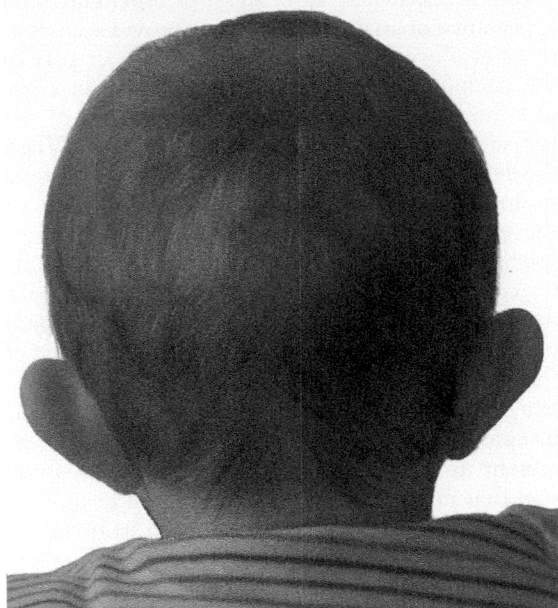

Figure 5.9. *Flared-out ears in association with external rotation of the temporal bones.*

attachments of the auricle allows one to assess temporal bone rotation relative to the sagittal plane. When the upper attachment is more anteriorly located than the inferior attachment it suggests a component of anterior rotation of the temporal bone. Conversely, when the upper attachment is posterior to the inferior attachment it is consistent with posterior temporal bone rotation. The anterior or posterior rotation of the temporal bone in the sagittal plane is the major component of external and internal rotation, respectively. Although the relative outflare of the ear is easily observed, the relative position of the upper and lower attachments of the auricle is a more reliable indicator of temporal bone somatic dysfunction.

Visual signs should be confirmed with palpation for function and tests of listening. A screening test for temporal bone position and motion consists of gently grasping the auricle and, with the gentlest of force, actively rotating the ear anteriorly and posteriorly in the sagittal plane. Comparison of compliance with these motions provides an indication of temporal bone movement. When the upper portion of the ear moves with greater ease anteriorly than it does posteriorly it is consistent with external rotation of the temporal bone; conversely, greater ease of posterior movement reflects internal rotation. Temporal procedures are described in Chapter 6.

Observation and palpation of the cranial base

The base of the skull is not totally accessible to observation or direct palpation. The lateral parts of the occiput or exocciputs, and the basilar part of the occiput, as well as the ethmoid, the body and lesser wings of the sphenoid and the petrous portions of the temporal bones, may be indirectly assessed by palpation for function.

Observe and palpate the shape, position and flexibility of the occipital squama below the nuchal line and external occipital protuberance. Pay particular attention to the most inferior aspect of the palpable occipital squama. Anterior displacement of one side as compared to the other may reflect an ipsilateral condylar compression of the occiput. Palpable asymmetry may also be indicative of either intraosseous dysfunction or occipital positional accommodation to somatic dysfunction of the SBS or the cervical spine below. Palpation for function, as described below, to assess the intraosseous relationship between occipital parts, as well as the interosseous relationship between the occiput, sphenoid and spine, provides the information to differentiate the causes of occipital asymmetry.

The mastoid process, the mastoid portion and the petrous portion of the temporal bone contribute to the cranial base. Mastoid processes are not present in newborns. They develop during the 1st year of life and, once present, should be assessed. Observe and palpate their size and position. The tip of the mastoid process moves posteriorly and medially with external rotation of the temporal bone and anteriorly and laterally with internal rotation. Palpation for function will differentiate between mastoid position that is a manifestation of dysfunction of the temporal bone as compared to mastoid position resulting from spinal sidebending and/or rotation. Asymmetric size of the mastoid processes may result from temporal intraosseous dysfunction or asymmetric pull of the sternocleidomastoid muscle.

Bilaterally palpate the mastoid portions of the temporal bones. Look for differences in position, size and flexibility. Asymmetry may reflect either intraosseous dysfunction of the temporal bone or accommodation to somatic dysfunction elsewhere. Occipitomastoid suture dysfunction is a common cause of such asymmetry.

The petrous portions of the temporal bones are not visible or directly palpable. Utilizing tests of listening, however, they may be indirectly evaluated, as may the lateral and basilar parts of the occiput, the ethmoid, and the body and lesser wings of the sphenoid. Tests of listening may be employed to assess the osseous components of the cranial base and their articular relationships. To effectively evaluate this area, a complete knowledge of the anatomy of the region and its mental visualization while palpating for function are of paramount importance.

The tests of listening to assess motion of the SBS may be performed. Utilize the fronto-occipital or vault hold to identify flexion, extension, torsions, sidebending–rotations, strains and/or compression.

While palpating the occiput, listen to the inherent motility of the bone and its relationship to surrounding structures. The presence of somatic dysfunction will manifest as decreased motility. At the same time, mentally visualize the occiput and its anterior and posterior intraoccipital synchondroses. The occipital condyles are located at the level of the anterior intraoccipital synchondroses and are often a site of intraosseous dysfunction. A condylar compression causes the sensation of tissue tension and restricted motility on that side of the occiput.

The relationship between the occipital and the temporal bones may be appreciated utilizing various handholds. Examine the occipitomastoid suture and, through its assessment, indirectly evaluate the jugular foramen. The petro-occipital suture should also be assessed. Because it remains unossified throughout life, it is normally an area where freedom of motion should always be present.

During palpation, mentally visualize the temporal bone and its synchondroses, and listen to their inherent motility and relationships. The assessment of the position and motion of the temporal petrous portion is also possible through mental visualization. Learn to visualize the structures associated with the temporal bone, such as the carotid artery or the trigeminal nerve, and to define any dysfunctional area that may affect such structures.

The principles described above may be applied to the sphenoid and the ethmoid. Tests of listening and mental visualization of the sphenoidal and ethmoidal synchondroses, as well as the relationship of the bones with surrounding structures, may be employed for diagnosis.

The membranous patterns of the cranial mechanism may be assessed at any time in the examination as determined by the infant's tolerance and cooperation. The fronto-occipital or vault hold may be utilized, in particular, to assess the falx cerebri, while the temporal five-finger hold may be utilized to assess the tentorium cerebelli.

Employ tests of listening to assess the global strain pattern of the reciprocal tension membranes. Dysfunctional tension of the membranous system can be responsible for maintaining osseous dysfunctional patterns and thus is of prime importance when diagnosing the skull. Furthermore, remember that, in the infant's skull, ossification is not complete and that completion of ossification follows the direction of strain present in the dural membranes. Consequently, the identification and treatment of membranous strain patterns is imperative. Particular attention should be given to the poles of attachment of the dura: the falx cerebri on the occipital squama and crista galli of the ethmoid, the tentorium cerebelli on the superior borders of the petrous portions of the temporal bones and the clinoid processes of the sphenoid. Listen for areas of dysfunctional tension within the dura mater. The dural membranes participate in the formation of structures of particular importance (e.g. the cavernous sinus or the petrosphenoidal ligament) and as such can dysfunctionally impact these structures. Once again, for diagnostic purposes, 'a knowledge of anatomy with its application covers every inch of ground that is necessary to qualify you to become a skillful and successful Osteopath . . .'.[11]

Observation and palpation of the viscerocranium

Observe the appearance and demeanor of the child. Do they appear to be happy or distressed? Somatic dysfunction is often uncomfortable, causing variable levels of unease.

The facial appearance of the infant provides information as to the presence and origin of asymmetry. Look for structural and functional asymmetries. Structural asymmetries – deformations as opposed to malformations – may be the result of intraosseous dysfunction. As such, they may be addressed with osteopathic manipulation. To avoid irreversibility, structural asymmetries should be recognized and treated as early as possible. This is particularly important in the viscerocranium, where the potential for growth after the first weeks and months of life is extremely high.

Functional asymmetries may be the result of interosseous or myofascial dysfunction; they may also follow structural asymmetries. Although structure and function are intimately associated, for purposes of treatment recognition of the primary cause of asymmetry is valuable.

Muscular asymmetries may also be due to paralysis (e.g. facial nerve paralysis). Subtle facial nerve paralysis may be recognized by observing the symmetrical fine motor control of the lips.

The observation part of the facial examination should be done before touching the child. Infants are extremely sensitive to touch in the facial area, requiring that the examiner use the lightest, most delicate contact. For this reason, it is important to obtain as much information as possible by observation.

Orofacial functions

Observe the diverse orofacial functions, such as breathing, sucking, swallowing and the utterance of sounds. If circumstances permit, observe the child's nursing habits: note agitation, the ease with which the child assumes neck and mandibular position, the coordination of the tongue and orofacial musculature, the rate of sucking and the ease with which the baby burps.

Enquire as to the use of a pacifier and how the child responds to the pacifier. Children with tongue thrust will commonly spit out their pacifier soon after it is placed in their mouth. If the child regularly refuses the pacifier (or bottle nipple), it is important to identify the shape of the pacifier (or nipple).

Observe the infant's resting respiration. Neonates are normally nasal breathers and breathing should be quiet. If noisy breathing is present without definitive upper respiratory tract pathology, the site of the origin of the noise should be identified. Upper nasal sounds resembling nasal congestion may reflect dysfunction of the frontal, ethmoid or nasal bones. Nasopharyngeal stertorous sounds may reflect dysfunction of the cranial base or maxillae. Laryngeal

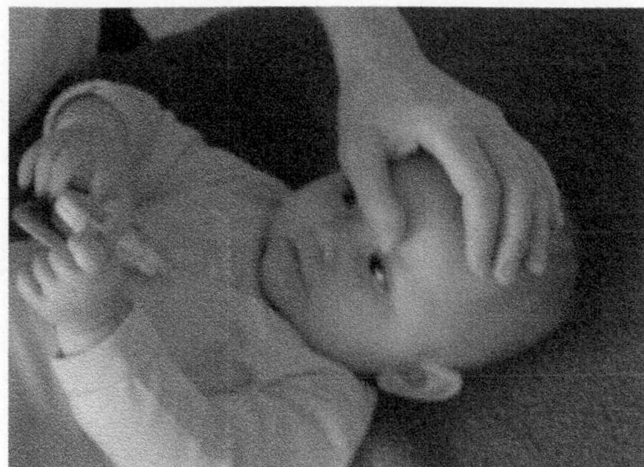

Figure 5.10. *Gentle palpation of the forehead assessing the metopic suture.*

stridorous sounds are associated with dysfunction of the cranial base, hyoid bone and cervical spine.

Frontal bone

Observe the forehead. Look for prominence of the metopic suture, an interosseous dysfunction between the two frontal bones resulting from bilateral compression, as can occur during forceps delivery. Observe asymmetry of the frontal bone. One side may be compressed more caudally or posteriorly compared to the other. This deformation of the frontal bone may be the result of a direct compression or it may be a compensation associated with SBS lateral strain dysfunction as is seen in the parallelogram-shaped head of non-synostotic posterior plagiocephaly.

Dysfunction of the frontal bone will manifest in the face below. Observe the relationship between the frontal and the facial bones. The face should be symmetrically suspended beneath the frontal bones and not deviated to one side or the other. The facial block should not be compressed under the frontal bone.

Gently palpate the forehead (Fig. 5.10). Note the shape and compliance of the frontal bones. Perform tests of listening to assess interosseous and intraosseous frontal dysfunction. During this procedure, mental visualization is helpful to precisely assess areas of restriction. Dysfunctional internal rotation of the frontal bone is of consequence because it causes the ethmoidal notch to be narrowed, restricting the movement of the ethmoid below, and affects the biphasic motion of the PRM in relation to the nasal cavities.

Orbital cavity and the eye

When a frontal dysfunction is present, it may affect the eyes. Observe the shape of the eyebrows and the shape and size of the orbital cavities, as well as the ocular globes. In the infant, the eyeball is normally large and projects slightly beyond the orbital rim. A downward displacement of the brow ridge with decreased height of the orbit is associated with frontal bone internal rotation or intraosseous dysfunction. On this side the eye will appear smaller and, in newborns, when the child wakes up, it will take more time for that eye to open compared to the other eye.

Changes in orbital diameter – the distance between the superior medial and inferior lateral angles of the orbit – may be reflective of a unilateral external or internal rotation pattern of the bones that constitute the orbital cavity. A cranial flexion–external rotation pattern increases the orbital diameter and results in an orbital cavity that is wider than normal. An extension–internal rotation pattern decreases the orbital diameter, resulting in an orbital cavity that is narrower than normal.

The zygomatic bone is the cheekbone. In zygomatic internal rotation, the cheek appears to be prominent, whereas in external rotation it appears to be recessed. Observe its position and note its effect on the orbital diameter – increased in external rotation and decreased in internal rotation. Palpation for function confirms the observation; if identified, treat any dysfunction.

To assess the function of the extraocular muscles, hold a toy or some other bright object before the child in order to catch their attention. Proceed to move the object before the child horizontally, vertically and in both diagonals. Comparatively note the speed and ease with which both eyes move to follow the object. Note asymmetry in these movements and in the neutral resting position of the eye. Varying degrees of asymmetry from the very slightest to overt strabismus may be observed as the result of cranial dysfunction of the bones of the orbit. The two most commonly encountered forms of strabismus are medial and medially upward deviations. Medial deviation of the eye can be associated with ipsilateral temporal bone dysfunction, affecting the abducent nerve (CN VI) as it passes under the petrosphenoidal ligament. Deviation of the eye in the superior–medial–oblique direction can reflect ipsilateral dysfunction of the frontal bone and its relationship to the superior oblique muscle at the trochlea, attached to the trochlear fossa of the frontal bone. Identification of functional abnormalities of the eye necessitates an in-depth ophthalmologic examination to rule out significant underlying pathologies. The presence of epicanthus – a vertical fold of skin extending down from the upper eyelid that covers the medial portion of the eye – may result in the appearance of medially deviated strabismus. This is a normal finding among some ethnic groups and does not require treatment; however, it may be indicative of genetic disorders such as Down's syndrome, necessitating further diagnostic evaluation.

Observe the infant in profile. Look at their eyes. Increased prominence of the globe may be present on the side of cranial external rotation. Conversely, on the side of internal rotation, the eye will appear to be less prominent.

Puffiness under the eyes may be associated with frontal bone dysfunction and is indicative of decreased lymphatic drainage from the region. Frontal bone dysfunction is also associated with nasolacrimal duct obstruction, where the dysfunction lies between the frontal bone, lacrimal bone and maxilla. Excessive lacrimation may be present in severe cases, whereas in milder presentations there may only be slight lacrimal puncta crusting. Indirect principles should be employed with great delicacy to treat nasolacrimal duct obstruction and, most of the time, result in excellent outcome.

Nose

Next, observe the global symmetry of the nose. Horizontal creases may be present across the base of the nose. The prominence of the nose makes it more vulnerable than any other facial structure; consequently, during delivery, nasal compression or subluxation often occurs. Very commonly the nose is posteriorly rotated under the frontal bones, with subsequent dysfunction at the level of the frontonasal suture and creases at the level of the nasion. This is generally associated with noisy breathing. Palpation of the region of the frontonasal suture reveals edematous tissue texture change.

Compare the size and shape of the nares. With the greatest delicacy, palpate the tip of the nose. Gently introduce nasal lateral displacement to the left and right and compare compliance. Asymmetry of compliance may result from nasal septal asymmetry. It may also reflect somatic dysfunction involving the ethmoid, maxillae, nasal bones and nasal cartilages. The mother may report increased nasal secretion and crusting of the naris on the dysfunctional side.

The relationships between the vomer and the sphenoid, ethmoid, maxillae and palatine bones, as well as the articulation between the two maxillae, should be evaluated. The nasal cartilages should be assessed in their relationship with the nasal bones and perpendicular plate of the ethmoid.

The columella that serves as a soft tissue anchor for the nasal cartilages and their intervening connective tissue is in continuity with the tissues surrounding the nasal apertures. The nasal apertures act as valves that open during nasal breathing. This valvular action is controlled to a significant extent by the dilatator naris muscles. Nasal breathing stimulates these structures. Conversely, mouth breathing is associated with hypotonicity of this region that may be palpable in the columella. Hypotonicity of the columella is associated with nasal septal dysfunction.

Apply indirect principles to treat any myofascial dysfunction of the nasal valve and columellar region. Use indirect cranial procedures to treat identified dysfunctions between the vomer and adjacent bones, as well as between the two maxillae, and between the nasal cartilages and the nasal bones and perpendicular plate of the ethmoid.

Maxillae and mouth

Assess the proportion of the lower portion of the face in the context of the complete face. In newborns this part of viscerocranium is normally smaller than in adults because the sinuses are not yet fully developed and the teeth have not yet erupted.

Observe the maxillae and compare size and shape. Like the nose, the maxillae very often seem to be impacted and posteriorly rotated under the frontal bones. Observe the position of the mandible; note the location of the gnathion that may be laterally displaced. Newborns normally demonstrate retrognathia.

When observing the mouth area, first look at the lips. Babies are normally nose breathers and, when not interacting, keep their mouths closed and their lips approximated. If the infant demonstrates an open mouth with their tongue positioned forward (Fig. 5.11), one should suspect dysfunction of the cranial base, possibly associated with dysfunction of the mandible and hyoid bone. Tongue forward position can result in excessive drooling.

The inside of the mouth should be carefully examined. Evaluate the length of the frenulum of the tongue. Clipping of the frenulum (frenuloplasty) may be necessary in cases of short frenulum linguae because it impairs the mobility of the tongue, resulting in speech impediment and disrupting the normal positioning of the teeth. Examine the teeth as to position and eruption consistent with the child's

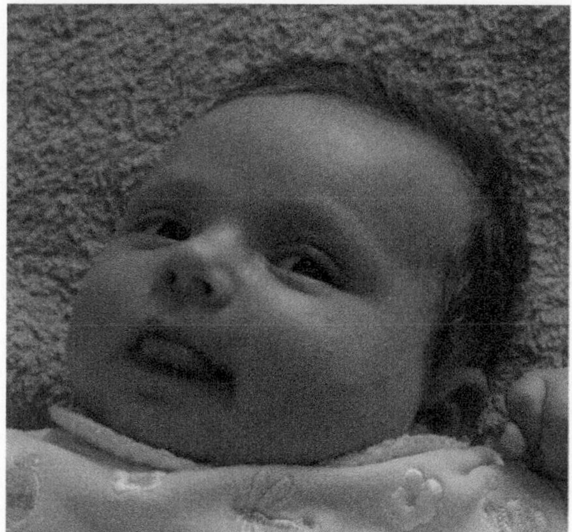

Figure 5.11. *Tongue thrust is frequently seen in association with cranial base and craniocervical dysfunction.*

age. At the same time, observe the shape and symmetry of the palate. A wide flattened palate is associated with external rotation of the maxillae, a narrow arched palate with internal rotation.

Palpation for function and treatment of identified dysfunction should follow. Sometimes addressing motion restriction and facilitating inherent motility, releasing tension in the osseous matrix, may overcome a functional delay in developmental progress. Delayed tooth eruption may be addressed by treating the SBS, vault and facial bones to ensure optimal freedom of movement.

PHYSICAL EXAMINATION OF THE CHILD

The basic principles of the physical examination of the child and the interpretation of the findings are similar to those described above in the section 'Physical examination of the infant'. The difference is that the child's musculoskeletal system has usually grown and is more developed. Skeletal areas that were unossified in the infant are now closer to ossification or are fully ossified. Muscular tone and coordination have progressed. The child is attaining developmental milestones and has acquired bipedal stance. This allows for the addition of the standing structural and functional evaluation to the examination process.

'Savoir-faire' in establishing the physician–patient relationship with toddlers and children is essential in order to gain the patient's trust and cooperation. In particular, younger children may come to be seen with a personal history of previous unpleasant encounters with healthcare providers. They have probably received injections and consequently past medical visits are associated with disagreeable memories. It is therefore necessary to diminish the patient's fears. Consequently, allow the child to stay close to their caregiver and approach them slowly. Pay close attention to the child's facial expression and body language. If at all possible, do not touch the child before they are willing to accept the contact. Give the child time to establish a sense of territorial security. Unless the child is emergently ill or injured, there is no benefit to be gained by forcing yourself upon them.

Toys are the secret. An excellent approach to the establishment of contact is to present the child with the opportunity to play. Toddlers and young children may be offered a basket of toys to discover. This should contain safe but intriguing objects with unusual shapes and bright colors, as well as more complex objects with moving parts or the potential to be assembled and taken apart. As the child begins to play, it provides the practitioner with an opportunity to evaluate the level of parental interaction, as well as the child's personality and temperament – shy, cautious, anxious, curious. Their speech, verbal skills, cognitive abilities, gross and fine motor skills and coordination may also be assessed. As the child begins to play, the caregiver (who may also probably be anxious) will relax, further facilitating the ease of the child. Most children will become engrossed in the activity of play and allow the examiner to establish the physical contact necessary for diagnosis and treatment. The creation of such an environment of comfort and relaxation is consistent with indirect principles and augments the efficacy of the osteopathic treatment.

The following description of evaluation follows an arbitrary sequence. The order may vary depending on the cooperation of the child and the area of complaint. It is sometimes preferable, if it is not too uncomfortable to palpate, to begin the evaluation by examining the area of complaint first, to communicate to the child that the intention of the treatment is to alleviate the complaint. The examination should be performed in such a fashion that the child perceives that the examiner is reliable and in control of the situation. This will set boundaries for the child and encourage them to cooperate with the process. Although it may seem paradoxical, it is entirely possible for the examiner to be both gentle and playful, and yet firmly in control. It is important to realize that the osteopathic examination and treatment of the patient is more than just palpation and manipulation. This necessitates a dynamic interchange between the patient and the osteopath. It is important to explain to these patients, in simple terms, what is being done and why.

Observation and palpation in the standing position

Whatever the chief complaint, the examination should always begin with the standing evaluation unless the child is unable to assume the position. This is because the standing evaluation provides a global perspective of the individual's body mechanics.

It is of value to have the child gowned in such a way that their back and bare legs may be observed. Although toddlers and small children may not voluntarily stand still for examination, their dynamic weight bearing and body mechanics may be assessed by observing them as they move about. This type of dynamic examination is of particular value when appraising the lower extremities. At this time, it is easy to note the alignment of their feet and assess for intoeing or out-toeing. Intoeing is more frequently encountered and the most common etiologies are internal tibial torsion and increased femoral anteversion. Further observe the feet for inversion or eversion. Young children commonly have a plantar fat pad giving the appearance of flat feet. A visible longitudinal arch is not apparent until between 2 and 6 years of age.[12] Before the arch develops completely, however, if the child stands on their toes, the presence of the medial longitudinal arch may be demonstrated.

Observe the alignment of the lower extremities and note any valgus or varus confi guration of the feet and knees (Fig. 5.12). Very commonly, children less than 2 years of age are bowlegged and after 2 years may demonstrate a knock-kneed appearance until the age of 5 or 6. Look for interosseous rotation between the tibia and femur, and for intraosseous torsion of either bone. Note the placement of the patella. Medial deviation of the patella is consistent with femoral torsion or pelvic bone imbalance. Enquire as to the ability of the child to squat, hop and run.

Next, observe the pelvis for asymmetry and inequity of the heights of the greater trochanters and iliac crests. Imbalance of these landmarks may indicate unequal growth of the long bones of the legs. Such imbalance can also result from asymmetric foot, ankle, knee, hip or sacroiliac dysfunction.

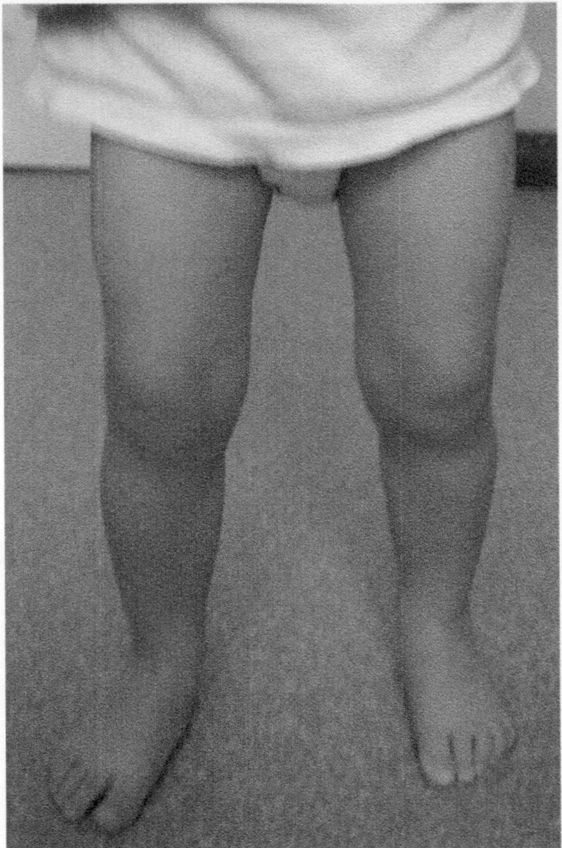

Figure 5.12. *Observe the alignment of the lower extremities and note any valgus or varus configuration. This figure illustrates right tibial torsion and right foot valgus.*

Observe the pelvis for increased anterior tilt, possibly the result of craniosacral extension of the sacrum, increased lumbar lordosis or abdominal distension often associated with gastrointestinal dysfunction. Decrease of the normal anterior pelvic tilt is consistent with craniosacral flexion of the sacrum or sacrococcygeal dysfunction.

Assess spinal alignment and curves. From behind the child observe the symmetry of the anatomic landmarks: the scapular angles, shoulder heights and mastoid processes (Fig. 5.13). Note the level of contact of the tips of the fingers as the child holds their arms in a relaxed position at their sides. Spinal sidebending curves result in compensatory asymmetry of these landmarks. Look for asymmetric paravertebral prominence, consistent with the rotational component of a group spinal curve. Such prominence will be located on the side of the convexity of the curve and may be more clearly observed with

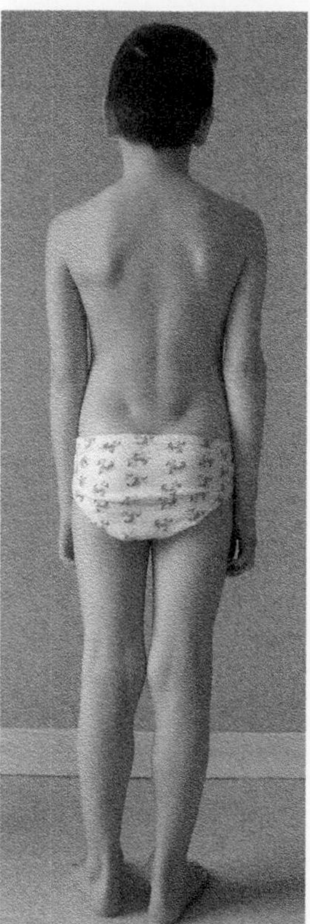

Figure 5.13. *Observe the symmetry of the anatomic landmarks. Note right sidebending of the head.*

the child bending forward at the hips. Although sidebending curves of the spine are usually primary somatic dysfunctions, they may also be secondary to craniocervical dysfunction affecting the spine from above or pelvic imbalance affecting the spine from below. As with infants, the dysfunction responsible for the curve may be intraosseous, interosseous or membranous.

From the child's side observe the spinal anterior–posterior (AP) curves. Lumbar lordoses are commonly encountered in young children, up to about the age of 7 years. An increased curvature that is limited to a portion of the spine may reflect dysfunction within the curve, in an adjacent spinal curve or at the adjacent junctions between the spinal AP curves. Forward displacement of the head is often seen in association with breathing dysfunctions, such as chronic rhinitis and mouth breathing. The child will likely demonstrate increased cervical and upper thoracic AP curves associated with somatic dysfunction of the craniocervical junction or upper thoracic vertebrae. A spinal pattern that involves all of the curves can be the result of cranial and sacral dysfunction. Decreased AP curves will be found with cranial flexion of the SBS and sacrum (Fig. 5.14) and increased curves with cranial extension (Fig. 5.15). Early detection of increased or decreased kyphotic and lordotic curves is desirable for the most effective treatment.

Assess the normal gross motions of the spine by having the child actively flex, extend, sidebend and rotate each region of the spine to confirm the previous observations. Tension within muscles, between anterior and posterior groups, will differ according to the compensatory response required by the spinal curve that is present. The hyperlordotic child will demonstrate increased tension of the hamstrings and hip flexors, and at the same time their abdominal muscles will lack tension. When such an individual is asked to bend forward, they will compensate by flexing their knees. This portion of the examination is ideally performed in front of a mirror so that the child may be made aware of their compensations. Treatment for these patients should include body awareness and proprioceptive training, as well as manipulation.

Observe the anterior thoracic cage, looking for pectus carinatum and pectus excavatum. Look for protraction or an associated asymmetric pattern of the pectoral girdle. Palpate the shape and alignment of the spinous processes of the vertebrae.

Proceed to the tests of listening to further identify previously recognized dysfunction and, if necessary, also assess the grosser range of motion. It should noted that, because of the flexibility of their myofascial structures, dysfunctional mechanics in young children differ from those of adolescents and adults in that definitive dysfunctional barriers are not encountered to the same extent.

A total body pattern tending toward eversion of the feet – and eventually flat feet and genu valgum, associated with increased sagittal curves, particularly the lumbar curve – may be correlated with a craniosacral extension–internal rotation dysfunctional pattern. Conversely, inversion of the feet with an increased medial longitudinal arch, genu varum and decreased sagittal curves may be found in association with a craniosacral flexion–external rotation pattern.

Further palpation for structure and function may be accomplished with the child in the supine position. In this fashion, any area of complaint may be studied additionally and in greater depth.

Observation and palpation of the pelvic girdle and lower limbs

With the child in the supine position, observe the feet. Look for deformation of the phalangeal

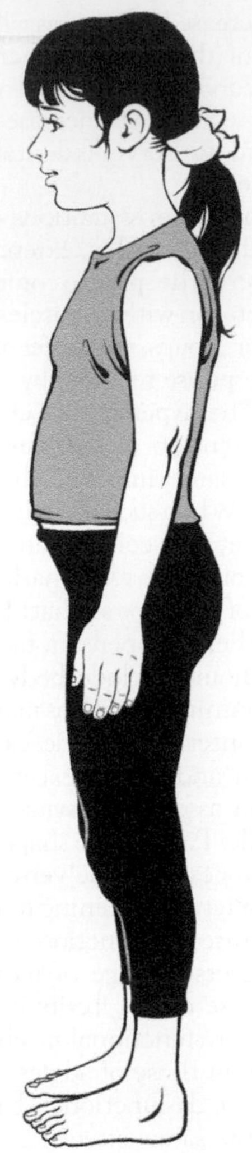

Figure 5.14. *Decreased AP curves may be found with craniosacral flexion.*

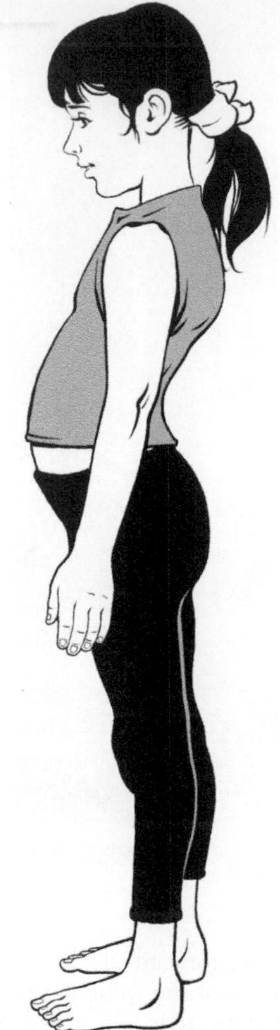

Figure 5.15. *Increased AP curves may be found with craniosacral extension.*

alignment of the toes. Utilizing tests of listening, check for any dysfunction of the tarsal bones. If necessary, palpate the position and range of motion of the bones of the foot, particularly the calcaneum, talus and cuboid, to provide additional information as to the functional status of the subtalar, calcaneocuboid and cuneocuboid articulations. Do not underestimate the dysfunctional significance of childhood ankle strains. Although post-traumatic pain frequently resolves rapidly in these young patients, dysfunctional mechanics commonly persist, with long-term effects on postural balance.

Note the comparative confi guration of the two knees. Often a dysfunctional knee will demonstrate visible malposition between the tibia, femur and patella. Next observe the alignment of the tibia and femur, looking for genu varum or genu valgum that persists in the supine position. Palpate the knee to assess for tibiofemoral rotation, lateral strain and abduction or adduction.

Observe the way the thighs rest on the table. Note the presence of asymmetric hip flexion and external or internal rotation. If rotational asymmetry of position of the thighs is present, determine if the rotation involves only the thigh or extends to involve the entire lower extremity. The rotational position of the entire lower extremity is indicative of ipsilateral pelvic bone dysfunction, where external rotation of the lower extremity follows external rotation of the pelvic bone and internal rotation demonstrates the same coupled relationship.

Assess the extent of the gross motion of internal and external rotation at the hip joints. Young children demonstrate approximately equal rotation in both directions, 45° ± 20°.

Observe the pelvis in relation to the examination table, the lower extremities below and torso above. Lateral deviation of the pelvis on the table from the midline can be indicative of lumbosacral dysfunction or, less often, intraosseous pelvic bone dysfunction. Look for asymmetry of the anatomic landmarks: anterior–superior iliac spines, iliac crests and greater trochanters. Palpate the pelvic bones, comparing size and shape.

Perform the test of listening on the pelvic bones and proceed to evaluate the sacrum and lumbar spine. The non-weight bearing assessment provides more precise information about the motion of the pelvis than does the standing evaluation. If pelvic dysfunction observed during the standing examination persists when the child is lying down, the site of the dysfunction is within the pelvis. If, however, dysfunction observed standing is not present during the non-weight bearing examination, the pelvic dysfunction is an accommodation to somatic dysfunction elsewhere. It is not rare to find sacroiliac dysfunction in children. It may have functional consequences and is frequently seen in association with constipation. In a similar fashion, dysfunction of the lumbar spine and sacrum may be responsible for functional abdominal pain.

The treatment of any identified dysfunctional areas should follow. Specific attention should be paid to areas of significant dysfunction using indirect principles. If the area of dysfunction fails to completely respond to the treatment, look for contributory tension in adjacent regions. Treatment of these dysfunctions using myofascial release will often facilitate a more complete response elsewhere, in the primary dysfunctional area.

Observation and palpation of the thoracoabdominal area

Observe the thoracic cage. Note the configuration of the ribs and sternum. Assess resting pulmonary respiratory motion, noting the frequency and amplitude of the respiratory movements. The motion of pulmonary respiration should involve all areas of the thoracic cage symmetrically. To the extent that diaphragmatic respiration is present, the abdomen will rise during pulmonary inspiration and sink back down during expiration. If diaphragmatic excursion is unencumbered, the lower thoracic cage and abdomen will be seen to move synchronously throughout the respiratory cycle. In the presence of diaphragmatic dysfunction, this motion will be restricted at the end of inspiration or expiration, depending on the diaphragmatic dysfunction. A diaphragmatic expiratory dysfunction demonstrates limitation of pulmonary inspiration, whereas an inspiratory dysfunction demonstrates limited pulmonary expiration. Observe for the use of accessory muscles of respiration, seen in association with conditions such as asthma.

Next, observe the contour of the abdomen. Note any abdominal obesity and, if present, take advantage of the opportunity to discuss good dietary habits with the child. Look for a slight depression in the abdominal wall immediately below the xiphoid process, often seen with digestive complaints related to diaphragmatic dysfunction.

Utilizing tests of listening, palpate the thoracic cage for dysfunction of the ribs, sternum and diaphragm and treat identified dysfunction. Palpate the abdominal wall and abdominal contents. Tests of listening may be employed to assess myofascial dysfunction and alteration of inherent motility affecting the viscera, as well as the abdominal wall. Employing indirect principles, treat dysfunctional structures.

Observation and palpation of the pectoral girdle and upper limbs

Observe the general contour and symmetry of the shoulders and clavicles. Difference in the rotational resting position of the upper extremities is often found in association with upper thoracic somatic dysfunction. Note the degree of myofascial tension in the extremities. Increased tone, associated with limitation of full extension of the elbows, wrists and hands, may be seen in conjunction with a craniosacral extension–internal rotation pattern anywhere in the cranium and axial skeleton.

Compare the two upper extremities for asymmetry. Look at the carrying angle of the elbows. Note any difference in the torsional pattern between the arms and forearms. Observe for activity of the hands that may indicate the level of nervousness of the child. If the child appears agitated, it is appropriate to reassure them.

Next, proceed to palpation for function, with tests of listening. If necessary, further document the active range of motion of the limbs and passively evaluate using gross motion testing. Beginning centrally and progressing peripherally, treat identified dysfunction.

Observation and palpation of the thoracic and cervical areas

With the child lying supine, observe the spontaneous position of the head. Look for gross sidebending and rotation, noting the level of involvement – cervicothoracic, mid-cervical or upper cervical. If the head is held with sidebending and rotation in the same direction, the responsible dysfunction is likely in the upper thoracic or cervical spine; if sidebending and rotation are in opposite direction, the origin may be dysfunction of the occipitocervical junction.

Palpate the upper thoracic and cervical regions for tissue texture change. Assess the upper thoracic and cervical vertebrae, noting the shape and alignment of the spinous processes. Vertebral somatic dysfunction is often found in association with a palpable increase or decrease of the space between adjacent spinous processes. Examine the first ribs.

Upper thoracic somatic dysfunction is commonly found and its diagnosis should not be overlooked. Left untreated it can be the source of many chronic problems. Mechanically, it affects the head and neck above, upper extremities and, through postural compensation, even the sacrum. Neurologically, it exerts significant influence on the sympathetic nervous system and consequently is the source of multiple somatovisceral and somatosomatic reflexes.

The thoracic region is initially evaluated during the standing examination. If somatic dysfunction has been identified in the mid to lower thoracic region, it may be further evaluated with the child seated or in the prone position. Observation, tests of listening, visualization and, if necessary, gross motion testing are applied.

Once the thoracic and cervical regions have been thoroughly screened, palpate for function using tests of listening to identify membranous, myofascial and ligamentous somatic dysfunction. Treat any somatic dysfunction that has been identified. Start with upper thoracic dysfunction followed by treatment of the ribs and cervical spine.

Observation and palpation of the neurocranium

Observe the general appearance of the skull. It should be balanced on the spine. Look globally for asymmetry and indications of flexion–external rotation or extension–internal rotation. Look at the skin. Dermatologic changes on the face and scalp can be indicative of underlying cranial somatic dysfunction.

Confirm previous findings and palpate aspects that may be appreciated more easily than with simple observation. The bony surfaces and prominences of the skull are easily identified by palpation. Palpation of the position of different structures offers information as to their relationship to the cranial mechanism. Knowledge of the normal positions and relationships of the cranial components is necessary in order to recognize dysfunction. The following is a basic list of the minimum that should be palpated:

- The occipital squama is lower in flexion–external rotation and higher in extension–internal rotation.
- The temporal fossa is full in flexion–external rotation and recessed in extension–internal rotation. Its palpation provides information as to the lateral-most aspect of the greater wing of the sphenoid.
- The tip of the mastoid process is posterior, medial and high in external rotation, and anterior, lateral and low in internal rotation.
- The medial edge of the parietal bone is flattened in external rotation and prominent in internal rotation.
- The lateral angle of the frontal bone is lateral in external rotation and medial in internal rotation. Prominence of the metopic suture indicates internal rotation.

Because of the fetal position and forces during the birth process, every individual's body is asymmetrically molded. All of the fasciae, the craniosacral membranes and all of the matrices of the future osseous structures are imprinted with this asymmetry. Therefore, it is not unusual to find one side of the patient in external rotation and the other side in internal rotation. Only palpation for function allows the differentiation between a functional asymmetric state, with complete quantity and quality of movement, and somatic dysfunction that demonstrates restricted mobility.

Palpation for function with tests of listening, utilizing the vault hold, begins with the appreciation of the global quality of the tissues of the head. It may feel heavy and compact. On the other hand, the PRM may be easily perceived, with movements of expansion of the skull during cranial inspiration (flexion–external rotation) and contraction during cranial expiration (extension–internal rotation).

It may be compared to the movement of the thoracic cage during pulmonary respiration but at a lower frequency.

Compare the sensations perceived on the right and left sides of the head. The skull ideally should demonstrate symmetrical unrestricted motility. In the presence of dysfunction, restriction of motility may affect the complete skull or be limited to one side. Sphenobasilar dysfunction is associated with global restriction of motility manifesting on both sides of the skull, whereas unilateral dysfunction, such as occipitomastoid or sphenosquamous compression, is associated with restriction limited to the side of the dysfunction. To further identify a unilateral dysfunction, compare the sensation in the anterior and posterior halves of the skull on the dysfunctional side. Once again, the restriction of motility is indicative of the location of the dysfunction.

Palpate the lateral aspects of the greater wings of the sphenoid and the occipital squama to evaluate the SBS for function. Note the presence of any particularly dominant movement. Assess flexion and extension. In flexion, the lateral aspects of the greater wings of the sphenoid expand laterally, while the superior–lateral portions of the occipital squama move posteriorly and laterally. During SBS extension, the opposite of these motions of the greater wings and occipital squama occurs. Palpation of the SBS for function may also be assessed using the fronto-occipital hold. In this instance, the movement is palpated to a greater degree in the sagittal plane.

It is easy to commit the error of palpating the superficial motion and assuming that what is being perceived is the SBS motion. It should be remembered that the contact points on the sphenoid and occiput are on bones of membranous origin and because of flexibility may demonstrate some degree of motion, even in the presence of SBS compression. Palpation of the superficial sphenoid and occipital components must be augmented by visualization to interpret the function of the SBS.

In SBS torsion, the greater wing of the sphenoid moves superiorly on one side and inferiorly on the other, while at the same time the reverse movement occurs with the squama of the occipital bone. In SBS sidebending–rotation, the greater wing and the lateral occipital squama move inferiorly on the same side and, most of the time, separate from one another on that side.

Vertical or lateral strains of the SBS consist of movement that is perceived in the anterior portion of the skull, which is opposite to that perceived posteriorly. Thus, in a superior vertical strain, the sphenoid is felt to move upward while the occiput moves downward; in an inferior vertical strain, the opposite motion is appreciated. In a right lateral strain, the sphenoid is felt to move with greater ease to the right and the occiput to the left; in a left lateral strain, the opposite motion is palpable. In the presence of compression of the SBS little or no biphasic movement is perceivable.

Palpation should be done to appreciate the state of tension in the intracranial and intraspinal membranes. The head, as in any other part of the body, is comprised of different layers. To specifically address the membranes, one must first know their anatomy. Hand placement on opposite sides of the head is followed by mental placement at the level of the membranes through visualization. When touching the head, mentally visualize the layer of the scalp; this is associated with very light touch. Then visualize the bony layer; the touch will be slightly firmer. Maintaining this amount of palpatory pressure, visualize the deeper layer of the membranes that will provide a less rigid feel. Assess the sensation of the different areas of reciprocal membranous tension and the quality of the PRM transmitted through the membranes. Note any areas of intracranial tension. Note the focal point of balance within these tensions. Dysfunction from a distant area, the spine or the sacrum creates the sensation that the membranes are being pulled in that direction. This may be felt in the presence of scoliosis with tethered intraspinal membranes.

At a deeper level, appreciate the motility of intracranial fluid. Assess the frequency and potency of the cranial rhythmic impulse. Note the regularity and dominant pattern of the waves, as well as the presence of stasis. Utilize indirect principles to treat any identified dysfunction. A possible sequence for the treatment of somatic dysfunction of the neurocranium is to begin by addressing membranous strain patterns. Next, the SBS may be treated, followed by other dysfunctions of the base and vault.

Observation and palpation of the viscerocranium

Observe the global shape of the face. It is wider with flexion–external rotation and narrower with extension–internal rotation. This should not be confused with ethnic variations of facial shapes. In an individual whose face is wide because of their ancestry, flexion–external rotation of the skull will result in a face that is wider yet. Palpation for function allows the examiner to recognize these differences.

Identify the midline of the face, consisting of the metopic suture, nose and symphysis menti. These structures should be aligned in a straight line. A curvature of this line, with the face relatively smaller on the side of the concavity, is consistent with SBS dysfunction. Alternatively, an angular disruption of the midline is typically consistent with local viscerocranial dysfunction affecting the individual bones. Observe the face for symmetry of the forehead, eyebrows, eyes, nares, cheeks, lips and jaw line. Note the quality of the skin – ruddiness, pallor, dryness, scaliness, eruptions and excoriations.

Frontal bone

Although the metopic suture is fused in the majority of individuals around the age of 6 years, it may be identified as the midline of the frontal bone and features on either side can be compared for symmetry. Observe the brow ridges as reflected by the eyebrows, the zygomatic processes and the frontal tuberosities. Decreased prominence of the frontal tuberosity and apparent lateral displacement of any of these landmarks is associated with frontal bone external rotation on that side. Conversely, increased prominence of the frontal tuberosity and apparent medial displacement of the landmarks indicates internal rotation. Palpate the frontal bone and employ tests of listening to confirm observational findings. Palpate the individual halves of the frontal bone for resilience of the bone and underlying dura. This area should be compliant in children. The frontal bone is of particular significance because of its influence on the viscerocranium that hangs beneath it. Anecdotally, frontal bone restriction is associated with belligerent behavior in children. The tests of listening may be blended seamlessly into indirect manipulative procedures to treat any dysfunctions of the frontal bone.

Orbital cavity and the eye

Observe the bony orbit for size and symmetry. Note if the pattern exhibited by the orbit corresponds with the functional pattern of the skull. A wider orbit reflects a pattern of flexion–external rotation. When the skull of the subject is also wider, the bony orbit fits the global pattern of the skull and the SBS should be tested to rule out underlying dysfunction. If the pattern of the orbit does not fit the global pattern of the skull, examine the constituent bones of the orbit for dysfunction.

Look at the eyes, noting any difference in size, shape and position. Observe for symmetry and quality of ocular movement. Note the neutral resting position of each eye as well as any tendency for deviation from bilateral ocular alignment. Bilaterally examine the medial ends of the frontal supraorbital margins for symmetry. These structures are located immediately anterior to the trochlear attachment of the superior oblique muscle. Frontal bone dysfunction affecting this area will, in turn, affect the function of the muscle. Assess the cheeks for position and prominence. Prominence of the cheek is indicative of internal rotation of the zygomatic bone. The orbital edge of the zygoma is everted in external rotation and inverted in internal rotation, whereas the posteroinferior edge of the zygomatic process is inverted in external rotation and everted in internal rotation. Any dysfunction of the zygoma will affect the lateral rectus muscle and the balance of the extraocular muscles.

Observe the temporal fossae for clues as to the position of the greater wings of the sphenoid. A fossa that is higher, lower, deep or shallow on one side is indicative of the position of the lateral aspect of the greater wing on that side. With the child's eyes closed, note the obliquity of the upper lid margins bilaterally. The lines formed by the lid margins typically reflect the position of the ipsilateral wings of the sphenoid.

Information obtained by observation must be further elucidated. Palpate and employ tests of listening to confirm observational findings. If somatic dysfunction is identified, treat it using indirect principles. After treating any dysfunction of the sphenoid and frontal bones, treat any dysfunction of the components of the orbit.

Nose

Look at the size, shape and position of the nose. Observe the alignment of the nasal crest with the midline of the frontal bone. Further observe the alignment between the different portions of the nose – the nasal bones, the nasal lateral cartilages and the tip of the nose. Assess the two nares for symmetry of size, shape and position. Deviation of the nose to one side is often accompanied by asymmetric size of the nares. The site of dysfunction responsible for the deviation should be identified. It may be externally located at the frontonasal suture or at the articulation between the nasal bones and the lateral cartilages, or the site may involve only the tip of the nose. It may be internally located and involve deeper structures within the viscerocranium, including the septal cartilage, the vomer or the perpendicular plate of the ethmoid. The attachment between the base of the columella and the philtrum reflects the nasal septal position and should be positionally consistent with the remainder of the nose. Lightly palpate the tip of the nose with one finger. Lift it in the midline, noting the ease with which this is possible. Observe the nasal septal position during this maneuver. Allow the nose to return to its original position and gently attempt to laterally displace the tip to the left and right, noting asymmetry of motion. Deviation of the nasal septum will result in impaired nasal airflow and mucociliary clearance.

The nose should also be observed in the context of its function during respiration. This is of particular importance in children because nasal breathing is a dynamic factor in the growth of the viscerocranium. Assess the route of respiration – nasal or mouth. If the child is mouth breathing, determine if it is a short-term or chronic condition. If nasal breathing, note patency and functional asymmetries of the nares and alar parts during the respiratory cycle. Note the presence of bilateral or unilateral nasal secretions or crusting. If unilateral, ask the caregiver if it is chronically on the same side.

Nasal patency and airfl ow may be assessed by having the child participate in breathing 'games'. The examiner or child gently compresses the naris opposite the side to be evaluated. The compressive force should be suffi cient to occlude the naris but not enough to displace the nasal septum and the child should be asked to breathe through the unobstructed side. This test is then repeated on the opposite side. The performance of this test should not cause the child respiratory discomfort. Both sides should demonstrate equal ease of unencumbered airfl ow The force of airfl ow may be assessed by holding a wisp of fi bers from a cotton ball beneath the child's nose and noting displacement during exhalation. The child can also exhale through the nose onto a chilled mirror that is held beneath the nares. Asymmetry in nasal expiratory airflow may be observed by the resulting condensation.

The above observation should be confi rmed by tests of listening. The functional obstruction of the nose can be the result of cranial somatic dysfunctions including torsion or sidebending of the SBS. It may also result from dysfunctions affecting the frontal bone such as internal rotation of one side that results in narrowing of the ethmoidal notch and restriction of the frontoethmoidal suture. Finally, nasal functional obstruction may be the result of dysfunction of the bones of the nose itself, including most often the nasal bones restricted at the frontonasal suture, or the ethmoid or vomer restricted in their relationships between themselves or with the sphenoid. Identifi ed dysfunction may be treated with indirect procedures. Dysfunction of the basicranium, if present, should be treated first, followed by treatment of any frontal bone dysfunction and finally dysfunctions of the viscerocranium.

Maxillae and mouth

Observe the mouth and lips for symmetry and tonicity. The upper lip refl ects the functional pattern of maxillae, while the lower lip refl ects the mandible. Note the alignment of the lips and their relationship to one another. When the mandible is approximated with the maxillae, the lips should be in soft contact without protrusion, tension of perioral muscles, retraction or pursing. Look at the chin. Note any indication of contraction of the mentalis muscles. Look for any scars on the chin that would indicate a fall or blow that might result in SBS, temporomandibular joint or occipitocervical extension dysfunction.

Compare the nasolabial sulci for depth and obliquity. Increased depth of the nasolabial sulcus on one side is indicative of external rotation of the ipsilateral maxilla and/or the zygoma, whereas decreased depth is consistent with internal rotation. Observe the philtrum – the groove above the upper lip – and the philtral ridges. The orientation of both the nasolabial sulci and the philtral ridges follows the pattern of the maxillae. The more horizontal these landmarks, the more external rotation is present; the more vertical, the more internal rotation. The majority of children demonstrate some degree of asymmetry, with external rotation of one maxilla and internal rotation of the other. On the side of external rotation, the maxilla will appear to be wider, the palate lower and flattened, and the teeth everted. With internal rotation, however, the maxilla appears narrow, the palate high and arched, and the teeth inwardly directed.

Observe the position of the mandible. Note the alignment of its midline with the midline of the face above and the suprasternal notch below. If the mandibular midline is not in alignment with the maxillae, compare the two halves of the mandible for symmetry of size and shape. Asymmetry of size or shape may be the consequence of intraosseous mandibular dysfunction or asymmetry of orofacial function such as mastication. It can also result from dental malalignment. Asymmetry of position typically results from asymmetry of the temporal bones. External rotation of the temporal bone is associated with posterior displacement of the mandibular fossa, where the mandibular condyle articulates. Temporal bone internal rotation results in anterior mandibular fossa displacement. As a result, the chin is displaced toward the side of temporal external rotation and away from the side of internal rotation.

Assess the position and function of the tongue. Have the child open their mouth. Observe the relative position of the tongue within the oral cavity. The tongue should be contained inside the mandibular arch and should not cover the lower teeth. Have the child slightly protract their tongue and look for the presence of dental imprints on the lateral aspects of the tongue, indicative of lingual malposition and/or dental malalignment. Inspect the tongue for deviation or limitation of movement. Check the length of the lingual frenulum. If the child is old enough, ask them to touch the tip of the tongue to the upper incisors. If the child is too young, encourage them to smile and laugh and take advantage of any time where the tongue is lifted to observe the ventral surface of the tongue. If the frenulum is too short, it anchors the tongue to the floor of the mouth and interferes with tongue movements and position, potentially resulting in mouth breathing and dental malocclusion. Children with dysfunctional tongue posture often demonstrate decreased tone and eversion of the lower lip.

Observe the child when swallowing and note, if possible, the action of the tongue and perioral muscles. Older children may be asked to describe the location of the tip of their tongue during swallowing. Normally, around 5 years of age, with mature deglutition, it should contact the hard palate behind the upper incisors. Immature deglutition is present when the tip of the tongue protracts between the upper and lower teeth. Therefore, each time the child swallows, they apply pressure to their front teeth, promoting overbite. Immature deglutition present after 5 years of age requires rehabilitation.

Have the child open their mouth and observe the teeth for progression of dental development. Have the child clench their teeth and observe the occlusion of the teeth. The midline between the upper and lower incisors should be in alignment. The upper incisors should slightly override the lower incisors and the upper molars should rest on the lower molars. Look for misalignment or protrusion of the upper or lower incisors, as well as crowding of teeth. Dental crowding can be associated with a dysfunctional cranial extension–internal rotation pattern. Asymmetric crowding will follow ipsilateral internal rotation. It has been associated with impaired ipsilateral nasal breathing and/or dysfunctional mastication.

Tests of listening and treatment of the maxillae and mandible should precede any orofacial procedures or rehabilitation to facilitate satisfactory results. Orofacial dysfunctions involving the maxillae and mandible are frequently associated with dysfunction elsewhere in the cranial base and craniocervical junction that should also be addressed.

PHYSICAL EXAMINATION OF THE ADOLESCENT

The principles of examination of the child, as discussed above, may be extended to include the adolescent, although these patients are progressively more and more like adults. The growth and maturation of their musculoskeletal system make them less malleable than infants and young children, but still more pliant than adults. Their ability to understand and cooperate with the examination and treatment process is more like that of the adult. This is a period often associated with great psychological stress, where the individual is searching to identify themselves and define their role within society. Evaluation of the adolescent's behavior in the context of affect (mood, self-esteem, relationships, risk-taking behaviors) and cognitive development (school performance, planning for the future) is important.[13] It is also a time of physical changes and, frequently, resultant sensitivity about their bodies. This requires that the practitioner be respectful about what is said and how the adolescent is touched. Adolescents are progressively seeking to control their own lives. As such, the empowerment of therapeutic counsel should be directed more toward them than toward the caregiver, as would be the case for infants and children. As with children, it is important to explain to these patients what is being done and why.

The sequence that follows is arranged for descriptive purposes. Clinical practice necessitates that the implementation of examination and treatment be fluid. The chief complaint and variability among patients will determine the sequence that is appropriate for each individual.

Observation and palpation in the standing position

Note the patient's overall demeanor and body language. Posturing is an expression of psychological state but the pattern of the posture is determined by body mechanics.

From the front, the side and from behind observe the pattern of weight-bearing mechanics in the context of symmetry and the positioning of the line of gravity.

Standing in front of the patient, look at the alignment of midline structures: mandibular symphysis

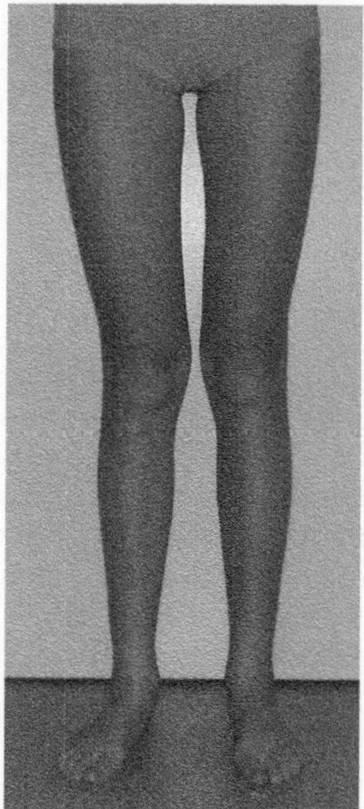

Figure 5.16. *Observe the symmetry of the anatomic landmarks. Note right knee valgus and right pes planus.*

menti, larynx and trachea, suprasternal notch, xiphoid process, umbilicus and pubic symphysis. The gravitational midline should fall through each of these structures to end at a point on the floor equidistant between the heels. Assess the position of the head, sternoclavicular joints, clavicles, acromioclavicular joints, coracoid processes, anterior axillary folds, lateral thoracic contour, lateral flanks, iliac crests, anterior superior iliac spines (ASISs), medial and lateral malleoli and the arches of the feet. Asymmetry of these structures may readily relate to the patient's chief complaint or it may represent an occult dysfunction from a previous forgotten injury that is now responsible for secondary dysfunction (Fig. 5.16).

Standing to the side of the patient, note the AP curves of the spine. Decrease of spinal lordosis and kyphosis is associated with craniosacral flexion and the inhalation of the PRM, whereas increased curves are associated with craniosacral extension and the exhalation of the PRM. Note if the spinal curves follow one another in a global pattern or if changes in the AP curvature are localized to an isolated area of the spine. Observe the lateral alignment of the line of gravity that should pass through the external auditory meatus, midline of the shoulder, greater trochanter, lateral condyle of the knee and lateral malleolus.

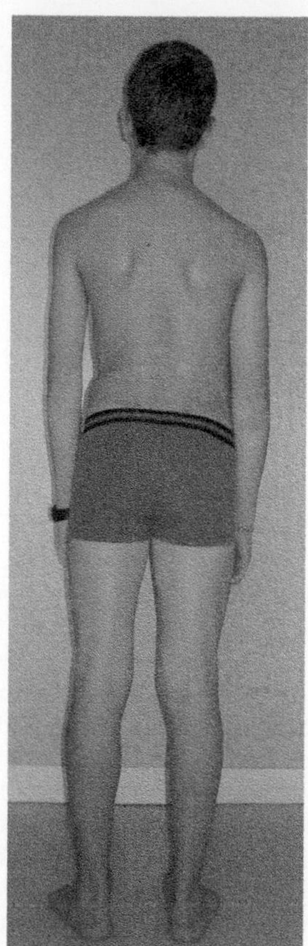

Figure 5.17. *Observe the symmetry of the anatomic landmarks. Note inequality of leg length and pelvic tilt.*

Observing from behind the patient, look at the alignment of midline structures: occipital protuberance (inion), spinous processes and intergluteal fold. As observed anteriorly, the gravitational midline should fall through each of these structures to end at a point on the floor equidistant between the heels. Look at the inferior hairline posteriorly which is indicative of the position of the occiput and basicranium. It reflects cranial or upper cervical somatic dysfunction that may have existed since birth, often representing a pattern of occipital sidebending and rotation. Observe the positional symmetry of paired landmarks, including the ears, mastoid processes, posterior axillary folds, acromion processes and inferior angles of scapulae, lateral torso contour, iliac crests and posterior superior iliac spines (PSISs) (Fig. 5.17). Additionally, observe any cutaneous signs – hyperemia, changes in pigmentation, telangiectasia and acneform lesions – commonly seen in the skin over somatic dysfunction affecting the upper thoracic and lumbosacral regions. Have the patient bend

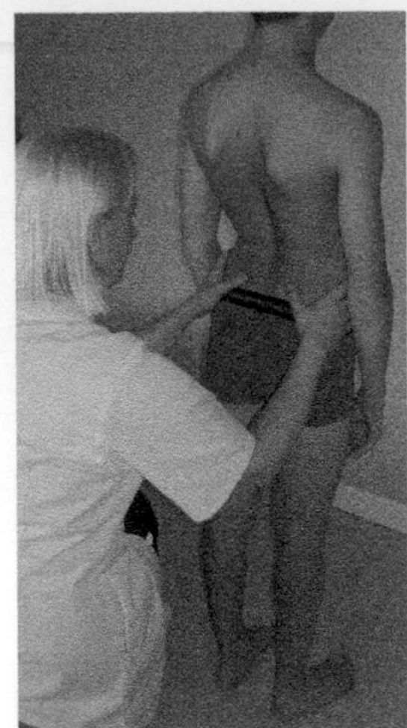

Figure 5.18. *Pelvic test of listening.*

forward from the hips. Observe for asymmetric paravertebral prominences found on the side of the convexity of minor spinal lateral curves and rib humping with scoliosis (curvature greater than 10°).

Follow with palpation and tests of listening. These tests are of interest during the standing postural assessment because much of the somatic dysfunction encountered in the axial skeleton is the result of the adjustment of the body to gravity. Tests of listening may be applied anywhere; however, when applied to the pelvis while the patient is standing, they provide information as to pelvic accommodation to forces from above and below.

From behind the subject, with the examiner's thumbs contacting the PSISs and the hands placed bilaterally on the iliac crests, palpate the PRM (Fig. 5.18). Ideally, both pelvic bones should demonstrate unrestricted external and internal rotation, with components of motion in each of the three cardinal planes and a sense of pelvic girdle unity where the two pelvic bones synchronously follow the biphasic PRM.

More often, because of the asymmetric pattern established by fetal posture and forces at birth, or following spinal dysfunction occurring in childhood, the pelvis will be felt to move in a torsional pattern. One pelvic bone moves more easily into external rotation and returns to demonstrate a less prominent internal rotation phase. Simultaneously, the other pelvic bone moves easily into internal rotation, with less prominence in the external rotation phase. It should be noted at this time that the sense of unity of pelvic girdle motion is still present, i.e. with the sensation that when one pelvic bone moves, the other side moves in synchrony, although in the opposite direction.[14] This asymmetric pattern most commonly is the result of dysfunction in the axial skeleton above, possibly including the cranial base. The pelvis in this case is not primarily dysfunctional, the pattern is an accommodation to dysfunction above. As a rule of thumb, the greater the torsional sensation, the lower the dysfunction in the axial skeleton.[15]

On the contrary, if during palpation the sense of pelvic girdle unity is absent, with the sensation that both pelvic bones are moving out of synchrony, the dysfunction is in the lower limbs.[14] This can include the pelvic bones or the sacroiliac joints.

The patterns of pelvic torsion commonly encountered in adults often have their origin in childhood or earlier. Although frequently a site of pain in adults, they are seldom painful in children and adolescents unless complicated by overuse, trauma or viscerosomatic reflexes.

The structural organization of the body is established early in life. Asymmetries of structure may be addressed prior to this time. Later, structure responds progressively less well to treatment and the balancing of function becomes the goal.

Adolescents demonstrate dysfunctional patterns that progressively resemble those of adults, requiring that treatment focus on the balance of function. However, because musculoskeletal growth and development are not yet complete, it is still appropriate to attempt to balance structure as well as function. Furthermore, effective treatment that establishes functional balance enhances the impact of physical activity on the adolescent's structural development. The reflex musculoskeletal response to proprioception is still malleable. The establishment of good postural habits and myofascial functional balance, before adult patterns are engrained, is an investment for the future.

With the patient standing, tests of listening may be employed to assess the weight-bearing response of the spine. With experience, tests of listening will also provide information relative to the functional status of individual vertebral segments. Palpate with the index and middle fingers on either side of the spinous process of the vertebra to be assessed while visualizing the complete vertebra and it articulations with adjacent segments. By listening to the inherent motility of the PRM in that segment, identify if it moves more easily in flexion or extension, in sidebending right or left and in rotation right or left.

If necessary, examination of the spine may continue with the patient seated. This allows the patient to relax more without interference from the lower limbs, such as occurs with an inequity of leg length. Palpate for lumbar and thoracic tissue texture changes over the spinous processes and paravertebrally over the transverse processes and rib angles. Palpate for alignment of the spinous processes and compare interspinous spaces, looking for irregularities. Tests of listening may then, if necessary, be followed by gross motion testing of the areas. Treat any identified vertebral somatic dysfunction.

Observation and palpation of the pelvic girdle and lower limbs

In the supine position evaluate leg length. Be sure that the patient is lying straight on the examination table. Grasp both feet with your hands in such a way that the patient's heels rest in your palms. Compare the levels of the distal medial malleoli. With smaller inequities this method does not effectively differentiate between functional and anatomic leg length differences. A difference of 1.5 cm or greater in leg length is considered to be signifi cant for a risk of postural deviation such as scoliosis. The clinical assessment of inequity of leg length is controversial and, if a difference is suspected, further radiological evaluation is required.[16] Smaller inequities of leg length, although they will produce functional imbalance, will typically not result in clinical symptoms until much later in life.[17] The functional impact of these relatively minor inequities should, however, not be ignored.

The lower extremities can be examined in the supine position. Utilizing tests of listening, evaluate the inherent motility of the PRM in the different bones. Being paired structures, all of the bones individually demonstrate biphasic external and internal rotation.

The motion of the bones of the feet is complex, demonstrating a combination of the motion in the three cardinal planes. Typically, this consists of a major component with two minor, but equally important, components resembling inversion of the foot in craniosacral external rotation and eversion during craniosacral internal rotation.

Apply tests of listening to the bones of the feet. Identify dysfunctional restriction in the major components of external or internal rotation, and in the minor components of adduction and supination or abduction and pronation. Proceed to gross motion testing if further information is necessary and treat any identifi de dysfunction utilizing indirect principles.

Using tests of listening, assess the motility of the PRM in the long bones that demonstrates craniosacral external and internal rotation around their long axes. Listen to motion between the tibia and fibula to assess any dysfunction in the proximal or distal joints. Assess posterior or anterior glide of the proximal fibula relative to the tibia that should be linked with the opposite motion of the distal fibula. Listen to motion at the knee, paying attention to the tibia relative to the femur in external or internal rotation, abduction or adduction, lateral or medial translation. If necessary, utilize gross motion tests. With indirect principles, treat any dysfunction. The fibula should be considered first in most cases before proceeding to the treatment of the knee or foot. Often physical complaints at the knee result from dysfunction at the ankle below or hip or pelvis above. Slipped femoral capital epiphysis – a condition necessitating orthopedic evaluation – commonly presents as knee pain and, as such, the examination of any lower extremity complaint must always include the assessment of the whole body and not just the site of the complaint.

Further assessment of the pelvis may be done in the supine position. Sacroiliac dysfunction may be tested and treated with indirect procedures, as described in Chapter 6. The lumbosacral junction and lumbar vertebrae can also be evaluated in this position, and treated as well. Additionally, in this position the adolescent is able to see what the practitioner is doing. This lets them interact verbally, giving the patient a sense of control and allowing them to be more relaxed.

Somatic dysfunction of the lumbar, sacral and pelvic regions in the adolescent should not be ignored, even when there is no associated pain complaint. Rapid growth and physiologic changes that occur in this age group make them vulnerable. Lumbopelvic dysfunction often results from athletic activities or, paradoxically, lack of physical activity. With menarche, girls may experience menstrual irregularities and discomfort coupled with lumbar, sacral and pelvic somatic dysfunction. The associated viscerosomatic and somatovisceral reflexes give good reason for osteopathic treatment. If not treated, the lumbar, sacral and pelvic dysfunctions in adolescence will be the ground for low back pain in adult life.

Observation and palpation of the thoracoabdominal area

Observe the thoracic cage and the ease with which the patient breathes. Note the symmetry and coordination of respiratory movement between the abdomen and thoracic cage. Diaphragmatic respiration should be unencumbered, with a coordinated alternation between the rise and fall of the abdomen during pulmonary inspiration and expiration. Diaphragmatic dysfunction causes these interdependent motions to be restricted in a fashion similar to that discussed above in 'Physical examination of the child'.

Diaphragmatic dysfunction may occur as a primary dysfunction of the diaphragm itself. It can also be the result of dysfunction of the lower thoracic cage, lumbar spine or temporal bones. Dysfunction of the lower ribs (6 through 12) can affect the diaphragm at its attachments, while the lower ribs may be dysfunctional as the result of lower thoracic spinal dysfunction. Dysfunction of the lumbar spine affects the diaphragm through its impact on the diaphragmatic crura, while diaphragmatic dysfunction is found associated with stiffness of the upper lumbar vertebrae. Additionally, dysfunction of the temporal bones that affects the PRM and the cranial diaphragm will, in turn, prevent full excursion of the thoraco abdominal diaphragm. On occasion, midcervical somatic dysfunction, through the phrenic nerve, will also affect diaphragmatic function.

Palpate the thoracic cage, looking for rib dysfunction in either inspiration or expiration. Assess the sternum and sternocostal joints and treat any dysfunctional areas, employing indirect principles. Listen to the diaphragm, compare its different portions and note any difference in tension and freedom of movement between the two sides, as well as the posterior and anterior portions. Release any diaphragmatic dysfunction.

Observe the abdominal contour and its movement during respiration. The contour and movement should be smooth and symmetrical. Note the muscular tone of the abdominal wall – firm and flat as with athletic adolescents or the presence of subcutaneous fat and poor muscle tone. In this latter circumstance it is appropriate to discuss dietary and exercise habits, stressing the fact that good habits in adolescence will lay the groundwork for health during the rest of their lives.

Observe the location of the umbilicus which should be centered. If not, it may indicate intra-abdominal dysfunction or somatic dysfunction at the level of the mid-lumbar spine. In males and some females note the pattern of hair that is seen extending from the pubic hair up to the umbilicus or above. This line reflects the functional status of the lumbar spine. Deviation from the midline may indicate lumbar somatic dysfunction at the same horizontal level. Palpate the abdominal wall and abdominal contents. Employ tests of listening to evaluate tone and symmetry of the myofascial components of the abdomen. Listen to the inherent motility of the abdomen globally, the abdominal wall and individual viscera within. Identified areas of dysfunctional tension or restricted motility should be treated.

Observation and palpation of the cervical spine

The diagnostic observation, palpation and treatment of the cervical region should be performed before treating any dysfunction of the skull. Cervical somatic dysfunction, resulting in neck pain or headache, is commonly encountered in adolescent patients. This is often the consequence of chronic postural stress, as when studying and working or playing on computers, or from athletic injury. Significant somatic dysfunction is frequently found in the upper cervical region and at the craniocervical junction.

This region is most appropriately examined with the adolescent supine. Observe the position of the head. Note the presence of sidebending and rotation and whether they occur in the same or opposite direction. The combination of sidebending and rotation in opposite directions is consistent with occipitoatlantal dysfunction, whereas sidebending and rotation in the same direction is associated with dysfunction in the typical cervical or upper thoracic vertebrae. Myofascial dysfunction involving the sternocleidomastoid or scalene muscles may also be present.

Next, palpate for superficial and deep tissue texture quality and myofascial tension. Palpate the vertebrae for function. Diagnostic palpation of the cervical spine, particularly its upper region, requires great palpatory precision. When examining the occiput and atlas, the movements induced are, too often, transmitted to the level of C3 or lower because of lack of precision in palpation and the utilization of force and amplitude that are too great.

When assessing occipitoatlantal motion it is necessary to visualize the location of the occipital condyles. When grasping the skull one has to recognize that the condyles are not caudal to the tips of the examiner's fingers but rather are located anteriorly deep and somewhat superior to the tips of the fingers. In similar fashion, precision of palpation is required in the examination of the atlas. The tips of the transverse processes of the atlas are palpable about 1 cm below and in front of the apex of the mastoid process. The transverse processes of the atlas may be barely palpable in small individuals and are highly sensitive, requiring delicacy of touch. The remainder of the cervical spine should be evaluated with the same level of sensitivity.

Use indirect methods to treat identified somatic dysfunction. The beauty of these procedures is that while addressing highly localized somatic dysfunction they simultaneously normalize other components participating in the maintenance of the global dysfunctional pattern.

Observation and palpation of the neurocranium

Begin by observing the global shape of the head. Different morphological skull types may be defined by the cephalic index obtained by multiplying the maximum transverse diameter by 100 and dividing the total by the maximum sagittal diameter:

(transverse diameter × 100)/sagittal diameter = cephalic index

The brachycephalic type, with a disproportionately short head, has an index greater than 80; the dolichocephalic type, with a disproportionately long head, has an index less than 75.

Cranial flexion produces an increase in the width of the skull, giving the appearance of brachycephaly; extension decreases skull width, resembling dolichocephaly. Only by testing mobility can one differentiate a dysfunction with restriction of movement from a morphologically wider or narrower skull in which motion is unimpaired.

Most of the time palpation is carried out with the patient supine and the operator seated at the head of the table. Observe any asymmetry of the skull and, using tests of listening and visualization, palpate the SBS for dysfunction. Compare the pattern identified in the skull with that of the rest of the body. Most of the observation and palpation of the adolescent is similar to that discussed above in 'Physical examination of the child'. Only points of particular interest will be discussed below, with a summary of the main characteristics of landmark observation being provided in Table 5.1.

The whole skull, including the membranes, is involved in the pattern of flexion, extension and torsion or sidebending–rotation. In adolescents, the SBS is beginning to fuse and therefore motion starts to be less prominent than that palpated in younger children. Bony compliance should still be present. The motions felt reflect both the available motion of the SBS and those dictated by the patterns of the membranous components of the skull. When listening, focus attention to differentiate between the bony layer of the skull and the membranous layer of the dural membranes. Assess for restriction of mobility and asymmetry of tension of the dural membranes.

Table 5.1

Observation of landmarks

Landmarks	External rotation	Internal rotation	Remarks
Vault	Lower	Prominent	
Sagittal suture	Flat	Projected	
Forehead	Wide	Narrow, more vertical	
Frontal eminence	Receding	Prominent	
Supranasal vertical folds	Smooth	Increased	
Transverse frontal folds	Wide	Narrow	Reflection of the sphenoid's position
Eyebrow	Longer	Curved, short	
Orbit	Open	Closed	Orbital diameter: from the superomedial angle of the orbit to the inferolateral angle
Eyeball	Protruded	Recessed	
Nares	Open	Closed	History of previous trauma to the nose could result in such changes
Nasiolabial sulcus	Deeper	Smooth	
Cheek bone	Receding	Prominent	
Palate	Wide, lower	Narrow, convex	Possibility of intraosseous dysfunctions at the level of the maxillae
Upper incisors	Separated distally	Approximated or overlapping	
Molars	Everted	Inverted	
Mandible	Displaced toward this side	Displaced on the opposite side	Bilateral internal rotation of the temporal bones = protruded mandible
Ear	Protruded	Close to head	

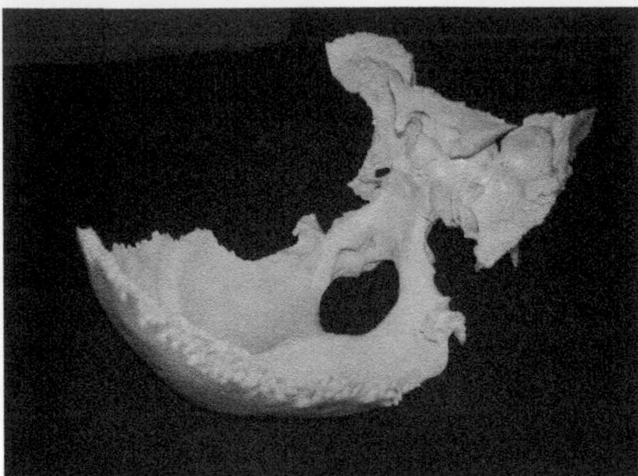

Figure 5.19. *Palpation of the sphenoid is through the greater wings and visualization of the sphenoidal body is necessary.*

It is easy to commit the error of palpating the superficial motion and assuming that what is being perceived is the motion of the SBS. It should be remembered that the contact points on the sphenoid and occiput are on bones of membranous origin which are capable of remaining flexible long after the cartilaginous SBS has fused (between the ages of 8 and 25).[18–23] It is particularly important to remember this when assessing the sphenoid. The first sensation when palpating the sphenoid is through the greater wings and what is felt is the motion of the greater wings and not necessarily the motion of the sphenoidal body (Fig. 5.19).

After palpating the SBS, assess the remaining articulations of the cranial base. By adolescence all of the intraosseous synchondroses of the occiput, temporal bone and sphenoid are fused, but bony compliance should remain. Diagnosis and treatment are consequently directed more at interosseous dysfunction, including occipitomastoid, petro-occipital sutures and sphenopetrosal synchondrosis. Dysfunction involving the occipitomastoid suture is frequently encountered as the result of blows to the occiput as might occur when an individual falls backward. This may present as headache, cervical pain and motion restriction, dizziness or occasionally vagal dysfunction because of CN X entrapment in the jugular foramen.

Disparate findings may be obtained when palpating the temporal bone if the examiner does not realize that the mastoid portion follows the occiput while the squamous portion is significantly influenced by the sphenoid. The presence of intraosseous dysfunctions at the petrosquamosal junction established prenatally or in infancy may be responsible for this discrepancy. In this case, the minor components of motion of the squamous and petrous portions of the temporal bone feel as if they move out of synchrony in external and internal rotation. As is often the case, the solution resides in the visualization of the anatomy of the portion of the bone and the layer of tissue being assessed or treated, i.e. superficialis fascia, muscle, bone, dura, fluid and nervous system.

Assess the relationship between the base and the vault. Palpate the sagittal, lambdoid and coronal sutures for structure and function to identify restriction of motion. Evaluate the freedom of intraosseous compliance of the frontal bone. Appraise the relationship between the frontal, sphenoid and parietal bones. Dysfunction of the frontal bone is associated with learning difficulties and behavioral problems. Frontal dysfunctions are also of significance when problem solving complaints involving the viscerocranium.

Treat dysfunctions identified in the SBS, cranial base, vault and intracranial dural membranes. Such dysfunction can affect the neurocranium, viscerocranium and, through the core link, the remainder of the body. Treatment applied to the skull can release the intraspinal dural membranes. Although this may be beneficial when treating scoliosis with tethered intraspinal membranes, it must be stressed that the treatment of scoliosis also includes attention directly to the spine and the use of rehabilitative exercises.

Observation and palpation of the viscerocranium

The shape of the face, like that of the cranial base, is determined by genetic factors. The development of the face, however, is also strongly influenced by epigenetic factors. These include the utilization of the musculature of the viscerocranium, as occurs with oral functions, respiration and visual functions. The face, therefore, is a manifestation of the functional impact of the facial musculature and surrounding fasciae.

Observe the facial expression of the adolescent. As the individual matures, the facial soft tissues begin to create a mask which indicates that person's habits of facial expression. An individual's emotional status becomes progressively more and more engrained into the structure of their face. Negative emotions and the stresses of life will produce a pattern of internal rotation in the soft tissues, whereas positive emotional events and a relaxed environment participate to produce external rotation of the facial tissues. A very secure adolescent will usually demonstrate an external rotation appearance with eyes wide open and a wide smiling mouth. These observations are consistent with what will be observed in the rest of the body, but are more prominent in the soft tissues of the face. The face allows us to communicate with the world. The status of this communication may be seen in the creases around sensory structures, such as the eyes, mouth and nose, that are interfaces between the outside world and the inner individual.

Orofacial functions also affect the observable structure of the face and the outside world plays a part in the development of these functions. Differences in facial structure are linked to the environment. An individual who lives in a humid environment will have a difference in nasal structure when compared to a person from a dry environment.[24] In addition, function affects structure as may be seen with an adolescent who has always been a chronic mouth breather and demonstrates underdevelopment of the nasal cavities. Emotional and physical experience are thus imprinted in the structures of the individual's face.

The remainder of the examination of the viscerocranium of the adolescent is essentially the same as discussed above in 'Physical examination of the child'. Pay attention to the zygomae, an area in the face that is frequently traumatized. Common adolescent complaints include rhinitis and sinusitis, and malocclusion. Osteopathic treatment may be employed to address pain, function and structure. It is appropriate to treat viscerocranial dysfunction in adolescents with indirect principles. Treatment of the adolescent viscerocranium is very similar of that of the child, bearing in mind that structural patterns become more engrained and are less readily influenced as the individual ages. Thus the treatment of the adolescent, like that of the adult, is more effective when addressing pain and functional issues, while attempting to modify structure is progressively less effective as the adolescent ages.

REFERENCES

1. Sutherland WG. Contributions of thought. Fort Worth, TX: Sutherland Cranial Teaching Foundation; 1998:1.
2. Nelson KE, Sergueef N, Glonek T. Recording the rate of the cranial rhythmic impulse. J Am Osteopath Assoc 2006;106(6):337–41.
3. Nelson KE. The primary respiratory mechanism. AAO Journal 2002;12(4):25–34.
4. Baum JD, Searls D. Head shape and size of pre-term low-birth-weight infants. Dev Med Child Neurol 1971;13:576–81.
5. Glass RB, Fernbach SK, Norton KI, Choi PS, Naidich TP. The infant skull: a vault of information. Radiographics 2004;24(2):507–22.
6. Amiel-Tison C, Gosselin J, Infante-Rivard C. Head growth and cranial assessment at neurological examination in infancy. Dev Med Child Neurol 2002;44(9):643–8.
7. Huang MH, Gruss JS, Clarren SK. The differential diagnosis of posterior plagiocephaly: true lambdoid synostosis versus positional molding. Plast Reconstr Surg 1996;98(5):765–74.
8. David DJ, Menard RM. Occipital plagiocephaly. Br J Plast Surg 2000;53(5):367–77.
9. Mulliken JB, Vander Woude DL, Hansen M, LaBrie RA, Scott RM. Analysis of posterior plagiocephaly: deformational versus synostotic. Plast Reconstr Surg 1999;103(2):371–80.
10. Oommen A. A study of the normal position of auricle in neonates. Clin Anat 1997;10(1):19–21.
11. Still AT. Philosophy of osteopathy. Kirskville, MO: A.T. Still; 1899:16. Reprinted: Indianapolis, IN: American Academy of Osteopathy; 1971.
12. Volpon JB. Footprint analysis during the growth period. J Pediatr Orthop 1994;14(1):83–5.
13. Algranati PS. Effect of developmental status on the approach to physical examination. Pediatr Clin North Am 1998;45(1):1–23.
14. Sergueef N. L'odyssée de l'iliaque. Paris: Spek; 1985.
15. Sergueef N. Normaliser la colonne sans 'manipulation vertébrale'. Paris: Spek; 1994.
16. Brady RJ, Dean JB, Skinner TM, Gross MT. Limb length inequality: clinical implications for assessment and intervention. J Orthop Sports Phys Ther 2003;33(5):221–34.
17. Nelson KE. The management of low back pain. AAO Journal 1999;9(1):33–9.
18. Irwin GL. Roentgen determination of the time of closure of the spheno-occipital synchondrosis. Radiology 1960;75:450–3.
19. Madeline LA, Elster AD. Suture closure in the human chondrocranium: CT assessment. Radiology 1995;196(3):747–56.
20. Mann SS, Naidich TP, Towbin RB, Doundoulakis SH. Imaging of postnatal maturation of the skull base. Neuroimaging Clin N Am 2000;10(1):1–21, vii.
21. Melsen B. Time of closure of the spheno-occipital synchondrosis determined on dry skulls. A radiographic craniometric study. Acta Odontol Scand 1969;27(1):73–90.
22. Okamoto K, Ito J, Tokiguchi S, Furusawa T. High-resolution CT findings in the development of spheno-occipital synchondrosis. Am J Neuroradiol 1996;17(1):117–20.
23. Williams PL (ed). Gray's anatomy, 38th edn. Edinburgh: Churchill Livingstone; 1995.
24. Irmak MK, Korkmaz A, Erogul O. Selective brain cooling seems to be a mechanism leading to human craniofacial diversity observed in different geographical regions. Med Hypotheses 2004;63(6):974–9.

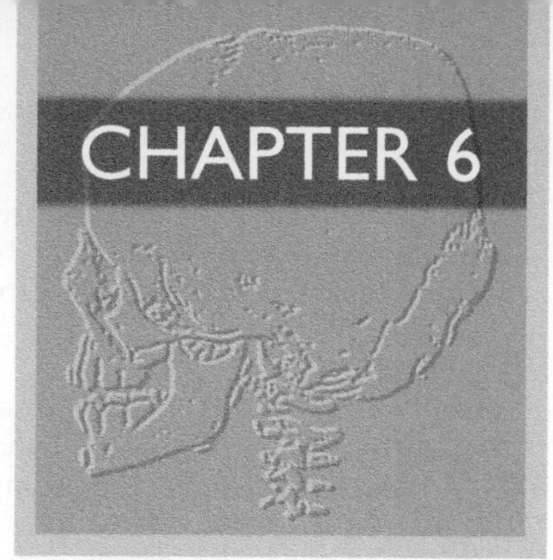

TREATMENT OF THE PATIENT

'Listen through the hands, not with the hands.' —RE BECKER[1]

The main principles

The procedures described hereafter are intended to provide the osteopathic practitioner with a collection of techniques that may be employed to treat infants, children and adolescents. These procedures follow the fundamental principles of classic osteopathy and, as always, are based on knowledge of anatomy. Thus, Still stated: 'An osteopath reasons from his knowledge of anatomy. He compares the work of the abnormal body with the work of the normal body.'[2]

These procedures should be considered as a foundation from which anyone can develop their own practice. It must be stressed that osteopathy is the treatment of the patient and not of the condition. Therefore, to consider these procedures only as a list of recipes for the treatment of the ailments that affect infants, children and adolescents is insufficient. In order for them to be effectively employed, precise diagnosis of the dysfunctional pattern of the individual is an absolute prerequisite.

The fundamental principles of osteopathy may be summarized as follows:

- The body is a unit. Dysfunction in any area will impact all other areas of the body through membranous, myofascial, bony articular, neurologic and vascular interactions, and through the primary respiratory mechanism (PRM). Consequently, the osteopathic treatment of somatic dysfunction affects the entire body.
- The body is a self-regulatory mechanism. Its function is directed toward homeostasis, i.e. the maintenance of physiologic balance resulting from a dynamic state of equilibrium between interdependent body functions. Somatic dysfunction impairs this mechanism.
- Structure determines function and is, in turn, influenced by function. Dysfunction – the impediment of normal function – will, over time, result in abnormal structure. What is unique in the treatment of infants and young children is that structure is responsive and consequently may be affected by osteopathic procedures. The modification of structure becomes progressively less successful as the individual ages, so that the treatment of adolescents is more effective when addressing functional issues.
- The body has the inherent capacity to heal itself that can be impaired by its inability to compensate for age, illness and somatic dysfunction. The progression of time is permanent, while illness may be treated to a greater or lesser extent by standard medical means and somatic dysfunction addressed by

osteopathic treatment. Effective treatment of somatic dysfunction, through the body's self-healing capacity, will enhance standard medical treatment of illness.

The objective of osteopathic practice, therefore, is to identify and treat somatic dysfunction at the various levels of fluid, membranous, myofascial, ligamentous, intra- and interosseous dysfunctions, thereby enhancing the whole body capacity for repair and maintenance of health.

The identification of somatic dysfunction is the result of observation, palpation for structure and palpation for function. Palpation for function is further subdivided into gross motion testing and tests of listening. Mastery of the tests of listening often provides sufficient information to eliminate the need for gross motion testing. To effectively employ touch to listen, the practitioner should focus on the inherent motility that is part of the PRM as it is expressed in the structure being examined. Every structure within the body manifests the biphasic PRM motion. Flexion–external rotation and extension–internal rotation are concomitant with the inspiratory and expiratory phases of the PRM, respectively. In the presence of somatic dysfunction, the symmetry and potency of this biphasic phenomenon is impaired. The impediment results in decreased motility, or restriction, in one phase of the mechanism and the sense of balance that is normally felt between the two phases shifts toward the unencumbered phase.

Listening for dysfunction within the PRM, its rate and potency in any given structure, or between structures, requires focus to obtain the desired information. As the practitioner masters the art of listening, the time and patience initially necessary for the novice will be replaced by rapid awareness that offers an efficient means of diagnosis. Tests of listening provide rapid identification of dysfunction while maintaining total respect for the patient. They are, most often, performed in the patient's position of comfort. Additionally, because the lightest possible touch is employed, infants and children are not disturbed, making these procedures of particular value.

There are as many different methods to treat a patient as there are osteopaths, and skilled practitioners regularly get positive results. Therefore, no category of treatment procedures should be considered to be a panacea. There are a multitude of treatment types that may be employed when treating infants, children and adolescents. They cover a broad spectrum from forceful articulatory to indirect cranial procedures. The more aggressive methods may be employed when treating adults and, to some extent, older adolescents; the more gentle procedures lend themselves to the treatment of infants, children and adolescents.

Ultimately, all manipulative treatment procedures may be classified as direct, indirect or combined. Subgroups exist but the main principles stay the same. The goal of manipulation is the alleviation of somatic dysfunction. The diagnosis of somatic dysfunction has been assigned a numeric identifier (739) in the *International Classification of Diseases*, ICD-9.[3] The classification is subdivided according to the anatomic region where dysfunction is diagnosed: somatic dysfunction cranial 739.0, cervical 739.1, thoracic 739.2, lumbar 739.3, sacrum/pelvis 739.4, ilium/pelvis 739.5, lower extremity 739.6, upper extremity 739.7, ribs 739.8 and abdomen/other 739.9. Somatic dysfunction is almost universally identified in the context of the impediment of normal motion of the dysfunctional structure. The resultant motion restriction may be treated using direct, indirect or combined procedures.

Direct procedures move the dysfunctional structure in the direction in which motion is restricted with the intention of overcoming that restriction. Indirect procedures take the dysfunctional structure away from the restriction. When treating infants, children and adolescents the use of indirect procedures is more appropriate. Also referred to as functional or sensorial techniques, in these procedures the operator follows the dysfunctional structure as it moves away from the restriction to a point of balance. This balancing is accomplished by listening for the direction of freedom of motion in the major and minor movements, and then by following it. This will lead to a point of balance where spontaneous pulmonary respiratory cooperation often occurs. Following this, the structure being treated will become unencumbered in all directions of the major and minor movements and the inherent motility of the PRM will be optimized.

Pulmonary respiration normally occurs at a frequency slightly greater than that of the PRM. Indirect procedures that are employed in accord with the PRM tend to induce patient relaxation. When the patient relaxes, the respiratory rate normally slows, approximating that of the PRM. The coming together of these two independent rhythms results in entrainment that is frequently heralded by a deep sighing pulmonary respiration. This may be intentionally accomplished in older individuals by instructing them to take a deep breath at a strategic point in the treatment. This occurs when, after having followed the freedom of motion in the major and minor movements, a point of balance is obtained but the tissues are not yet ready to release. This is what is palpated when a still point – the temporary cessation of the rhythmic motion of the PRM – is reached but the ensuing response from the PRM is restrained. For very young children who cannot be instructed to breathe deeply, the practitioner must be patient and, when the still point is reached, wait for the PRM to respond. A still point should never be held or restrained. This is contrary to the principles of indirect treatment.

The perception of following the dysfunctional motion pattern may be enhanced by employing visualization of the anatomic area being treated, paying attention to anatomic layers from the most superficial movement and tension of the skin through to the movements of the deepest structures in the region being addressed. The palpatory contact is always light but following indirect principles the firmness of touch is dictated by the depth of the dysfunction being treated. It is important to remember that the goal of treatment should be focused on the optimization of the quality, potency and fluidity of the motion, rather than the quantity.

It must be recognized, when treating infants and children, that the flexibility of the tissues results in palpable motion patterns that are potentially very fluid in nature. As such, the suggestion that the various bones move upon specific axes of motion is an artificial construct used to communicate how they move. The patterns described in this text are global descriptions of dysfunctional mechanics. They are intended to provide the practitioner with a model with which to interpret their observations. In practice it is important to follow the pattern that the patient presents and not attempt to force the patient into some preconceived pattern. The utilization of tests of listening and indirect treatment procedures requires that the practitioner trusts their perceptions.

Cranial osteopathy addresses the total body, not just the skull and sacrum; as such, the reciprocal is also true. The dysfunction of the skull is as inseparably linked to the functional pattern of the entire body as dysfunction within the body is linked to the pattern of the skull. Utilizing indirect principles, the patient must be allowed to position themselves in a manner that affords total ease and relaxation. They should be allowed to reposition themselves spontaneously as necessary throughout the course of the treatment. This principle may be readily observed when treating infants and young children who, unlike adults, will not consciously assume a position that is deemed to be appropriate for treatment. They will move with the treatment process, at which time the interrelationship of the various parts of the body is readily apparent.

Treating the whole body means that all involved anatomic components – membranes, ligaments, fasciae, muscles, bones, joints and viscera, as well as the PRM – should be addressed during the treatment. Manipulative treatment utilizing the cranial model impacts the patient through its effect on the anatomy and physiology of the area. It further results in a global response through the action of the autonomic nervous system (ANS). Any treatment that influences the PRM influences the ANS. That, in turn, affects the inherent biodynamic forces of the individual, causing the body to balance itself globally and also at the precise level of the treated dysfunction.

When treating infants and small children, it may be more effective to allow them to rest either in their mother's arms or, in the case of toddlers, to have them seated with some toys to put them at ease. In order to follow indirect principles, the child should be comfortable and should accept the practitioner's touch. It is important to realize that if the child is comfortable, the caregiver will also be at ease. The comfort of the caregiver further reinforces the comfort of the child. The search for functional balance should be a harmonious experience for all involved, and the child, if at all possible, should not cry. Sometimes crying might act as a form of respiratory cooperation with the manipulative treatment, but this should in no way be used as an excuse to be insensitive to the child. In essentially every instance treatment can be successfully completed without causing the child to cry.

To employ indirect treatment procedures effectively, the practitioner must also be relaxed and comfortable. They should be seated on a stool with adjustable height and wheels that allow them to readily shift their position. Their hands must be relaxed and warm. Their fingers should conform to the contour of the area being treated. Tension of the fingers occludes the proprioceptive cues from the interphalangeal and metacarpophalangeal joints that are necessary to follow the PRM and the patient's response to the treatment process. The focus of touch should be bilateral. It is easy to become focused on proprioceptive input from the practitioner's dominant hand. Hand placement need not be restricted to the position of initial contact or that preordained by a formal technique description. The practitioner should feel free to shift their hand position according to the response of the area being treated.

A variation of an indirect treatment approach is the application of pumping and molding. This is particularly indicated for intraosseous and chronic dysfunctions and consists of following the freedom of the major and minor movements of the dysfunctional area in association with the movement of the PRM. The movement of the PRM within the dysfunctional pattern may be augmented to gently pump the area being treated in the direction of the restriction. This is not in the pure sense a direct procedure because the barrier imposed by the dysfunction is never engaged. The process occurs in the position of ease but employs the rhythm and potency of the PRM to remove the dysfunctional restriction. The operator continues this pumping action up to the point of release. This procedure is very effective when the minor movements and PRM are specifically employed in conjunction with the more readily identifiable major movements. Techniques of molding may be applied to address the intraosseous dysfunctions of a bone. They consist of balancing the different portions of the bone that constitute the dysfunction in accordance with the principles of indirect techniques and pumping described above. Very often the two procedures are associated, thus speaking of 'pumping–molding'.

If you utilize tests of listening you will identify the site of greatest restriction. This should be treated first. However, individuals with limited experience are often uncertain where to begin and appreciate treatment protocols. Such recipes are of limited value because no two patients, even though they share the same anatomy, are the same. Consequently, treatment protocols, in the broadest sense, can be identified, but they should be used only as imperfect models and the treatment, when applied, must always take individual patient variations into consideration first.

A safe beginning is to start with the area of chief complaint, always bearing in mind that the area of complaint may be secondary to adjacent or distant dysfunction. Additionally, if the chief complaint is one of pain it may not be appropriate to begin there with infants and young children. It is important to build trust with these patients and commencing the patient encounter by manipulating a painful area is not advisable. In this case it is appropriate to begin these sessions by addressing general body mechanics with myofascial release procedures intended to induce relaxation and then to progress to more specific treatment interventions. Often it may be useful to treat areas surrounding the area of complaint to attain relaxation.

It is good practice to begin treating the pelvis and spine, particularly the upper thoracic and upper cervical regions, before commencing treatment of the skull. Treatment of infants, children and adolescents is best done using indirect procedures and principles. If an area of somatic dysfunction is reticent to treatment it is not appropriate to continue working on that area but rather to move to another area of dysfunction, treat it, and when it responds, return to the resistant area and assess for changes. Even then it may not be appropriate to treat the resistant area at that time.

When treating the skull, first address the membranous strain patterns and then the cranial base with specific attention to the sphenobasilar synchondrosis (SBS). When the membranes have been released and the SBS has been satisfactorily treated, unless there is reticence as discussed above, address any interosseous dysfunctions between the occiput and sphenoid with the temporal bones. Treat intraosseous dysfunctions of the occiput and temporal bones and, if the patient is young enough and the synchondroses are not yet fused, the sphenoid.

If the complaint is one of viscerocranial dysfunction, treat the relationship between the sphenoid and frontal bones, the frontal bones themselves and the specific areas of dysfunction in the viscerocranium. Temporomandibular joint (TMJ) complaints may be treated after the cranial base, with attention to temporal bone dysfunction, has been addressed.

The duration of treatment of any given area is dictated by the response of the patient. Once a response has occurred, even if that response is not complete resolution, treatment of that area should be stopped and the intervention should move to another area if necessary.

Hand placement for the treatment procedures described below is the same as that employed for the diagnostic tests of listening. This offers the advantage that once experience has been garnered, diagnosis and treatment can blend seamlessly into one another. Although useful procedures are described below, the best techniques are the ones that the practitioner creates according to anatomy, physiologic motion, the patient's dysfunctions and the practitioner's internal balance and technical ability. The practitioner must have the ability to adapt and to be creative. No technique can be repeated identically from one patient to another and often not in the same patient from visit to visit.

Ideally, a child should be normalized at the time of birth. This requires some skill with procedures, but equally as important is great patience and the ability to establish respectful contact with the infant.

The reward is that infants respond quickly and sometimes with what might be interpreted by individuals unacquainted with osteopathic principles of treatment as miraculous results.

Equilibration of intracranial and intraspinal membranes

EQUILIBRATION OF INTRACRANIAL MEMBRANES

Global equilibration of intracranial membranes

Indications

Equilibration of intracranial membranes is part of every cranial treatment, whatever other procedures are utilized, and is often the first cranial procedure to employ. It is also indicated to promote venous sinus drainage.

Procedure (Fig. 6.1)

Patient supine; practitioner seated at the head of the patient when using a vault hold or to the side of the table when using a fronto-occipital hold.

For the vault hold, the thumbs are interlocked over the sagittal suture, the hands contacting the lateral parts of the skull so that the tips of the index fingers are on the top of the greater wings of the sphenoid, the middle fingers are on the temporal squamae anterior to the external auditory meatus, the ring fingers are on the temporal bones behind the external auditory meatus and the little fingers are on the occipital squama. A patient will relax so that the cranial rhythmic impulse can be observed in an unencumbered fashion only if the practitioner's hand placement is comfortable. The practitioner should, therefore, contact the skull with the lightest possible pressure.

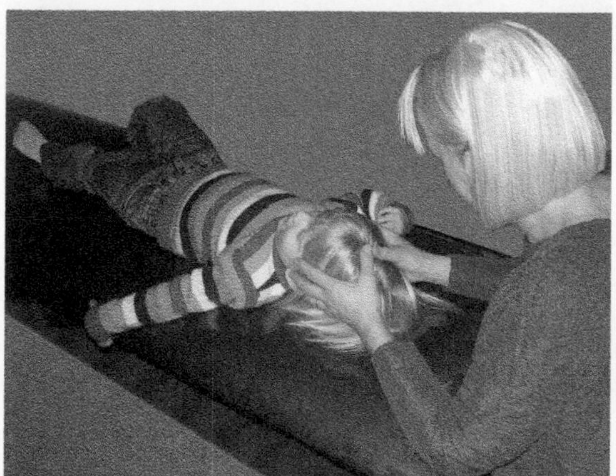

Figure 6.1. *Equilibration of intracranial membranes using the vault hold.*

For the fronto-occipital hold, one hand is transversely placed under the occiput (Fig. 6.18). The other hand is placed in contact with the frontal portion of the patient's skull, such that the tip of the thumb is on the superior aspect of one greater wing and the tip of the middle finger is on the corresponding spot on the other side. In infants and young children, it is best to position the hand on the frontal bone in such a fashion as not to cover the patient's eyes.

Visualize the membranes, listen and follow in the direction of ease, paying attention to the PRM until a release occurs. At this point a spontaneous respiratory cooperation frequently takes place in the form of a deep breath. If this does not occur, or the release is incomplete, patients who are old enough to follow instructions may be asked to breathe deeply, inhale and hold to augment the release of a flexion–external rotation dysfunctional pattern, or to exhale and hold for extension–internal rotation.

Remarks

As the practitioner follows the imbalance of membranous tension they may need to modify their hold, always respecting the minor movements within the dysfunction so that release can occur. When release occurs, it is accompanied by a sensation of the tissues becoming warmer, softer and more flexible.

Full membranous release always requires treatment of inter- and intraosseous dysfunction.

Equilibration of the tentorium cerebelli

Indications

Temporal bone imbalance; CN III, IV, V and VI entrapment; promotion of venous sinus drainage; balance of the hypophysial fossa.

Procedure (Fig. 6.2)

Patient supine; practitioner seated at the head of the patient, holding the temporal bones, with the thumbs superior and index fingers inferior to the zygomatic processes. The middle fingers contact the area of the external auditory meatus, the ring fingers are on the tips of the mastoid processes and

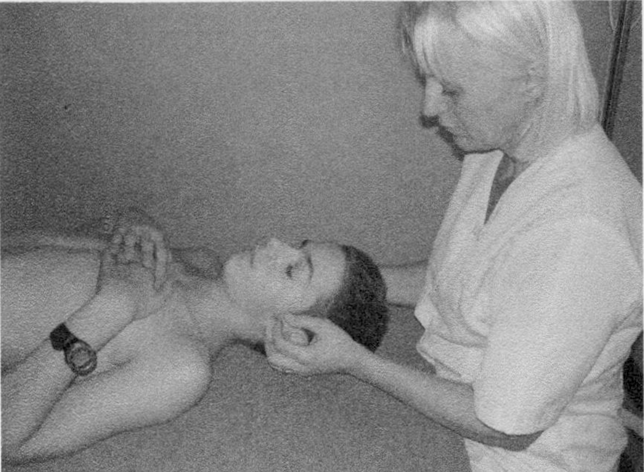

Figure 6.2. *Equilibration of the tentorium cerebelli holding the temporal bones.*

the little fingers are on the occiput posterior to the asterion.

Visualize the tentorium cerebelli, listen and, paying attention to the PRM, follow in the direction of ease of the tentorium cerebelli and the motion pattern of the temporal bones until a release occurs. Respiratory cooperation may be employed. The patient can inhale and hold to augment the release of temporal bone external rotation, or exhale and hold for internal rotation.

Remarks

Infants can become uncomfortable with this procedure if the external auditory meatus is blocked by the examiner's middle finger. By moving the thumbs to contact the lateral aspects of the greater wings of the sphenoid (Fig. 6.3), the practitioner may add the control of the sphenoid to this procedure. This allows them to focus attention on the anterior portions and attachments of the tentorium cerebelli, particularly the roof and lateral wall of the cavernous sinus as they relate to the sphenoid. The petrosphenoid ligament, sometimes considered to be a thickened portion of the anterior tentorium cerebelli, may also be addressed with this procedure.

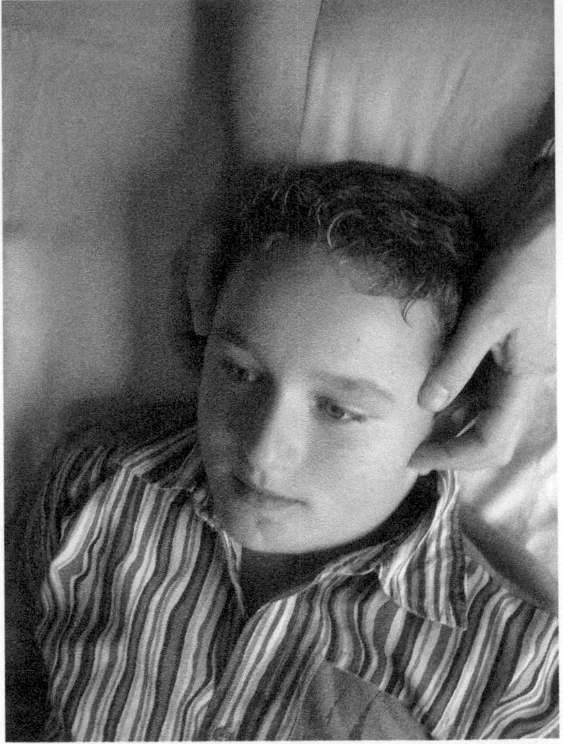

Figure 6.3. *Equilibration of the tentorium cerebelli holding the temporal and sphenoid bones.*

EQUILIBRATION OF INTRASPINAL MEMBRANES

Indications

Facilitation of harmonious function between the three diaphragms: cranial, thoracoabdominal and pelvic. Equilibration of intraspinal membranes is part of every spinal treatment.

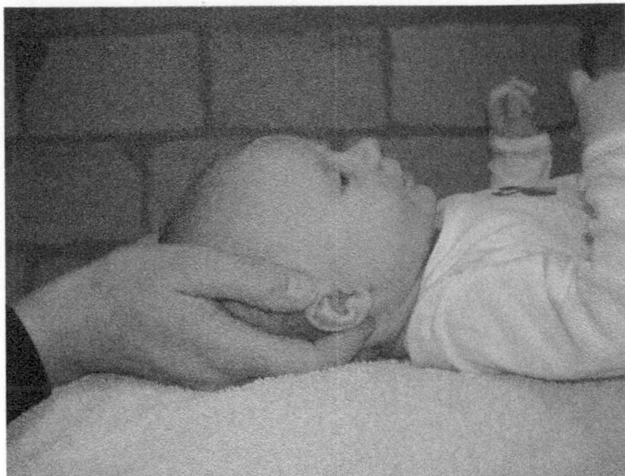

Figure 6.4. *Equilibration of intraspinal membranes: one-practitioner procedure.*

One-practitioner procedure

Procedure (Fig. 6.4)

Patient supine; practitioner seated at the patient's head with both hands placed in a relaxed fashion beneath the occiput in such a way that the pads of the fingers contact the occipital squama just below the superior nuchal line.

While palpating the occiput, visualize the intracranial dural attachments and the core link, the continuity of the intracranial dura with the spinal dura and its attachment to the sacrum and coccyx. Listen and, paying attention to the PRM, follow in the direction of ease to the point where a sensation of occipital balance is felt. Balance may be enhanced by instructing older children to dorsiflex their feet and/or place their legs in external rotation to facilitate sacral flexion and augment the release of a flexion dysfunctional pattern, or to plantar flex and/or internally rotate the legs for extension. Patterns of torsion and sidebending demonstrate external rotation on one side and internal rotation on the other. This procedure can, therefore, be carried out by requesting dorsiflexion and external rotation on the side of the external rotation, and plantar flexion and internal rotation on the other side. At this point spontaneous respiratory cooperation may occur in the form of a deep breath. If not, the patient can be asked to take a deep breath and briefly hold it in inhalation to augment flexion or in exhalation to augment extension.

Two-practitioner procedure

Procedure (Fig. 6.5)

Patient supine; one practitioner is seated at the patient's head as described above and the other practitioner stands at the level of the patient's pelvis, putting one hand under the patient's sacrum with the fingers directed cephalad toward the sacral base and the middle finger extending up to the spinous process of L5. The index finger contacts one sacroiliac articulation and the ring finger contacts the other sacroiliac articulation. Employing indirect principles, both practitioners should follow the tissues they are palpating until a release occurs.

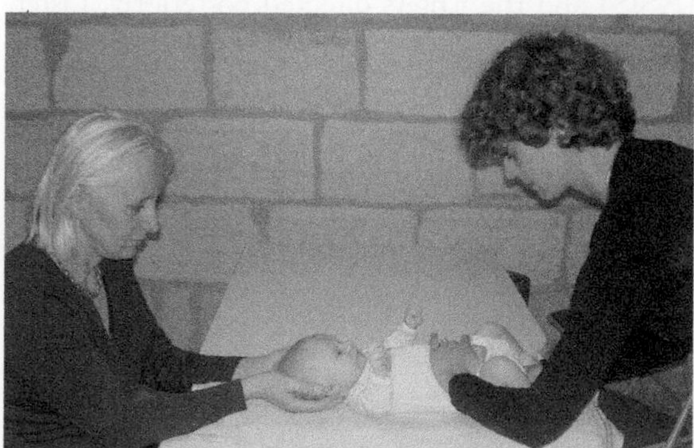

Figure 6.5. *Equilibration of intraspinal membranes: two-practitioner procedure.*

Remarks

This procedure allows efficient craniosacral equilibration but the two practitioners must cooperate. With experience, it is possible for one practitioner to appreciate the effect on the mechanism that is being exerted by the other practitioner.

When treating infants, one practitioner may perform this procedure by placing one hand beneath the sacrum and the other hand under the head (Fig. 6.6). The patient may be supine on the table, held in the practitioner's lap or held upright facing the practitioner. The procedure may be employed to address the dysfunctional patterns associated with fetal position.

STERNAL EQUILIBRATION PROCEDURES

Indications

Functionally, within the PRM, the sternum is balanced between the occiput and sacrum and its normalization is essential for optimal function of the PRM as well as local function of the thoracic cage.

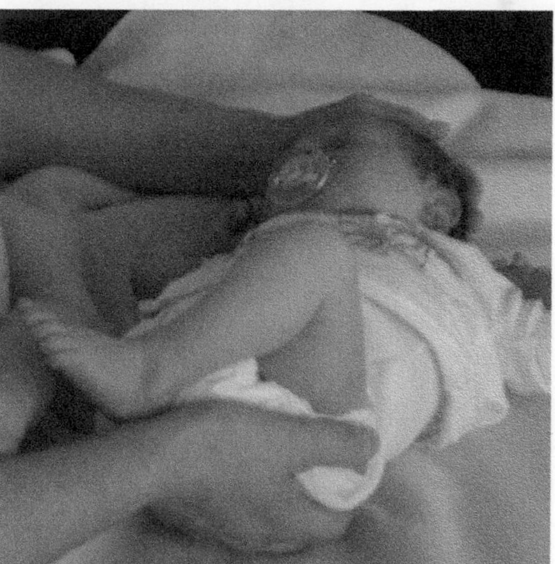

Figure 6.6. *Equilibration of intraspinal membranes in infants.*

Sterno-occipital equilibration procedure

Procedure (Fig. 6.7)

Patient supine; practitioner seated at the head of the patient with one hand cradling the occiput, the other resting on the sternum with the palm over the sternal body and the fingers directed inferiorly. Listen and, paying attention to the PRM, follow the sternum and occiput, allowing them both to move into the position of ease where spontaneous respiratory cooperation will frequently occur in the form of a deep breath. If this does not occur, or the release is incomplete, ask the patient to breathe deeply, inhale and hold to augment the release of a flexion dysfunctional pattern, or to exhale and hold for extension.

Sternosacral equilibration procedure

Procedure (Fig. 6.8)

Patient supine; practitioner either seated or standing at the level of the pelvis with one hand on the sternum and the other under the sacrum, palm up, with the fingers directed cephalad toward the sacral base and the middle finger extending up to the spinous process of L5. The index finger contacts one sacroiliac articulation and the ring finger contacts the other sacroiliac articulation. Listen and, paying attention to the PRM, allow the sternum and sacrum to move into the position of ease until spontaneous respiratory cooperation occurs in the form of a deep breath. If this does not occur, or the release is incomplete the patient who is old enough may be asked to breathe deeply, inhale and hold to augment the release of a flexion dysfunctional pattern, or to exhale and hold for extension.

Remarks

Obtaining a total body release results in synchronous motion between the three diaphragms: cranial, thoracoabdominal and pelvic.

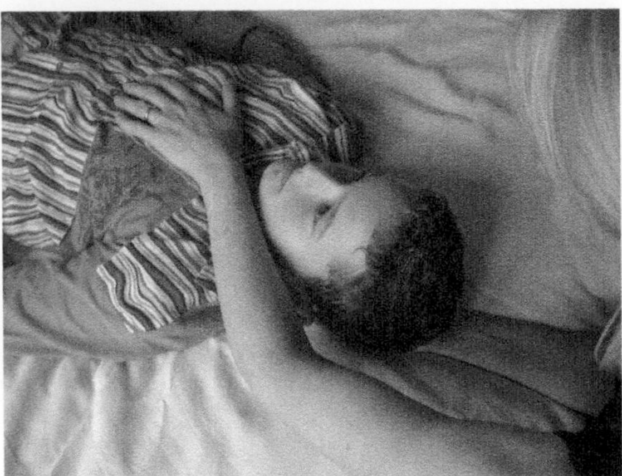

Figure 6.7. *Sterno-occipital equilibration procedure.*

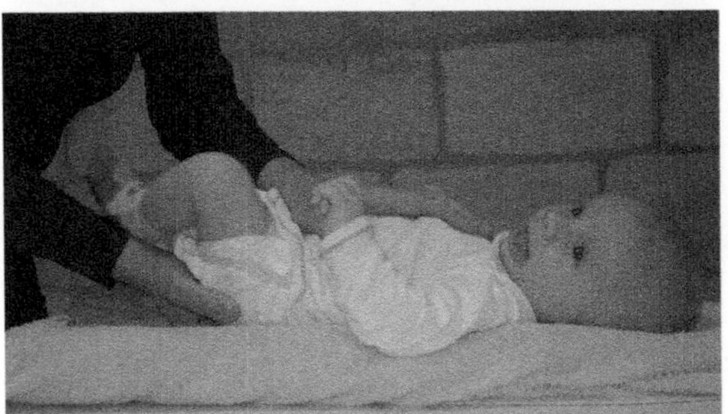

Figure 6.8. *Sternosacral equilibration procedure.*

Myofascial procedures

LOWER EXTREMITY MYOFASCIAL PROCEDURES

Global lower extremity myofascial procedure

Indications

Intoeing or out-toeing; varus or valgus deformities of the knee; patellar disorders; toewalking.

Procedure (Fig. 6.9)

Patient supine; practitioner seated beside the patient on the side of the dysfunction. Grasp the foot with one hand such that the thumb contacts the lateral aspect of the foot and the fingers the medial aspect. Place the other hand on the iliac crest, with the thumb contacting the anterior superior iliac spine (ASIS) and the fingers directed posteriorly. Listen and, paying attention to the PRM, allow the

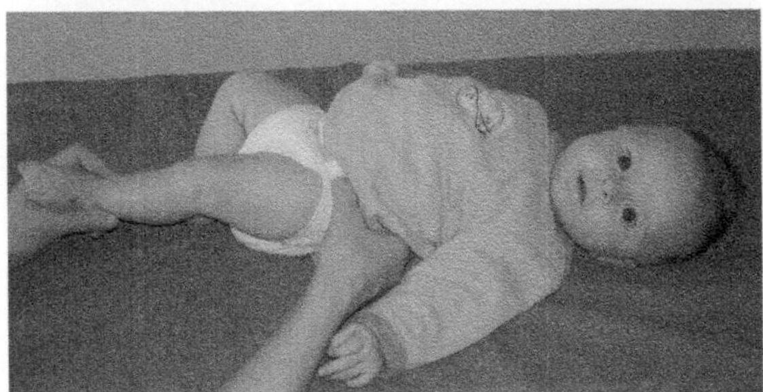

Figure 6.9. *Global lower extremity myofascial procedure.*

myofascial structures of the entire extremity to move into the position of ease. This is most often a torsional pattern along the long axis of the limb and may require various combinations of positioning of the ankle, knee and hip to augment the release. Because myofascial patterns are total body phenomena it is necessary to position the entire body in the position of comfort.

Remarks

The total body position of comfort is most often the position that infants and children will spontaneously assume when lying on the treatment table, and as such it is important not to attempt to force these patients into some preconceived position for treatment.

This procedure is most effective when employed in infants and children. When treating adolescents, the size of the lower extremity may necessitate that the procedure be performed by two practitioners.

Segmental lower extremity myofascial procedure

Indications

Intraosseous tibial and femoral torsions; gait disorders; intoeing or out-toeing.

Procedure (Fig. 6.10)

Patient supine; practitioner seated beside the patient on the side of the dysfunction. Grasp the proximal and distal ends of the segment to be treated, most commonly the tibia, occasionally the femur, with your hands. Listen and, paying attention to the PRM, allow the myofascial structures to move into the position of ease. This is most often a torsional pattern along the long axis of the segment. Await a release.

Foot myofascial procedure

Indications

Metatarsus adductus; pes cavus; pes planus; toewalking; in adolescents, plantar fasciitis.

Procedure (Fig. 6.11)

Patient supine; practitioner seated beside the patient on the side of the dysfunction at the level of the foot. Grasp the distal foot between the thumb and fingers of one hand and cradle the heel with the other hand. Listen and, paying attention to the PRM, allow the myofascial structures of the foot to move into the position of ease. This is most often a torsional pattern involving internal rotation of the distal foot. Await a release.

UPPER EXTREMITY MYOFASCIAL PROCEDURE

Indications

Brachial plexus injury; nursemaid's elbow; writer's cramp.

Procedure (Fig. 6.12)

Patient supine or seated; practitioner seated beside the patient on the side of the dysfunction. Grasp the wrist with the caudal hand, such that the thumb contacts the extensor surface and the fingers the flexor surface proximal to the wrist. Place the cephalic hand on the shoulder, with the thumb

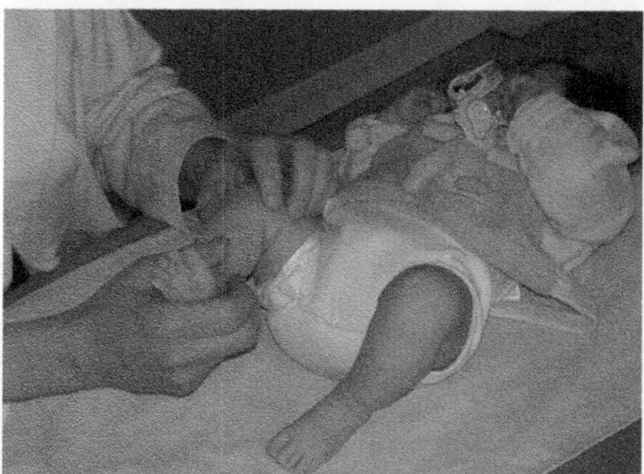

Figure 6.10. *Segmental lower extremity myofascial procedure.*

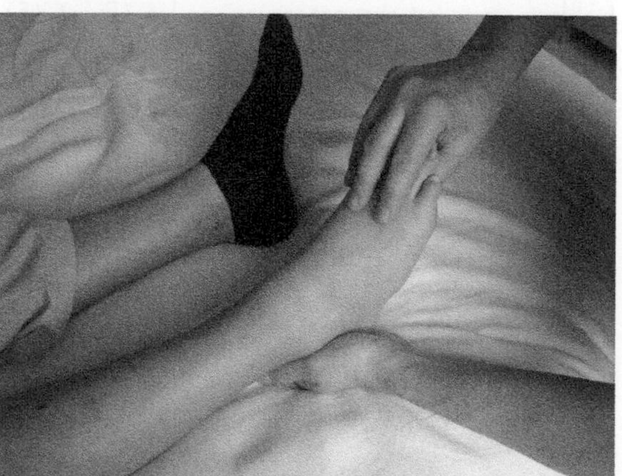

Figure 6.11. *Foot myofascial procedure.*

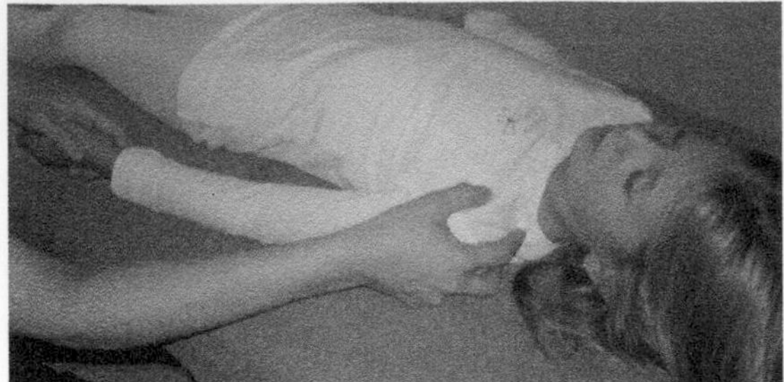

Figure 6.12. *Upper extremity myofascial procedure.*

contacting the clavicle and the fingers directed posteriorly. Listen and, paying attention to the PRM, allow the myofascial structures of the entire extremity to move into the position of ease. This is most often a torsional pattern along the long axis of the limb and may require various combinations of positioning of the wrist, forearm (pronation or supination), elbow and shoulder to facilitate the release. Because myofascial patterns are total body phenomena it is necessary to allow the entire body to assume the position of comfort. Await a release.

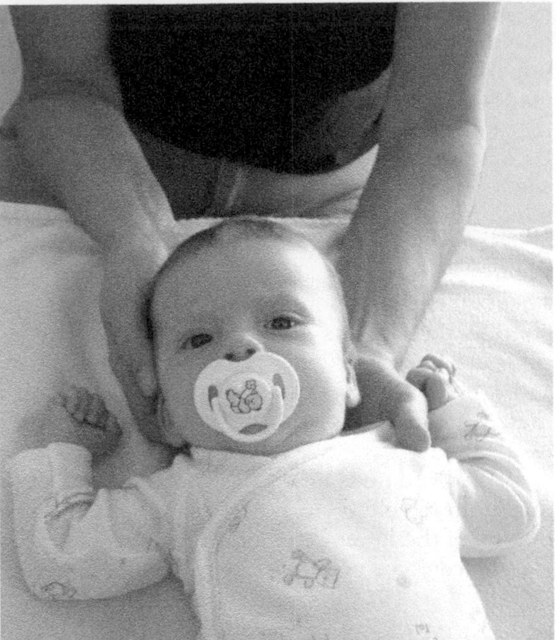

Figure 6.13. *Occipitoscapular procedure.*

AXIAL MYOFASCIAL PROCEDURES

Occipito scapular procedure

Indications

Myofascial tensions found in association with brachial plexus injury; torticollis; plagiocephaly.

Procedure (Fig. 6.13)

Patient supine; practitioner seated at the patient's head with one hand cradling the occiput and the other on the shoulder. Infants may be treated holding them on the practitioner's lap (Fig. 6.15). Listen and, paying attention to the PRM, allow the myofascial structures of the area to move into the position of ease. It may be necessary to shift the position of the shoulder to obtain the release. Await a release.

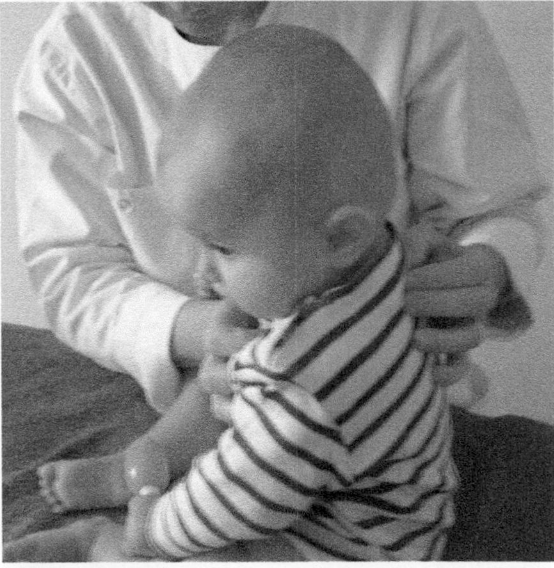

Figure 6.14. *Sternovertebral procedure.*

Sternovertebral procedure

Indications

Myofascial tensions found in association with thoracic cage; pulmonary dysfunctions.

Procedure (Fig. 6.14)

Patient supine or seated; practitioner seated at the patient's side with one hand on the sternum and the other on the upper thoracic spine. Listen and, paying attention to the PRM, allow the thoracic myofascial structures to move into the position of ease. Most of the time the anterior and posterior fasciae will move in opposite directions. Await a release.

Remarks

A similar procedure may be employed to address the myofascial relationships between the scapula and thoracic spine by placing one hand on the scapula and the other on the thoracic spine.

Molding procedures

SACRAL MOLDING PROCEDURE

Indications

Intraosseous sacral somatic dysfunction; facilitation of release of the intracranial and spinal membranes; to affect pelvic splanchnic autonomic tone in the treatment of visceral conditions such as enuresis, constipation and dysmenorrhea.

Procedure (Fig. 6.15)

Patient supine; practitioner standing or seated beside the patient at the level of the pelvis. Place one hand beneath the patient, palm up, with the fingers directed cephalad and cradle the sacrum. Note the patterns of craniosacral flexion–extension, torsions and/or sidebending of the sacrum. Using indirect principles, follow these patterns to facilitate listening to the PRM and assess the intraosseous motility of the sacrum to identify restricted motion between the sacral segments. Following the freedom of the major and minor movements of the sacrum, employ the inherent forces of the PRM to gently pump the intraosseous dysfunction, molding the sacrum.

Remarks

This is a very relaxing procedure. It increases parasympathetic tone and may be employed to begin treatment.

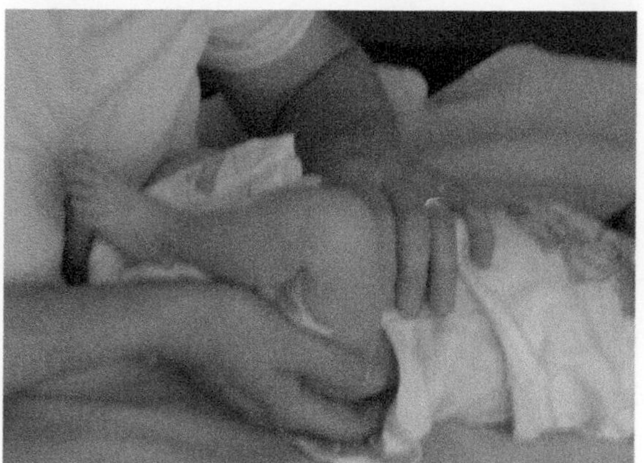

Figure 6.15. *Sacral molding procedure.*

OCCIPITAL MOLDING PROCEDURE

Indications

Intraosseous occipital somatic dysfunction as seen in plagiocephaly; facilitation of release of the intracranial and spinal membranes; to affect vagal autonomic tone.

Procedure (Fig. 6.16)

Patient supine; practitioner seated at the head of the patient. Place one hand beneath the patient's head, palm up, and cradle the occiput. Note the patterns of cranial flexion–extension, torsions and/or sidebending as they affect the occiput and the relationship between the occiput and atlas. Follow these patterns using indirect principles to facilitate listening to the PRM and assess the intraosseous motility of the occiput to identify motion restriction within the occiput. Follow the freedom of motion and employ the inherent forces of the PRM to gently pump the occipital intraosseous dysfunction.

Remarks

Important cranial base dysfunctions should be addressed first in order to facilitate occipital molding. Molding of the occiput may be employed alone or in association with other procedures such as sphenobasilar release. Following the PRM in this process increases tissue relaxation and results in intraosseous molding.

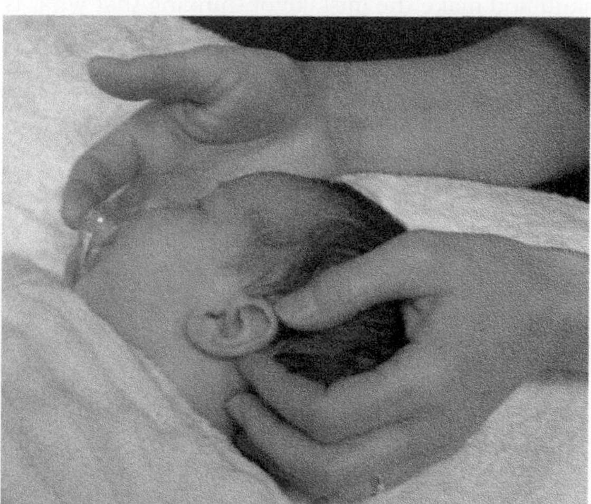

Figure 6.16. *Occipital molding procedure.*

VAULT MOLDING PROCEDURE

Indications

Intraosseous somatic dysfunction of the vault bones: parietal bones, frontal bones, and occipital or temporal squamae. Among others things, intraosseous parietal dysfunctions are associated with sleep disorders and cognitive disorders such as dyslexia, frontal with behavioral disorders and temporal with speech disorders.

Procedure (Fig. 6.17)

Patient supine; practitioner seated at the head of the patient. Place the dominant hand on the part of the vault to be molded and the other hand such that it allows the skull to be comfortably held. Note the pattern of cranial motion, flexion–external rotation and extension–internal rotation. Using indirect principles, follow this cranial pattern, listening to the PRM. Assess the intraosseous motility of the parietal bones, frontal bones, and occipital or temporal squamae to identify motion restriction within. Follow the freedom of motion and employ the inherent forces of the PRM to gently pump the dysfunctional bone.

Equilibration of the sphenobasilar synchondrosis

The three procedures that follow are intended to address dysfunction of the SBS. The points of palpatory contact on the skull are, however, distant from the SBS. Consequently, it is easy to palpate the superficial motion of the membranous portion of the skull and make the mistake of thinking that what is being perceived is the motion of the SBS. Thus the palpation of the superficial skull must be augmented by a thorough knowledge of the anatomy involved and the use of visualization to interpret the deep motion, or lack of motion, of the SBS.

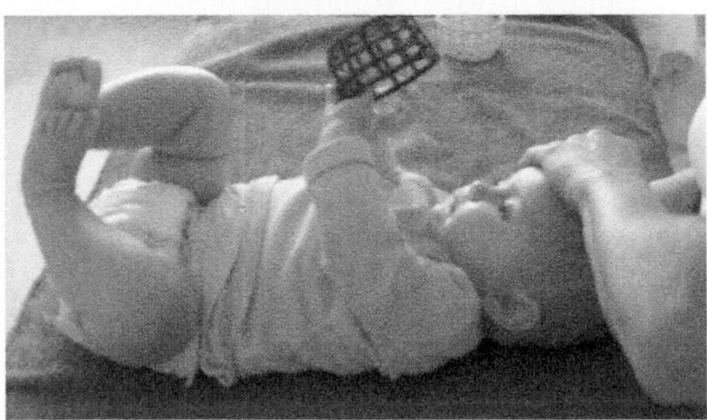

Figure 6.17. Vault molding procedure.

FRONTO-OCCIPITAL HOLD

Indications

SBS dysfunction, membranous strains.

Procedure (Fig. 6.18)

Patient supine; practitioner seated at the head of the table, toward one side. One hand lies palm up transversely under the occiput. The other hand is placed on the anterior portion of the patient's skull, such that the tip of the thumb is on the superior aspect of one greater wing of the sphenoid and the tip of the middle finger is on the corresponding spot on the other side. Listen to the SBS and determine the dysfunctional pattern. Utilize indirect principles in conjunction with the inherent forces of the PRM and treat what has been found.

Using the inherent forces of the PRM, it is sometimes necessary to initiate a gentle pumping of the SBS. When doing this, both occiput and sphenoid should be maintained in their positions of greatest ease until release occurs. This modification is especially recommended in chronic SBS dysfunctions and compression.

The response may be augmented by attention to the cervicothoracic region. Often the patient's cervical spine demonstrates extension that should be specifically treated. In any case, this area should be placed in the position of ease. Similarly, positioning the lower body to accommodate the position of the sacrum facilitates the release.

Remarks

The practitioner may place one hand under the occiput and the other hand on the sphenoid. The

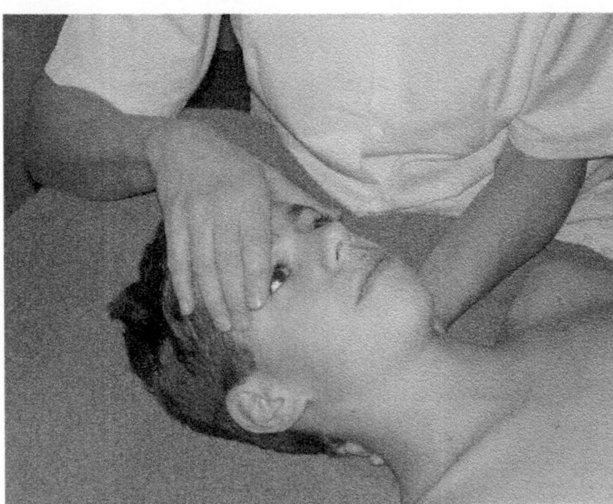

Figure 6.18. Fronto-occipital hold.

comfort of the practitioner and the patient determines the choice of position. However, when the hand that is palpating the sphenoid is placed in such a way that the palm is over the infant's or child's face covering their eyes, they often resist.

Alternatively, if the hand that is palpating the sphenoid is placed in such a way that the palm is over the infant's or child's forehead, it allows the examiner to monitor the sphenoid additionally through the frontal bone. This is because the posterior borders of the orbital plates of the frontal bone articulate with the lesser wings of the sphenoid. The lesser wings and the sphenoidal body are part of the cartilaginous cranial base. Therefore, by visualizing the relationship between the frontal bone and lesser wings, and considering this area as a functional unit, the examiner is given an additional sense of the function of the sphenoidal body.

An alternative hand placement for the fronto-occipital hold is to place one hand palm up longitudinally under the occiput with the fingers extending caudally. The other hand, also oriented longitudinally with fingers directed caudally, is placed on the frontal bone such that the tip of the thumb is on the superior aspect of one sphenoidal greater wing and the tip of the little finger is on the corresponding spot on the other side.

VAULT HOLD

Indications

SBS dysfunction; membranous strains.

Procedure (Fig. 6.19)

Patient supine; practitioner, seated at the patient's head, uses a four-finger vault hold. Contact the skull with the lightest possible pressure. The thumbs are interlocked over the sagittal suture, but not touching it, the hands contacting the lateral parts of the skull so that the tips of the index fingers are on the top of the greater wings of the sphenoid. The middle fingers are on the parietal bones and temporal squamae anterior to the external auditory meatus. The ring fingers are on the parietal and temporal bones behind the external auditory meatus and the little fingers are on the occipital squama. Listen to the SBS. Determine the dysfunctional pattern and, utilizing indirect principles in conjunction with the inherent forces of the PRM, treat what has been found.

Remarks

An infant or child will relax so that the cranial rhythmic impulse may be optimally palpated only if the practitioner's hand placement is comfortable. This procedure has the advantage of positioning the practitioner out of the direct line of sight of the infant or child. It may be easily performed with the patient cradled in the arms of the caregiver. For these reasons, it is a good approach if the child is having difficulty relaxing in the presence of the practitioner.

CRADLING THE SKULL

Indications

SBS dysfunction; membranous strains.

Procedure (Fig. 6.20)

Patient supine; practitioner seated at the patient's head, hands under the occiput in such a way that the distal pads of the index, middle and ring fingers

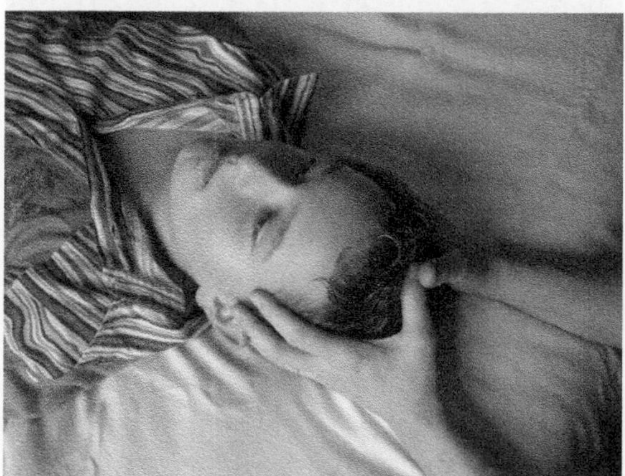

Figure 6.19. *Vault hold.*

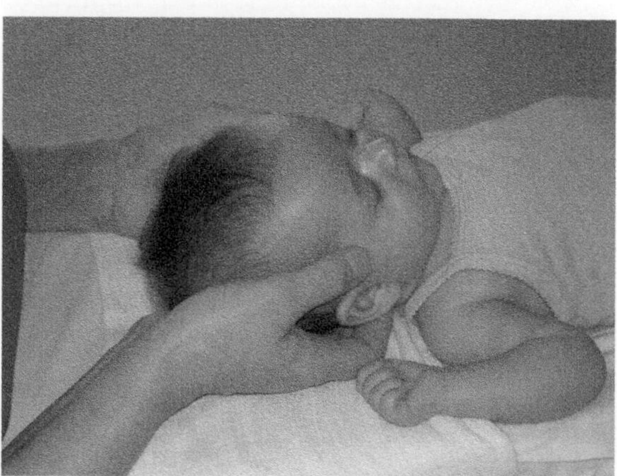

Figure 6.20. *Cradling the skull.*

are in contact with the squamous portion of the occiput along and inferior to the superior nuchal line. The lateral aspects of the distal phalanges of the thumbs contact the greater wings of the sphenoid bilaterally. Listen to the SBS and determine the pattern of ease. Utilizing indirect principles in conjunction with the inherent forces of the PRM, treat the identified dysfunction.

Remarks

This procedure provides an alternative hand placement for that of the vault hold. It offers similar advantages in that the child can be treated in many positions, including lying in the caregiver's lap or, if necessary, seated. Additionally, many individuals find this hand placement to be more ergonomically satisfactory than that of the vault hold.

Occipital procedures

BILATERAL CONDYLAR DECOMPRESSION

Indications

To restore the normal functional relationship between the occipital condyles and the atlas.

Procedure (Fig. 6.21)

Patient supine; practitioner seated at the head of the table holding the patient's head with their hands, palm up, under the occiput in such a way that the distal pads of the index, middle and ring fingers are in contact with, and extending as low as possible on, the squamous portion of the occiput. Care must be exerted to keep the hands fully in contact with the occiput and medial to the occipitomastoid suture. Compressive forces over the occipitomastoid suture are to be avoided. The occipital condyles are not accessible for direct palpation; therefore, their relationship with the atlas should be visualized during the entire procedure. Visualizing each condyle, listen to its motion on the atlas. The presence of condylar compression results in limitation of motion. Identify unilateral or bilateral compression. Utilizing tests of listening, identify the pattern of occipitocervical flexion–extension sidebending and rotation, and follow it into the position of greatest ease. Employ the inherent motility of the PRM to gently pump the area of compression to induce release.

Remarks

It must be remembered that in infants the occipital condyles are not ossified and consist of two parts separated by the cartilaginous anterior intraoccipital synchondrosis. This procedure should be performed in the gentlest possible fashion to avoid the introduction of an intraosseous condylar dysfunction. During the procedure, the child should not manifest discomfort.

BASE EXPANSION

Indications

Dysfunction between the occiput and atlas, occiput and temporals and compression of the foramen magnum and jugular foramina.

Procedure (Fig. 6.22)

Patient supine; practitioner seated at the head of the table with their hands beneath the occiput in such

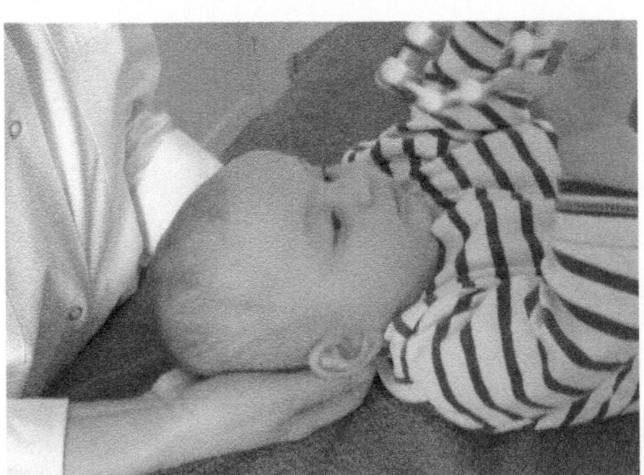

Figure 6.21. *Bilateral occipital condylar decompression.*

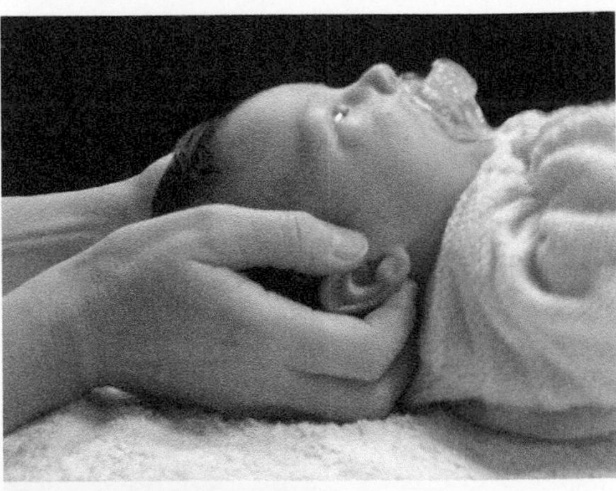

Figure 6.22. *Base expansion.*

a fashion that the ring and little fingers contact the occipital squama, the tips of the middle fingers are placed at the level of C1, the index fingers are contacting the posterior aspect of the mastoid processes and the thumbs rest lightly on each side of the head. Listen and identify the pattern of occipito-atlantal flexion–extension sidebending and rotation, and follow it into the position of greatest ease. In this position, listen next to the bilateral relationship between the occiput and temporal bones, and, with the index fingers, follow the temporal bones into their position of ease. Employ the inherent motility of the PRM to reinforce the previous two steps and wait for a release.

Foramen magnum decompression may be accomplished at this point in the procedure by utilizing the biphasic PRM to gently pump and mold the foramen magnum and its surrounding tissues.

Remarks

This procedure offers potential benefit to almost every patient, improving postural balance. It is important to remember the significant attachment of the dura mater on the circumference of the foramen magnum as well as C2 and C3 below.

The application of this procedure requires the harmonious and simultaneous use of all the fingers. The middle finger, at the level of C1, is employed to monitor the procedure, keeping it focused on the cranial base and avoiding its extension into the spine below. The practitioner must be constantly aware of the patient's position; the most frequent error is to flex excessively the occiput on the atlas.

Many patients demonstrate an anterior dysfunction of the occiput on the atlas. It is imperative when performing base expansion to follow respectfully the dysfunctional occipitoatlantal position in order to avoid reactions such as nausea, vomiting and headache.

Very often the patients place themselves in a position of sidebending–rotation of the occiput, i.e. sidebending to one side, rotation to the opposite side. The practitioner should not alter this resting position lest they increase the tension of the intracranial, intraspinal membranes and fasciae. Rather they should position themselves to the side of the patient as much as necessary.

This procedure may be modified to include diagnosis and treatment of the SBS by placing the lateral aspect of the thumbs on the superior portions of the greater wings of the sphenoid in a hand placement similar to that described above in the procedure 'Cradling the skull'.

INTRAOSSEOUS PROCEDURE

Indications

Dysfunction affecting the occipital synchondroses and the contour of the squamous portion.

Procedure (Fig. 6.23)

Patient supine; practitioner seated at the head of the table supporting the occiput in their hands with the distal index, middle and ring fingers on the squamous portion. It is important to keep the hands in contact only with the occiput, avoiding the occipitomastoid suture. The intraoccipital synchondroses are not accessible for direct palpation and, therefore, should be visualized during the entire procedure. Visualize the different components of the occiput and listen to their motion within the global motion pattern of the occiput. Identify possible unilateral or bilateral compression of the synchondroses as well as restriction of compliance of the occipital squama in response to the biphasic PRM. Intraosseous dysfunction affecting any of these areas of the occiput will result in limitation of motion. Utilizing tests of listening, identify the pattern of occipitocervical flexion–extension sidebending and rotation, and follow it into the position of greatest ease in order to reduce myofascial and dural tension on the occiput. Employ the inherent motility of the PRM to gently pump the area of intraosseous dysfunction to induce release.

Remarks

It should be remembered that muscles, aponeurosis, dural and spinal membranes that collectively constitute myofascial components blend into and are in

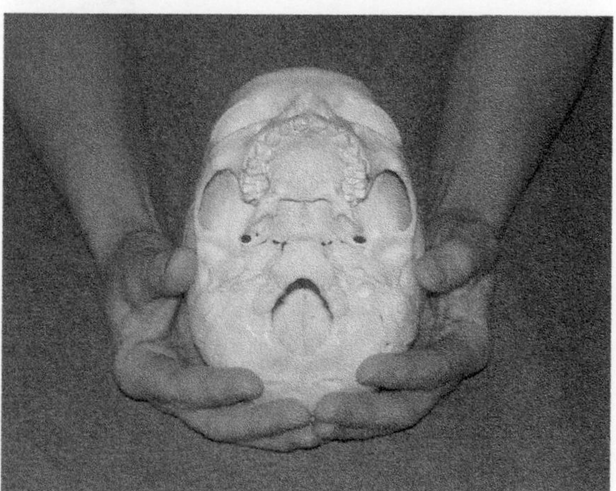

Figure 6.23. *Occipital intraosseous procedure.*

continuity with the periosteum at the site of their attachment. Therefore, any dysfunctional tension within these tissues will interfere with the release of an intraosseous dysfunction. Consequently, tension within surrounding tissues as well as those within the bones must be addressed in order to treat these dysfunctions effectively. In fact, every tissue of the body should and can be addressed, which is one of the advantages of indirect procedures in that by respecting the patient's position of comfort their effect is global as well as local.

Sphenoidal procedures

SPHENOID AND ZYGOMA

Indications

Interosseous dysfunction between the sphenoid and zygomatic bone. This dysfunction is commonly the result of blows to the face that occur during rough play and athletic activity. It is also seen in association with ocular and maxillary sinus dysfunctions.

Procedure (Fig. 6.24)

Patient supine; practitioner seated at the head of the table with the hands bilaterally contacting the sphenoid and zygomae. The lateral aspects of the distal thumbs contact the top of the greater wings of the sphenoid and the index and middle fingers contact the orbital border and the inferior border of the zygomae, respectively. Listen to the movement of the sphenoid and zygomae, noting their inherent motility and the relationship between them. Move in the direction of ease to treat any identified dysfunction.

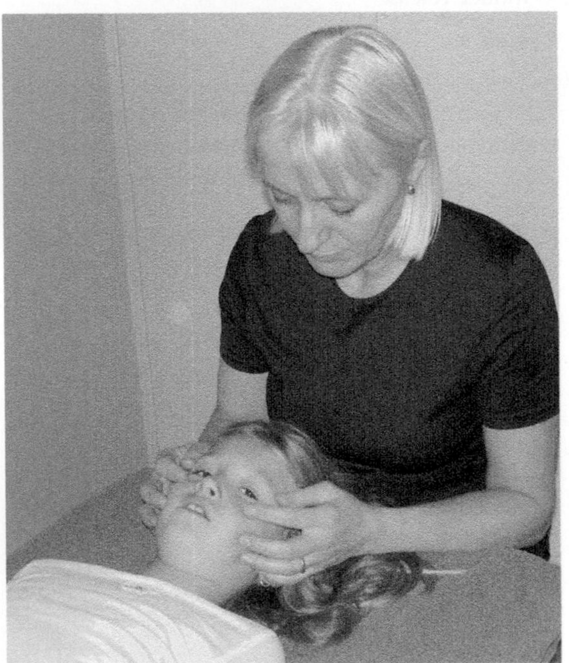

Figure 6.24. *Sphenozygomatic suture procedure.*

Remarks

The above procedure may be performed unilaterally or bilaterally.

SPHENOID AND FRONTAL BONE

Indications

Interosseous dysfunction between the sphenoid and frontal bones; also the result of blows to the face and seen in association with ocular dysfunctions.

Procedure (Fig. 6.25)

Patient supine; practitioner seated at the head of the table with the hands bilaterally contacting the sphenoid and frontal bones. The tips of the middle fingers contact the top of the greater wings of the sphenoid and the tips of the index fingers contact the zygomatic processes of the frontal bones bilaterally. Listen to the movement of the sphenoid and frontal bones and their interosseous relationship and note the inherent motility of the PRM. Using indirect principles, follow the motion in the direction of ease and await a release.

Remarks

The above procedure may be performed unilaterally or bilaterally.

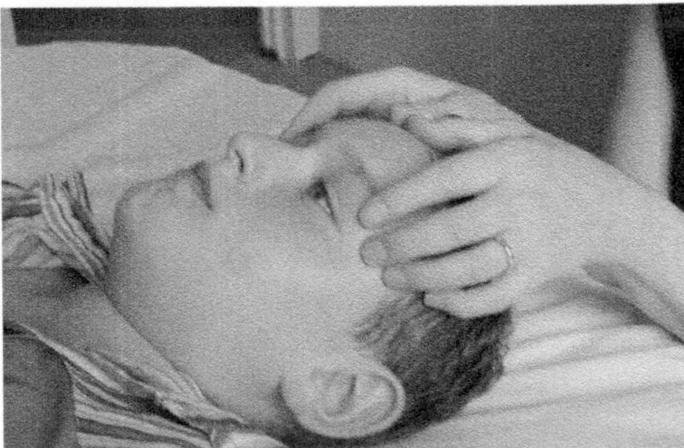

Figure 6.25. *Frontosphenoidal suture procedure.*

SPHENOID AND SQUAMOUS TEMPORAL BONE

Indications

Compression of the sphenosquamosal suture.

Procedure (Fig. 6.26)

Patient supine; practitioner seated at the head of the patient with both hands in opposition to one another along the sphenosquamosal suture. The pads of the index and middle fingers of one hand are on the anterior border of the squamous portion of the temporal bone, the pads of the index and middle fingers of the other hand are on the lateral border of the greater wing of the sphenoid. Listen to the quality of inherent motility at the suture which is reduced by compression of the suture. Employ the inherent forces of the PRM to gently pump the area to induce release.

Remarks

The precise location of the sphenosquamosal suture is often difficult to palpate. In infants after difficult labor, however, the sense of density that accompanies the compression is palpable.

SPHENOID AND PETROUS TEMPORAL BONE

Indications

Entrapment of CN III, IV, V and VI; dysfunction of the sphenopetrosal synchondrosis; balancing of the tentorium cerebelli.

Procedure (Fig. 6.27)

Patient supine; practitioner seated at the head of the patient, the hands bilaterally contacting the sphenoid and the temporal bones. The lateral aspects of the distal thumbs contact the superior portion of the greater wings of the sphenoid. The index fingers are inferior to the zygomatic processes, the middle fingers contact the area of the external auditory meatus and the ring fingers are on the tips of the mastoid processes. Listen to, and visualize, the movement of the sphenoid and temporal bones. Note the inherent motility of the PRM and any restriction of motility of the sphenopetrosal synchondrosis. Utilize the principles of indirect treatment and await a release.

Remarks

This procedure requires precise visualization of the sutures involved in the dysfunction. The middle finger is oriented along the line of the petrous ridge. Focusing on this finger allows the identification of the major and minor components in the pattern of cranial external and internal rotation of the petrous portion of the temporal bones. This facilitates identification of dysfunction at the sphenopetrosal synchondroses.

CN VI passes beneath the petrosphenoidal ligament that is situated at the anterior end of the petrous ridge. The middle finger should be continuously reoriented to follow the petrous portion of the temporal bone, allowing the practitioner to influence the petrosphenoidal ligament. This is greatly facilitated by visualization.

Unilateral variation (Fig. 6.28)

Patient supine; practitioner seated at the head of the patient slightly to the side. One hand is on the

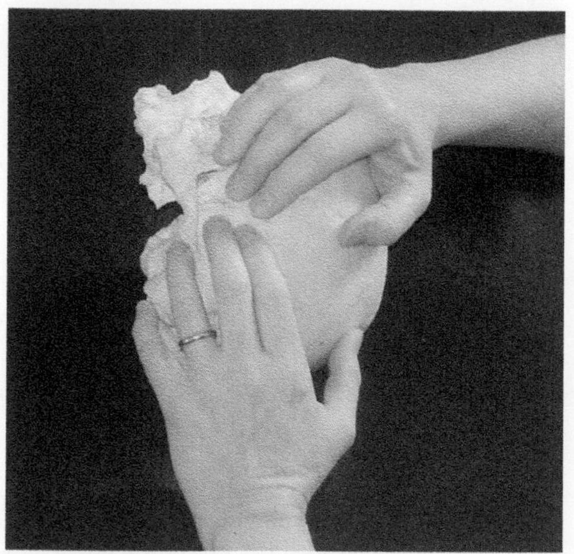

Figure 6.26. *Sphenosquamosal suture procedure.*

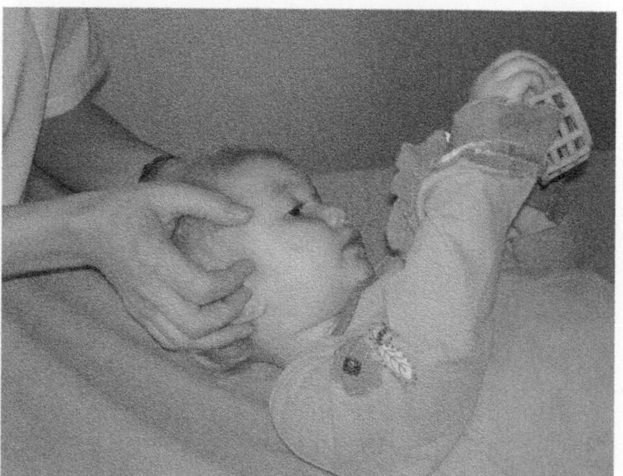

Figure 6.27. *Bilateral sphenopetrosal synchondrosis procedure.*

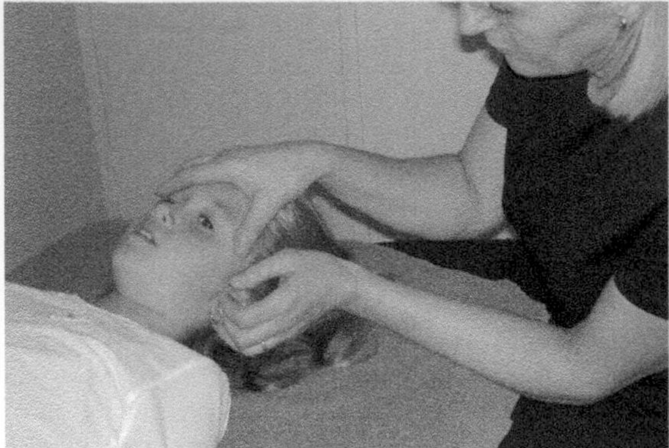

Figure 6.28. *Unilateral sphenopetrosal synchondrosis procedure.*

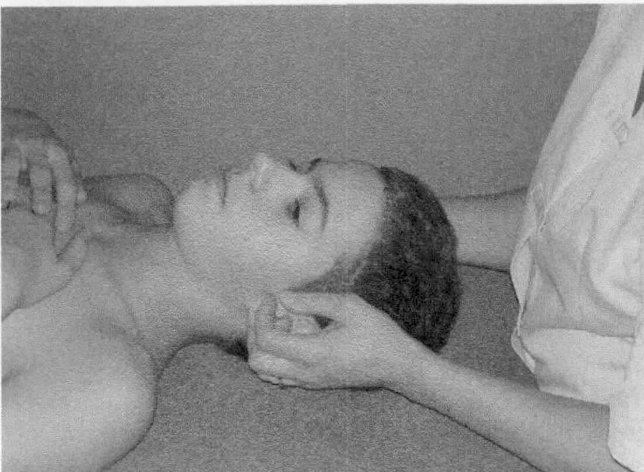

Figure 6.29. *Balancing of the temporal bones.*

temporal bone, with the thumb superior and the index finger inferior to the zygomatic process. The middle finger contacts the area of the external auditory meatus and the ring finger is on the tip of the mastoid process. The other hand is placed on the anterior portion of the patient's skull, such that the tip of the thumb contacts the superior aspect of one greater wing on the side being treated, while the tip of the middle finger is on the corresponding spot on the other side. This hand creates a functional unit between the frontal bone and the sphenoid. Visualize as above, utilize the principles of indirect treatment and await a release.

Temporal bone procedures

BALANCING OF THE TEMPORAL BONES

Indications

Imbalances between the temporal bones, often in association with dysfunction of the tentorium cerebelli; vestibular dysfunctions.

Procedure (Fig. 6.29)

Patient supine; practitioner seated at the head of the table, with the thumbs and index fingers superior and inferior to the zygomatic processes, the middle fingers if possible at the external auditory meatus, the ring fingers on the tip of the mastoid processes and the little fingers on the superior part of the mastoid portions. After a period of listening, follow the pattern in the direction of the dysfunction to the point of balance and await a release. Respiratory cooperation again can be employed to facilitate the release, using inhalation for external rotation dysfunction and exhalation for internal rotation.

Remarks

Extreme care should be used when placing the tip of the finger in the external auditory meatus of infants and young children. An alternative hand placement may be employed by contacting the squamous portion of the temporal bone with the thumb and by curling the index finger beneath the ear so that the lateral aspect of the tip of the finger approximates the mastoid portion. (*Note*: In infants the mastoid process is not yet fully developed and precision is essential.) Additionally, it is easy to misinterpret the slightest amount of active rotation of the head by the child as motion of the temporal bone.

WITH SURROUNDING BONES

Temporal and occiput: occipitomastoid suture

Indications

Restriction between the temporal bone and the occiput at the level of the occipitomastoid suture; dysfunction affecting the jugular foramen and its contents, often the result of blows to the back of the head.

Procedure (Fig. 6.30)

Patient supine; practitioner seated at the head of the table, with one hand palm up, transversely oriented beneath the occiput, with the tips of the index and middle fingers contacting the squamous portion of

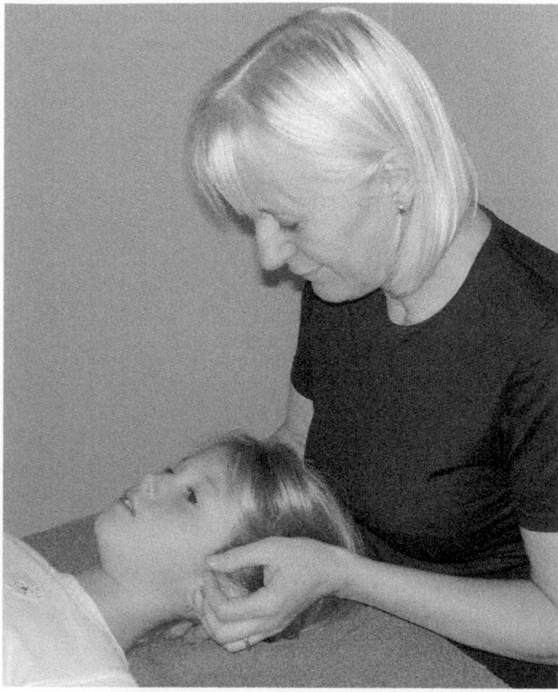

Figure 6.30. *Occipitomastoid suture procedure.*

the occipital squama, immediately medial to the occipitomastoid suture. The other hand is placed on the temporal bone with the thumb and index finger superior and inferior to the zygomatic process, the middle finger if possible at the external auditory meatus, the ring finger on the tip of the mastoid process and the little finger on the mastoid portion. Listen to the quality of inherent motility at the suture. Using indirect principles, follow the dysfunctional pattern and, if necessary, employ the inherent forces of the PRM to gently pump the area and induce release.

Remarks

Because of the importance of the content of the jugular foramen caution should be exerted when performing this procedure in order to avoid adverse reactions such as nausea, vomiting and headache.

Temporal and occiput: petrobasilar suture

Indications

Restriction between the temporal bone and the occiput at the level of the petrobasilar suture; dysfunction affecting the jugular and lacerum foramina and their contents; pharyngeal and soft palate dysfunctions.

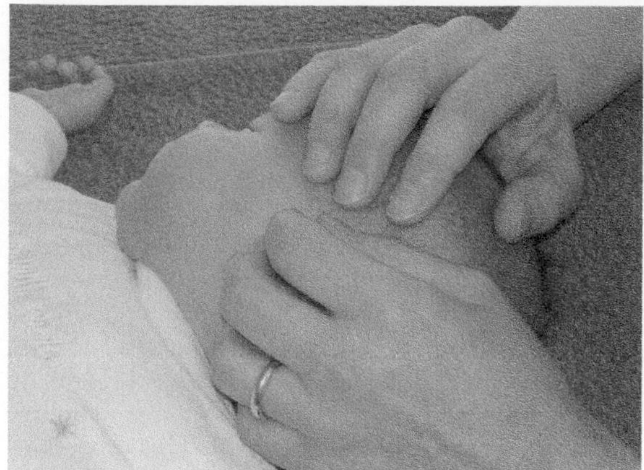

Figure 6.31. *Squamous suture procedure.*

Procedure

Patient supine; practitioner seated at the head of the table, as described above in the procedure for the occipitomastoid suture. In this procedure, focus attention on the petrous portion of the temporal bone and visualize the petrobasilar suture. The middle finger over the external auditory meatus and its orientation along the line of the petrous ridge provides information as to the status of the petrobasilar suture. Listen to the quality of inherent motility at the suture and follow the dysfunctional pattern in indirect fashion. Gently pump the area employing the inherent forces of the PRM to induce release if necessary.

Remarks

The petrobasilar suture remains patent throughout life and as such should demonstrate motility in all individuals. The attachment of the upper portion of the pharynx is in part located on both sides of this suture.

Temporal and parietal

Indications

Overlapping of the squamous suture at birth.

Procedure (Fig. 6.31)

Patient supine; practitioner seated at the head of the table with one hand palm transversely oriented over the calvaria, with the tips of the index, middle and ring fingers contacting the inferior border of the parietal bone, immediately above the squamous suture. The other hand is placed on the temporal bone with the thumb curled over the ear in such a fashion that its lateral aspect contacts the temporal squama below the squamous suture. The index finger is inferior to the zygomatic process, the middle finger is over the external auditory meatus, the ring finger is on the tip of the mastoid process and the little finger is on the mastoid portion. Listen to the motility of the suture. Using indirect principles, follow the dysfunctional pattern to induce release. If overlapping of the squamous suture is present, it may be necessary to gently pump the area, employing the inherent forces of the PRM. This procedure may be employed to affect the entire suture or specific areas of restriction within the suture as illustrated in Figure 6.31.

Temporal and zygoma

Indications

Dysfunction of the temporozygomatic suture frequently following blunt facial traumas.

Procedure (Fig. 6.32)

Patient supine; practitioner seated at the head of the table, slightly to the side. The thumb and index finger of one hand are placed superior and inferior to the zygomatic process of the temporal bone, while the thumb and index finger of the other hand are placed superior and inferior to the temporal process of the zygoma. Listen and follow the dysfunctional pattern in the direction of ease to the point of balance and wait for a release.

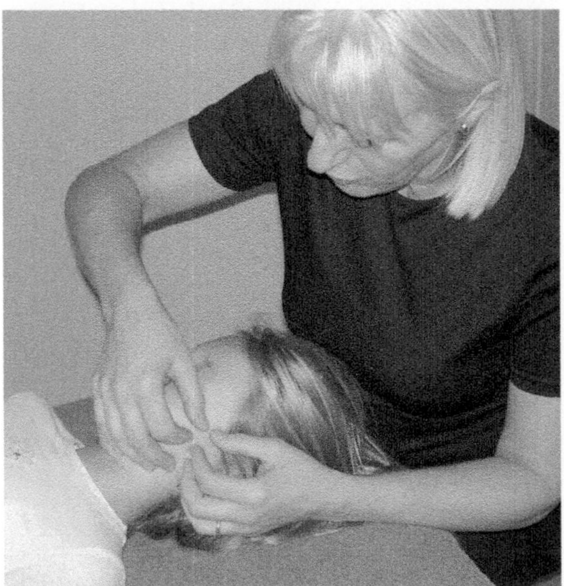

Figure 6.32. *Temporozygomatic suture procedure.*

Temporal and mandible

Indications

Temporomandibular joint (TMJ) dysfunction; orofacial dysfunctions and orthodontic-related disorders.

Procedure (Fig. 6.33)

Patient supine; practitioner seated at the head of the table, on the side opposite to the dysfunction. One hand is placed on the temporal bone with the tips of the thumb, index and middle fingers above the mandibular fossa. The tips of the thumb and index finger of the other hand are placed on either side of the vertical ramus of the mandible near the condyle. Listen to the motility of the TMJ and, utilizing indirect methods, follow the dysfunctional pattern to the position of ease and await a release. Employing the inherent forces of the PRM to gently pump the area can facilitate the treatment of chronic dysfunction.

Remarks

The significance of TMJ dysfunction in children and adolescents should not be underestimated. Although they may not present with a pain complaint, this dysfunction provides the foundation for significant difficulties later in life.

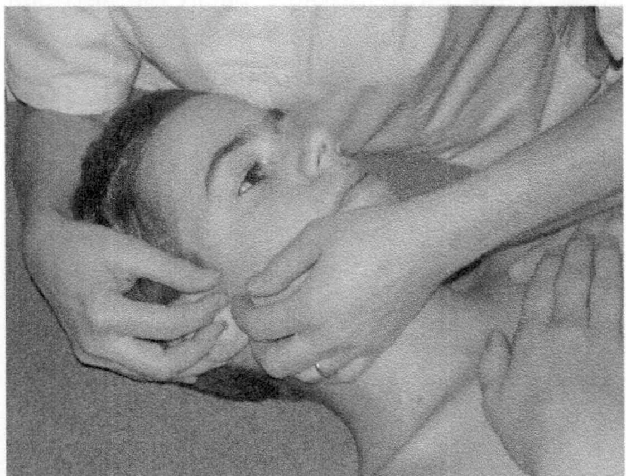

Figure 6.33. *Temporomandibular joint procedure.*

INTRAOSSEOUS PROCEDURES

Indications

Intraosseous dysfunction between the squamous, petromastoid and tympanic portions of the temporal bone, seen in conditions such as plagiocephaly and otitis.

Procedure (Fig. 6.34)

Patient supine; practitioner seated at the head of the table, with the thumbs and index fi ngers superior and inferior to the zygomatic processes, the middle fi ngers if possible at the external auditory meatus, the ring fi ngers on the mastoid processes and the little fingers on the superior part of the mastoid portions. With visualization, focus your attention on the area to be treated. Listen for impairment of the intraosseous inherent motility in the area of the dysfunction. Utilizing the inherent forces of the PRM, follow the different portions of the temporal bone to the point of balance to allow the PRM to demonstrate maximum potency.

Remarks

The mastoid portion of the temporal bone develops from the squamous and petrous portions and as such is subject to intraosseous dysfunction. It is frequently compressed in infants, resulting in functional ENT impairments. A specifi c intraosseous pumping procedure may be performed on the mastoid portion to enhance the drainage of the mastoid air cells.

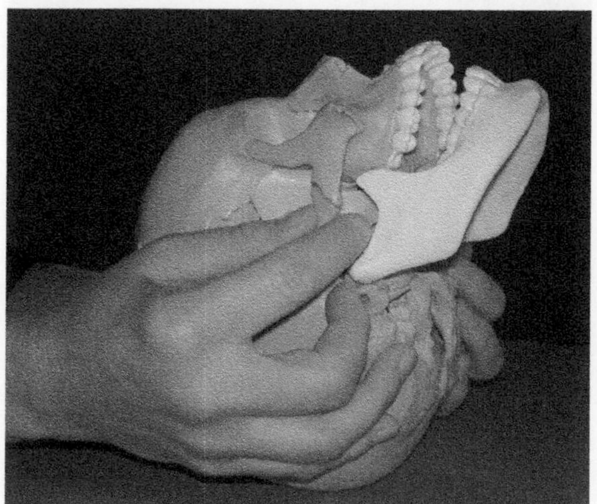

Figure 6.34. *Temporal intraosseous procedure.*

GALBREATH[4] PROCEDURE

Indications

Improve function of pharyngotympanic tube and decongestion of the middle ear.

Procedure (Fig. 6.35)

Patient supine with their head slightly elevated and turned so that the dysfunctional side is up; practitioner stands to the side of the table, in front of the patient. With the cephalic hand, stabilize the patient's head in such a way that the tips of the fingers approximate the TMJ. With the caudal hand, grasp the mandible with the index and middle fingers on either side of the vertical ramus near the condyle, the palm resting on the mandibular body. Rhythmically pull and release the mandible for about 1 minute. The pull should be body but fi rm in an inferior medial direction. This process can be repeated by caregiver at home.

Remarks

This procedure was described in 1929 prior to Sutherland's original publication of *The Cranial Bowl*.[5] Although it is not in the purest sense a 'cranial' procedure, principles of cranial manipulation may be employed to add an additional dimension to this classic treatment.

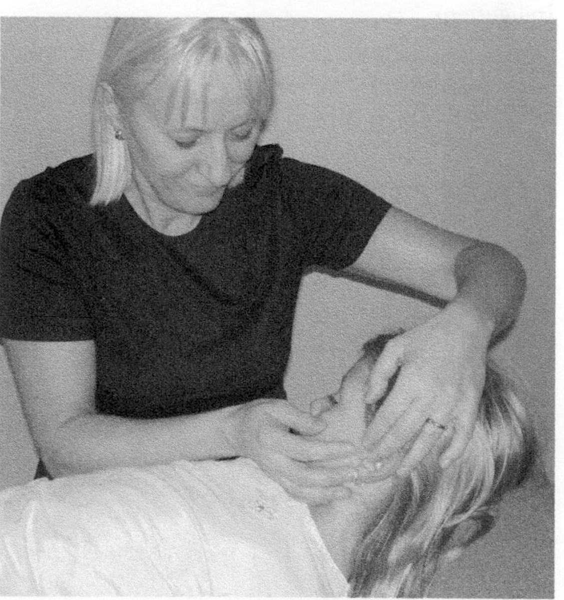

Figure 6.35. *Galbreath procedure.*

Frontal procedure

Indications

Dysfunction of the falx cerebri and viscerocranium, eyes and nasal cavities; behavioral problems.

Procedure (Fig. 6.36)

Patient supine; practitioner seated at the head of the table. Place the tips of both index fingers on either side of the metopic suture, with the middle and ring fingers resting on the frontal bones so that the tips of the ring fingers contact the zygomatic processes bilaterally. Listen to the movement within and between the two frontal bones. Note the inherent motility of the PRM and any restriction of motility. Follow indirect, pumping and molding principles to obtain a release.

Remarks

This procedure is very relaxing and is generally highly appreciated by the patient. It may be the primary focus of treatment for patients with behavioral or cognitive problems. It is also an excellent starting point when addressing facial disorders. The descriptions of the facial bone procedures are provided below.

Vault procedures

RELEASE OF THE SAGITTAL SUTURE

Indications

Congestion of the superior sagittal sinus; dysfunction of the sagittal suture, often compression; dysfunction of the falx cerebri.

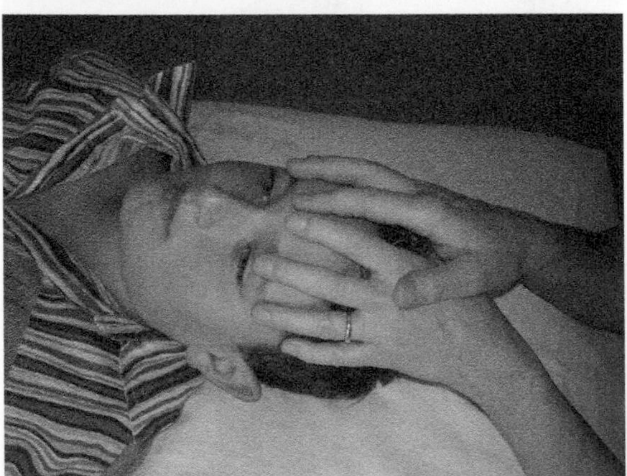

Figure 6.36. *Frontal procedure.*

Procedure (Fig. 6.37)

Patient supine; practitioner seated at the head of the patient with the thumbs interlocked on each side of the sagittal suture as far posterior as possible, the other fingers lightly placed on the parietal bones. Listen and note the movements of the two parietals, the PRM and any imbalance of membranous tension. Follow indirect principles to obtain a release. In chronic dysfunction or to improve circulatory stasis, pumping and molding principles may be used.

Remarks

Pumping the sagittal suture facilitates venous circulation in the superior sagittal sinus. It is indicated to produce increased venous drainage of the vault. Prior to facilitating the cranial venous circulation, it is important to address dysfunction affecting the jugular foramen.

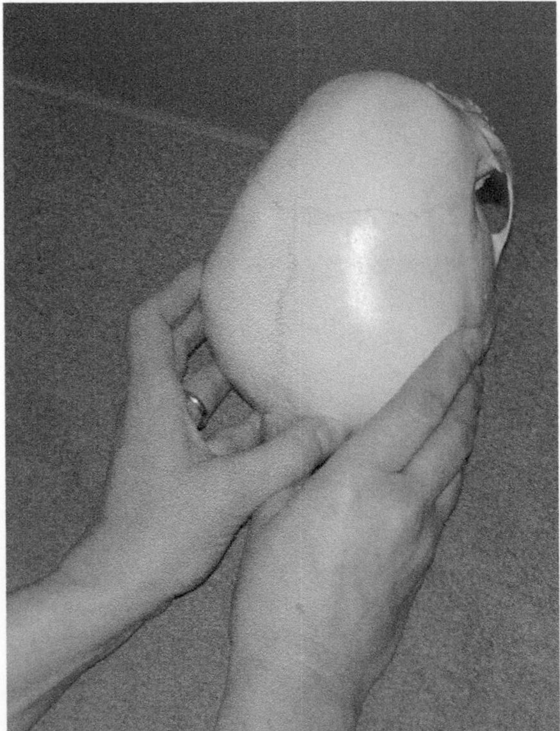

Figure 6.37. *Release of the sagittal suture.*

DECOMPRESSION OF THE CORONAL AND LAMBDOID SUTURES

Indications

Restricted motion in the sutures as may be seen in non-synostotic plagiocephaly.

Coronal procedure (Fig. 6.38)

Patient supine; practitioner seated at the head of the patient with the thumbs on either side of the sagittal suture as far anterior as possible, the tips of the other fingers placed anteriorly to the coronal suture on the lateral portions of the frontal bone. The practitioner's thumbs may or may not be interlocked. Listen, follow the dysfunctional pattern and, if necessary, utilize the potency of the PRM in a pumping fashion to increase the motion present at the suture.

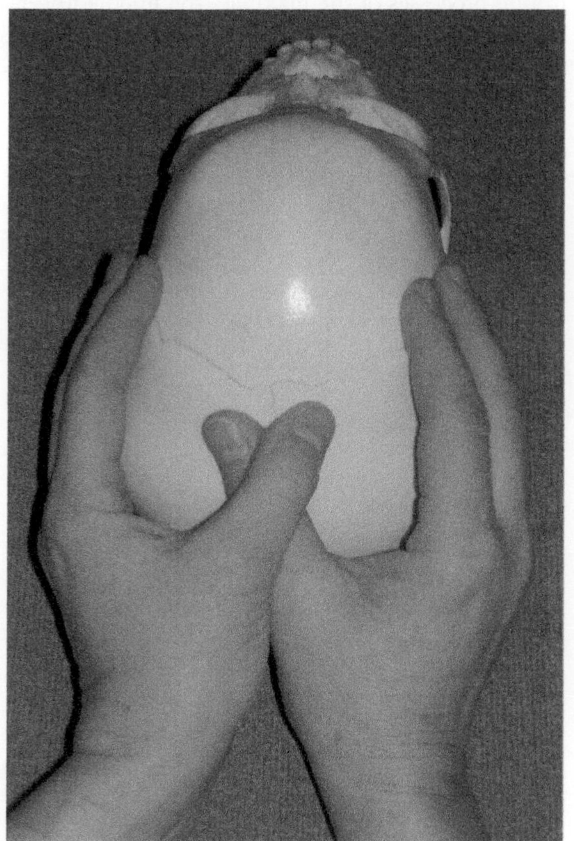

Figure 6.38. *Coronal suture procedure.*

Lambdoid procedure (Fig. 6.39)

Patient supine; practitioner seated at the head of the patient with the thumbs on either side of the sagittal suture as far posterior as possible and the tips of the little fingers placed on the occipital squama in its lateral portion. Treat using the same principles as above.

Remarks

An alternative hand placement for either of the above procedures is to place the tips of the fingers of each hand on either side of the suture to be treated, in which case the practitioner should be seated at the side of the patient.

In severe dysfunctions, stiffness is observed in the entire cranium and addressing the dysfunction of the vault may be a starting point for the introduction of motion. Be aware of the beveling of the coronal and lambdoid sutures. Pressure should never be applied over an internal bevel. Note that the anterior and posterior borders of the parietal bones have the same beveling, i.e. an external bevel for their medial portions and an internal bevel for their lateral portions. The corresponding parietal border of the frontal bone and lambdoidal border of the occiput demonstrate an internal bevel in their medial portions and

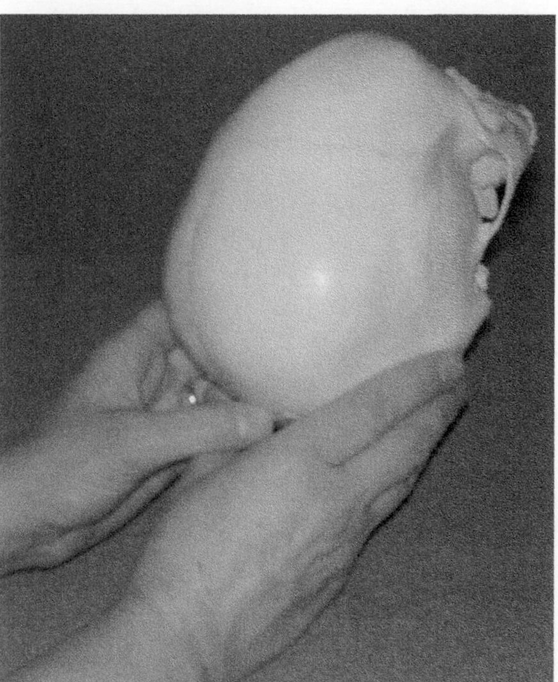

Figure 6.39. *Lambdoid suture procedure.*

an external bevel for their lateral portions. Thus, in order to disengage one bone from another, pressure should be placed on the side of the suture of the externally beveled bone to be disengaged. (*Note*: In infants, although bevels are not yet present, the relationships are the same.)

Facial procedures

BALANCING OF THE FACE

Indications

Dysfunction of any of the components of the viscerocranium; sinusitis; preparation for orthodontia.

Procedure (Fig. 6.40)

Patient supine; practitioner seated to one side of the head of the table. Place the cephalic hand across the frontal bone, such that the tips of the index finger and thumb are placed bilaterally on the zygomatic processes of the frontal bone. The caudal hand monitors the maxillae under the nose with the metacarpophalangeal articulation of the index finger and the zygomae with the thumb on one side and the index and middle fingers on the other side. Listen and visualize the relationship between the frontal bone and bones of the viscerocranium below. The relationship may be one of torsion, sidebending or compression between these two blocks. Utilizing indirect principles, follow the pattern to a point of ease and await a release. This procedure may be further augmented by employing the inherent motility of the PRM to pump the two blocks.

Remarks

The practitioner must be able to change finger position in response to the pattern of dysfunction. This procedure is very relaxing, facilitates sinus drainage and improves circulation of blood and lymph to and from the viscerocranium.

FRONTO-MAXILLO-ZYGOMATIC PROCEDURE

Indications

Sinusitis; rhinitis; functional nasal airway obstruction; nasolacrimal duct obstruction.

Procedure (Fig. 6.41)

Patient supine; practitioner seated at the head of the table, with both hands on the patient's face such that the tips of the thumbs rest on the glabella, the tips of the index fingers contact the frontal processes of the maxillae, the middle fingers are on the maxillae, and the ring and little fingers are on the zygomae. Listen, visualizing the global pattern of motion between the frontal bones and the maxillae and zygomae. Follow this pattern, noting fine details in the relationship between these individual bones. Utilizing indirect principles and the PRM, follow the fine details of motion in relation to the global pattern to the position of ease and await a release.

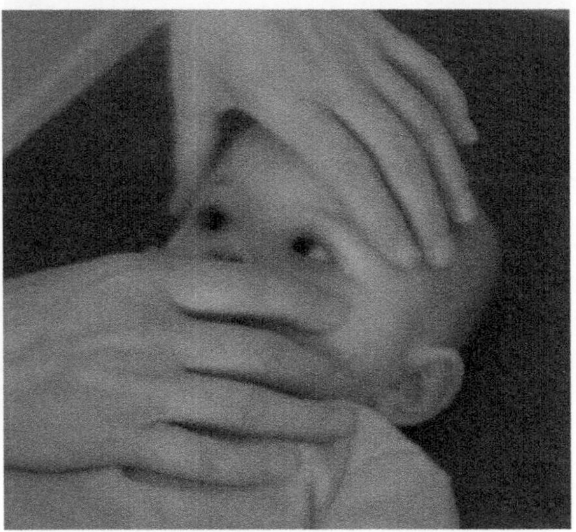

Figure 6.40. *Balancing of the face.*

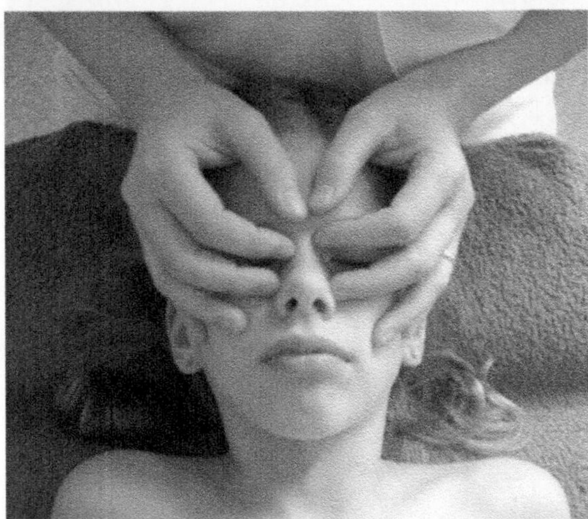

Figure 6.41. *Fronto-maxillo-zygomatic procedure.*

Remarks

The tips of the index fingers can be placed on the nasal bones if necessary to further assess the relationship between the nasal bones and the frontal bones and maxillae as shown in Figure 6.41.

An alternative hand placement is to contact the frontal bones with one hand placed transversely. The maxillae are monitored between the thumb and index finger of the other hand. This procedure also allows the practitioner to have a more specific effect on the premaxilla.

OCCIPITO-FRONTO-FACIAL BALANCING

Indications

Restriction of motion in the anterior attachment of the falx cerebri affecting the ethmoid and structures surrounding it.

Procedure (Fig. 6.42)

Patient supine; practitioner seated at the head of the table, one hand cradling the occipital bone, the other on the frontal bone with the fingers oriented caudally. Listen and visualize the motion at the level of, and between, the occiput and frontal bones. Visualize the falx cerebri and note tension within. Follow the motion of the frontal and occipital bones to release the membranous strain pattern within the falx. Next, follow the direction of ease of the frontal bone in relation to the facial bones, noting fine details. This may be accomplished by moving the hand slightly so that the fingertips contact the facial bones. Utilizing indirect principles and the PRM, follow the various components to the position of ease and await a release.

Remarks

The last part of this procedure is not the procedure of choice for infants and children because the hand placement covers their eyes and is consequently not readily accepted. It works well for older children and adolescents and may be employed to accomplish many things. It balances the intracranial membranes as it normalizes the face. It can be employed to improve results in cases of recalcitrant neck pain.

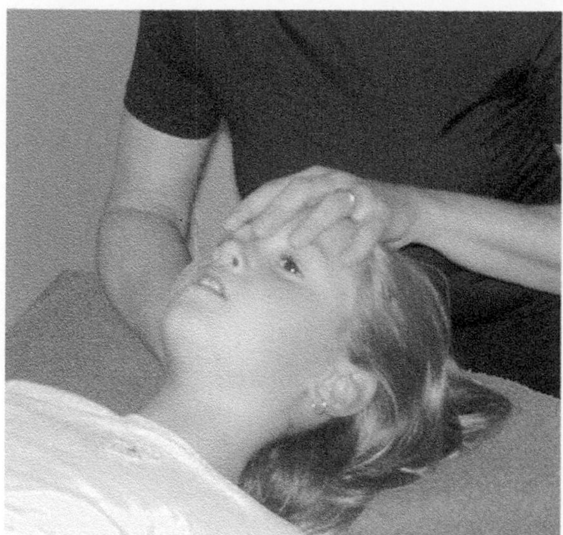

Figure 6.42. *Occipito-fronto-facial balancing.*

BALANCING OF THE ZYGOMAE

Indications

Dysfunction of the zygomae, commonly found as the result of a blow to the face.

Procedure (Fig. 6.43)

Patient supine; practitioner seated at the head of the table. Bilaterally place the index fingers on the orbital borders and the middle fingers on the inferior borders of the zygomae. Listen to the motion of the zygomae and follow it to the position of ease. In cases of chronic dysfunction the indirect procedure may be augmented with pumping that follows the rhythm of the PRM.

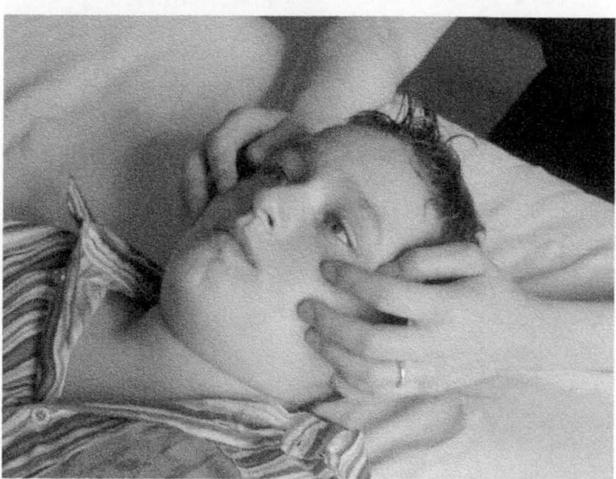

Figure 6.43. *Balancing of the zygomae.*

Remarks

An alternative hand position may be employed (Fig. 6.44). The thumbs are placed on the orbital borders and the index fingers on the inferior borders of the zygomae.

The zygomae may be considered as anterior extensions of the greater wings of the sphenoid and as such may be employed as levers to affect the sphenoid.

FRONTOZYGOMATIC NORMALIZATION

Indications

Frontozygomatic dysfunctions as seen with ocular dysfunctions.

Procedure (Fig. 6.45)

Patient supine; practitioner seated at the head of the table on the opposite side of the dysfunction. Place the thumb and index finger of the cephalic hand on either side of the zygomatic process of the frontal bone. The thumb and index fi nger of the caudal hand are placed on either side of the frontal process of the zygoma. Listen and follow the motion in the direction of ease, frequently compression, between the two bones. Await a release.

Remarks

An alternative hand position may be employed (Fig. 6.46). Instead of using the thumbs and index fingers, the same hold may be accomplished between the index and middle fingers. In both cases, it is important to establish contact as close to the frontozygomatic suture as possible.

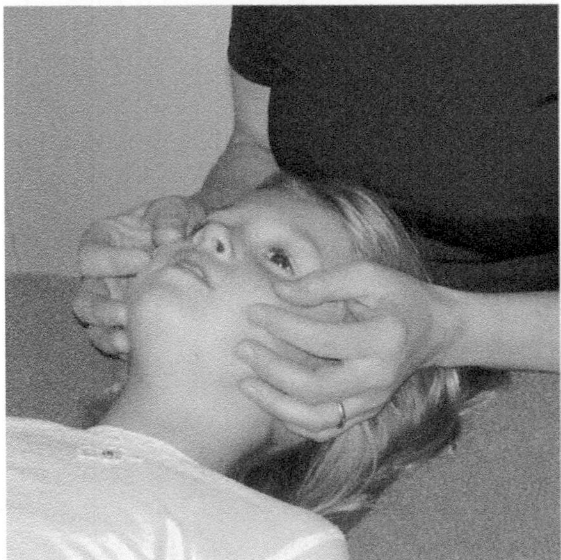

Figure 6.44. *Alternative hand placement for balancing of the zygomae.*

NORMALIZATION OF THE FRONTO-SPHENO-ZYGOMATIC COMPLEX

Indications

Dysfunction between the sphenoid, frontal bone and zygoma, often encountered as the result of blunt facial trauma.

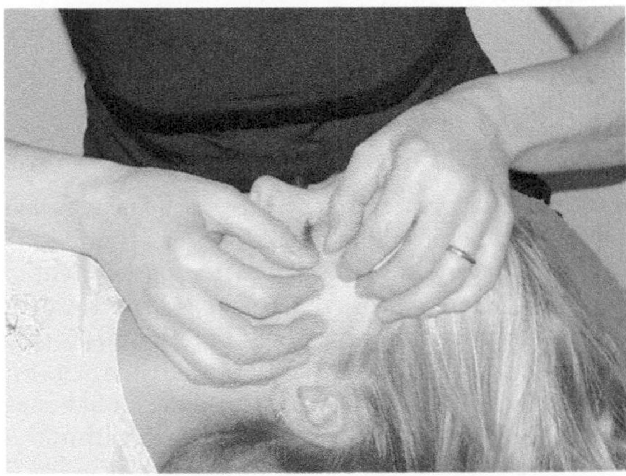

Figure 6.45. *Frontozygomatic suture normalization.*

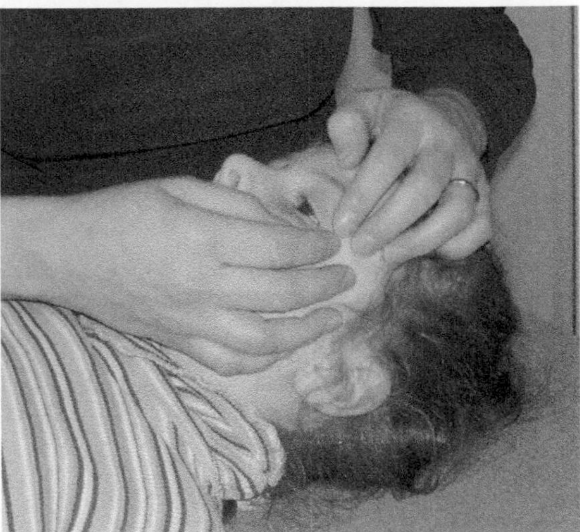

Figure 6.46. *Alternative hand placement for frontozygomatic suture normalization.*

Procedure (Fig. 6.47)

Patient supine; practitioner seated at the head of the table on the opposite side of the dysfunction. Place the caudal hand on the zygoma such that the index finger is on the orbital border and the middle finger is on the inferior border. The cephalic hand is placed on the frontal bone, the index finger on the zygomatic process and the tip of the middle finger on the top of the greater wing of the sphenoid. Listen and follow the frontal bone, the sphenoid and the zygoma according to their major and minor movements in the direction of ease. Await a release. In cases of compression a pumping action that follows the PRM may be employed.

Remarks

The dysfunction of this area may be traumatic, demonstrating compression, and may precede the development of ocular dysfunction.

BALANCING OF THE ETHMOID

Indications

Dysfunction of the ethmoid; sinusitis; rhinitis; functional nasal airway obstruction; noisy breathing; nasolacrimal duct obstruction.

Procedure (Fig. 6.48)

Patient supine; practitioner seated to the side of the head of the table. Place the cephalic hand on the frontal bones with thumb and index finger on either side of the nasal notch. The thumb and index finger of the caudal hand are on either side of the nasal bones. Visualize the ethmoid located behind the nasal bones and, through the nasal bones, listen and follow the motion of the ethmoid in the direction of ease, often in a pattern of compression beneath the frontal bone. Await a release. The PRM may be employed to assist the release.

Remarks

Prior to treating the ethmoid, it is necessary to be certain that the ethmoidal notch of the frontal bone is free from dysfunction. When treating the ethmoid an alternative hand position may be employed that utilizes the nasal septum (Fig. 6.49). The tips of the

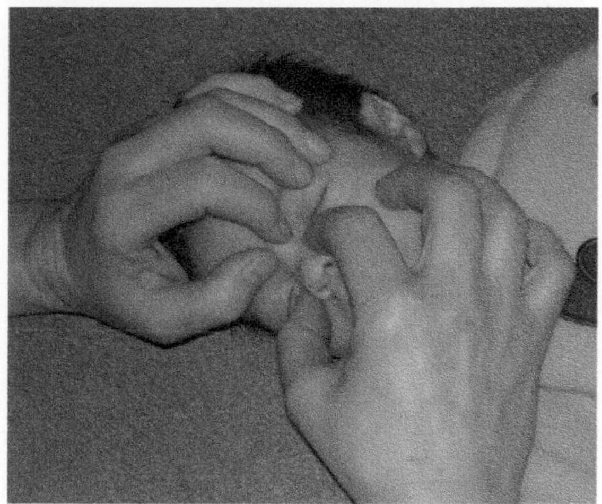

Figure 6.48. *Balancing the ethmoid.*

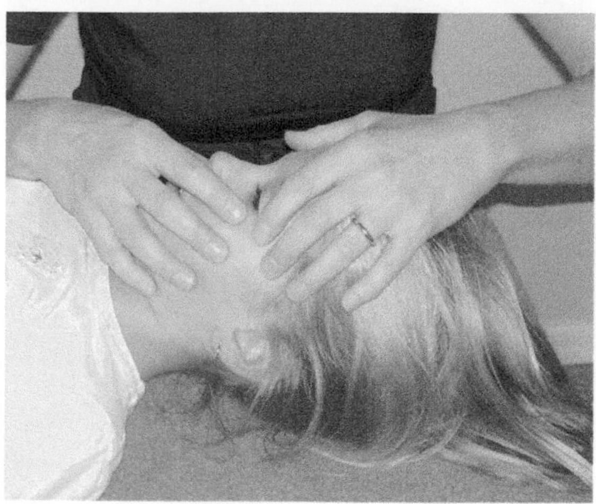

Figure 6.47. *Normalization of the fronto-spheno-zygomatic complex.*

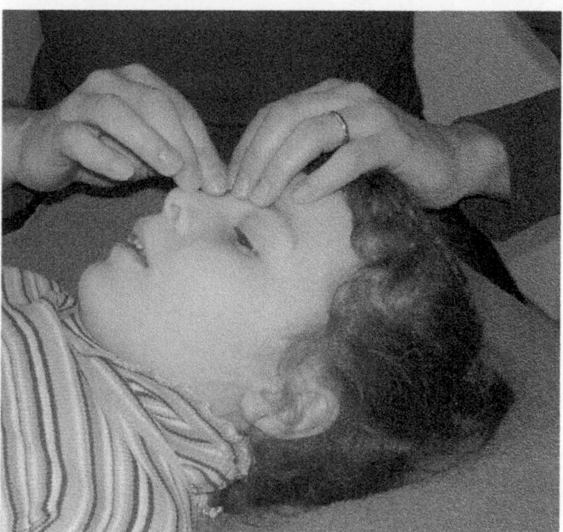

Figure 6.49. *Alternative hand placement for balancing the ethmoid.*

index and middle fingers may be placed on the nose and the ethmoid is visualized through the nasal cartilage.

In both these examples, the hold should be as light as possible.

BALANCING OF THE NASAL BONES

Indications

Dysfunction of the nasal bones; functional nasal airway obstruction; noisy breathing; nasolacrimal duct obstruction.

Procedure (Fig. 6.50)

Patient supine; practitioner seated to the side of the head of the table. Place the thumb and index finger of the caudal hand on either side of the nasal bones. The cephalic hand reaches down over the frontal bone such that the middle finger is on the metopic suture, the other fingers resting comfortably on either side. Listen and follow the motion of ease, with the help of pumping from the PRM, up to the point of release.

Remarks

This is not a traction procedure where the nasal bones are pulled away from the frontal bones. The most commonly encountered dysfunction is that of compression, often complicated by other minor movements.

External rotation of the frontal bone may be facilitated using a slight pressure on the metopic suture by the middle finger of the cephalic hand.

BALANCING OF THE MAXILLAE

Indications

Dysfunction of the maxillae; maxillary sinusitis; teething difficulties; dental malalignment and malocclusion.

Procedure (Fig. 6.51)

Patient supine; practitioner seated at the head of the table. Place the tips of the thumbs on the glabella, extending the other fingers in a caudal direction such that the tips of the index, middle and ring fingers lie on the alveolar processes of the maxillae. Listen and follow the motion of ease. Pay attention to the inherent intraosseous motility of the maxillae. With the tips of the fingers produce minor accommodations to the motions of the maxillae in order to facilitate the release. Await a release.

Remarks

The pressure on the glabella facilitates external rotation of the maxillae.

In the case of a narrowed palate, an intraoral procedure can be performed between the two maxillae. The practitioner places their flexed index fingers in contact with the palatal surfaces of the maxillae and with the palatal side of the alveolar processes of the molars. Care should be taken not to exert pressure directly on the molars. Listen to the inherent

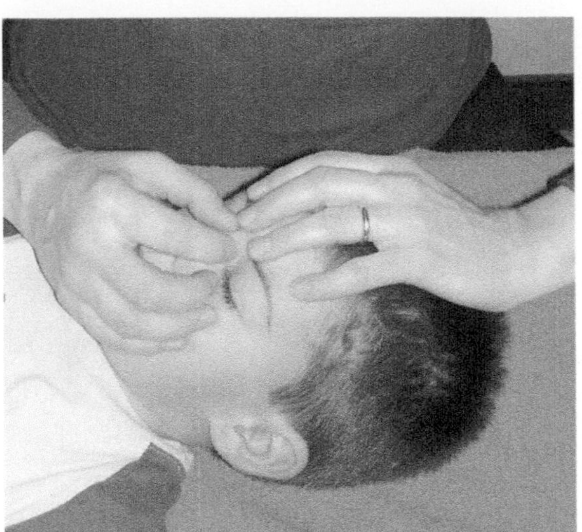

Figure 6.50. *Balancing the nasal bones.*

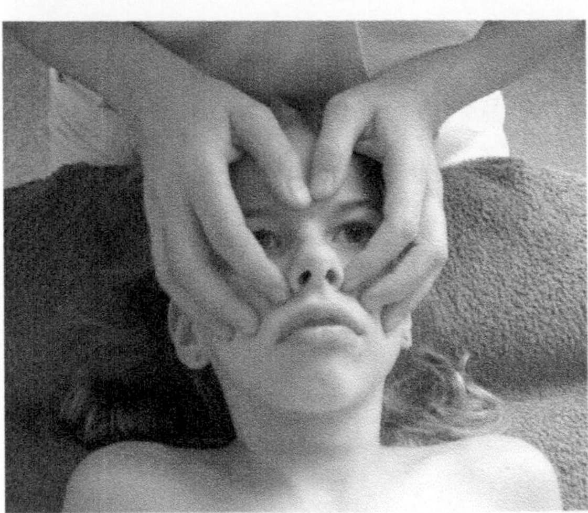

Figure 6.51. *Balancing the maxillae.*

motility of the two maxillae. Using indirect principles, follow the maxillae to their positions of ease and with the inherent pumping action of the PRM await a release.

The patient may be instructed to do the following exercise. Put the thumbs in contact with the palatal side of the alveolar processes approximating the molars (Fig. 6.52) and apply laterally directed forces during inhalation, releasing during exhalation; repeat this several times a day.[6]

BALANCING OF THE VOMER

Indications

Dysfunction of the vomer and sphenoid; functional nasal airway obstruction; noisy breathing; sinusitis; dysfunction of the maxillae.

Procedure (Fig. 6.53)

Patient supine; practitioner seated at the head of the table, toward one side. The cephalic hand is placed on the frontal bones such that the tip of the thumb is on the superior aspect of one greater wing and the tip of the middle finger is on the corresponding spot on the other side. Place the pad of the little finger of the caudal hand inside the mouth of the patient, in contact with the intermaxillary suture. Visualize the vomer oriented posteriorly and superiorly in the direction of the body of the sphenoid. Listen and note the dysfunctional pattern. Follow the motion of the greater wings of the sphenoid, as well as that of the vomer. Utilize indirect principles in conjunction with the inherent forces of the PRM and treat what has been found. A pumping motion between the vomer and sphenoid may further enhance the release.

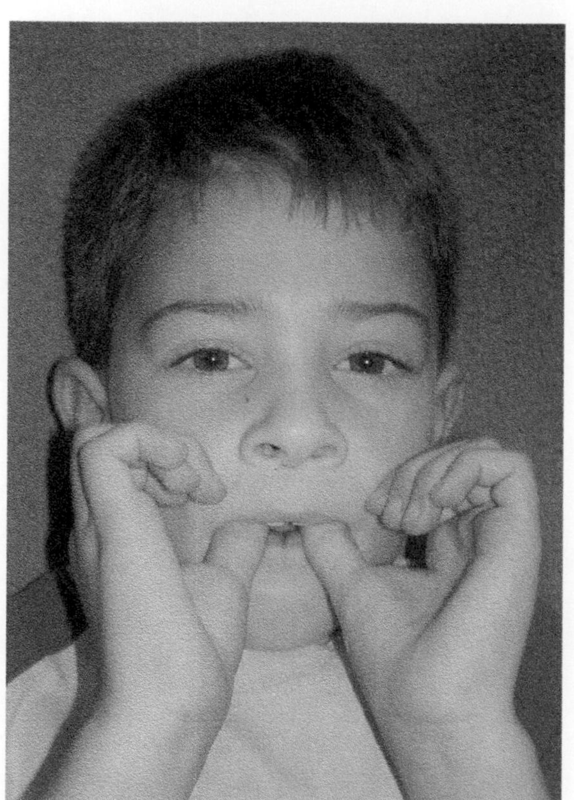

Figure 6.52. *Autobalancing the maxillae.*

Remarks

This is a procedure that, like all intraoral procedures, necessitates the very lightest of touch.

In older children and adolescents whose mouth will tolerate two fingers, by keeping the sphenoid hold and putting the index and middle fingers of the caudal hand on either side of the intermaxillary suture, the practitioner can act on that suture (Fig. 6.54) and, if the fingers are placed more posteriorly, on the interpalatine suture. This is indicated in the case of a narrowed palate.

Pelvic procedures

GLOBAL BALANCING OF THE PELVIS

Indications

Pelvic somatic dysfunctions; pelvic visceral dysfunctions, including constipation, enuresis and

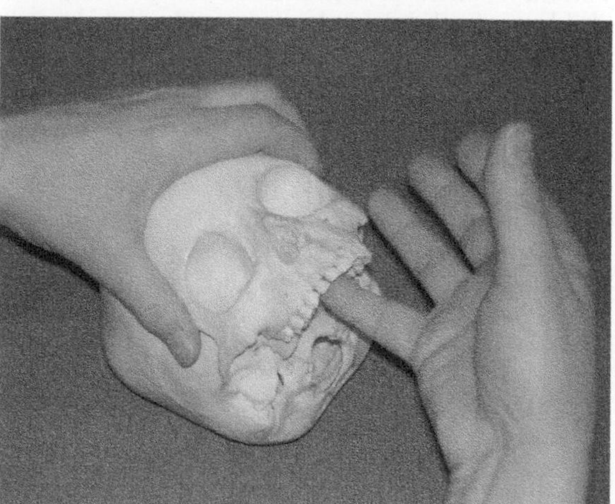

Figure 6.53. *Balancing the vomer.*

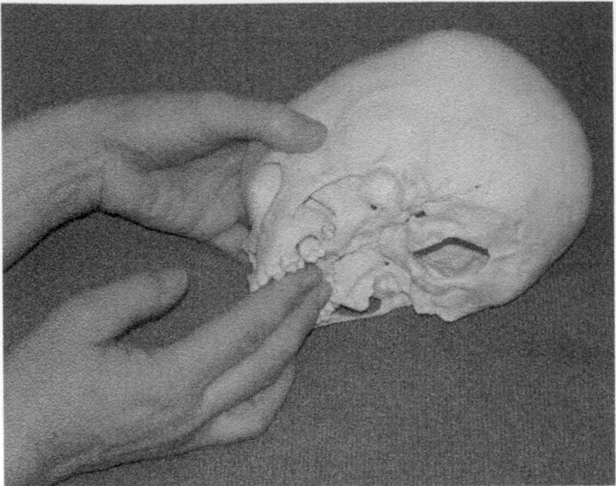

Figure 6.54. *Balancing the intermaxillary suture.*

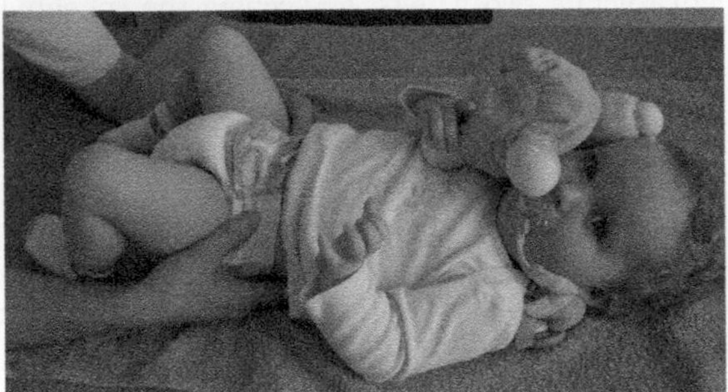

Figure 6.55. *Global balancing of the pelvis.*

dysmenorrhea; patellar disorders; functional leg length inequity.

Procedure (Fig. 6.55)

Patient supine; practitioner standing facing the child, at the level of the pelvis. Place the hands bilaterally on the child's pelvis in such a way that the thumbs contact the ASISs, the index fi ngers curl laterally around the iliac crests and the pads of the middle fingers contact, if possible, the child's PSISs. Listen to the pelvic bones, their position and inherent motion. Feel for internal or external rotation in the context of the major and minor motions. Using indirect principles, follow the motion pattern. Dysfunctions of the pelvis often demonstrate asymmetric motion patterns with greater motion restriction on one side. Release of the side of greater restriction can be enhanced by the use of the inherent forces of the PRM as a pumping procedure. The goal of treatment is to have both sides moving as freely as possible, with external–internal rotation occurring in synchrony with the biphasic motion of the PRM.

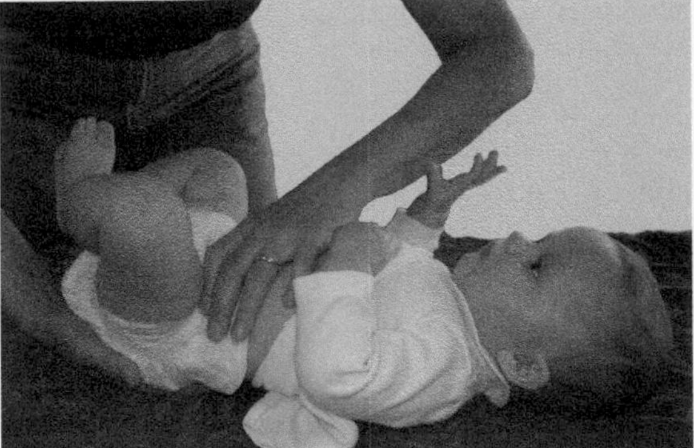

Figure 6.56. *Sacrum procedure.*

Remarks

If dysfunction of the hips is identifi ed, it should be treated before treatment of the pelvis (see hip procedure described below).

The diagnosis and global balancing of the pelvis should always precede treatment of spinal dysfunction.

SACRUM PROCEDURE

Indications

Sacral somatic dysfunction; scoliosis; pelvic autonomic dysfunction.

Procedure (Fig. 6.56)

Patient supine; practitioner standing facing the child, at the level of the pelvis. Place the dominant hand palm up under the child's sacrum in such a way that the fi ngers are directed cephalad. The index and little fi ngers each contact one of the child's PSISs and the middle and ring fingers are in contact with the base of the sacrum. Position the other hand transversely, contacting the anterior pelvis, using the forearm as well if the size of the child necessitates. Listen, and feel if the sacral motion is the same on both sides as the sacral base moves into the hand in craniosacral flexion or moves anteriorly in craniosacral extension. Note the presence of asymmetric patterns such as torsion with components of sidebending and rotation. Follow the motion in the direction of ease and, using indirect principles, treat any dysfunctional pattern. Toddlers and adolescents may be instructed to utilize respiratory cooperation by inhaling to augment craniosacral fl exion and exhaling for craniosacral extension.

Remarks

The hand placement beneath the sacrum may be modified to use three fingers when treating infants.

If greater restriction is palpable between the sacrum and PSISs on one side, it is indicative of sacroiliac dysfunction and should be treated as discussed below.

SACROILIAC PROCEDURE

Indications

Sacroiliac dysfunction; pelvic visceral dysfunctions, including constipation and enuresis; pelvic autonomic dysfunction.

Procedure (Fig. 6.57)

Patient supine; practitioner standing or seated facing the child, at the level of the pelvis on the side of the dysfunction. Place the caudal hand palm up under the child's sacrum in such a way that the fingers are directed cephalad and the index, middle and ring fingers are in contact with the base of the sacrum. Place the cephalic hand such that the thumb contacts the ASIS and the index finger curls around the iliac crest with the pad of the middle finger contacting the child's PSIS. Listen and follow the motion in the direction of ease. Pay particular attention to the minor components of innominate bone motion. Await a release.

Remarks

The lower extremity may be employed as a lever to move the pelvic bone in relation to the sacrum (Fig. 6.58).

Small children may be treated in a seated position on the practitioner's lap (Fig. 6.59). Using indirect principles the practitioner adjusts the relative position of their thighs to affect the relationship between the sacrum and pelvic bones while their hands monitor the sacrum and pelvic bones.

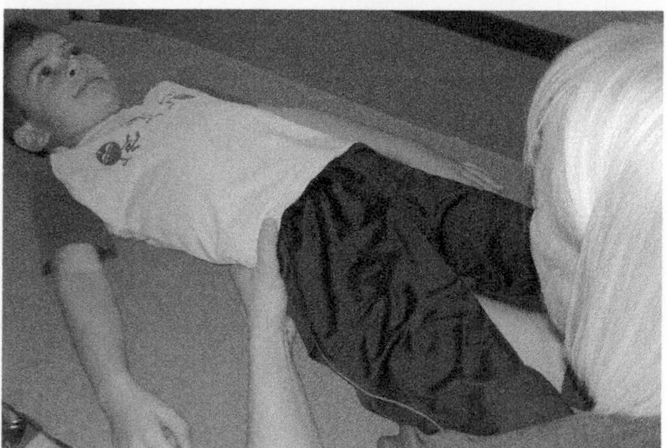

Figure 6.57. *Sacroiliac procedure.*

INNOMINATE INTRAOSSEOUS PROCEDURE

Indications

Intraosseous dysfunction of the innominate; dysplasia of the acetabulum.

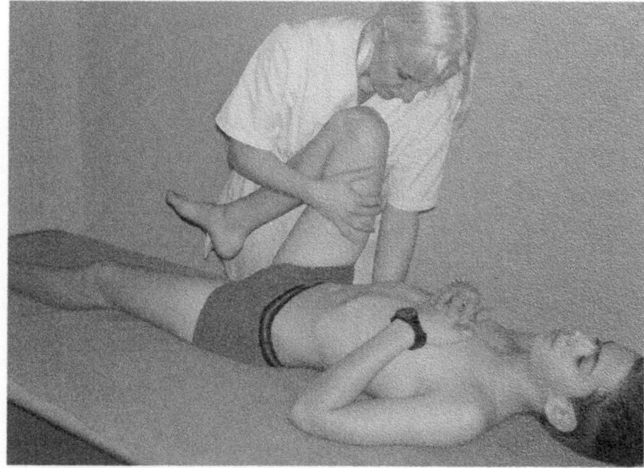

Figure 6.58. *Alternative hand placement for sacroiliac procedure.*

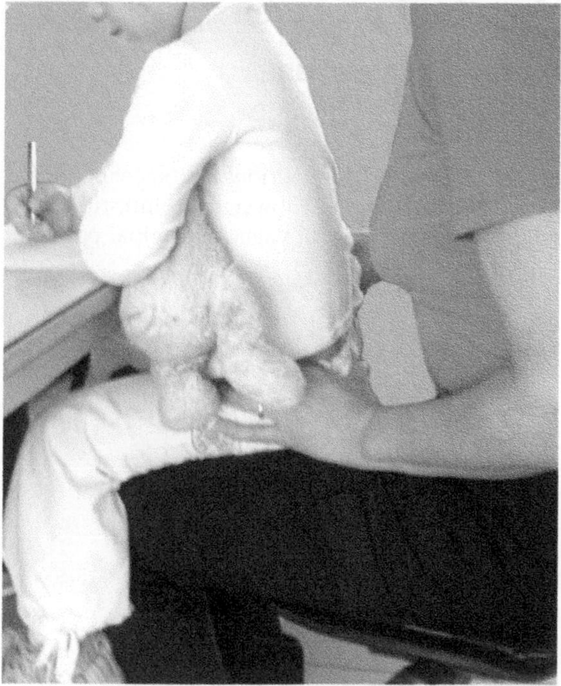

Figure 6.59. *Alternative position for sacroiliac procedure.*

Procedure (Fig. 6.60)

Patient supine; practitioner standing or seated facing the child, at the level of the pelvis on the side opposite the dysfunction. Place the cephalic hand such that the thumb or index finger contacts the ASIS on the side of the dysfunction. With the caudal hand, flex the hip on the dysfunctional side to a comfortable position and use your forearm to support the leg. Place the caudal hand beneath the innominate with the pad of the index or middle finger contacting the PSIS and the hypothenar eminence contacting the ischial tuberosity. Listen to the respective inherent motility of the three intraosseous components of the innominate bone. Follow the intraosseous relationships and utilize indirect principles and the inherent forces of the PRM to obtain a release.

Remarks

Any of the three component parts of the innominate, ilium, ischium and pubes may demonstrate intraosseous dysfunction. As such, the practitioner should have a clear knowledge of their anatomic relationship in order to diagnose and treat this dysfunction. When treating hip dysplasia, it is important to treat dysfunction of the femoroacetabular relationship as well (see 'Hip balancing', below).

Vertebral procedures

LUMBAR PROCEDURE

Indications

Lumbar somatic dysfunctions; thoracoabdominal diaphragm dysfunction; lower gastrointestinal dysfunction; dysmenorrhea; vague abdominal pain.

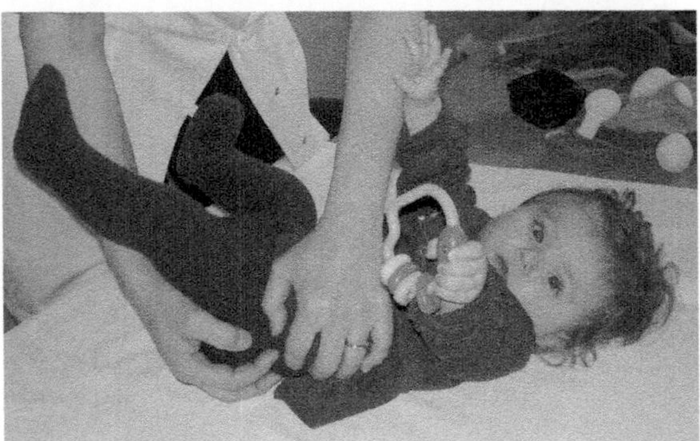

Figure 6.60. *Innominate intraosseous procedure.*

Procedure (Fig. 6.61)

Patient supine; practitioner standing facing the child, at the level of the pelvis, close to the patient. Bilaterally flex the patient's legs and, using the caudal arm, surround them and hold them in contact with the practitioner's lateral chest wall. Place the cephalic hand palm up transversely beneath the lumbar spine in such a way that the pads of the index, middle and ring fingers are in contact with the spinous processes of the dysfunctional area. Listen to the spinal segments and identify any restriction of the PRM's inherent motility, indicative of somatic dysfunction. If necessary, further assess lumbar dysfunction by introducing motion from below through the legs. Gently increase and decrease hip flexion to produce lumbar flexion and extension. Use the legs as a lever to produce lumbar sidebending and rotation. Follow the dysfunctional pattern and, through the legs, position the dysfunctional area to enhance the position of ease. Await a release.

Remarks

This is a gentle and relaxing procedure that should be done slowly in order to maintain appreciation of the palpatory cues arising from the dysfunctional area.

THORACIC PROCEDURE

Indications

Thoracic somatic dysfunctions; dysfunction of pulmonary respiration; dysfunction of the thoracoabdominal diaphragm; thoracic autonomic dysfunction.

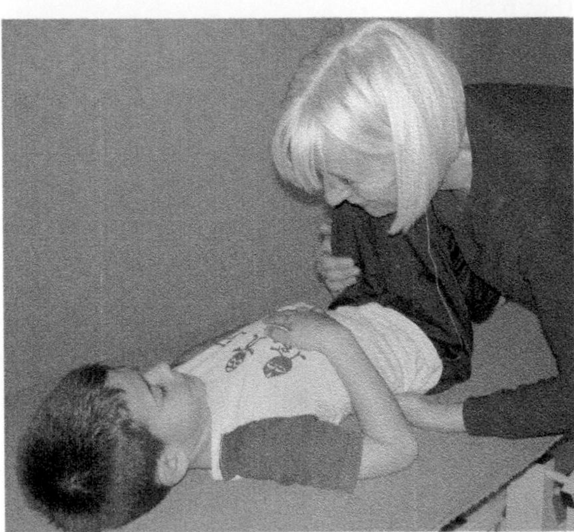

Figure 6.61. *Lumbar procedure.*

Procedure (Fig. 6.62)

Patient seated; practitioner seated behind or beside the patient. Place one hand transversely on the thoracic spine in such a way that the pads of the index, middle and ring fingers are in contact with the spinous processes of the dysfunctional area. Listen to the spinal segments and identify any restriction of the PRM's inherent motility, indicative of somatic dysfunction. If necessary, further assess thoracic dysfunction by introducing motion from above through the shoulders, head and neck. Gently increase and decrease cervical flexion to produce thoracic flexion and extension. Use the shoulders as a lever to produce thoracic sidebending and rotation. Follow the dysfunctional pattern and, from above, position the dysfunctional area to enhance the position of ease. Await a release.

Remarks

An alternative to the lumbar or thoracic procedure may be performed with the patient in the prone position (Fig. 6.63). Fine intersegmental treatment may be accomplished by placing the index and middle fingers of each hand on either side of the spinous processes of two adjacent vertebral segments, listening and employing indirect principles to treat.

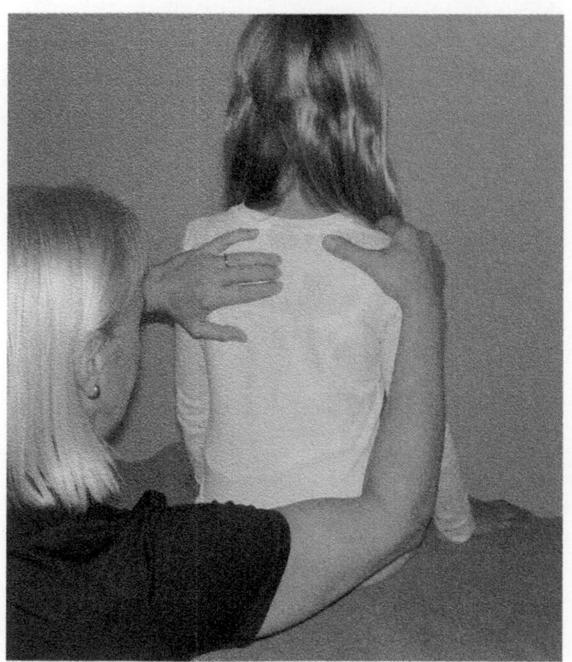

Figure 6.62. *Thoracic procedure.*

CERVICAL AND UPPER THORACIC PROCEDURE

Indications

Upper thoracic and cervical somatic dysfunctions; headaches. Because of the significance of upper thoracic sympathetic and upper cervical parasympathetic reflexes, a myriad of viscerosomatic and somatovisceral dysfunctions are found in these areas.

Procedure (Fig. 6.64)

Patient supine; practitioner seated at the head of the table. Place the pads of the index and middle fingers of one hand in contact with the spinous processes of the dysfunctional area. Cradle the occiput with the other hand. Listen to the spinal segments and identify any restriction of the PRM's inherent motility, indicative of somatic dysfunction of those segments. If necessary, further assess upper thoracic or cervical dysfunction by introducing motion from above

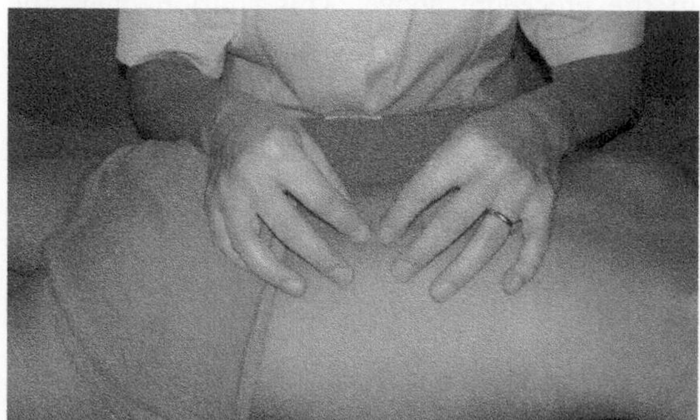

Figure 6.63. *Alternative hand placement for lumbar procedure.*

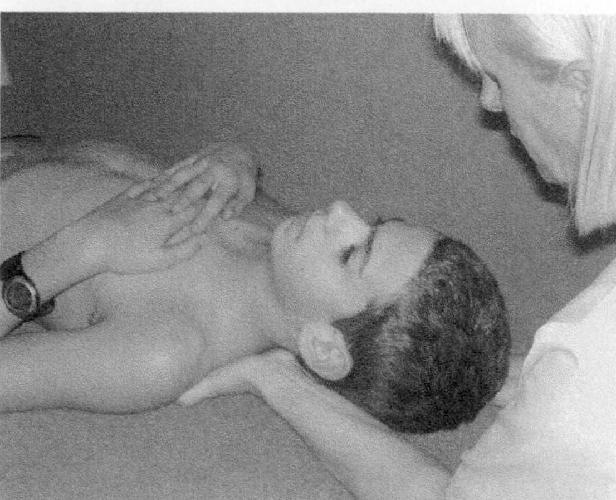

Figure 6.64. *Cervical and upper thoracic procedure.*

through the head. Most of the time, it is enough to visualize the motion to be introduced. The introduction of motions that are too gross will result in loss of localization. Gently increase and decrease occipital flexion to produce cervical or upper thoracic flexion and extension. Use the head to further induce sidebending and rotation. Using indirect principles, follow the dysfunctional pattern and, from above, position the dysfunctional area to enhance the position of ease. Await a release.

Remarks

If resistance to release is encountered during treatment, assess the spinal segments above and below the dysfunctional area for contributory dysfunction and, if found, treat it and return to the initial area.

An alternative procedure for the treatment of infants is to hold the child in the practitioner's lap with one hand contacting the spinous processes of the dysfunctional area and the other hand supporting the occiput (Fig. 6.65). Listen to the dysfunctional area and follow indirect principles as described in the procedure above. This position offers the advantage of being able to move the infant in an almost infinite combination of positions to recreate the fetal position. Because the infant is lying face up in the practitioner's hands, this position also allows the establishment of interpersonal connection between the infant and practitioner. This permits the practitioner to readily adjust the treatment intervention to the response of the infant.

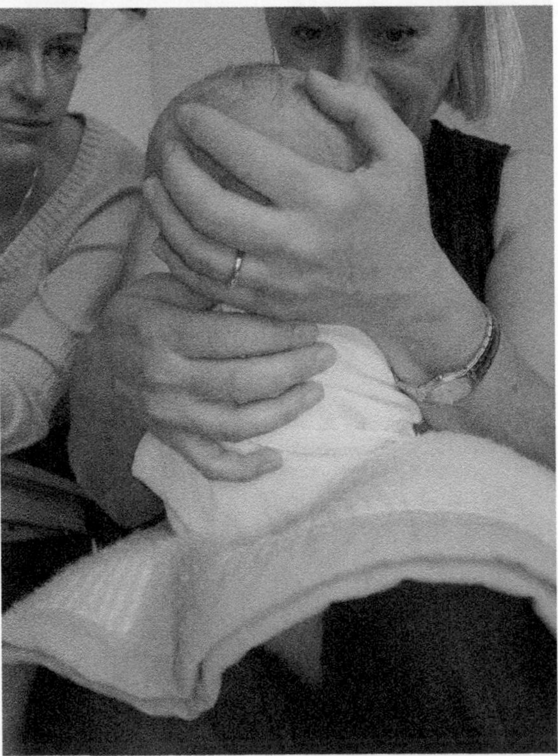

Figure 6.65. *Alternative hand placement for cervical and upper thoracic procedure.*

Appendicular procedures

LOWER EXTREMITY PROCEDURES

Global foot balancing

Indications

Metartarsus adductus; intoeing; pes cavus or pes planus.

Procedure (Fig. 6.66)

Patient supine; practitioner seated at the foot of the table. The cephalic hand grasps the calcaneus between the index finger medially and the thumb laterally. The caudal hand holds the forefoot between the thumb and fingers with the thumb resting transversely across the dorsum of the foot. Listen to the global pattern of the foot, noting external or internal rotation and any dominant component of motion within that pattern. Using indirect principles, follow the motion within the foot and allow the pumping action of the PRM to release the myofascial dysfunction.

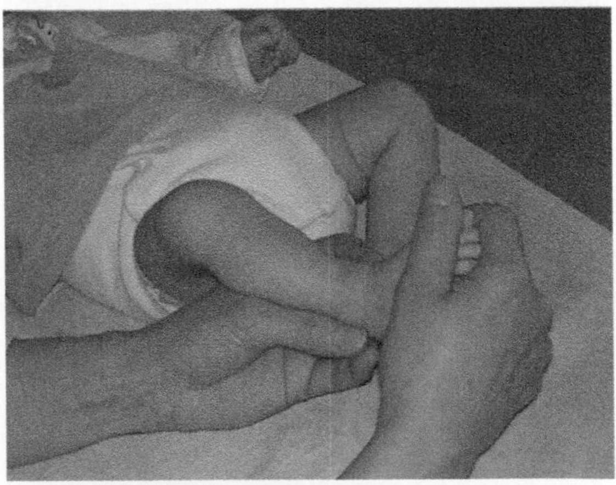

Figure 6.66. *Global foot balancing.*

Remarks

This procedure should be part of a total body approach, with specific consideration of the pelvis and the remainder of the lower extremity as well as the foot.

Fibular balancing

Indications

Dysfunction involving the knee and ankle; leg cramps; ankle sprains and strains.

Procedure (Fig. 6.67)

Patient supine; practitioner seated at the side of the table adjacent to the dysfunctional lower extremity. Place a small cushion beneath the knee to induce a small amount of flexion. With the cephalad hand grasp the proximal fibula between the thumb and index finger while holding the lateral malleolus between the thumb and index finger of the other hand. Using tests of listening, visualize the tissues surrounding the proximal and distal tibiofibula articulations and the interosseous membrane between the two bones. Follow the fibula to the position of ease and, with the aid of the pumping action of the PRM, await a release.

Remarks

This procedure may be employed globally to balance the relationship between the tibia and fibula It is important to remember that these dysfunctions almost always involve the interosseous membrane between the two bones. In practice, however, the distal, or more often proximal, fibula will demonstrate greater motion restriction. In this case, attention should focus on the area of restricted motion.

For ankle sprains and strains, experience has shown that the proximal fibula should be manipulated first. After the tibia and fibula have been normalized, the dysfunction of the ankle may be addressed.

Subtalar balancing

Indications

Ankle sprains and strains; pes cavus or pes planus.

Procedure (Fig. 6.68)

Patient supine; practitioner seated at the foot of the table. The cephalic hand grasps the calcaneus, cradling it in the palm of the hand or between the index finger medially and the thumb laterally. The caudal hand rests on the dorsum of the foot, monitoring the talar neck between the thumb and index finger. Listen and visualize the relationship between the talus and calcaneus. Note any dysfunction involving external or internal rotation and the minor components of these movements. Using indirect procedures, follow the dysfunction to the position of ease and, with the aid of the pumping force of the PRM, await a release.

Remarks

Although this procedure may be included as part of the global balancing of the foot, when employed it should be performed precisely between the talus and calcaneus.

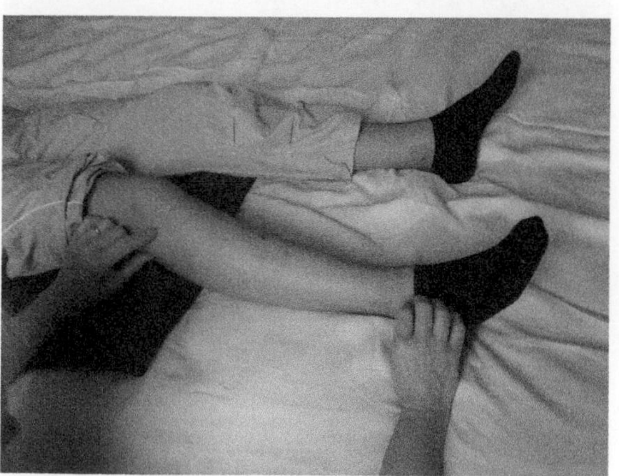

Figure 6.67. *Fibular balancing.*

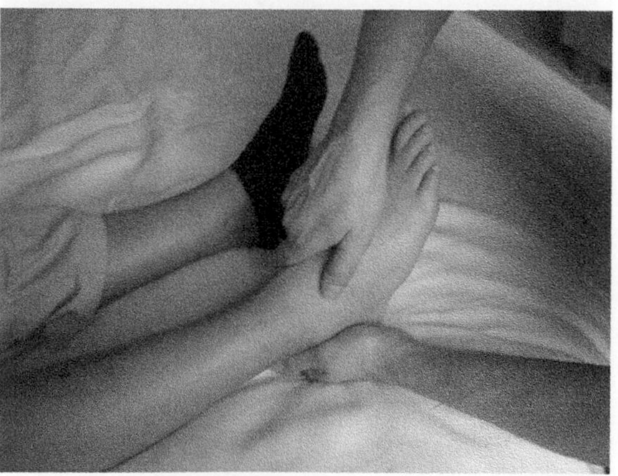

Figure 6.68. *Subtalar balancing.*

Intraosseous tibial balancing

Indications

Intraosseous tibial torsions; gait disorders, intoeing or out-toeing.

Procedure (Fig. 6.69)

Patient supine; practitioner seated beside the patient on the side of the dysfunction. Grasp the proximal and distal ends of the tibia with your hands. Listen and visualize the intraosseous dysfunctional pattern within the tibia, commonly torsional. Employ indirect procedures, follow the pattern into the position of ease and use the pumping action of the PRM to facilitate a release.

Remarks

For this procedure to be most effective, it is best done before the child begins to stand.

Knee balancing

Indications

Knee dysfunctions; knee sprains and strains.

Procedure (Fig. 6.70)

Patient seated in a relaxed position, on the side of the treatment table; practitioner seated in front of the patient, to the side of the dysfunction. Grasp the medial and lateral epicondyles of the femur with one hand while the other hand holds the proximal end of the tibia. Listen and visualize the pattern of motion that is present with attention to the minor components of the motions of the knee. Employ indirect principles and follow the pattern into the position of ease. Utilize the pumping action of the PRM to facilitate a release.

Remarks

When done properly this procedure is comfortable for both the patient and the practitioner.

Performing this procedure with the knee flexed provides the opportunity to modify knee position and most closely approximates the position in which the dysfunction originated.

Alternatively, the knee can be treated with the patient supine or prone with variable degrees of knee flexion.

Hip balancing

Indications

Dysfunction of the hip.

Procedure (Fig. 6.71)

Patient supine; practitioner seated facing the patient, at the level of the pelvis on the side of the

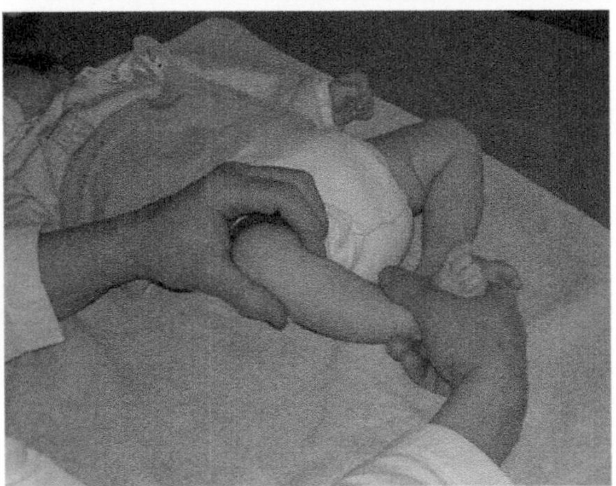

Figure 6.69. *Intraosseous tibial balancing.*

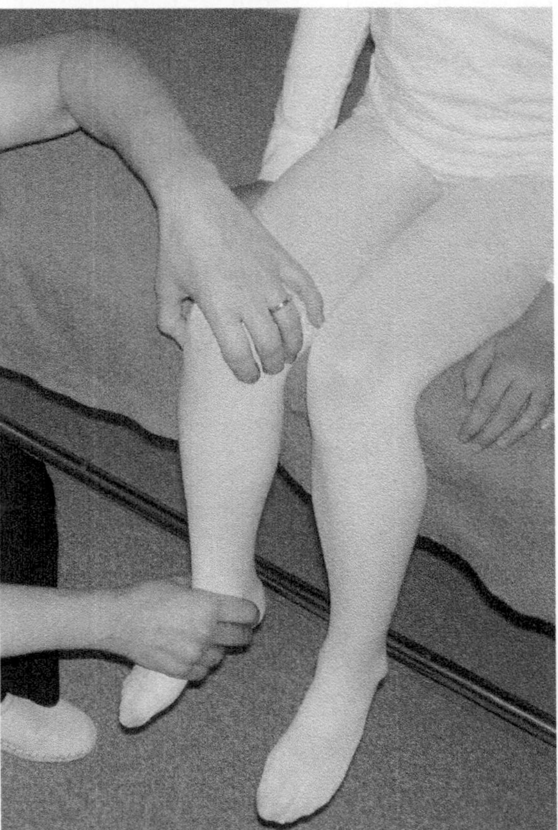

Figure 6.70. *Knee balancing.*

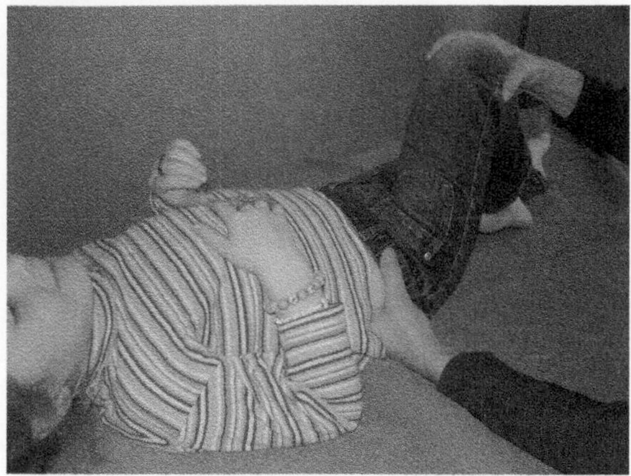

Figure 6.71. *Hip balancing.*

dysfunction. Grasp the patient's knee with the caudal hand and flex the hip to a position where the periarticular soft tissues are optimally relaxed, often approximately 90°. Place the cephalic hand on the ipsilateral pelvis, such that the thumb contacts the ASIS and the index finger curls around the iliac crest with the pad of the middle finger contacting the patient's PSIS. Listen and visualize the relationship between the femur and the acetabulum. Follow the motion in the direction of ease. Employ the inherent forces of the PRM and await a release.

Remarks

In infants, this procedure should be employed as part of the total approach to the treatment of hip dysplasia. It allows the femoral head to be recentered and stabilized. This is facilitated by flexing the hip, thus reducing tension of the iliopsoas, a muscle group that is often shortened because of the fetal position.

UPPER EXTREMITY PROCEDURES

Shoulder balancing

Indications

Dysfunction of the shoulder; brachial plexus injury; athletic injuries and overuse of the shoulder.

Procedure (Fig. 6.72)

Patient supine or seated; practitioner seated facing the child, at the level of the shoulder on the side of the dysfunction. Place the cephalic hand on the dysfunctional shoulder, with the index or middle finger at the level of the spine of the scapula and the thumb on the clavicle. With the other hand gently grasp the child's arm above the elbow, cradling their forearm with your forearm. Listen to the shoulder and follow the motion in the direction of ease. Employ the biphasic PRM to facilitate a release.

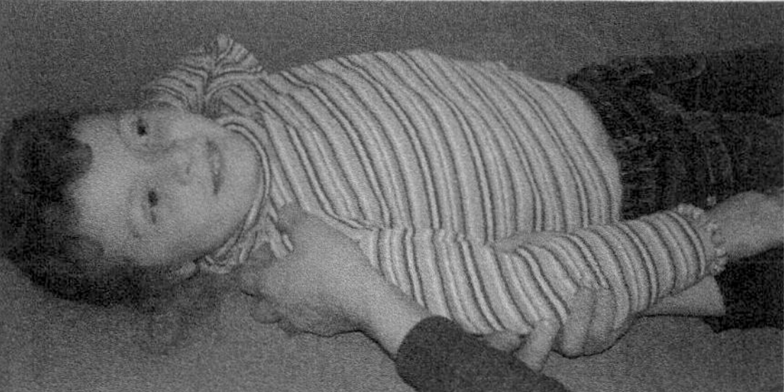

Figure 6.72. *Shoulder balancing.*

Remarks

When addressing brachial plexus injury with this procedure it is of the utmost importance that extraneous movement be minimized. Traction is particularly to be avoided.

When treating adolescents the principles apply as described above but the range of motion employed in treatment is proportionately larger.

It is good practice to identify and treat upper thoracic and cervical dysfunction prior to treating the shoulder.

Nursemaid's elbow procedure

Indications

Subluxation of the developing radial head from the annular ligament of the elbow joint.

Procedure (Fig. 6.73)

Patient seated; practitioner standing facing the patient. With one hand, grasp the patient's wrist on the dysfunctional side, with your thumb contacting the distal radius and your middle finger contacting the ulna. With your other hand, contact the radial head with your thumb. Listen and visualize the relationship between the radius, ulna and humerus, paying attention to the annular ligament and the interosseous membrane. Using flexion or extension, abduction or adduction, and pronation or supination, follow the elbow into the position of ease. Employ the PRM to facilitate the release of the radial head.

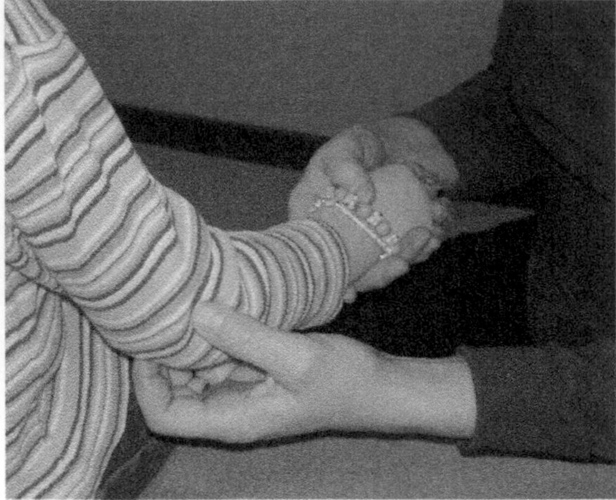

Figure 6.73. *Nursemaid's elbow procedure.*

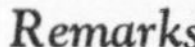

Remarks

Because nursemaid's elbow is of traumatic origin and the tissues of children are elastic, indirect principles lend themselves particularly well to its treatment. Placing the dysfunction in the position of ease is comforting for the child and consequently will alleviate their fears and not be met with resistance. Normally it should not be necessary to pry, pull or twist to treat this condition effectively.

Visceral procedures

GASTROESOPHAGEAL PROCEDURE

Indications

Gastroesophageal reflux; regurgitation.

Procedure (Fig. 6.74)

Patient supine; practitioner standing or seated beside the patient at the level of the abdomen. Place the caudal hand over the abdomen, with the thenar eminence lying in the midline and the thumb resting over the xiphoid process. The fingers are directed laterally with the fifth finger over the left hypochondrium. With this hand placement the gastric body will be cradled by the palm while the esophagus is monitored by the thumb. The cephalic hand contacts the anterior chest wall with the thumb on the sternum and the fingers directed laterally over the lower thoracic cage and thoracoabdominal diaphragm. Listen and visualize the stomach and gastroesophageal junction, noting the presence of torsion between the stomach and esophagus in the horizontal, frontal and sagittal planes. Follow the dysfunctional pattern using indirect principles and await a release. The caudal hand is employed to release the gastroesophageal junction while the cephalic hand releases the thoracoabdominal diaphragm.

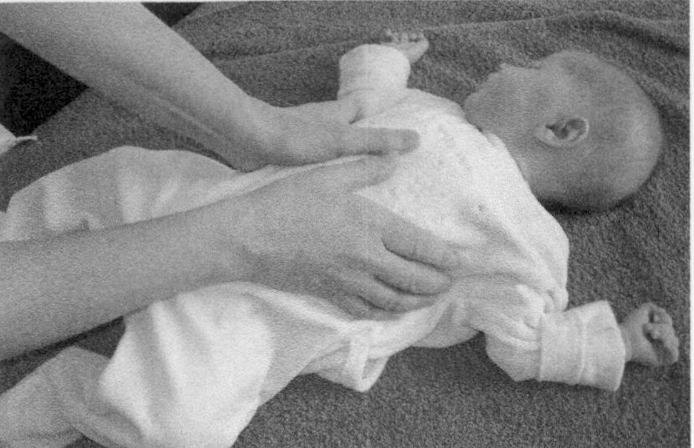

Figure 6.74. *Gastroesophageal procedure.*

Remarks

For infants, the child may be held facing forward in such a way that the cephalic hand monitoring the lower thoracic cage and diaphragm also supports the child's weight while the caudal hand is free to address the lower torso as well as the gastroesophageal junction.

An alternative position is to hold the infant in the practitioner's lap with the tips of the fingers of one hand contacting the spinous processes of the lower thoracic area and the ulnar border of the hand contacting the left lower ribs at the level of the posterior costal attachments of the diaphragm (Fig. 6.75). This hand monitors the diaphragm, gastroesophageal junction and lower thoracic spine. The other hand supports the occiput. Listen to the relationship between the two hands and move with the infant into the position of greatest ease. Following indirect principles, await a release. This position allows the practitioner to observe the infant's face, providing immediate feedback as to the infant's comfort.

TREATING COLIC

Indications

Colic, abdominal pain and distension.

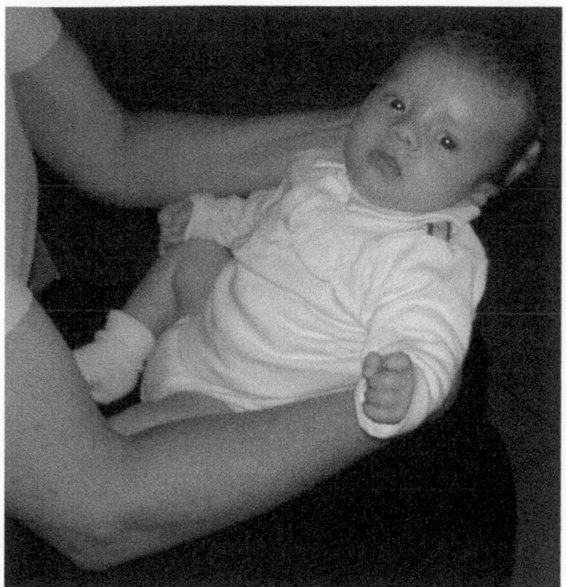

Figure 6.75. *Alternative hand placement for gastroesophageal procedure.*

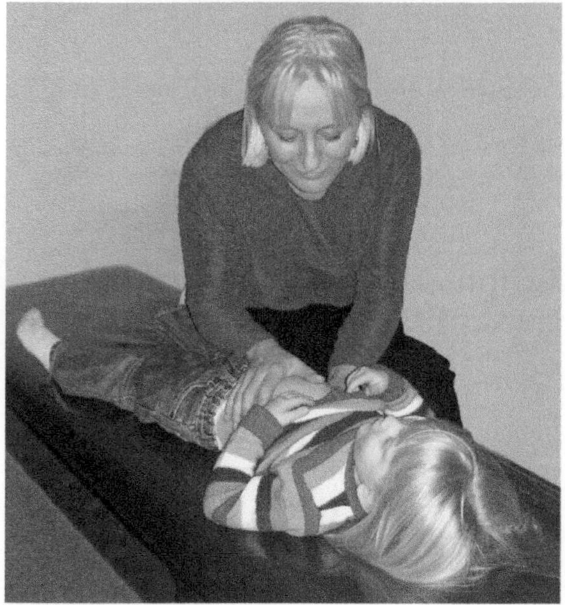

Figure 6.76. *Treating colic.*

Procedure (Fig. 6.76)

Patient supine; practitioner seated beside the patient at the level of the abdomen. Place the caudal hand on the abdomen with the palm centrally located over the periumbilical region. Listen and visualize the abdominal contents. The different layers of the abdomen should be appreciated through the palpatory contact. Identify the area of greatest tension within the abdomen. The cephalic hand lies beneath the spine, palm up, with the fingertips contacting the lower thoracic and lumbar spinous processes. Listen and identify the tissue texture and motion pattern of any thoracolumbar spinal somatic dysfunction. Working between the two hands and using indirect principles, follow the tissues to their position of greatest ease and await a release.

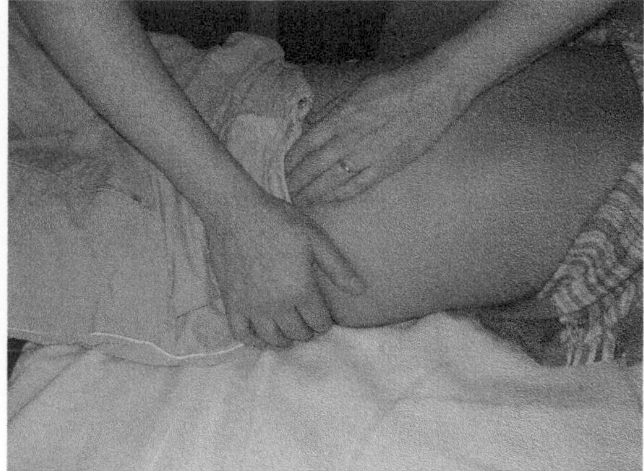

Figure 6.77. *Treating constipation.*

Remarks

It is important to remember that the spinal regions associated with viscerosomatic and somatovisceral reflexes of the small intestine are found in the lower thoracic region and those of the colon are found in the thoracolumbar and upper to mid lumbar regions.[7,8]

TREATING CONSTIPATION

Indications

Constipation.

Procedure (Fig. 6.77)

Patient supine; practitioner seated or standing on the right side of the patient at the level of the abdomen. Place the cephalic hand on the abdomen with the fingers contacting the left lower quadrant. Listen and visualize the abdominal contents. With the pads of the fingers identify the area of greatest tension within the descending and sigmoid colon. The caudal hand lies on the left innominate with the fingers directed posteriorly along the iliac crest. Listen and visualize the inherent motility of the innominate. With both hands, using indirect principles, follow the innominate and colon to a position of balance and await a release.

Remarks

Before using the above procedure it is imperative that somatic dysfunction of the innominate and sacrum be thoroughly identified and treated as described above.

Diaphragmatic procedure

Indications

Thoracoabdominal diaphragmatic dysfunction; lower respiratory tract dysfunction, bronchiolitis, asthma; upper respiratory tract dysfunction, sinusitis, mouth breathing.

Procedure

Patient supine; practitioner seated at the side of the patient at the level of the abdomen. Place both hands such that they encircle the lower thoracic cage bilaterally. The thumbs contact the inferior costal cartilages lateral to the xiphoid process. The fingers are directed posteriorly contacting the lower ribs. The hand placement in this procedure must be fluid, in accordance with the dysfunctional mechanics. In larger individuals, it may be necessary, during the procedure, to move the hands posteriorly so that the fingers contact the costotransverse articulations. Alternatively, the practitioner may place one hand under the thoracolumbar junction and the other over the xiphoid process and epigastrium as illustrated (Fig. 6.78). With either hand placement, apply a very light compressive force, just the amount of pressure necessary to reach the level of the diaphragm. Assess the motion of the diaphragm during pulmonary respiration. Listen and note any asymmetry or restriction of motion. Moving with respiratory excursion and using indirect principles, accompany the diaphragm in its position of ease and await a release. When the patient is relaxed, the pulmonary respiration will frequently become entrained with the PRM.

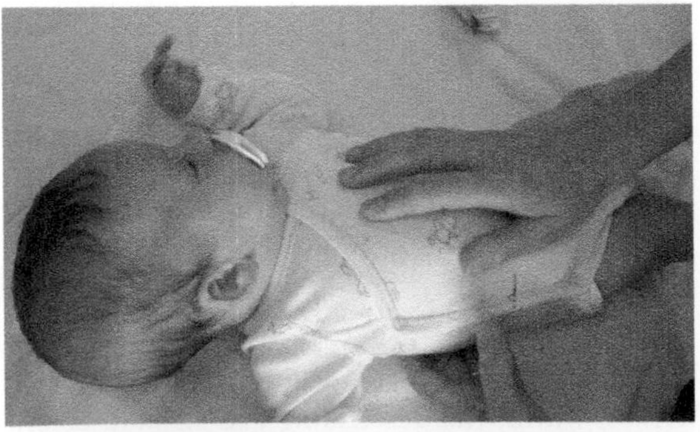

Figure 6.78. *Diaphragmatic procedure.*

Remarks

When treating a dysfunctional diaphragm it is imperative to first identify and treat dysfunction affecting the anatomic areas of diaphragmatic origin: lumbar vertebrae L2, L3, occasionally L1 and L4; ribs 7–12 and their respective vertebral segments, sternum and xiphoid process.

The phrenic nerve that arises essentially from the fourth cervical nerve, and receives a branch from the third and the fifth, innervates the diaphragm. Dysfunction of the corresponding cervical vertebrae should consequently be addressed.

An alternative position is to hold the infant seated, facing forward, on the practitioner's lap. Supporting the infant, the practitioner's hands encircle the lower thoracic cage, thumbs contacting the costotransverse area posteriorly and fingers directed anteriorly over the lower ribs. The diaphragm may then be treated following the sequence described in the procedure above.

Amplification of the cranial rhythmic impulse

When employing the principles of cranial manipulation it is imperative that the practitioner always employs the inherent forces of the biphasic PRM in every procedure, both in diagnosis and treatment. There are some procedures, however, that may be employed to increase the amplitude of the biphasic cranial rhythmic impulse (CRI), the palpable manifestation of the PRM.[9–11]

SACRAL APPROACH

Indications

Low amplitude CRI; initial approach to pelvic dysfunction when treating conditions such as enuresis, constipation and dysmenorrhea.

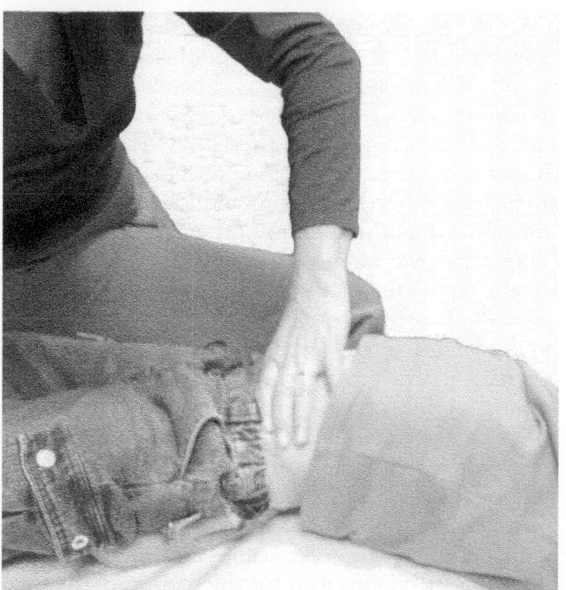

Figure 6.79. *Amplification of the cranial rhythmic impulse with a sacral approach.*

Procedure (Fig. 6.79)

Patient supine; practitioner seated at the level of the patient's pelvis. Put one hand beneath the patient's sacrum, fingers directed cephalad toward the sacral base. The middle finger rests in the midline. Both the index and ring fingers contact the sacral base medial to the sacroiliac articulations; the other hand rests in contact with the anterior pelvis. If the child is small enough, the practitioner's thumb can be placed on one ASIS and the index or middle finger on the other. If the child is larger, with the hand and forearm resting transversely across the pelvis, the fingertips should contact one ASIS and the forearm the other. Listen to the rhythm of the PRM and follow the inhalation and exhalation phases. Using indirect principles, allow these phases to reach their optimal amplitude. As this process occurs the child will relax and the PRM will amplify.

Remarks

This procedure may be employed when palpation of the skull is difficult and prior to the treatment of specific pelvic dysfunctions.

VAULT APPROACH

Indications

Low amplitude CRI; irritability and sleep disorders.

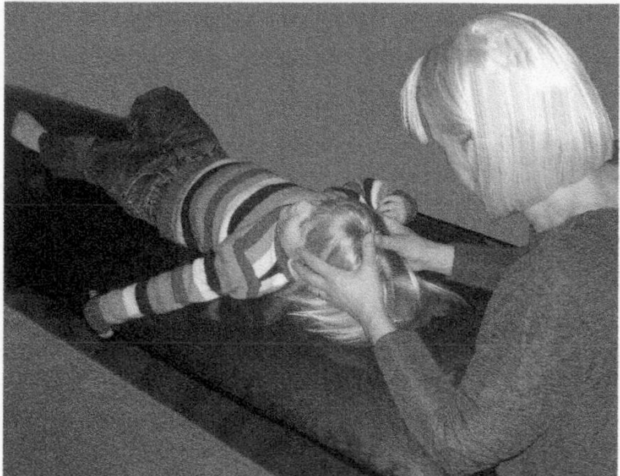

Figure 6.80. *Amplification of the cranial rhythmic impulse with a vault hold.*

Procedure (Fig. 6.80)

Patient supine; practitioner seated at the head of the table. Using a vault hold hand placement, listen to the rhythm of the PRM and follow the inhalation and exhalation phases. Using indirect principles, allow these phases to reach their optimal amplitude. As this process occurs the child will relax and the PRM will amplify.

Remarks

Infants and small children may be resistant to having their heads touched. If the child resists, the practitioner should never insist. The sacral approach described above may then be employed.

TEMPORAL APPROACH

Indications

To increase the CRI using a transverse bitemporal approach.

Procedure (Fig. 6.81)

Patient supine; practitioner seated at the head of the patient. Cradling the occiput in both hands, place the thumbs bilaterally on the anterior edges of the mastoid processes. Listen to the movement of each temporal bone. Listen to the rhythm and follow external rotation during the inhalation phase and internal rotation during the exhalation phase. Using indirect principles, allow these phases of the PRM to reach their optimal amplitude. As this process occurs the PRM will amplify.

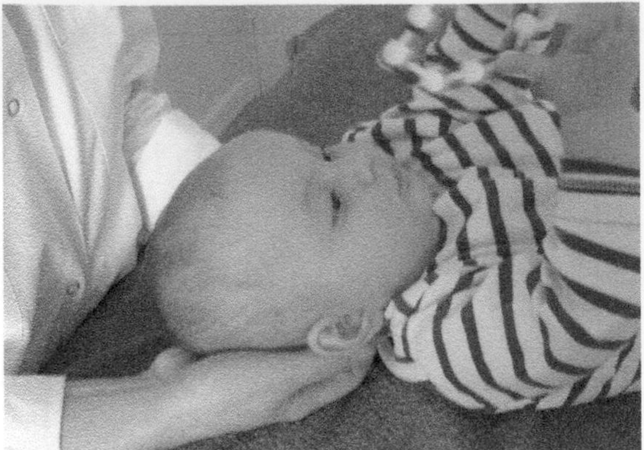

Figure 6.81. *Amplification of the cranial rhythmic impulse with a temporal approach.*

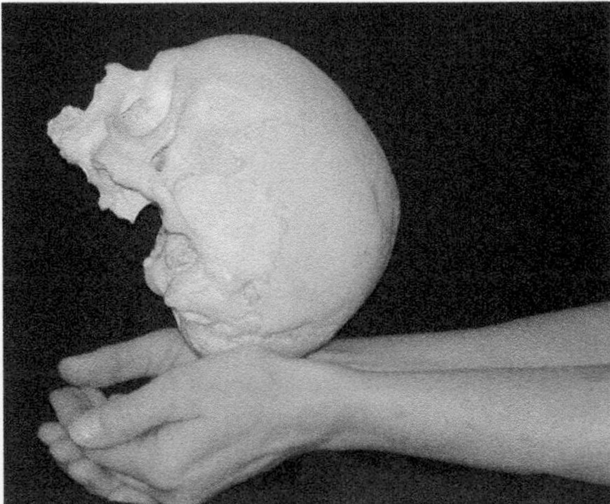

Figure 6.82. *Amplification of the cranial rhythmic impulse with an occipital approach.*

Remarks

This procedure necessitates the very lightest of touch.

OCCIPITAL APPROACH, COMPRESSION OF THE FOURTH VENTRICLE (CV4)

Indications

To increase the CRI using an occipital approach.

Procedure (Fig. 6.82)

Patient supine; practitioner seated at the head of the patient. Place the hands, palms up, beneath the patient's head. One hand rests in the palm of the other in such a manner that the thenar eminences are parallel to one another and contact the lateral angles of the occiput, medial to the occipitomastoid suture. The patient's head rests on the physician's thenar eminences, producing pressure on the lateral angles. Listen to the rhythm and follow the inhalation and exhalation phases of the PRM. Follow the occiput into the extension phase of the CRI (primary respiratory exhalation) and gently increase the medially directed pressure of the thenar eminences on the lateral angles. When the occiput reaches full extension, gently resist the flexion phase (primary respiratory inhalation) of the cycle and hold the occiput in extension. This process is repeated with each progressive cycle of the CRI. Track the amplitude of the CRI as it becomes progressively lower until a still point is reached, the still point being the moment when the CRI seems to palpably stop.[12] After the still point, wait for the motion of the CRI to return and follow it into the next flexion and extension.

Remarks

At the still point the patient will frequently sigh deeply.

This procedure may be employed in the treatment of adolescents. It is contraindicated in the treatment of infants and children where there is a risk of inducing intraosseous dysfunction of the occiput.

As an alternative procedure for the treatment of infants and children, the hand placement may be the same as for CV4, using indirect principles to allow the biphasic PRM to reach its optimal amplitude. As this process occurs the child will relax and the PRM will amplify. At no time apply compressive force to the occiput.

REFERENCES

1. Becker RE. Life in motion. Portland, OR: Rudra Press; 1997.
2. Still AT. Osteopathy research and practice. Seattle, WA: Eastland Press; 1992:7.
3. ICD-9CM, International classification of diseases, 9th revision: clinical modification, 5th edn. Salt Lake City, UT: Medicode; 1999.
4. Galbreath WO. Acute otitis media, including its postural and manipulative treatment. JAOA 1929;28:377–9.
5. Sutherland WG. The cranial bowl. Mankato, MN: Free Press, 1939.
6. Magoun HI. Osteopathy in the cranial field, 2nd edn. Kirksville, MO: The Journal Printing Company; 1966.
7. Beal MC. Viscerosomatic reflexes: a review. J Am Osteopath Assoc 1985;85(12):786–801.
8. Van Buskirk RL, Nelson KE. Osteopathic family practice: an application of the primary care model. In: Ward RC (ed)

Foundations for osteopathic medicine, 2nd edn. Philadelphia: Lippincott Williams and Wilkins; 2003:289–97.
9. Sergueef N, Nelson KE, Glonek T. The effect of cranial manipulation upon the Traube–Hering–Meyer oscillation. Altern Ther Health Med 2002;8(6):74–6.
10. Nelson KE, Sergueef N, Glonek T. Cranial manipulation induces sequential changes in blood flow velocity on demand. AAOJ 2004;14(3):15–7.
11. Nelson KE, Sergueef N, Glonek T. The effect of an alternative medical procedure upon low-frequency oscillations in cutaneous blood flow velocity. J Manipulative Physiol Ther 2006;29(8):626–36.
12. King HH, Lay E. Osteopathy in the cranial field. In: Ward RC (ed) Foundations for osteopathic medicine, 2nd edn. Philadelphia: Lippincott Williams & Wilkins; 2003:985–1001.

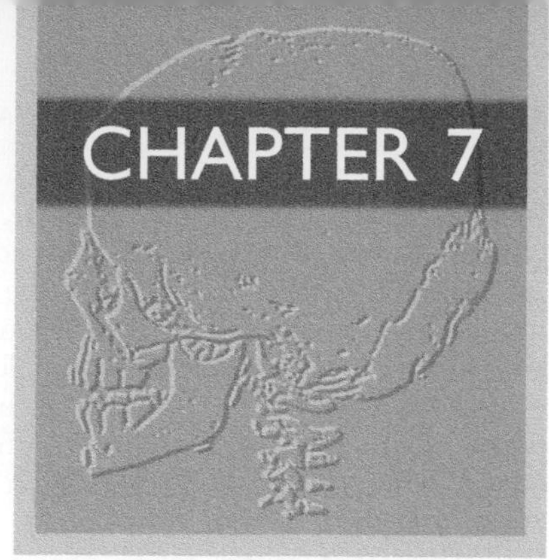

CLINICAL CONDITIONS

This chapter addresses some clinical conditions than can be effectively treated using manipulative procedures. Such treatment, however, is not intended to replace definitive medical or surgical treatments. Rather this therapeutic option is offered as a gentle, alternative, non-invasive approach, with essentially no untoward side effects, to be employed as a first line of therapy. Patients respond quickly to a specific technique when it is appropriately applied following a precise diagnosis.

It is the responsibility of the practitioner to ensure that underlying pathologies requiring more aggressive medical or surgical treatment have been ruled out or appropriately addressed. It should also be borne in mind that when a patient fails to respond to treatment as anticipated, they should be completely reassessed. If the osteopathic practitioner does not see a significant functional change in the patient's condition by the third to fifth treatment, the probability of misdiagnosis is likely.

For each clinical condition, the specific features of the condition are addressed. For the basic treatment protocols and descriptions of individual procedures, see Chapters 5 (Examination of the patient) and 6 (Treatment of the patient).

7.1 IMBALANCES OF THE AXIAL SKELETON

Congenital muscular torticollis and plagiocephaly are the most frequently occurring asymmetries of infancy. Brachial plexus injury, fracture of the clavicle, pectus excavatum and carinatum, scoliosis, kyphosis and vertebral somatic dysfunctions are other commonly encountered conditions with structural and functional consequences that can be addressed with osteopathic manipulative treatment.

TORTICOLLIS

Torticollis may be subdivided into congenital torticollis and congenital muscular torticollis (CMT). The patient with congenital torticollis presents at birth with their head tilted toward the involved side and rotated toward the opposite side. They commonly have associated medical conditions, such as osseous malformations, basilar impression or atlanto-occipital anomalies, and neurologic disorders such as Arnold–Chiari malformations.[1] These underlying conditions should be diagnosed and appropriate treatment initiated before osteopathic manipulation is considered.

The patient with CMT, on the other hand, is symmetric at birth, and the asymmetry develops in the first weeks of life. CMT presents with a tight sternocleidomastoid (SCM) muscle, causing the child's head to be tilted toward the side of the tight muscle and rotated in the opposite direction. A mass, or fibromatosis colli, can eventually be palpated within the muscle. The incidence of CMT ranges from 0.3 to 1.9%, but is as high as 3.92% when cases are diagnosed sonographically.[2] CMT occurs more often among boys than girls.[2,3] Some authors report a higher incidence on the right side,[1,4] whereas others report that it is more frequently encountered on the left.[2] Primiparity, assisted delivery[2,3] and breech presentation[3,5] frequently appear in the birth history. The larger the infant, birth body length and shoulder width, with more associated delivery trauma, the higher the incidence of CMT.[2]

Multiple theories to explain the etiology of CMT have been proposed. Van Roonhysen (1670) postulated abnormal uterine pressure as a cause of torticollis.[4] Pommerol, in the 19th century, attributed the unilateral shortening of the SCM to abnormal fetal position.[6] These 'intrauterine' theories have also attempted to explain the presence of several other deformities present at birth. Many authors have commented on aberrant constraint of the infant within the uterus and the association between torticollis, plagiocephaly, bat ears, scoliosis and congenital hip dislocation,[7–10] or hip dysplasia.[3]

Other theories link CMT to birth trauma. The high incidence of breech presentation associated with CMT may document the role of birth trauma in its occurrence. Others suggest that intrauterine torticollis predisposes the infant to breech presentation or forceps delivery.[11] It has been proposed that birth trauma with injury of the SCM and a resultant hematoma, which is then replaced with fibrous tissue, causes CMT. Histologic studies have, however, failed to support this proposition. Proposed compressive arterial occlusion as an etiology[12] has also been dismissed. Vascular compromise does not occur because there is abundant arterial and venous supply to the SCM that follows no regular or segmental pattern and has multiple anastomoses.[13]

Among more recent theories, CMT is proposed as the sequela of an intrauterine or perinatal compartment syndrome.[14] A bilateral imbalance of structures responsible for control of head posture may play a role – for example, as may be the case for the interstitial nucleus of Cajal, a neural integrator for head posture.[15]

Because the torticollis is not present at birth but appears later, it is possible that it results from improper handling of the child or incorrect positioning as in a car seat. Resultant dysfunction of the occipito-atlanto-axial joints may, therefore, occur and has been proposed as a cause for CMT.[16]

Several clinical variants are observed. The SCM mass is not always present.[17] Smaller masses may be found on the occipital bone below the superior nuchal line. When an SCM mass is palpable, usually in the first 2 months of life, it appears well circumscribed within the muscle, is located in the midportion of the SCM and ranges in size from 8 to 15.8 mm on maximal transverse diameter and from 13.7 to 45.8 mm in length (measured with ultrasound).[18] This mass typically disappears during the 1st year of life without any correlation with the resolution of the CMT.[3]

Although the findings of head tilt toward the involved side with head rotation toward the opposite side are consistent, the amount of rotation can differ between subjects. Contractures of the semispinalis capitis and the splenius capitis are sometimes present. CMT is probably the consequence of several concomitant factors. The problem may begin with a faulty intrauterine position that weakens the SCM, making it vulnerable to birth trauma and thus creating the dysfunction.

Osteopathic practitioners use their knowledge of anatomy to develop a rationale for treatment. The SCM arises, by two heads, from the sternum and clavicle (Fig. 7.1.1). The medial (or sternal) head has its origin on the upper part of the anterior surface of the manubrium sterni and the lateral (or clavicular) head arises from the anterior surface and superior border of the medial third of the clavicle. Initially, the two heads are separated from one another. They gradually join, below the middle of the neck, to form the body of a thick, rounded muscle. The SCM is inserted into the lateral surface of the mastoid process by a strong tendon and into the lateral half of the superior nuchal line of the occipital bone by a thin aponeurosis.

The two heads of the SCM consist of different types of fiber, the sternal head being more tendinous and the clavicular head being composed of fleshy and aponeurotic fibers. The clavicle is more mobile than the sternum and is subject to significant stress during the birth process, which may explain a different strain being put on the two parts of the SCM. A distinction between 'sternal torticollis' and 'clavicular torticollis' has been proposed.[19]

The insertion of the SCM covers the occipitomastoid suture; therefore, SCM tightness should be released whenever attempting to treat this suture. Conversely, somatic dysfunction between the temporal and the occipital bones will affect the SCM. The jugular foramen – located at the anterior end

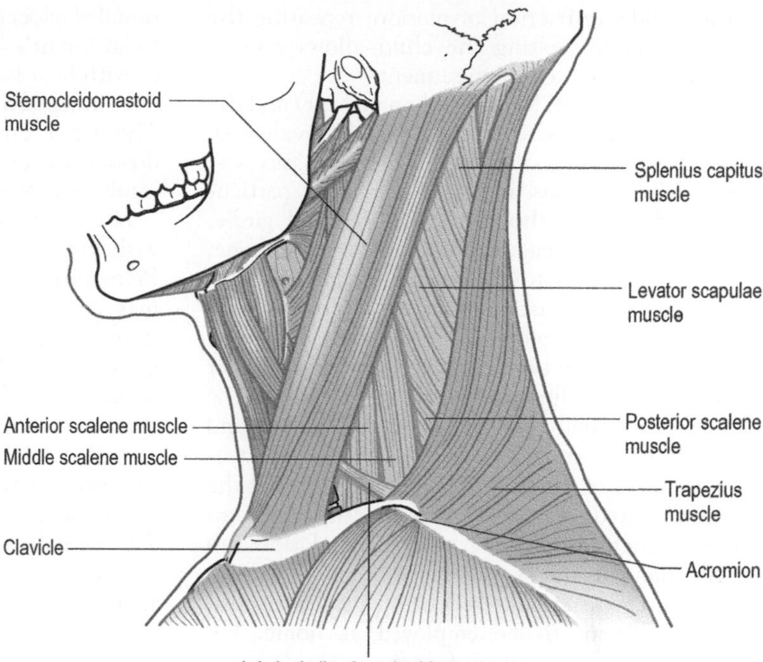

Figure 7.1.1. *Sternocleidomastoid muscle.*

of the occipitomastoid suture, between the petrous portion of the temporal bone and the occiput – will also be affected. The jugular foramen contains the inferior petrosal sinus and the sigmoid sinus that unite to form the internal jugular vein. It also contains the glossopharyngeal (CN IX), the vagus (CN X) and the accessory (CN XI) nerves. CN XI provides the motor supply to the SCM, its proprioceptive fi bres passing through branches from the anterior divisions of the second and third cervical nerves to innervate the SCM. Thus, Sutherland stated: 'You will probably fi nd the source of the torticollis to be entrapment neuropathy of the eleventh cranial nerve at the jugular foramen.'[20] Jacquemart and Piedallu, in 1964, recommended that osteopathic manipulation for CMT be directed at somatic dysfunction of the occiput and upper cervical spine.[16]

The mastoid process is not fully developed in the newborn and is totally covered by the tendon of the SCM from its apex to its superior border. The development of the mastoid process is linked to the traction of the SCM; asymmetric sidebending and rotation of the head, as in CMT, will cause the mastoid processes to develop asymmetrically. Cephalometric analysis demonstrates that, left untreated, persistent torticollis can lead to skull and facial asymmetry.[21] When it occurs, the cranial base deformation appears early, the changes being more significant in the posterior cranial fossa, whereas the facial deformity will develop later in childhood. Both the cranial base and facial deformities tend to increase with age.[22] Furthermore, the asymmetric function of the neck muscles stresses the mechanisms of postural control. Abnormal sensory input to the CNS and a sense of instability occurs that has to be compensated for with vision.[23] This can affect the infant's developing visual function. To prevent these sequelae, osteopathic procedures should be employed to address CMT as early as possible.

Physical examination and treatment

Observe the child for spontaneous rotation and sidebending of the cervical region. A good way to evaluate the range of motion in rotation and sidebending is to have the baby visually follow a toy moved in the directions to be tested. The child can also be held in the arms of the practitioner, facing the parents. The practitioner then pivots to the right and to the left, holding the infant in such a way that, in order to continue to observe their parents, the child must actively turn their head fi rst to the left in response to the practitioner's pivoting right, and then to the right in response to the practitioner's pivoting left. Having the parents participate in this procedure allows them to understand the extent of the child's restriction of motion; repeating the procedure after treating the child allows one to evaluate the effect of the treatment.

The size of the SCM mass (when present) and the tension of the muscle fibers should be evaluated. Palpate the infant to identify membranous, myofascial and interosseous somatic dysfunction, particularly in the upper thoracic spine, pectoral girdle, cervico-occipital area and cranium (temporal bone, occiput, occipitomastoid suture and jugular foramen). Treatment should use indirect principles. Because the mass associated with CMT often develops at the conjunction of the two heads of the SCM, in order to release the dysfunction the bones to which the muscle is attached (clavicle, sternum, occiput and temporal bone) should be balanced. Indirect myofascial release of the SCM may be employed. If the infant is treated early, before a dysfunctional pattern becomes engrained, osteopathic manipulation can rapidly alleviate the asymmetry of SCM.

The caregiver should be taught an active positioning program to be employed at home. For example, approaching the infant from the side opposite the rotation during daily activities, such as feeding and playing, head turning and lengthening of the SCM can be facilitated. The infant should be placed in a sleeping position that avoids reinforcement of the SCM shortening. It is improper to attempt to accomplish this by propping the infant's head with a pillow in such a way as to lengthen the SCM. Although this may appear to hold the head in the desired position, it induces a stretch reflex in the tight muscle, maintaining the shortening.

Gentle stretching exercises that induce active SCM stretching can be taught. These should be employed to rotate the head toward, and sidebend the neck away, from the side of the tight SCM. Such exercises are indicated until a full range of movement has been obtained.

PLAGIOCEPHALY

The term plagiocephaly – derived from the Greek *plagios* (oblique) and *kephalê* (head) – indicates distortion of the head and refers clinically to cranial asymmetry. Cranial deformations have been (and still are) produced intentionally, depending on the period and country, as signs of distinction, beauty, health, courage, freedom and nobility. The oldest known example is from Iraq, *c*.45 000 BC, and the earliest written reference is from Hippocrates, around 400 BC (*Airs, Waters, Places*), describing the Macrocephales who practiced head deformation.[24] Intentional plagiocephaly was obtained by pressure applied to an infant's skull, either through manual molding or with boards, pads or stones. Different deformities were induced depending on the methods employed.[25] The use of cradleboards and the wearing of headdresses are examples of other traditions that also resulted in head deformation.

Non-intentional plagiocephaly can be associated with premature sutural closure or craniosynostosis. Premature synostosis of one or several cranial sutures may be the result of genetic or metabolic conditions.[26,27] The fused suture does not allow bone growth and the shape of the skull reflects this anomaly: a brachycephaly develops when the coronal suture fuses, a dolichocephaly or a scaphocephaly when the sagittal suture fuses, and a trigonocephaly when the metopic suture fuses. Unilateral synostosis of the lambdoid or coronal suture (Fig. 7.1.2) results in a posterior or anterior plagiocephaly, respectively. Although any suture may be involved in synostotic plagiocephaly, true lambdoid synostosis with posterior plagiocephaly rarely occurs[28] and represents only 3.1% of all synostoses.[29] In the general population, the incidence of craniosynostosis has been estimated to be as low as 1 in 2100–3000 live births;[27,30] however, it is imperative that the diagnosis of synostotic plagiocephaly, which is most specifically accomplished by radiologic means, be made when the condition is present.

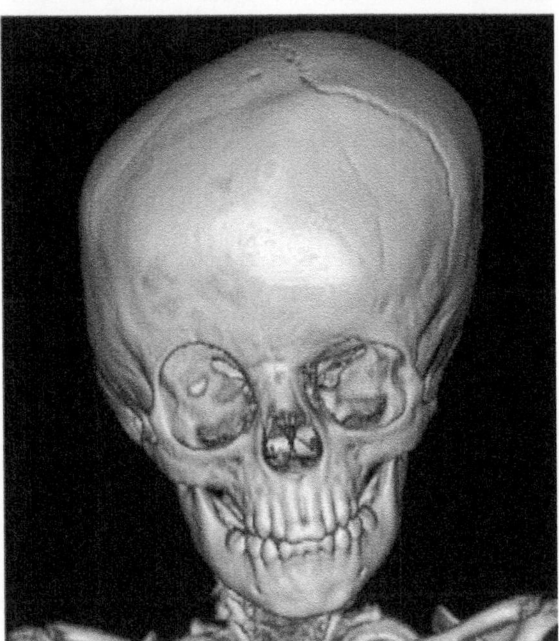

Figure 7.1.2. *Synostosis of right coronal suture.*

Children presenting with craniosynostosis should be monitored closely by a pediatric neurosurgeon for signs and symptoms of increased intracranial pressure. Treatment may require surgery, particularly for severe cases.

Non-synostotic plagiocephaly (NSP), also referred to as functional plagiocephaly, must be differentiated from craniosynostosis. The prevalence of NSP is estimated to be as high as 9.9% of all children under the age of 6 months.[31] NSP is identified as either frontal[32] or occipital[33] (Figs 7.1.3 and 7.1.4) depending on the site of the deformation. In 1992, the 'Back to Sleep' campaign was instituted in the USA for prevention of sudden infant death syndrome (SIDS). Parents were encouraged to put infants to sleep in the supine position. Following this, a shift occurred in the location of the deformity of NSP, from frontal plagiocephaly being more frequently encountered before the 'supine' directive, to occipital plagiocephaly more commonly encountered now.

Etiologies

NSP results from a variety of extrinsic and intrinsic factors affecting the infant before, during and after birth. These various factors may be isolated or may exert a cumulative effect. Associated risk factors for NSP include premature birth,[34] firstborn,[31,35] prolonged labor, unusual birth position,[35] use of forceps and vacuum extraction.[36] Male gender is also a risk factor because fetal distress during labor, with a consequently higher incidence of operative delivery, is more common with males than with females.[37]

Before birth, NSP may result from abnormal constraint on the fetal head in the intrauterine environment, as with a unicornuate uterus, uterine fibroids or oligohydramnios.[9] Multiple births are another risk factor, with deformational plagiocephaly being frequently encountered in these children.

Extrauterine constraints placed on the fetus can be responsible for NSP. This may be the result of pressure from neighboring abdominal organs. With athletic mothers, increased tonus of the abdominal muscles can compress the uterus back against the spine. Lack of abdominal muscle strength, on the other hand, will produce an increase in the already increased lumbar lordosis that is very common in late pregnancy. The increased lordosis is associated with anatomic flexion of the sacrum that displaces the sacral promontory forward, with resultant external pressure on the uterus.

During the birth process, the uterus contracts regularly to allow the descent of the fetus through the birth canal. Prolonged periods of uterine contraction may increase the mechanical forces applied to the infant's head. When the head enters the pelvic cavity, anatomic extension between the sacrum and the pelvic bones normally occurs to

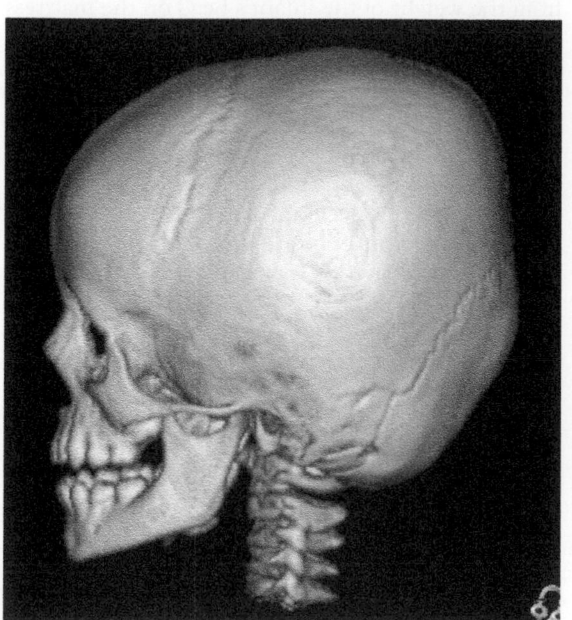

Figure 7.1.3. *Occipital non-synostotic plagiocephaly.*

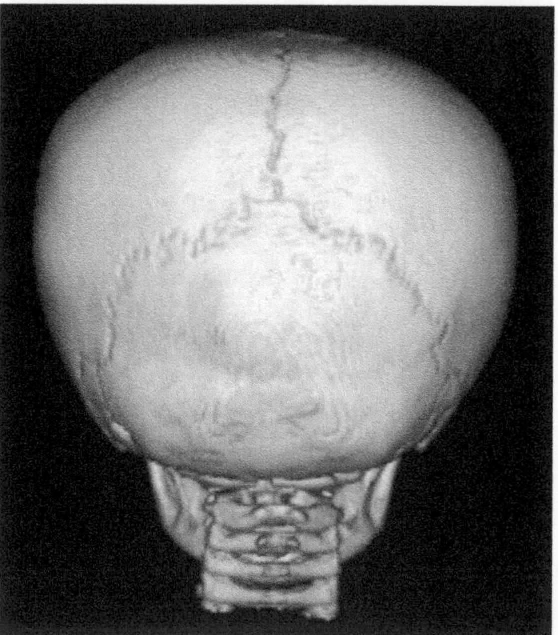

Figure 7.1.4. *Occipital non-synostotic plagiocephaly.*

increase the diameters of the pelvic outlet. Dysfunction of the maternal sacroiliac joints can result in a reduction of that increase and further constraint on the infant's head.

In the left occiput-anterior position – the most frequent birth presentation – the right side of the infant's occipital bone is in contact with the maternal pubic symphysis while the left frontal bone is compressed against the sacrum (Fig. 7.1.5). Asynclitism further increases the pressure of the infant's head against the pelvic bones with resulting occipital flattening on the right and frontal flattening on the left. The reverse – occipital flattening on the left and frontal flattening on the right – would result from the left occiput-posterior position. At the end of the descent, the head contacts the pelvic floor and turns in such a way as to position the occiput under the pubic symphysis. In the left occiput-anterior position, the right side of the occiput and the occipitomastoid area can be exposed to greater pressure. Later, during expulsion, compressive forces are applied on the occiput by the pubic symphysis.

After birth the pressure of the mattress on the infant's head is thought to contribute to occipital flattening.[38] Sleeping habits affect the cranial shape. When infants consistently sleep supine, as in Asiatic countries, posterior flattening of the skull occurs.[35]

Babies should be able to turn their head symmetrically to both sides. Asymmetric cervical rotation should be considered anomalous[39] and, if present, should be resolved by 12 weeks of age.[40] Although a preferred rotation of the head to the right side is present at birth in 59% of infants, this does not seem to be related to the fetal position. Often, infants may demonstrate asymmetric preferential motions, but a preferred motion should be differentiated from somatic dysfunction. Concern should arise when a rotational dysfunction is present. Early restriction of cervical motion is an identified risk factor for positional plagiocephaly,[41] particularly if the child is less active, staying in the same position to the point where an area of alopecia develops on the scalp. Upper thoracic and cervical restrictions, and SCM imbalance or torticollis, very often accompany plagiocephalies.[34,42,43] Furthermore, when the flattening has developed, it reinforces the preferential positional pattern with automatic positioning of the head on the flat area.

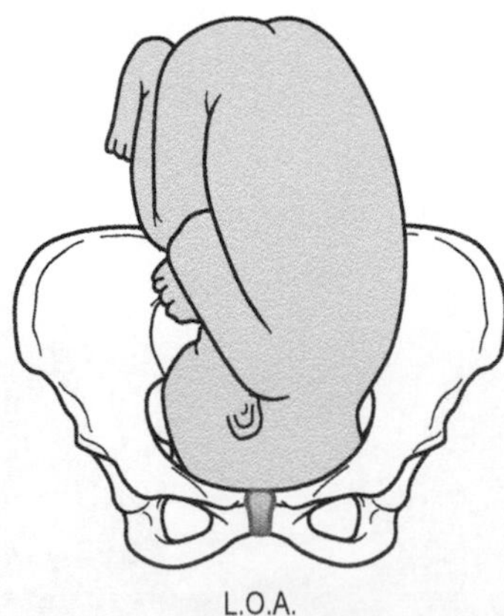

Figure 7.1.5. *Left occiput-anterior (LOA) presentation.*

Clinical aspect

By definition, plagiocephalic children have irregularly shaped heads. Since infants now sleep supine because of the 'Back to Sleep' campaign, the most commonly encountered forms of plagiocephaly are posterior, with either medial or lateral occipital deformity.

When compressive forces are applied to the squamous portion of the occiput, usually in the area of the lambda (superior angle of the occiput), the posterior portion of the head is flattened and assumes a brachycephalic shape. In severe cases, the flattening can demonstrate a slight depression, usually near the superior part of the occiput.

An asymmetric plagiocephaly results when dysfunctional rotation of the head is associated with the compressive forces. Because of the rotation, pressure from the weight of the infant's head on the mattress is asymmetric, and the occipitoparietal area on the side toward which the head is chronically rotated becomes flattened, while the other side develops excessively. This results in occipital flattening on one side and occipital bossing on the other. Anteriorly, the skull demonstrates frontal bossing on the same side as the occipital flattening, with frontal flattening on the opposite side. When the head is seen from above, it has a 'parallelogram' shape (Fig. 7.1.6).

The parallelogram cranial shape is commonly described in allopathic medical literature[28,33,44–47] as well as in osteopathic medical literature.[48–50] This pattern is also referred to as 'cranial obliquity'.[51] In the cranial concept, the parallelogram cranial shape is associated with a pattern of lateral strain in the sphenobasilar synchondrosis (SBS) (Fig. 4.10). Shearing between the posterior part of the body of the sphenoid, which is displaced laterally, and the anterior part of the occiput, displaced in the opposite direction, is lateral strain of the SBS and is found in children with NSP.[36] This results in the parallelogram shape of the head, with the basilar portion of the occiput displaced away from the side of the posterior flattening.

The relationship between the cranial bones is disturbed, as described in lateral strain of the SBS, but this is not the only dysfunction associated with NSP. The compressive forces responsible for NSP can affect the relationship between different portions of the cranial bones, producing intraosseous dysfunctions. The occiput and temporal bones are the most common bones that demonstrate intraosseous dysfunction in the presence of NSP. At birth, the occipital bone is composed of four parts and each of the temporal bones of three parts. When occipital flattening occurs, the deformity is obvious in the squamous portion of the occiput where the compression has occurred; however, the compressive forces have also been directed against the non-visible parts of the occipital bone, i.e. the anterior intraoccipital synchondrosis that lies between the two parts of the condylar facets. When such a compression of the occipital condyles occurs, it most often occurs asymmetrically.

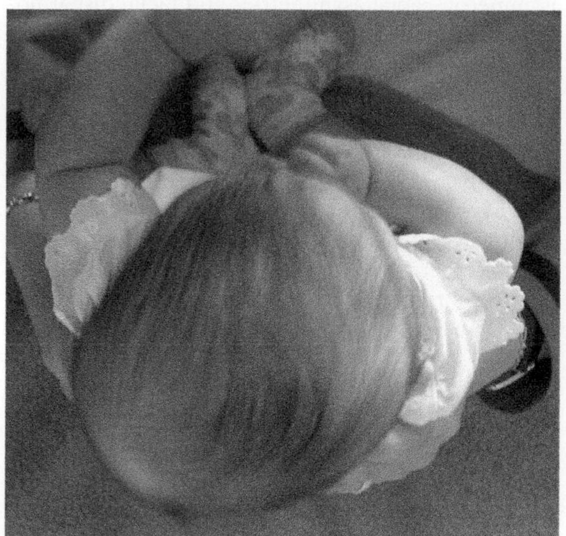

Figure 7.1.6. *Asymmetric posterior plagiocephaly.*

The hypoglossal canals are located bilaterally in the anterior intraoccipital synchondroses, between the basiocciput and the bilateral exocciputs. They contain the hypoglossal nerves that provide the motor supply to the tongue. Compressive force on one side can have an impact on tongue motor function, with resultant problems such as suckling difficulties.

Asymmetry of the cranial base can also affect the shape of the foramina therein, with potential for various entrapment neuropathies and vascular compressions. The jugular foramen, the right usually being larger than the left, contains the glossopharyngeal nerve (CN IX), the vagus nerve (CN X), the accessory nerve (CN XI) and the inferior petrosal and sigmoid venous sinuses. A broad spectrum of functions depends on these structures. Compression of CN IX is associated with altered sensation of the pharynx, fauces, palatine tonsil, pharyngotympanic tube (PT) and the posterior third of the tongue. Disturbances of CN X result in a wide range of symptoms including dysautonomia, colic and regurgitation. According to Magoun, 'the occipitomastoid suture and the jugular foramen should be considered as of significance with "pukey"

Figure 7.1.7. *Forceps delivery can be a risk factor for the development of asymmetric phlagiocephaly.*

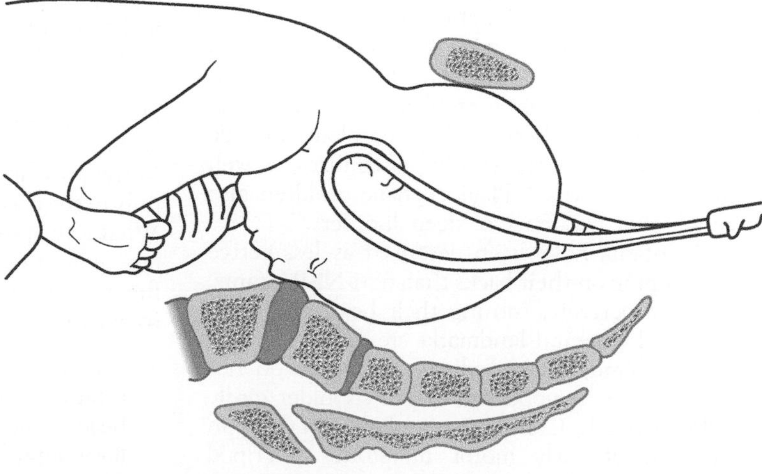

babies'.[52] Compression of CN XI can compromise the motor supply to the upper and middle portions of the trapezius and to the SCM. The trapezius receives a portion of its motor supply from CN XI; the SCM depends mainly on CN XI. CN XI can also affect swallowing through its impact on the pharyngeal constrictor muscles that receive their nervous supply from the cranial portion of the accessory nerve.

With the resultant asymmetry in the cranial base, a difference in tension between the two SCM muscles is palpable. There are multiple myofascial attachments on the cranial base that can be similarly affected, resulting in a multiplicity of dysfunctional patterns in distant areas. Asymmetric tensions in the trapezius and semispinalis capitis muscles can cause thoracic spine dysfunction, asymmetries of the stylopharyngeus and stylohyoideus muscles can affect the pharynx, and the styloglossus muscle can dysfunctionally influence the tongue.

The compressive forces applied to the fetal head also affect the temporal bones. When occipital flattening occurs on one side, the ipsilateral temporal bone and attached ear are moved forward and the mastoid portion is compressed. This deformation can be demonstrated with computerized tomography of the skull base. The long axis of the petrous portion of the temporal bone is displaced in the direction of the coronal plane,[53] thus placing the temporal bone in a position resembling external rotation.

Embedded in the petrous portion of the temporal bone are the bony portion of the PT and the vestibular apparatus. Compressive forces affecting the temporal bone may increase the risk of otitis. The bony portion of the PT, the vertical portion of the tensor veli palatini and the mastoid air cell system have been found to be smaller than normal in children with secretory otitis.[54]

Temporal bone dysfunction may have further implications. Children with NSP present with a higher risk of auditory processing disorders, which is thought to lead to subtle problems of cerebral dysfunction later at school.[55] These problems include language disorders and learning disabilities, as well as attention deficits.[56] Plagiocephalic children also have a higher incidence of sleep disorders.[36]

NSP infants have been described as less active when sleeping on their backs than non-NSP infants, who move actively, turning their head and torso when developmental landmarks are achieved.[56] On the other hand, infants who sleep supine do not need to use their upper trunk and shoulder girdle muscles as much. Consequently, there is a delay in acquisition of early motor milestones.[57] Tripod sitting, creeping and crawling are particularly delayed, which contributes further to weakening of the core muscles. Scoliosis has been associated with plagiocephaly where sleeping supine was identified as a causative factor.[51,58,59] In The Netherlands, where the supine sleeping position has been encouraged since 1989, approximately 2.4% of 2–3-year-old children have cervical restriction of motion and/or plagiocephaly.[31] Interestingly, the habit of always bottle feeding a child on the same side seems to contribute to the pattern of asymmetric cervical rotation. Alternating right- and left-sided bottle feeding is consequently an imperative for every baby, particularly NSP infants.

The facial skeleton adapts to the cranial base asymmetry. Facial asymmetries and facial disharmonies are associated with NSP.[44,60,61] On the side of the occipital flattening, the maxillary bone develops less well, with less distance separating the nasion and the temporomandibular joint. This reduction is proportional to the amount of posterior occipital deformation.[62] The growth of the neurocranium and the viscerocranium occurs at different rates. Consequently, compensatory developmental disorders of the viscerocranium will appear later in childhood than the original NSP, and the association, therefore, is not commonly recognized.

Physical examination and treatment

It is a common observation that infants will sleep preferentially with their head turned toward one side, and that will be the side of the occipital flattening of the NSP. Daily activities such as difficulty nursing or accepting bottle feeding bilaterally will also reflect dysfunctions because of difficulty in turning the head to both sides. Associated disorders such as regurgitation, colic or sleep disorders are also often present. Otitis media can be part of the picture if the child is over 3 months of age.

While taking the history, the infant's appearance, posture and range of motion are studied. When observing the child, the osteopathic practitioner assesses what dysfunctional mechanics are involved in the present NSP. Where is the dysfunction? Is it only in the cervical spine or are other areas involved? What is the primary dysfunction? Three mechanisms are quite frequent: occipitocervical somatic dysfunction, thoracic somatic dysfunction and cranial somatic dysfunction:

1. Is there a pattern of restricted cervical spinal rotation that has obliged the child to lay their head on one side that explains the head flattening? If the head moves freely in all

directions, no cervical spinal dysfunction is present.
2. Is there a pattern of thoracic somatic dysfunction? Does the child rotate their head with a movement involving only one side of the pectoral girdle, indicative of thoracic dysfunction? In this case, asymmetry of the movements of the arms may also be present.
3. Is there a cranial dysfunction, such as a lateral strain of the SBS that explains the parallelogram shape of the head?

These questions should be kept in mind in the following examination.

Observe the relationship between the head and the pelvis. In the presence of a 'total body' dysfunctional pattern, the pelvis and the head of the child are rotated in opposite directions on the vertical axis of the spine. Palpation and motion testing will confirm these observations and treatment should be applied accordingly.

Evaluate the skull. Infants usually do not present with thick hair as encountered in most adults, making observation of the neurocranium easier. Look for any bald spots that indicate chronic contact between that area of the head and the bed during sleep. Look for posterior and anterior flattening; in the presence of posterior plagiocephaly these are usually on opposite sides. This results in a parallelogram-shaped head that is easier to see from above when the child is held on the practitioner's or parent's lap.

Observe the child's face and frontal bones. A pattern of compressive forces applied directly to the frontal bone, with no occipital deformity, would indicate a frontal dysfunction. Frontal flattening opposite to the occipital flattening is consistent with a pattern of lateral strain of the SBS. Symmetry of the frontal bone with occipital deformity on one side is an indication of synostotic posterior plagiocephaly, where the forehead may be symmetric or flattened on the side of the occipital flattening.[63]

When a frontal dysfunction is present, this may affect the eyes. Observe the size and shape of the orbital cavities, as well as the ocular bulbs. The orbital diameter is the distance between the superior medial and inferior lateral angles of the orbit. An increase in the orbital diameter results in an orbital cavity that appears to be wider than it is high and is associated with a cranial flexion–external rotation pattern. Conversely, if the orbital cavity appears to be narrower, this is associated with a cranial extension–internal rotation pattern. Frontal dysfunction, in turn, affects the rest of the facial bones and is particularly important when problem solving dysfunctions of the nasal bones and the maxillae.

Observe the positions of the ears. They are very indicative of the positions of the temporal bones. In cases of NSP, the ear located on the side of the occipital flattening is displaced more anteriorly than the contralateral ear. If the ear is displaced more posteriorly on the flattened side, further diagnostic investigation is warranted because the displacement might be a sign of synostotic plagiocephaly.[29] This sign, however, is not an exclusive indicator and synostotic plagiocephaly may also present with an anterior ear position.[28,63]

Observe the size and shape of the ears. Usually, on the side of the occipital flattening of NSP, the ear may, for example, have been compressed against the uterine wall and, therefore, may be smaller. In this instance, expect to find intraosseous dysfunctions of the temporal bone on that side. This is the ear that the child will usually rub and that eventually may present with an otitis media.

After observation, the osteopathic practitioner gently palpates (i.e. caresses) the child's head, looking for depressions, bossing and irregularities of contour. Sutures are palpated for ridges, overlapping or irregularities in shape. A thick ridge over a suture calls for attention, because it may be a sign of a synostotic suture. Flattenings are the result of compressive forces. Tissues are palpated to evaluate for tissue texture abnormality and increased tenderness. Palpation of osseous tissues gives a sense of density that might be different between the two sides of the suture; increased tenderness is usually proportional to the strength of the compressive forces. Posterior occipital muscles are evaluated by palpation for tension and asymmetry.

Although the vault and the back of the head, the parietals and the squamous portion of the occiput are quite accessible to palpation, palpation of the frontal and facial bones necessitates a little more patience and delicacy in order to avoid disturbing the child. The base of the skull is not directly accessible to palpation for structure. The lateral parts of the occiput or exocciputs and the basilar part, as well as the sphenoid bone and the petrous portions of the temporal bones, should be assessed by palpating for function. To visualize these areas correctly while palpating them, knowledge of anatomy is of paramount importance.

Motion testing will confirm the findings of palpation and observation. Dysfunctional head rotation is a treatment priority. It is of considerable importance that the child leaves the office with a freer range of motion and an increased ability to turn their head. If not treated, the dysfunctional rotation will maintain the NSP. Look for any somatic dysfunction of the occipitocervical junction and the cervical and thoracic spine, and treat utilizing indirect principles. Structure will follow function, and if bilateral rotation is recovered, the traction of the muscles that insert on the occipital squama will help to reshape the flattened areas.

Membranous patterns of the cranial mechanism should be assessed and dysfunctions balanced. Particular attention should be given to the poles of attachment of the dura, the falx cerebri on the occipital squama and the tentorium cerebelli on the superior borders of the petrous portions of the temporal bones.

Motion of the SBS, occipitomastoid and lambdoid sutures should be assessed and treated accordingly. Check the frontal bones and their relationships with the facial bones. Any dysfunction should be treated.

Special attention should be directed at the cranial base, with the assessment and treatment of the compressed occipital condyles and compressed jugular foramina, when present. Molding procedures can be applied, with intraosseous balancing of the occiput, temporal bones, frontal bones, sphenoid and parietal bones as dictated by the patient's needs.

Advice to caregivers

Very often parents will comment on the fact that the flattening was not present at birth and say that they do not understand why NSP has developed. To succeed in the treatment of plagiocephaly, it is worthwhile explaining the mechanism of NSP and stressing the importance of parental participation in the following months. Explain that the initial asymmetry may have been present at birth in a very subtle way that has been exacerbated by a persistent positional preference. Explain that it is of paramount importance to encourage the child in activities that promote bilateral cervical rotation, as well as promoting sleeping positions that avoid pressure on the already flattened area. Successful treatment depends on this. Proper sleeping position may be obtained by elevating one side of the bed approximately 5 cm (2 inches). This can be accomplished by placing a rolled bath towel beneath the entire length of the mattress, on the side of the occipital flattening. This will encourage the infant to turn their head in the other direction. Toys and other attention-getting objects, soliciting the rotation of the child's head when lying supine, should be placed on the side opposite to the occipital flattening.

Encourage play in the prone position. It can be explained to the parents that activities in the prone position stimulate the posterior axial musculature. Muscular extension of the neck results in traction on the squamous portion of the occiput, helping to create a round head.

To stimulate the child's curiosity and open them to the world, while encouraging them to turn their head symmetrically left and right, carry the child facing forward, held in the midline of the parent's chest. One parental hand should support the child's bottom while the other hand contacts the front of the child's torso, holding them against the parent's chest. The prolonged use of a car seat or other similar such carrying device should be discouraged because it tends to maintain the child in a chronic position, usually that of the dysfunctional asymmetry.

Thumb sucking should be discouraged because the child assumes an asymmetric position while preferentially sucking one thumb. If oral gratification is necessary, an orthodontically shaped pacifier should be employed. Encourage the parents to gently caress the child's head bilaterally, behind the ears, in the areas over the occipitomastoid sutures and over the superior nuchal line of the occiput. This will help to reduce any dysfunctional tenderness.

SCOLIOSIS

Scoliosis is a lateral deviation of the spine. A structural scoliosis is a spinal deformation that is not totally reducible, while a functional scoliosis is totally reducible. The diagnosis of scoliosis is confirmed by radiographic analysis. A functional scoliosis is usually associated with pelvic or postural asymmetry, a difference in the length of the lower limbs or vestibular or visual disorders. A structural scoliosis presents a spinal deformation in the three planes of space involving sidebending, rotation and flexion or extension of the vertebrae. The side of convexity of the spinal curve defines the scoliosis – for example, a left scoliosis consists of a spinal curve that is convex on the left side.

Cobb's angle is a measurement of the degree of scoliosis between the most tilted vertebrae above and below the apex of the curve. This angle is obtained by measuring the angle of intersection between lines drawn perpendicular to the top of the most superior vertebra, and the bottom of the most inferior vertebra, of the curve.

A scoliosis is identified as idiopathic when no recognizable pathology explains its origin. It is identified as secondary in the presence of spinal anomaly or neuromuscular dysfunction. The classification of scoliosis is based on the age of the patient when the spinal curvature is first identified: congenital scoliosis is present at birth, infantile scoliosis is diagnosed under the age of 3 years, juvenile idiopathic scoliosis between 3 and 10 years, and adolescent idiopathic scoliosis (AIS) between 10 years and the end of skeletal growth.

Etiologies of idiopathic scoliosis

The cause of idiopathic scoliosis has not been established, but seems to be a multifactorial interaction of environmental and genetic factors. Studies have shown scoliosis as a single-gene disorder that follows the simple patterns of Mendelian genetics.[64,65] Traits can be dominant or recessive. Genetic links exist, with 3% of parents and 3% of siblings having a scoliosis.[64] Further, a correlated incidence of scoliosis has been described in twins.[66] Older maternal age is a risk factor for greater progression of the curve of AIS.[58] Maternal age of 27 years or more at the time of the child's birth is associated with a higher incidence of AIS, whereas paternal age has no significant effect.[67]

Changes in the extracellular matrix of the connective tissues (e.g. collagen distribution and elastic fibers) have been found among patients with scoliosis, but most researchers do not consider these changes to be the etiology of the deformity.[68] Similarly, a change in muscle fiber composition or chronic muscle overuse might explained the hyperintense signal intensity shown on MRI in the multifidus muscle on the concave side of the scoliosis associated with greater degrees of curve severity.[69] Myopathy involving impaired calcium pump activity is among other proposed etiologies that require further study.

The progression of AIS is associated with increased calmodulin (calcium-binding receptor protein) levels in platelets, with a possible modulation of the calcium-activated calmodulin by melatonin.[68] The level of melatonin has been proposed as a predictor for progression of spinal curvature in idiopathic scoliosis.[70] Melatonin is produced and released by the pineal body at night, and its production is inhibited by environmental light. It is proposed that a deficiency of melatonin could disturb equilibrium and postural mechanisms.[71]

Neurologic origins have also been proposed as etiologies of scoliosis. Hearing-impaired children who have a high incidence of vestibular dysfunction have significantly less idiopathic scoliosis than children with normal hearing, resulting in the suggestion that idiopathic scoliosis has a neural etiology.[72] A sensory input deficiency of the spatial orientation system, involving visual and vestibular dysfunction, is believed to cause motor cortex and axial posture control disturbances.[73,74] Another hypothesis is that developmental disorders in the central nervous system, followed by asymmetry of the spinal rotators and other trunk muscles, results in AIS. A less efficient postural regulation system with a diminished quality of standing stability has been demonstrated in some scoliotic patients.[75]

Developmental disorders have also been considered at the level of the spinal cord. Differences between the growth of the vertebral column and the growth of the spinal cord – 'uncoupled neuro-osseous growth' – either with asymmetric nerve root tension or with reduced growth of the cord, are suggested etiologies for scoliosis.[76] More rapid growth of vertebral bodies that occurs through endochondral ossification, as well as slower circumferential growth of the vertebral bodies and pedicles that occurs through membranous ossification, is observed in AIS patients.[77] Furthermore, the length of the vertebral canal is shorter than the length of the vertebral column. This leads to the hypothesis that the thoracic spine is tethered by a tight spinal cord, with a resultant diminution of the kyphosis. This, in turn, results in a displacement of the spinal cord to one side of the vertebral canal with an associated sidebending of the spine and lastly a rotation of the vertebral bodies to allow for their growth while the vertebral canal stays in the midline.[78] The base of the vertebral canal remains at a right angle to the sagittal plane of the patient, in its original position, and does not follow the rotation of the vertebral body.[78] The tension of the core link – the strong dural membranes covering the cord, between the pelvic and cranial bowls[79] – may play a role in this mechanism. The relationships between the different parts of the craniosacral mechanism, therefore, should be considered, and any dysfunction of the dura and/or the vertebral ligaments should be treated.

Biomechanical factors can affect spinal alignment. Sidebending–rotation and torsion of the SBS, for example, can modify the level position of the orbits through the sphenoid and thereby modify the occipital neutral position, again altering balance mechanics in the spine below.

Pelvic obliquity is considered a cause of imbalance in the axial skeleton. Pelvic obliquity has been associated with unequal leg length. If this imbalance appears early in the growth process, it will result in abnormal asymmetric weight-bearing pressures on the vertebrae. A 'dangerous triad' of joint laxity, delayed growth and persistence of asymmetric overloading of the spine has been described in rhythmic gymnasts who develop scolioses.[80] This group shows an incidence of scoliosis of 12%, compared to 1.1% in the general population of the same age group. Pelvic obliquity has also been associated with the 'molded baby syndrome', where intrauterine molding determines a vertebral curve, having a sacral tilt inferiorly on the side of the spinal convexity. Mechanical compressive forces acting on the infant during the prenatal, perinatal and postnatal periods have been proposed as an etiology for scoliosis. More breech presentations have been found among infants developing scoliosis during the first 6 months of life.[58] Plagiocephaly is frequently associated with infantile scoliosis.[58,81–84] A facial and cranial distortion, always on the side of the curve of the scoliosis and linked to the intrauterine position, has been described.[85]

McMaster noted that the scoliosis was rarely present at birth and, like plagiocephaly, develops very often within the first months of life. He proposed an explanation for the association between plagiocephaly and scoliosis, as follows. Infants prefer to turn toward their right side when in a supine position. Light but asymmetric pressures from the mattress on the skull as well as on the growing spine can create asymmetries, particularly when applied over a prolonged time or during a critical period of growth. With chronic right rotation of the head, the back of the head will flatten on the right, allowing growth of the skull on the left. The thorax follows the same pattern, the left side expanding freely backwards with a left rotation of the thoracic vertebrae.[83]

Infantile scoliosis is sometimes found in association with imbalance of the occiput or with dysfunction of the SBS. Intraosseous dysfunction of the occiput can produce asymmetry of the occipital condylar parts, resulting in altered balance mechanics in the spine below. The compressive forces applied to the occipital bone at the time of delivery have been described and suggested to be the causes for future compensatory scoliotic curves.[59,86] Thus, the child may prefer to sidebend their head slightly to one side and, as time goes on, with potential new injuries and therefore more difficulties for compensation, the adolescent will develop a scoliosis. Ventura et al. state: 'Even small deformities present at, or soon after, birth may get worse in infants whose connective tissues do not have a potential for recovery.'[84] To this we could add one or more of the components described above – the etiology is multifactorial.

Congenital and infantile scoliosis

Congenital scoliosis may be associated with neurologic pathology or a vertebral structural defect (failure of formation and/or segmentation), as well as associated abnormalities of the head, neck, pelvis and hips. A thorough medical examination should be performed to rule out these disorders. Hemivertebra is the most common anomaly that causes non-idiopathic congenital scoliosis[87] and is sometimes associated with posterior midline cutaneous abnormalities. Neural axis abnormalities have been demonstrated in 21.7% of otherwise asymptomatic patients with infantile scoliosis.[88] Congenital scoliosis is more common in females than in males, occurring in the ratio of 1.27 : 1.[87] Among children with congenital spinal anomalies, 30–60% have other anomalies located most commonly in the genitourinary tract, cardiovascular system, spinal cord or cervical spine.[89]

Since the time of Hippocrates, congenital and infantile scolioses have been described as potentially the result of mechanical factors operating during fetal life.[9] These scolioses are more common in males, presenting more often as a left thoracic curve.[83,85] Some resolve spontaneously, while others progress. Harrenstein in 1930,[90] quoted by Mehta,[91] stated: 'Spontaneous correction does occur without treatment but at the moment it is not possible to distinguish between the two at the time of the diagnosis.' Thus, in order to differentiate between progressive and non-progressive congenital and infantile idiopathic scoliosis, Mehta proposed a method of measurement of the rib–vertebra angle (RVA).[91] In an anteroposterior radiograph, the RVA is 'the angle formed between each side of the apical thoracic vertebra and its corresponding rib'. The RVAs are equal on a normal spine and a gap of 2–4 mm normally separates the head of the rib and the upper corner of the adjacent vertebra. Mehta states that the most progressive infantile scoliosis presents an RVA difference between the two sides equal to or greater than 20°. When this radiographic measurement is repeated after 3 months, the RVA remains unchanged or increases with a progressive scoliosis, whereas it decreases with a resolving curve. Furthermore, with time, in the anteroposterior radiograph, a progressive scoliosis demonstrates overlap of the rib shadow with the upper corner of the vertebra. The relationship between the rib and the vertebra and the tissue response to any stress during growth periods is of great importance.

Curve progression is the major concern in every type of scoliosis, and the differentiation between progressive and non-progressive congenital scoliosis and infantile idiopathic scoliosis has been confirmed through sequential comparisons of RVAs over time.[84,92] When spontaneous resolution occurs in non-progressive infantile scoliosis, it does so between the ages of 12 and 18 months.[84] Spontaneous resolution of infantile idiopathic scoliosis varies between 17%[93] and 92%.[94] Therefore, it is appropriate to detect the scoliosis at its earliest stage and to treat all affected babies within the first 6 months of life.[95] It is typical to employ a wait-and-watch approach to the progressive category because orthopedic treatment is complex and difficult to initiate before the age of 18 months.[96] Osteopathic procedures, on another hand, may be begun immediately, with potentially good results being obtained in cases of congenital and infantile idiopathic scoliosis.

Physical examination and treatment

Observe the baby for spontaneous positioning and areas of restricted mobility. Look for positional asymmetries of the torso, head and neck, arms and legs. Look also for a bulky back on the convex side of the thorax and creases in the skin laterally on the concave side. Skin creases are a sign of fixed scoliosis.[97] Observe the baby for clumsy movement in the maintenance of head position and in general coordination.

Palpate the infant to identify membranous, myofascial and interosseous somatic dysfunction contributing to the visually observed functional restrictions. The infant may be treated utilizing indirect principles to release any restriction of motion, particularly in the pelvis, upper thoracic spine, ribs, sternum, thoracic diaphragm, pectoral girdle, cervico-occipital area and cranium. Intraosseous dysfunctions – most commonly encountered in the sacrum, lumbar and thoracic vertebrae and occiput – may be addressed using molding procedures.

At home, following treatment, it is important to avoid movements and positions that will reinforce the scoliotic pattern. In considering daily activities, such as feeding and play, and when putting the infant to sleep, encourage the parents to position the infant correctly and to solicit movement from the infant that promotes symmetry. A child should sleep on their back to prevent SIDS, but should play in the prone position to develop the vertebral musculature of tonic posture.

Prevention is the best therapy. Osteopathy, as a non-invasive treatment, facilitates the spontaneous recovery process or regression as quickly as possible. This allows the child to progress through the developmental milestones of infancy without interference from a dysfunctional musculoskeletal system.

Juvenile and adolescent idiopathic scoliosis (AIS)

Scoliosis is present between 10 and 16 years of age in 2–4% of children.[98] These patients differ from those with infantile scoliosis in that there is predominance among females and for the curvature to be a right thoracic curve.[83,85] The vertebral rotation is associated with a 'rib hump' on the side of the convexity, with most curves convex on the right in the thoracic area and on the left in the lumbar area. Cobb's angle is sometimes debated as a true assessment of the scoliosis. AIS is a three-dimensional deformity of the spine, with morphologic changes in the trunk and rib cage. Vertebral rotation should be considered in the evaluation. The presence of severe pain or neurologic symptoms would be atypical for idiopathic scoliosis and should raise concern for spinal cord pathology.

Idiopathic scoliosis, if left untreated, increases in adult life. The period of puberty should be considered as a high-risk interval, and regular screening is recommended. A significant correlation between growth in height and progression of Cobb's angle has been found, with a possible increase until 2.5 years after menarche.[99] Current studies have indicated that the younger the patient at the time of diagnosis by pubertal or skeletal maturation landmarks, the greater the chance of curve progression. A curve measuring less than 30° at skeletal maturity is least likely to progress, whereas curves measuring 30–50° may gain another 10–15°.[65] Thoracic curves deteriorate most, followed by thoracolumbar curves and double curves.[100]

Less than 25% of adolescent idiopathic scoliosis resolves without treatment.[101] Orthopedic treatment with a cast or a brace might be indicated to limit the progression of the curve and to employ surgery to correct the scoliosis. Bracing for at least 23 hours per day appears to be optimal for interdicting progression of the curve.[102] Watchful waiting is suggested as an alternative treatment to bracing because bracing does not decrease the incidence of surgery and often results in adverse psychological effects.[103]

Manipulative treatment associated with exercise has been shown to stop curve progression in AIS.[104,105] Exercise may be used to effectively reverse the signs and symptoms of scolioses and to prevent progression of spinal curves in children and adults.[106] As scoliosis is a risk factor for the impairment of physical wellbeing and quality of life, treatment is important.

Physical examination and treatment

The physical examination begins with observation of the patient standing. Observe placement of the feet for asymmetries. From behind, note the level of the iliac crests and the symmetry of the pelvis and waist triangles. Leg length discrepancy as a contributing factor should be considered. Further, observe the relationship between the pelvic and pectoral girdles, and look for shoulder and scapular asymmetries. Elevation of the right shoulder compared to the left is associated with a thoracic curve convex on the right. Note the position of the patient's head. A vertical line dropped from the external occipital protuberance should fall in the middle of the intergluteal crease. The patient is next observed in profile for increased or decreased thoracic kyphosis, forward head posture and lumbar lordosis.

The Adam's forward bending test is employed to help identify scoliosis. The child bends forward, holding palms together with arms extended. The examiner looks from behind and from the side, along the horizontal plane of the back, to detect an asymmetry as a rotational deformity or 'rib hump' (Fig. 7.1.8). This deformity is associated with spinal curves and may be further delineated with radiographic evaluation. With the child remaining forward bent, observe the distance between tips of the fingers and the ground as an indication of general spinal flexibility.

The palpatory examination of the patient with AIS is directed at the identification of membranous, myofascial and interosseous somatic dysfunction. The patient may be treated utilizing indirect principles to address any identified dysfunction. Begin by treating the area of greatest motion restriction. This will often be in the upper thoracic and craniocervical regions. The presence of proprioceptive sensory endings in the ligaments and fascia of the upper cervical area contributes to postural balance. Primary high cervical somatic dysfunction can consequently

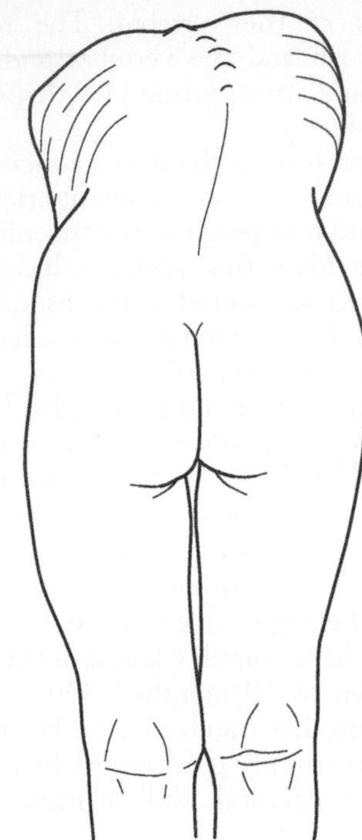

Figure 7.1.8. *The Adam's forward bending test allows the examiner to detect an asymmetry as a rotational deformity or 'rib hump'.*

impact postural balance. Somatic dysfunction in the upper thoracic region can result in compensatory dysfunction in the upper cervical spine. Once these areas have been treated, dysfunction of the thoracic spine, ribs, lumbar spine, sacrum and pelvis should be addressed.

Normalization of the diaphragm, to increase vital capacity, should always be part of the treatment of scolioses. Dysfunction of the thoracic diaphragm, because of the attachments of the crura on the lumbar spine, affects the mobility of the spine and may be linked to dysfunction in the pelvic and cranial diaphragms through the core link.

Any dysfunctional pattern present in the skull should be treated. Dysfunction in the occiput can affect the proprioceptive input from the craniocervical region. The vestibular apparatus located inside the petrous portions of the temporal bones contributes to balance mechanics and symmetric muscle tension. Dysfunction between the sphenoid, occiput and temporal bones should, therefore, be treated. By virtue of the fact that fusion of the SBS does not typically occur before late adolescence, there remains mobility in the base of the skull of younger AIS patients, making them particularly receptive to cranial treatment.

Cranial dysfunction may also affect the scoliotic patient through the reciprocal tension membranes. Dysfunctional tensions in the dura have been proposed as an etiology of scoliosis.[76] Equilibration of intracranial and intraspinal membranes should, therefore, be employed. In younger patients where active bone growth is still present, intraosseous dysfunctions – most commonly encountered in the sacrum, lumbar and thoracic vertebrae and occiput – may be addressed using molding procedures.

Exercises are an important component of the treatment protocol. A properly employed exercise program should teach the patient to breathe effectively, increasing vital capacity and enhancing thoracic cage mobility. It should facilitate the establishment of the fullest range of motion possible and the development of symmetry of movement, particularly spinal rotation, while strengthening the core musculature and stabilizing the spine. It should allow the patient to develop proprioception and establish good postural habits.

KYPHOSIS–LORDOSIS

Kyphosis is an increase of the spinal curve in the sagittal plane that results in a greater than normal posterior convexity (anterior concavity). An increased kyphotic curve is encountered more often in the thoracic spine, where it produces a rounded upper back, or 'humped back'. In the cervical and lumbar spines, normal curves present with posterior concavity or lordosis. Under dysfunctional circumstances, the lumbar and cervical curves are reversed and become kyphotic. At the lower portion of the spine, a kyphosis can be ascribed to the sacrum, when its usual posterior convexity is increased.

A thoracic kyphosis of >45° is considered pathologic. Congenital kyphotic deformities are infrequent and can be caused by a failure of formation of the vertebral body or a failure of segmentation, for which the treatment is surgical.[107] In the infant, tumor of the spine is also a potential cause of kyphosis that requires specific medical attention.

In the juvenile period, Scheuermann's disease is a cause of kyphosis resulting from an alteration of the vertebral development. Wedging of the vertebral bodies, the posterior height being greater than the anterior height, produces the kyphotic deformity. Boys are more frequently affected and the resultant back pain might be the trigger for an X-ray where the diagnosis is made. Irregularities in the endplates of the vertebrae can be observed, particularly at the level of the lower thoracic and upper lumbar spine. Scheuermann's disease may also be associated with scoliosis.[108]

Because kyphosis is a spinal deformity, it should not be confused with poor posture. When examining an infant who is seated without support, it is normal to find a kyphosis of the thoracic and lumbar spine. Proprioception and muscular tone develop with age to maintain adequate sagittal balance. Sagittal spinal curves change as a child grows.[109,110] The thoracic kyphosis is more pronounced in males,[111] at a mean age of 12.8 years.[112]

More often, the exaggerated kyphotic curve is associated with dysfunctional posture. Juvenile and adolescent kyphosis can be the result of poor posture, as a compensatory pattern to an extension dysfunction elsewhere. Anterior displacement of the occipital bone on the superior articular surface of the atlas will project the chin forward, and the ensuing postural compensation will result in an increased thoracic kyphosis. This pattern is commonly found in individuals who demonstrate oral breathing.

When encountered in a child, an apparent kyphosis may also be the result of protraction of the pectoral girdle. In this case, the thoracic curve is not fi xed in the kyphotic position and spinal backward bending can be achieved on demand, although lack of flexibility is common. The child is usually shy, and an extension–internal rotation pattern may be present, either at the level of the pelvis or at the level of the SBS, the temporal or occipital bones. A thoracoabdominal diaphragmatic dysfunction is very often associated with diminished thoracic fl exibility and reduced vital capacity. The areas of the diaphragmatic attachments onto the inferior portion of the sternum and adjacent ribs might be the causative dysfunctional agents.

An increased thoracic kyphotic curve is usually compensated for by an increase in the lumbar lordosis. Kyphosis and lumbar lordosis generally compensate each other. A correlation between these two spinal curves has been found in most age groups.[113]

The cervical and lumbar regions are normally lordotic. Hyperlordosis is an increase of the lumbar lordosis and is considered pathologic. It can be associated with other conditions, such as developmental dysplasia of the hip or neuromuscular disorders. There may be a family history of hyperlordosis, but it can also follow trauma, commonly from athletic activities, particularly highly competitive sports, during periods of growth. Adolescents may also present with hyperlordosis as a consequence of a developmental spondylolisthesis. With this disorder, studies have shown an increase of hyperlordosis and sacral inclination, but a decrease of thoracic kyphosis.[114]

The degree of lumbar lordosis is correlated with sacral position. Sacral anatomic extension (craniosacral flexion) is normally associated with decreased lordosis; sacral anatomic flexion (craniosacral extension) is associated with increased lordosis. The global amplitude of the vertebral curves, cervical lordosis, thoracic kyphosis and lumbar lordosis changes with growth, but the association with the position of the sacrum is constant under normal conditions.

The relationship between the cranial and the pelvic bowls, through the core link, is a fundamental principle within the cranial concept. Cranial flexion is associated with sacral craniosacral flexion, and cranial extension is associated with sacral craniosacral extension. The vertebral anteroposterior curves are decreased when flexion of the cranial base is present; conversely, there is an increase of the lordotic or kyphotic curves with extension of the cranial base.[115]

Physical examination and treatment

Early detection of kyphotic and lordotic curves is important for successful treatment. The child should be considered from a total body approach and the posture of the whole body should be evaluated in the standing position:

- Observe the pattern of weight-bearing mechanics.
- Observe the feet for a pattern of inversion or eversion. A pattern toward eversion of the feet, and eventually flat feet, is consistent with increased sagittal curves and cranial extension–internal rotation.
- Observe the knees. Genu valgum is consistent with increased sagittal curves and cranial extension–internal rotation.
- Observe the pelvis for an increase of anterior tilt, with the sacrum in craniosacral extension.
- Observe for pelvic asymmetry and any difference in the greater trochanter and innominate crest heights.
- Observe the spine for an increase of the anterior–posterior curves. A pattern involving all of the curves might be the consequence of a cranial or sacral dysfunction with extension and internal rotation. A pattern of increased curvature limited to a portion of the spine may be associated with a dysfunction within the curve, in an adjacent spinal curve or adjacent junctions between the spinal AP curves.
- Observe the pectoral girdle for protraction or an associated asymmetric pattern. A difference in shoulder heights is common. This suggests somatic dysfunction in the thoracic spine with associated sidebending and rotational components.
- Observe the position of the head in relation of the rest of the body, in both the frontal and the sagittal plane. Forward displacement of the head is often associated with somatic dysfunction of the craniocervical or upper thoracic vertebrae.

Next, observe the child while they are moving. If necessary, have the child demonstrate active flexion–extension, sidebending and rotation of the spine to confirm previous observations. Muscles may show a difference in tension between anterior and posterior groups. Hyperlordotic children will present with increased tension in the hamstrings and hip flexors, while at the same time their abdominal muscles will lack tension.

Tests of listening are performed on the innominates, the sacrum, the lumbar and cervical vertebrae and the cranium. The treatment of any identified dysfunctional areas should follow using indirect principles. The postural response to effective manipulation is almost immediate. You should be able to see improvement in the posture of the child after the first treatment.

Simple exercises may be recommended, particularly if poor posture is present. Pelvic tilt is useful, as are stretching the hamstrings and proprioceptive exercises to increase body posture awareness. The child should be encouraged to judiciously practice athletic activities, such as swimming and tai chi, which will strengthen and balance the core muscles and improve flexibility and coordination.

Advice should be given that appropriately addresses daily living conditions. For example, the patient should avoid carrying a backpack on one shoulder; rather, they should carry it using both shoulders. They should avoid reading and writing on a flat horizontal surface and should work instead on a surface that is tilted approximately 20° to limit cervicothoracic flexion.

Once the problem has been effectively addressed, the child may then be treated as needed, but they should be followed on a regular basis, at least annually, until they have stopped growing.

PECTUS EXCAVATUM AND CARINATUM

Pectus excavatum is a deformity of the anterior thoracic cage in which the sternum is depressed in a concave shape, whereas in pectus carinatum the sternum is protruded in a convex shape. These deformities may or may not be associated with genetic disorders or with scolioses. Decreased thoracic cage compliance and reduced vital capacity may be present, although the heart and lungs develop normally. Pectus excavatum and pectus carinatum are present at birth, but the parents usually do not become aware of the deformity until it becomes more apparent with growth. Severe cases often result in significant psychological impact, usually in early adolescence.

Pectus excavatum is frequently associated with an SBS extension pattern. This results in internal rotation of the paired structures, specifically the pectoral girdle. These individuals may also demonstrate direct mechanical derangement of the internal fascial structure of the thoracic cage and intraosseous dysfunction of the ribs and sternum. A diaphragmatic dysfunction is almost always associated with this condition. In pectus carinatum, similar mechanisms exist but with a tendency for SBS flexion.

Physical examination and treatment

The evaluation of the patient commences by examining the interrelationship between the sternum and the thoracic spine, and between the sternum and the occiput. Next, examine all myofascial structures attached to the sternum, including the pectoral girdle and the diaphragm. The anterior abdominal wall should be evaluated for dysfunctional tension, and, if present, contributory mechanics should be sought out in the lumbar spine, sacrum and pelvis. Visceral abdominal dysfunction should also be considered.

Treatment consists of myofascial release applied to identified dysfunctions. If possible, molding procedures directed at the sternum should be employed simultaneously with the myofascial release modalities to enhance the efficacy of both. The application of these procedures should be done in synchrony with, and with the intent to enhance, the inherent motility of the body. The younger the patient when treatment is initiated, the greater the potential for positive outcome.

VERTEBRAL SOMATIC DYSFUNCTION

Vertebral somatic dysfunction in infants and children can be found at any level of the spine. It will, however, be more commonly encountered in the lumbar, upper thoracic and cervical regions. It usually results from the day-to-day physical activities and traumas of childhood. In younger children, dysfunction in the cervical region will often present as cervical pain and, eventually, as torticollis. In the lumbar region, somatic dysfunction may remain quiescent for a protracted period, in time manifesting through a somatovisceral mechanism as abdominal pain. In older children and adolescents, the initial complaint from vertebral dysfunction is usually localized or referred musculoskeletal pain. Because of the young patient's ability to compensate for somatic dysfunction, any vertebral somatic dysfunction should be thoroughly evaluated to rule out a viscerosomatic origin.

The mechanics of vertebral somatic dysfunction manifest in children and adolescents is the same as that encountered in adults, showing the coupled relationships between flexion–extension, sidebending and rotation as described by Fryette.[116] However, because of the flexibility of the soft tissues in these young patients, dysfunctional barriers are more compliant, lending to the application of indirect techniques in their treatment.

Somatic dysfunction may also exist as a reflex manifestation of visceral dysfunction and disease. Although the precise locations of viscerosomatic reflexes in infants and young children have not been specifically reported, it is reasonable to anticipate locations similar to those in adults. The facilitated state of the segmental spinal cord in the presence of visceral input can, in turn, result in a somatovisceral response. A listing of viscerosomatic locations as they have been reported in the osteopathic literature is summarized in Box 7.1.1.

Because of the growth potential of these patients, vertebral somatic dysfunction can exert disproportionate impact on their developing posture as well as on the viscera through somatovisceral reflexes.

Box 7.1.1

VISCEROSOMATIC REFLEXES

The following locations are summarized from a review of the osteopathic literature.[117–123]

- *Eyes, ears, nose, and throat*: The sympathetic reflex is T1–T5. The trigeminal nerve is the final common pathway for both sympathetic and parasympathetic innervation of the upper respiratory tract. The muscles of mastication, commonly the temporalis muscles, receive motor innervation from the trigeminal nerve and serve as the somatic component for the upper respiratory tract sympathetic and parasympathetic reflexes. An additional reflex site is occiput–C2. This results from a reflex between the trigeminal nerve and upper cervical nerves.[123]
- *Heart*: The sympathetic reflex is T1–T5, left-sided greater than right. The parasympathetic reflex is vagal, occiput, C1, C2.
- *Lung*: The sympathetic reflex is bilateral from T1 to T4. Conditions involving both lungs result in bilateral reflex findings. Conditions involving one lung result in a reflex on the same side as the involved lung. The parasympathetic reflex is vagal, occiput, C1, C2.
- *Gastrointestinal tract*:
  - — The parasympathetic reflex from the gastrointestinal tract proximal to the mid-transverse colon is vagal, occiput, C1, C2; the parasympathetic reflex from the distal half of the transverse colon to the rectum is sacropelvic S2–S4
  - — The esophagus has a right-sided sympathetic reflex from T3 to T6
  - — The stomach has a left-sided sympathetic reflex from T5 to T10
  - — The duodenum has a right-sided sympathetic reflex from T6 to T8
  - — The small intestine sympathetic reflex is bilateral from T8 to T10
  - — The appendix and cecum sympathetic reflex is from T9 to T12 on the right
  - — The ascending colon sympathetic reflex is from T11 to L1 on the right
  - — The descending colon to rectum sympathetic reflex is from L1 to L3 on the left.
- *Pancreas*: The sympathetic reflex may be left-sided or bilateral and is T5–T9. The parasympathetic reflex is vagal, occiput, C1, C2.
- *Liver and gallbladder*: The sympathetic reflex is right-sided from T5 to T10. The parasympathetic reflex is vagal, occiput, C1, C2.
- *Spleen*: The sympathetic reflex is left-sided from T7 to T9.
- *Kidney*: The sympathetic reflex is on the same side as the involved kidney, from T9 to L1. The parasympathetic reflex is vagal, occiput, C1, C2.
- *Urinary bladder*: The sympathetic reflex is bilateral from T11 to L3. The parasympathetic reflex is sacropelvic, S2–S4.
- *Ovaries (and testes)*: The sympathetic reflex is on the same side as the involved organ from T10 to T11.
- *Adrenal glands*: The sympathetic reflex is on the same side as the involved gland from T8 to T10.

REFERENCES

1. Lincoln TL, Suen PW. Common rotational variations in children. J Am Acad Orthop Surg 2003;11(5):312–20.
2. Chen MM, Chang HC, Hsieh CF, Yen MF, Chen TH. Predictive model for congenital muscular torticollis: analysis of 1021 infants with sonography. Arch Phys Med Rehabil 2005;86(11):2199–203.
3. Cheng JC, Tang SP, Chen TM. Sternocleidomastoid pseudotumor and congenital muscular torticollis in infants: a prospective study of 510 cases. J Pediatr 1999;134(6): 712–6.
4. Macdonald D. Sternomastoid tumour and muscular torticollis. J Bone Joint Surg 1969;51B(3):432–43.
5. Hsieh YY, Tsai FJ, Lin CC, Chang FC, Tsai CH. Breech deformation complex in neonates. J Reprod Med 2000; 45(11):933–5.
6. Todd TW, Lyon DW. Endocranial suture closure. Its progress and age relationship. Part I. Adult males and white stock. Am J Phys Anthropol 1924;7:325–84.
7. Chapple CC, Davidson DT. A study of the relationship between fetal position and certain congenital deformities. J Pediatr 1941;18:483–93.
8. Watson GH. Relationship between side of plagiocephaly, dislocation of hip, scoliosis, bat ears and sternomastoid tumors. Arch Dis Child 1971;46:203–10.
9. Dunn PM. Congenital postural deformities. Br Med Bull 1976;32(1):71–6.
10. Good C, Walker G. The hip in the moulded baby syndrome. J Bone Joint Surg 1984;66B(4):491–2.
11. Coventry MB, Harris LE. Congenital muscular torticollis in infancy; some observations regarding treatment. J Bone Joint Surg 1959;41A(5):815–22.
12. Brooks B. Pathologic changes in muscle as a result of disturbances of circulation. Arch Surg 1922;5:188–216.
13. Chandler FA, Altenberg A. 'Congenital' muscular torticollis. JAMA 1944;125(7):476–83.
14. Davids JR, Wenger DR, Mubarak SJ. Congenital muscular torticollis: sequela of intrauterine or perinatal compartment syndrome. J Pediatr Orthop 1993;13(2):141–7.
15. Klier EM, Wang H, Constantin AG, Crawford JD. Midbrain control of three-dimensional head orientation. Science 2002;295(5558):1314–6.
16. Jacquemart M, Piedallu P. Le torticolis 'congénital' est-il simplement un torticolis obstétrical? Le Concours Médical 1964;36:4867–70.
17. Cheng JC, Wong MW, Tang SP, Chen TM, Shum SL, Wong EM. Clinical determinants of the outcome of manual stretching in the treatment of congenital muscular torticollis in infants. A prospective study of eight hundred and twenty-one cases. J Bone Joint Surg 2001;83A(5): 679–87.

18. Dudkiewicz I, Ganel A, Blankstein A. Congenital muscular torticollis in infants: ultrasound-assisted diagnosis and evaluation. J Pediatr Orthop 2005;25(6):812–4.
19. Jahss SA. Torticollis. J Bone Joint Surg 1936;18A:1065–8.
20. Sutherland WG. Teachings in the science of osteopathy. Fort Worth, TX: Sutherland Cranial Teaching Foundation; 1991:222.
21. Chate RA. Facial scoliosis due to sternocleidomastoid torticollis: a cephalometric analysis. Int J Oral Maxillofac Surg 2004;33(4):338–43.
22. Yu CC, Wong FH, Lo LJ, Chen YR. Craniofacial deformity in patients with uncorrected congenital muscular torticollis: an assessment from three-dimensional computed tomography imaging. Plast Reconstr Surg 2004;113(1): 24–33.
23. Schieppati M, Nardone A, Schmid M. Neck muscle fatigue affects postural control in man. Neuroscience 2003; 121(2):277–85.
24. Gerszten PC, Gerszten E. Intentional cranial deformation: a disappearing form of self mutilation. Neurosurgery 1995; 37(3):374–81.
25. Gosse LA. Essai sur les déformations artificielles du crâne. Ann Hyg Publique Méd Lég Paris 1855;3:317–93.
26. Cohen MM Jr. Sutural biology and the correlates of craniosynostosis. Am J Med Genet 1993;47:581–616.
27. Hehr U, Muenke M. Craniosynostosis syndromes: from genes to premature fusion of skull bones. Mol Genet Metab 1999;68:139–51.
28. David DJ, Menard RM. Occipital plagiocephaly. Br J Plast Surg 2000;53(5):367–77.
29. Huang MH, Gruss JS, Clarren SK. The differential diagnosis of posterior plagiocephaly: true lambdoid synostosis versus positional molding. Plast Reconstr Surg 1996;98: 765–74.
30. Warren SM, Longaker MT. The pathogenesis of craniosynostosis in the fetus. Yonsei Med J 2001;42(6):646–59.
31. Boere-Boonekamp MM, Van Der Linden-Kuiper LT. Positional preference: prevalence in infants and follow-up after two years. Pediatrics 2001;107(2):339–43.
32. Bruneteau RJ, Mulliken JB. Frontal plagiocephaly: synostotic, compensational or deformational. Plast Reconstr Surg 1992;89:21–31.
33. Captier G, Leboucq N, Bigorre M et al. Etude clinicoradiologique des déformations du crâne dans les plagiocéphalies sans synostose. Arch Pediatr 2003;10:208–14.
34. Kane AA, Mitchell LE, Craven KP, Marsh JL. Observations on a recent increase in plagiocephaly without synostosis. Pediatrics 1996;97(6 Pt 1):877–85.
35. Peitsch WK, Keefer CH, Labrie RA, Mulliken JB. Incidence of cranial asymmetry in healthy newborns. Pediatrics 2002;110(6):e72.
36. Sergueef N, Nelson KE, Glonek T. Palpatory diagnosis of plagiocephaly. Complement Ther Clin Pract 2006;12(2): 101–10.
37. Bekedam DJ, Engelsbel S, Mol BW, Buitendijk SE, Van Der Pal-De Bruin KM. Male predominance in fetal distress during labor. Am J Obstet Gynecol 2002;187(6):1605–7.
38. Moss ML. The pathogenesis of artificial cranial deformation. Am J Phys Anthropol 1958;16:269–86.
39. Vles J, Van Zutphen S, Hasaart T, Dassen W, Lodder J. Supine and prone head orientation preference in term infants. Brain Dev 1991;13(2):87–90.
40. Hopkins B, Lems YL, Van Wulfften Palthe T, Hoeksma J, Kardaun O, Butterworth G. Development of head position preference during early infancy: a longitudinal study in the daily life situation. Dev Psychobiol 1990;23(1):39–53.
41. Hutchison BL, Hutchison LA, Thompson JM, Mitchell EA. Plagiocephaly and brachycephaly in the first two years of life: a prospective cohort study. Pediatrics 2004;114(4): 970–80.
42. Golden KA, Beals SP, Littlefield TR, Pomatto JK. Sternocleidomastoid imbalance versus congenital muscular torticollis: their relationship to positional plagiocephaly. Cleft Palate Craniofac J 1999;36(3):256–61.
43. Sergueef N. Approche ostéopathique des plagiocéphalies avec ou sans torticolis. Paris: Spek; 2004.
44. Biggs WS. Diagnosis and management of positional head deformity. Am Fam Physician 2003;67(9):1953–6.
45. O'Broin ES, Allcutt D, Earley MJ. Posterior plagiocephaly: proactive conservative management. Br J Plast Surg 1999;52:18–23.
46. Pollack IF, Losken HW, Fasick P. Diagnosis and management of posterior plagiocephaly. Pediatrics 1997;99: 180–5.
47. Persing J, James H, Swanson J, Kattwinkel J. Prevention and management of positional skull deformities in infants. Pediatrics 2003;112(1 Pt 1):199–202.
48. Magoun HI. Osteopathy in the cranial field. Kirksville, MO: The Journal Printing Company; 1951:203.
49. Magoun HI. Osteopathy in the cranial field, 2nd ed. Kirksville, MO: The Journal Printing Company; 1966:133.
50. King HH, Lay EM. Osteopathy in the cranial field. In: Ward RC (ed). Foundations for osteopathic medicine, 2nd edn. Philadelphia: Lippincott, Williams & Wilkins; 2003: 993–6.
51. Arbuckle BE. The selected writings of Beryl E. Arbuckle, D.O., F.A.C.O.P. Newark OH: American Academy of Osteopathy; 1971:188.
52. Magoun HI. Osteopathy in the cranial field, 2nd edn. Kirksville, MO: The Journal Printing Company; 1966:186.
53. Rekate HL. Diagnosis and management of plagiocephaly. Barrow Quarterly 1986;2:69–75.
54. Kemaloglu YK, Goksu N, Ozbilen S, Akyildiz N. Otitis media with effusion and craniofacial analysis – II: 'Mastoid–middle ear–Eustachian tube system' in children with secretory otitis media. Int J Pediatr Otorhinolaryngol 1995;32: 69–76.
55. Balan P, Kushnerenko E, Sahlin P, Huotilainen M, Naatanen R, Hukki J. Auditory ERPs reveal brain dysfunction in infants with plagiocephaly. J Craniofac Surg 2002; 13(4):520–5; discussion 526.
56. Miller RI, Clarren SK. Long-term developmental outcomes in patients with deformational plagiocephaly. Pediatrics 2000;105(2):e26.
57. Davis BE, Moon RY, Sachs HC, Ottolini MC. Effects of sleep position on infant motor development. Pediatrics 1998;102:1135–40.
58. Wynne-Davies R. Infantile idiopathic scoliosis: causative factors, particularly in the first six months of life. J Bone Joint Surg 1975;57B:138–41.
59. Magoun HI Sr. Idiopathic adolescent spinal scoliosis: a reasonable etiology (1975). In: Peterson B (ed). Postural balance and imbalance. Indianapolis, IN: American Academy of Osteopathy; 1983:94–100.
60. Kawamoto HK. Torticollis versus plagiocephaly. In: Marchac D (ed). Cranio-facial surgery. International Society for CranioMaxilloFacial Surgery. New York: Springer; 1987:105–9.
61. Kelly KM, Littlefield TR, Pomatto JK, Ripley CE, Beals SP, Joganic EF. Importance of early recognition and treatment of deformational plagiocephaly with orthotic cranioplasty. Cleft Palate Craniofac J 1999;36(2):127–30.

62. Björk A, Björk L. Artificial deformation and cranio-facial asymmetry in ancient Peruvians. J Dent Res 1964;43(3): 353–62.
63. Mulliken JB, Vander Woude DL, Hansen M, LaBrie RA, Scott RM. Analysis of posterior plagiocephaly: deformational versus synostotic. Plast Reconstr Surg 1999;103(2): 371–80.
64. Wynne-Davies R. Familial (idiopathic) scoliosis. J Bone Joint Surg 1968;50B:24–30.
65. Miller NH. Cause and natural history of adolescent idiopathic scoliosis. Orthop Clin North Am 1999;30(3):343–52, vii.
66. Murdoch G. Scoliosis in twins. J Bone Joint Surg 1959; 41B:736–7.
67. Henderson MH Jr, Rieger MA, Miller F, Kaelin A. Influence of parental age on degree of curvature in idiopathic scoliosis. J Bone Joint Surg 1990;72A(6):910–3.
68. Lowe TG, Edgar M, Margulies JY et al. Etiology of idiopathic scoliosis: current trends in research. J Bone Joint Surg 2000;82A(8):1157–68.
69. Chan YL, Cheng JC, Guo X, King AD, Griffith JF, Metreweli C. MRI evaluation of multifidus muscles in adolescent idiopathic scoliosis. Pediatr Radiol 1999;29(5):360–3.
70. Machida M, Dubousset J, Imamura Y, Miyashita Y, Yamada T, Kimura J. Melatonin: a possible role in pathogenesis of adolescent idiopathic scoliosis. Spine 1996;21(10): 1147–52.
71. Machida M, Saito M, Dubousset J, Yamada T, Kimura J, Shibasaki K. Pathological mechanism of idiopathic scoliosis: experimental scoliosis in pinealectomized rats. Eur Spine J 2005;14(9):843–8.
72. Woods LA, Haller RJ, Hansen PD, Fukumoto DE, Herman RM. Decreased incidence of scoliosis in hearing-impaired children. Implications for a neurologic basis for idiopathic scoliosis. Spine 1995;20(7):776–80; discussion 781.
73. Herman R, Mixon J, Fisher A, Maulucci R, Stuyck J. Idiopathic scoliosis and the central nervous system: a motor control problem. Spine 1985;10(1):1–14.
74. Wiener-Vacher SR, Mazda K. Asymmetric otolith vestibulo-ocular responses in children with idiopathic scoliosis. J Pediatr 1998;132(6):1028–32.
75. Nault ML, Allard P, Hinse S et al. Relations between standing stability and body posture parameters in adolescent idiopathic scoliosis. Spine 2002;27(17):1911–7.
76. Roth M. Idiopathic scoliosis caused by a short spinal cord. Acta Radiol Diagn (Stockh) 1968;7(3):257–71.
77. Guo X, Chau WW, Chan YL, Cheng JC. Relative anterior spinal overgrowth in adolescent idiopathic scoliosis. Results of disproportionate endochondral–membranous bone growth. J Bone Joint Surg 2003;85B(7):1026–31.
78. Porter RW. Idiopathic scoliosis: the relation between the vertebral canal and the vertebral bodies. Spine 2000; 25(11):1360–6.
79. Magoun HI. Osteopathy in the cranial field. Kirksville, MO: The Journal Printing Company; 1951:112.
80. Tanchev PI, Dzherov AD, Parushev AD, Dikov DM, Todorov MB. Scoliosis in rhythmic gymnasts. Spine 2000; 25(11):1367–72.
81. Dunn PM. Congenital postural scoliosis. Arch Dis Child 1973;48(8):654.
82. James JI. The management of infants with scoliosis. J Bone Joint Surg 1975;57B(4):422–9.
83. McMaster MJ. Infantile idiopathic scoliosis: can it be prevented? J Bone Joint Surg 1983;65B(5):612–7.
84. Ventura N, Huguet R, Ey A, Montaner A, Lizarraga I, Vives E. Infantile idiopathic scoliosis in the newborn. Int Orthop 1998;22(2):82–6.
85. James JI. The etiology of scoliosis. J Bone Joint Surg 1970;52B(3):410–9.
86. Arbuckle BE. 'Scoliosis capitis'. J Am Osteopath Assoc 1970;70(2):131–7.
87. Mohanty S, Kumar N. Patterns of presentation of congenital scoliosis. J Orthop Surg (Hong Kong) 2000;8(2):33–7.
88. Dobbs MB, Lenke LG, Szymanski DA et al. Prevalence of neural axis abnormalities in patients with infantile idiopathic scoliosis. J Bone Joint Surg 2002;84A(12):2230–4.
89. Jog S, Patole S, Whitehall J. Congenital scoliosis in a neonate: can a neonatologist ignore it? Postgrad Med J 2002;78(922):469–72.
90. Harrenstein RJ. Die Skoliose bei Säuglingen und ihre Behandlung. Z Orthop Chir 1930;52:1–40.
91. Mehta MH. The rib–vertebra angle in the early diagnosis between resolving and progressive infantile scoliosis. J Bone Joint Surg 1972;54(2):230–43.
92. Diedrich O, von Strempel A, Schloz M, Schmitt O, Kraft CN. Long-term observation and management of resolving infantile idiopathic scoliosis: a 25-year follow-up. J Bone Joint Surg 2002;84B(7):1030–5.
93. James JIP, Lloyd-Roberts GC, Pilcher MF. Infantile structural scoliosis. J Bone Joint Surg 1959;41B:719–35.
94. Lloyd-Roberts GC, Pilcher MF. Structural idiopathic scoliosis in infancy: a study of the natural history of 100 patients. J Bone Joint Surg 1965;47:520–3.
95. Stehbens WE, Cooper RL. Regression of juvenile idiopathic scoliosis. Exp Mol Pathol 2003;74(3):326–35.
96. Guillaumat M, Khouri N. Scoliose idiopathique en période de croissance. Encycl Méd Chir (Editions Scientifiques et Médicales, Elsevier SAS, Paris), Pédiatrie 2000;4–007-B-20.
97. Browne D. Congenital postural scoliosis. Br Med J 1965; 5461:565–6.
98. Reamy BV, Slakey JB. Adolescent idiopathic scoliosis: review and current concepts. Am Fam Physician 2001; 64(1):111–6.
99. Escalada F, Marco E, Duarte E et al. Growth and curve stabilization in girls with adolescent idiopathic scoliosis. Spine 2005;30(4):411–7.
100. Edgar MA, Mehta MH. Long-term follow-up of fused and unfused idiopathic scoliosis. J Bone Joint Surg 1988;70B(5): 712–6.
101. Morin C. Traitement des scolioses idiopathiques chez l'enfant en période de croissance. Bull Acad Natl Med 1999; 183(4):731–5.
102. Rowe DE, Bernstein SM, Riddick MF, Adler F, Emans JB, Gardner-Bonneau D. A meta-analysis of the efficacy of nonoperative treatments for idiopathic scoliosis. J Bone Joint Surg 1997;79(5):664–74.
103. Donnelly MJ, Dolan LA, Weinstein SL. How effective is bracing for treatment of scoliosis? Am Fam Physician 2003;67(1):32, 35; author reply 35.
104. Niesluchowski W, Dabrowska A, Kedzior K, Zagrajek T. The potential role of brain asymmetry in the development of adolescent idiopathic scoliosis: a hypothesis. J Manip Physiol Ther 1999;22(8):540–4.
105. Morningstar MW, Woggon D, Lawrence G. Scoliosis treatment using a combination of manipulative and rehabilitative therapy: a retrospective case series. BMC Musculoskelet Disord 2004;5:32.
106. Hawes MC. The use of exercises in the treatment of scoliosis: an evidence-based critical review of the literature. Pediatr Rehabil 2003;6(3–4):171–82.
107. Lonstein JE. Congenital spine deformities: scoliosis, kyphosis, and lordosis. Orthop Clin North Am 1999;30(3):387–405, viii.

108. Deacon P, Berkin CR, Dickson RA. Combined idiopathic kyphosis and scoliosis. An analysis of the lateral spinal curvatures associated with Scheuermann's disease. J Bone Joint Surg 1985;67B(2):189–92.
109. Mac-Thiong JM, Berthonnaud E, Dimar JR 2nd, Betz RR, Labelle H. Sagittal alignment of the spine and pelvis during growth. Spine 2004;29(15):1642–7.
110. Cil A, Yazici M, Uzumcugil A et al. The evolution of sagittal segmental alignment of the spine during childhood. Spine 2005;30(1):93–100.
111. Poussa MS, Heliovaara MM, Seitsamo JT, Kononen MH, Hurmerinta KA, Nissinen MJ. Development of spinal posture in a cohort of children from the age of 11 to 22 years. Eur Spine J 2005;14(8):738–42.
112. Nissinen M. Spinal posture during pubertal growth. Acta Paediatr 1995;84(3):308–12.
113. Willner S, Johnson B. Thoracic kyphosis and lumbar lordosis during the growth period in children. Acta Paediatr Scand 1983;72(6):873–8.
114. Labelle H, Roussouly P, Berthonnaud E, Dimnet J, O'Brien M. The importance of spino-pelvic balance in L5–S1 developmental spondylolisthesis: a review of pertinent radiologic measurements. Spine 2005;30(6 Suppl): S27–34.
115. Magoun HI. Osteopathy in the cranial field. Kirksville, MO: The Journal Printing Company; 1951:184.
116. Fryette HH. Principles of osteopathic technic. Carmel, CA: Academy of Applied Osteopathy (American Academy of Osteopathy, Indianapolis IN); 1954.
117. Pottenger FM. Symptoms of visceral disease, 5th edn. St Louis: Mosby; 1938.
118. Owens C. An endocrine interpretation of Chapman's reflexes, 2nd edn. 1937. Reprinted: Indianapolis, IN: Academy of Applied Osteopathy (American Academy of Osteopathy); 1963.
119. Beal MC. Viscerosomatic reflexes: a review. J Am Osteopath Assoc 1985;85(12):786–801.
120. Kuchera ML, Kuchera WA. Osteopathic considerations in systemic dysfunctions, 2nd edn. Columbus, OH: Greyden Press; 1994.
121. Dowling DJ. Neurophysiologic mechanisms related to osteopathic diagnosis and treatment. In: DiGiovanna EL, Schiowitz S (eds) An osteopathic approach to diagnosis and treatment, 2nd edn. Philadelphia: JB Lippincott; 1997:29.
122. Van Buskirk RL, Nelson KE. Osteopathic family practice: an application of the primary care model. In: Ward RC (ed). Foundations for osteopathic medicine, 2nd edn. Philadelphia: Lippincott Williams and Wilkins; 2002:289–97.
123. Sumino R, Nozaki S, Kato M. Central pathway of trigemino-neck reflex [abstract]. In: Oral-facial sensory and motor functions. International Symposium, Rappongi, Tokyo. Oral Physiol 1980:28.

7.2 APPENDICULAR IMBALANCE

Upper extremity

FRACTURES OF THE CLAVICLE

The clavicle is the bone most frequently fractured during the birth process. Clavicular fractures occur in about 1.6% of all vaginal deliveries[1,2] and 0.5% when considering all live births.[3] Both males and females are affected equally, with equal left versus right-sided incidence.[3] There is, however, a slightly increased incidence of right-sided fractures in left occiput-anterior deliveries.[4]

Reported risk factors for clavicular fractures include increased duration of the second stage of labor, increased birth weight and neonatal length (macrosomia), instrumental delivery[2] and shoulder dystocia.[3] In cephalic presentation, the compression of the infant's anterior shoulder against the maternal symphysis is responsible for the trauma.[4] Direct pressure or torsion applied to the clavicles to facilitate delivery can also result in fracture.

Complete or incomplete greenstick fractures are most frequent. They present with edema, crepitus, a palpable bony bump and tissue texture changes over the fracture site. Decreased or absent movement of the affected arm is present, as may become apparent when eliciting the Moro reflex. Asymptomatic or incomplete clavicular fractures may not be initially identified until after discharge from the hospital. Usually, the caregiver will notice that the child demonstrates irritability with discomfort and pain when putting the child's arm through the sleeve of a garment or when lifting the child by holding them under their arms. They are also liable to report that the child cries when positioned on the affected side.

Shoulder dislocation, humeral fracture and brachial plexus injury are part of the differential diagnoses. The diagnosis is confirmed radiographically. Associated complications, such as Erb's palsy, are present in 11.3% of newborns with fractures of the clavicle,[2] although clavicular fracture may actually reduce the potential nerve injury from traction on the brachial plexus.[4]

Usually no orthopedic treatment is necessary for asymptomatic and incomplete clavicular fractures. When the neonate presents with pain or discomfort, the affected arm may be immobilized by pinning the sleeve to the front of the shirt for 7–10 days.[5] A large callus typically forms at the fracture site within a week, and recovery is usually considered to be complete. Osteopathic procedures may be employed to assist the recovery process and address the dysfunctions usually associated with a fracture of the clavicle.

The clavicle is of importance because of its myofascial attachments. It serves as a junction between the fasciae of the thorax, arm and neck. The investing layer of the deep cervical fascia completely surrounds the neck. Superiorly, it is attached to the external occipital protuberance and the superior nuchal line, the mastoid processes, zygomatic arches and the inferior borders of mandible. It splits to surround the trapezius and sternocleidomastoid muscles. Inferiorly, it is attached to the manubrium of the sternum, the acromion and the spine of the scapula.

The clavicle is the link in the fascial continuity between the investing layer of the deep cervical fascia and the fascia of the thorax and the arm. The clavipectoral fascia attaches on the clavicle, as does the deltoid fascia. The deltoid fascia is in continuity with the brachial fascia. The clavicle, therefore, plays an important role in the equilibrium of the fascia of the thorax, arm and neck, and should be balanced, as should the myofascial structures attached to it.

Forces applied during the delivery that are great enough to fracture the clavicle also affect the neck and upper thoracic vertebrae of the neonate. Therefore the osteopathic practitioner should evaluate these structures and treat any dysfunctions accordingly, using indirect principles.

Furthermore, because of pain from the fractured clavicle, the child will prefer to lie on the opposite side, thereby fostering the development of asymmetric fascial tensions. These asymmetries can, in turn, induce the child to select a chronic position of comfort, long after the clavicle has healed. The chronic asymmetric positioning can then predispose the child to the development of plagiocephaly.

Fractures of the clavicle that occur during childhood are usually the result of rough play or athletic activities. In childhood, the forces that result in clavicular fractures are usually violent, most often involving impact on the hand with the arm extended or impact on the shoulder. In 75% of cases the site of fracture involves the medial third of the bone. The standard orthopedic treatment reduces the displacement at the fracture site by maintaining the shoulder in an upward and backward position with a bandage or plaster.

Physical examination and treatment

Osteopathic procedures applied to the older child follow the same anatomic principles as for the infant, i.e. to alleviate myofascial imbalances and upper thoracic and cervical dysfunction. The acromioclavicular junction may demonstrate somatic dysfunction; it should, therefore, be evaluated and treated following indirect principles. It is of importance to allow for normal function of the growing upper extremity. Acromioclavicular dysfunction is the source of many adult shoulder disorders.

BRACHIAL PLEXUS INJURY

A brachial plexus injury occurs most commonly as a result of a difficult birth, fetal malpresentation,[5] shoulder dystocia, macrosomia[6] or assisted vaginal delivery.[7] Fracture of the clavicle(s) or humerus,[8] shoulder dislocation, torticollis, hematomas of the sternocleidomastoid muscle or paralysis of the diaphragm may be associated with injury of the brachial plexus.[5]

A commonly believed etiology of brachial plexus injury is excessive traction on the fetal head during birth. In vaginal delivery, during the attempt to deliver the anterior shoulder, the applied downward traction can damage the brachial plexus. This theory, however, is questionable because, in almost half the cases of brachial plexus injury, delivery of the shoulders occurs without difficulty. Therefore, an in utero, atraumatic theory is also proposed.[8] When asymmetry and diminished movement of the arm are observed on the fetal ultrasound, a vulnerable plexus may be injured without traction during delivery.[9]

The brachial plexus is formed by the union of the anterior divisions of the lower four cervical nerves and part of the anterior division of the first thoracic nerve. In addition, the fifth cervical nerve frequently receives a branch from the fourth cervical, and the first thoracic a branch from the second thoracic. The plexus extends from the inferior aspect of the side of the neck to the axilla. The fifth and sixth cervical nerves unite to form the upper trunk; the eighth cervical and first thoracic nerves form the lower trunk, while the seventh cervical nerve runs out alone as the middle trunk. These three trunks pass beneath the clavicle and split into the anterior and posterior divisions. The plexus is attached to the first rib and to the coracoid process by the costocoracoid membrane and is subject to any force that disturbs the relationship between the cervical vertebrae, the first thoracic vertebra and ribs, the clavicle and the scapula (Fig. 7.2.1).

Most of the time brachial plexus injury is unilateral and immediately recognizable. Brachial plexus injury can affect different spinal nerve roots and is identified as follows:

- *Upper type*, with involvement of C5 and C6, or Erb–Duchenne palsy that affects muscles of the shoulder and elbow. The child presents with adduction of the upper extremity and internal

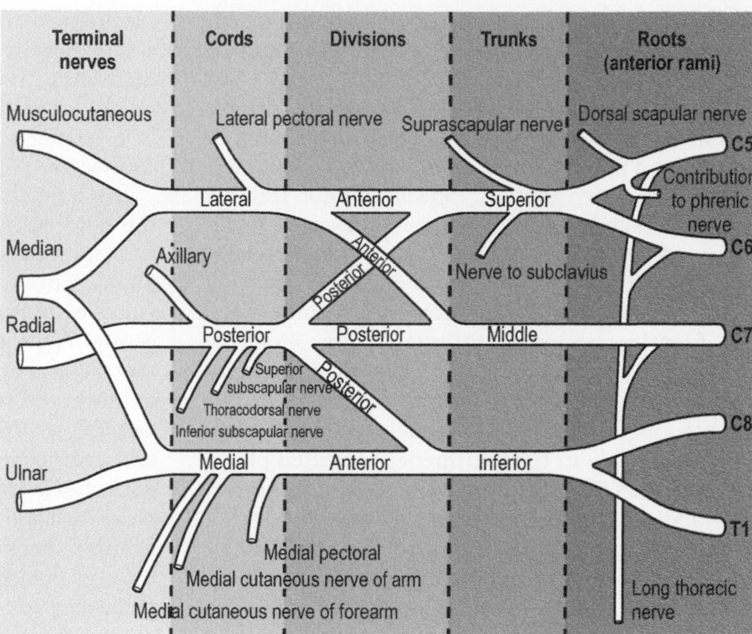

Figure 7.2.1. *Branches of the brachial plexus.*

rotation of the shoulder, but grasp remains intact. It represents most of the brachial plexus paralyses[10] and is considered to have a good prognosis.

- *Lower type*, with involvement of C7, C8 and T1, or Klumpke's palsy that affects muscles of the forearm and hand. The child presents with a paralysis of the hand and wrist. The presence of an ipsilateral Horner's syndrome (anhidrosis, miosis and ptosis) indicates an involvement of the sympathetic fibers associated with an intraspinal avulsion of the root of T1.
- *Whole arm type*, with involvement of C5–T1, with no movement of the upper extremity and often associated with sensory loss.

Extreme lateral flexion and traction of the head may be responsible for the stretch applied to the brachial plexus. The injury results in anything from a mild edema or hemorrhage within the affected nerves, to tearing of the nerve(s) that could be as extensive as to produce a total avulsion of the complete plexus. The C5 and C6 spinal nerves are located in the sulcus nervi spinali of the transverse processes. In that location they are strongly attached by various fibrous slips as extensions of the prevertebral fascia and surrounding structures attached to the spinous processes, and are, therefore, more likely to be ruptured.[11] The C8 and T1 spinal nerves may, more often, be subject to avulsion.[11]

Neuronal injury associated with brachial plexus injury may be of different degrees of severity:

- Neuropraxic lesions are failure of conduction without the axon having been affected, and are reversible.
- Axonotmetic lesions involve disruption of both the myelin sheath and the axon, but with the surrounding neuronal elements kept intact. Wallerian degeneration of the axon distal to the injury occurs.
- Neurotmetic lesions are total sectioning of the nerve with its myelin sheath and supporting connective tissue.
- Avulsion is a separation of the plexus from the spinal cord.

Obstetric brachial plexus palsy occurs in 0.4–2.5 per 1000 live births with an upper root (C5–C6) involvement in 50% of cases; C5, C6 and C7 involvement in 25%; and the whole plexus in 25%.[6,8,12] Neuropraxic and axonotmetic lesions have better prognoses.

Physical examination and treatment

The diagnosis is made by physical examination. The Moro reflex is asymmetric and the biceps' deep tendon reflex is absent. The grasp reflex is, however, normal. The child should be moved very gently: the injuries are painful and the tissues very fragile. Initial treatment is usually conservative with regular assessment. If the patient fails to show significant improvement by 3 months of age, surgical opinion should be sought.[13]

Physical therapy, consisting of gentle passive mobilization, may be employed to maintain range of motion and prevent contractures while the infant is recovering active motion. Specific motor training can be initiated within the first 2 weeks, with facilitation of active movement. The persistent neurologic deficits may result in the development of internal rotation and adduction contractures of the arm. Gentle stretching of internal rotators should be performed to reduce this risk while avoiding reinforcement of forearm supination.

Osteopathic procedures should be employed as early as possible in the treatment of brachial plexus injury. Traumatic forces may have injured the brachial plexus, but other areas, such as the upper thoracic spine, the first rib, the cervical spine, clavicle and all of the myofascial components of the thoracic outlet, have been stressed as well. Dysautonomia may also be present because somatic dysfunction of the cranial base and occipitoatlantal region can affect the parasympathetic tone through the vagus nerve, while somatic dysfunction in the upper thoracic spine can affect sympathetic nervous function. Direct compression of the venous and lymphatic drainage of the brachial plexus, as well as somatovisceral reflexes, should be considered when attempting to facilitate nerve regeneration. Osteopathic procedures aim to promote fluid, electrolyte and metabolic exchange within the tissues to facilitate drainage of edema and to prevent or reduce tissue scarring. Treatment is intended to optimize nerve regeneration and prevent the development of muscular imbalance. Recuperation of the common motor deficits, such as the absence of active external rotation, flexion and abduction of the shoulder, and function of the biceps should be addressed to minimize bony deformities and joint contractures.

The neonate with possible brachial plexus injury may be examined on the treatment table. Observe for spontaneous movements of the head, trunk, pelvis and limbs. Check for subtle facial palsy that may be found as a concomitant result of birth trauma. Inspect shoulders and limbs for deformities. Evaluate range of motion of every joint of the affected limb. Palpate for tissue texture changes in the upper extremities. Look for signs of shoulder instability such as a palpable or audible click during movement. Palpate for tissue texture changes in the suboccipital, neck and upper thoracic areas. The connective tissues are responsible for the maintenance of shape against both external and internal stresses.[14] Mechanical forces contribute to the development and evolution of the extracellular matrices found in the connective tissues.[15] As tissue texture changes follow trauma, osteopathic procedures should help in resetting structure and function of traumatized connective tissues.

Evaluate, through tests of listening, the function of the humerus, scapula, clavicle, sternum, upper thoracic spine, first ribs, cervical spine and craniocervical joints. This method of assessment is of particular value with this type of pathology because it is so gentle. Anatomic visualization is, as always, important. As you evaluate the patient, visualize the different layers of soft tissue: fascia superficialis, cervical fascia, costocoracoid membrane, sternocleidomastoid and scalene muscles. Evaluate and visualize the different bones involved. Listen to the inherent motions in order to define the dysfunctional area. Study the relationship between the shoulder and the vertebral column. For instance, in the case of a Klumpke's palsy, place the pad of the fingers of one hand on the spinous processes of C6, C7, T1 and T2, and place the other hand on the ipsilateral shoulder. Listen, and look for dysfunctional motion. One vertebral segment may be more dysfunctional than others. The relationship between the humerus and the shoulder should also be balanced. Treat the dysfunctions you identify by applying indirect principles.

Improvement should be rapid and most cases have a favorable prognosis. Injuries involving the fifth and sixth cervical nerve roots have the best prognosis, whereas lower plexus and total plexus injuries have a poorer prognosis. Significant deficit persisting after 3 months should be explored surgically. Prognosis is excellent if antigravity movement of biceps and shoulder abductor is present by 3 months of age. Assessment may be performed by testing the biceps' strength in a supine position while simultaneously palpating the muscle. Bicipital activity should not be confused with flexion of the elbow obtained by the action of the supinator muscle. Surgery is considered by some authors when antigravity movement of the biceps is not present by 3 months of age.[16] Surgery is considered to be justified by others when an initial involvement of the C7 nerve root is present, with a birth weight above the 90th percentile and there is only poor elbow flexion at 6 and 9 months of age.[12]

SHOULDER DYSPLASIA

The plasticity of the glenohumeral joint in the newborn makes it subject to shoulder dysplasia and, in more severe cases, dislocation. These disorders may be compared to similar disorders occurring in the hip joint – hip dysplasia and hip dislocation – and in some cases the etiology may be similar.

Intrauterine forces applied to the fetus can result in shoulder dysplasia. During the latter part of pregnancy any compression of the upper fetal torso within the uterus may affect the glenohumeral joint and the surrounding soft tissues.

Stresses during the birth process can also contribute to the development of shoulder dysplasia. Increased duration of the second stage of labor, greater than 2 hours, has been described as a factor contributing to shoulder dystocia.[17] Additionally, macrosomia that results in a size discrepancy between the fetal shoulders and the maternal pelvic inlet can, in severe cases, lead to significant neonatal morbidity including asphyxia and trauma, particularly to the brachial plexus. A large fetal trunk, or increased bisacromial diameter, prevents the rotation of the fetal shoulders into the oblique pelvic diameter during delivery.[18] As a consequence, certain obstetrical maneuvers may have to be employed to alleviate the impaction of the fetal shoulders within the maternal pelvis.[19] As stressful as such a disproportionate relationship between the fetus and the maternal pelvis can be, it does not always result in overt trauma to the brachial plexus. It can, however, cause injury to the shoulder that can lead to shoulder dysplasia. This type of injury to the shoulder can occur even from the stresses of an otherwise normal delivery.

Dysplasia of the shoulder may also result from postpartum conditions. The presence of dysfunctional asymmetries in the newborn, congenital muscular torticollis, non-synostotic plagiocephaly and brachial plexus injuries may contribute to abnormal development of the glenohumeral joint. Contractures of the muscles of internal rotation in neonatal brachial plexus palsy are responsible for posterior dislocation of the humerus from the glenoid fossa,[20–22] requiring orthopedic repair.

Physical examination and treatment

Milder cases of dysplasia without dislocation may be treated using osteopathic procedures. If untreated, these glenohumeral dysfunctions can increase with age, becoming the cause of adult scapulothoracic problems. Therefore, the scapula and the glenohumeral joint should be evaluated at birth for any signs of dysplasia, as precisely as the pelvis is evaluated. Particular attention should be directed at the identification of signs of shoulder instability, such as a palpable or audible click during movement. Observe and compare the size and shape of both shoulders. The examination may reveal asymmetry in the number of skin folds in the proximal part of the arms. Observe the freedom and range of motion of both shoulders. Note any restriction, stiffness of movement and asymmetry in movement, particularly external rotation and abduction of the arm. The malposition of the humeral head may result in an apparent difference in the length of the arms, with the arm on the side of the dysplasia appearing to be shorter. Compare the anterior and posterior aspects of the shoulders and look for any posterior fullness that may be indicative of a posteriorly displaced humeral head, necessitating orthopedic attention.

Treat any somatic dysfunction identified using indirect principles. Stabilization of the humeral head in the glenoid fossa may be facilitated when myofascial procedures are applied to the periarticular muscles of the shoulder.

NURSEMAID'S ELBOW

Nursemaid's elbow, also called pulled elbow, is a radial head subluxation that occurs in younger children when traction is applied suddenly to their hand or forearm. This commonly occurs when an adult is attempting to lift a child up by pulling upward while holding the child's hand. Traumas such as falls or when the infant initiates rolling over are other possible causes of this condition.

The head of the radius articulates with the radial notch of the ulna and the surrounding annular ligament. Under normal conditions, the annular ligament encircles the head of the radius with a certain amount of tension that maintains the contact with the radial notch. The normal movements of the head of the radius, within the ring formed by the annular ligament and the radial notch of the ulna, are anterior and posterior motion. Pronation is associated with posterior radial motion and supination with anterior radial motion.

In nursemaid's elbow a subluxation of the developing radial head from the annular ligament of the elbow joint occurs. A combination of pronation and traction on an extended elbow causes a proximal slip of the annular ligament over the top of the radial head with resultant interposition of some fibers of the anterior joint capsule between the two bones.[23]

Physical examination and treatment

The most common symptoms of nursemaid's elbow are immediate pain and an inability to move the arm. The child will have a partially flexed elbow with pronation of the forearm. Most of the time anxiety is also present.

The intention of osteopathic treatment is to restore motion between the head of the radius and the radial notch of the ulna and surrounding annular ligament. Ligamentous articular strains may be balanced utilizing indirect principles that apply perfectly to this condition. Balancing the annular ligament and the radial collateral ligament of the elbow may prevent recurrence of a posterior radial head subluxation. The caregiver should be told to avoid pulling or lifting their child by the arms or hands.

Lower extremity

A frequent complaint in an osteopathic practice is intoeing, i.e. the child's feet turn in when walking or running. Malposition of the feet, developmental dysplasia of the hip and toe walking are among the other complaints encountered with infants, while sprains are more frequently encountered with the older children and teenagers.

DYSFUNCTIONS OF THE FEET

Metatarsus adductus

Metatarsus adductus is an adduction of the forefoot that occurs in 1 : 5000 live births.[24] The classic view of it resulting from intrauterine positioning is debated, since genetic factors may contribute.[25] Sleeping in the prone position also seems to promote it. This is a frequent cause of intoeing during the first year of life and is more frequently encountered on the left side.[24] Normally, in the neutral position, the heel-bisector line drawn through the midline axis of the hindfoot passes through the forefoot at the second web space. In cases of metatarsus adductus, the line passes lateral to the third toe. Therefore, an angulation exists medially between the forefoot, or metatarsals, and the hindfoot. Sometimes a transverse crease is present on the medial side of the foot and the lateral border of the foot is convex (Fig. 7.2.2).

Metatarsus adductus associated with an inversion of the foot is named metatarsus varus and adduction of the first metatarsal is metatarsus primus varus. Metatarsus adductus is frequently associated with internal tibial torsion. Metatarsus adductus associated with retracted equinus – the inability to dorsiflex at the ankle – is indicative of a diagnosis of clubfoot.

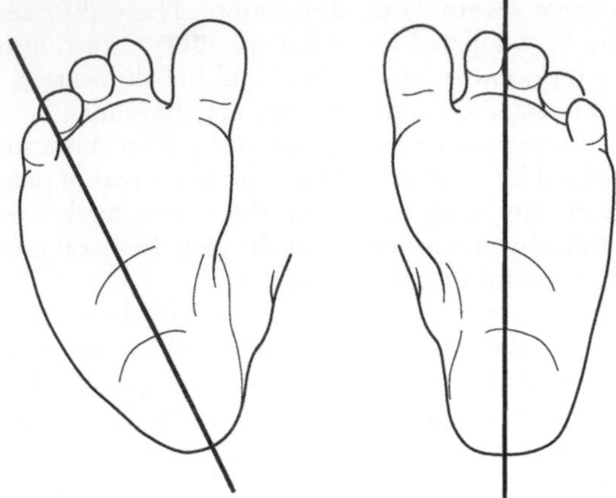

Figure 7.2.2. *Metatarsus adductus of the right foot.*

Dysfunctions of the feet might not seem grave, but left untreated they will lead to postural dysfunctions and compensatory dysfunctions of the feet, with difficulty wearing shoes and the development of bunions and hammer toes. A group of children with metatarsus varus, followed an average of 7 years, showed that 10% maintained a moderate, although asymptomatic, deformity and 4% demonstrated residual deformity and dysfunction (stiffness).[25] The opinion is that metatarsus adductus left untreated will persist into adulthood in 4–5% of cases.[26,27] Furthermore, some cases only appear to be clinically improved because of a compensatory pronation of the midtarsal joints and rearfoot.[28]

Metatarsus adductus is classified according to its flexibility. Normally, an infant should extend and abduct the foot when being tickled (e.g. with a toothbrush) along the lateral border of the foot, particularly over the fifth metatarsal head. The inability of the infant to react in such a way is indicative of metatarsus adductus. The physician should consider the total body approach and treat any dysfunctional mechanics, particularly of Lisfranc's joints (tarsometatarsal) following the principles of functional procedures. The parents should be encouraged to stimulate abduction of the forefoot, using a toothbrush or similar stimulus, as described above. In more severe cases it should be proposed that stretching exercises be practiced several times a day (e.g. at each diaper change). The calcaneus is maintained between the thumb and index finger, while the forefoot is gently pulled into a corrected position, holding the correction for 10 seconds and repeating the process about five times. It should be stressed that this exercise should be done properly, without creating a valgus of the hindfoot. If these treatments fail, and also in cases of severely rigid feet, a series of casts are used to gradually straighten out the deformity.

Congenital idiopathic talipes equinovarus (CTEV)

CTEV, or clubfoot, is a complex deformity of unknown pathogenesis with several etiologic hypotheses that range from genetic to intrauterine factors.[29] The head–body angle of the talus (declination angle) which normally increases after the 16th week of gestation has been found to be decreased in CTEV, associated with hypoplasia of the talus.[30] More recently, studies indicate that talar deformity is not the primary lesion, but follows loss of spatial orientation of the deltoid and spring ligaments and tibialis posterior tendon insertion, with contracted soft tissues.[31]

CTEV is a relatively common congenital deformity that occurs with geographical differences ranging from 0.5 : 1000 live births in Japan to 7 : 1000 in the South Pacific (1.2 : 1000 live births among Caucasians).[32] About 50% of the cases are bilateral. The male-to-female ratio for affected children is 2.5 : 1.[32,33]

Clubfoot deformity presents with different components: hindfoot equinus (inability to dorsiflex), hindfoot varus and metatarsus adductus. The flexibility of the deformity is important to determine the degree of severity. Classic treatment consists of manipulation of the foot followed by casting.[34] Generally, casting is attempted for 3 months; if unsuccessful, surgery is planned.

Osteopathic procedures should be employed as early as possible for best results. Every bone of the hindfoot – the calcaneus, talus, navicular and cuboid bones – should be evaluated and treated to release any dysfunctional relationships between them and to equilibrate the soft tissues surrounding them. The deltoid and plantar calcaneonavicular (spring) ligaments are of particular importance and should be balanced with gentle fascial release procedures.

Pes cavus

Pes cavus, or high-arched or hollow foot, should first make you think of ruling out an underlying neurologic disorder as the primary etiology. Anterior pes cavus, where both the medial and lateral longitudinal arches are high, is benign. Medial pes cavus is more severe, often with claw foot deformity of the toes. The two may be differentiated by dorsiflexing the foot. In the presence of medial pes cavus the claw foot deformity of the toes increases with dorsiflexion of the foot.

The position and range of motion of the hindfoot bones, particularly the talus, should be evaluated. Hollow foot is often associated with a flexion–external rotation pattern of the craniosacral mechanism.

You must differentiate total flat foot or total hollow foot from partially flat foot or partially hollow foot. In the latter, only the posterior portion of the longitudinal arch is involved, resulting from an imbalance of the subtalar, calcaneocuboid or cuneocuboid articulation.

Pes planus (flat feet)

A rigid pes planus is a pathologic flat foot, also named tarsal coalition, in which one or more of the tarsal bones that should have a joint between them become fused. In infants the fused joints are cartilaginous and are still relatively flexible. Thus the condition is typically not symptomatic before adolescence.

Physiologic pes planus is a loss or reduction of the longitudinal arch (Fig. 7.2.3) that can be reestablished when the child stands on their toes. Physiologic pes planus is flexible and often associated with generalized ligamentous laxity. In a sample of primary school children, 2.7% demonstrated flat feet, and being overweight was shown to increase the prevalence of the condition.[35] Because of ligamentous laxity and/or obesity, the child's ankles cave in.

The plantar calcaneonavicular ligament plays an important role in maintaining the arch of the foot (Fig. 7.2.4). It supports the head of the talus and is part of the astragalonavicular joint. Any dysfunction of the plantar calcaneonavicular ligament affects the head of the talus that tends to be displaced downward, medially and forward by the weight of the body. The tibialis posterior, an inversion muscle, lies directly below the plantar calcaneonavicular ligament and participates considerably in maintaining the longitudinal arch of the foot. In cases of dysfunction of these structures, the foot becomes flattened, expanded and turned laterally.

This condition has been suggested as a cause for tarsal tunnel syndrome.[28] It has also been suggested as contributing to back and knee problems later in life, but no evidence supports this contention. Flat feet and dysfunction of the spine are, however, very often two components of the same problem, where postural mechanics are involved. Flat foot is usually

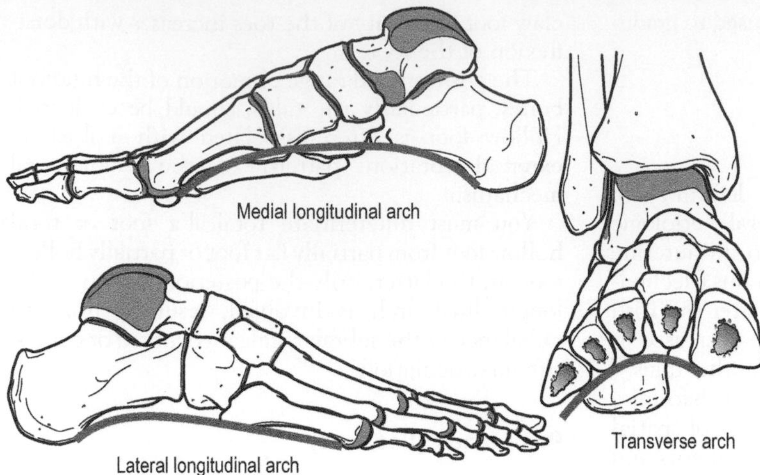

Figure 7.2.3. *Arches of the right foot.*

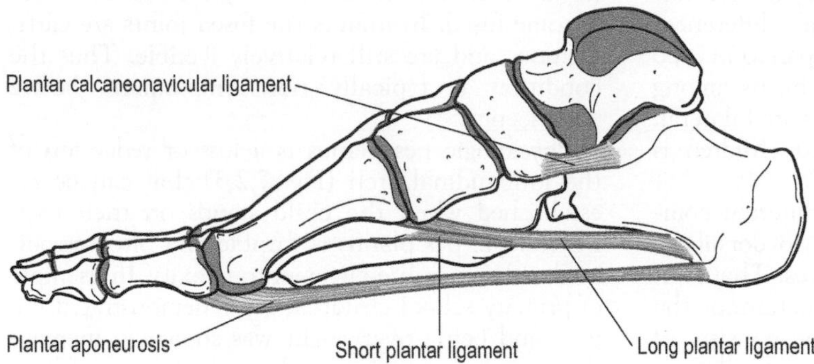

Figure 7.2.4. *Support for the arches of the foot.*

associated with an extension–internal rotation pattern of the craniosacral mechanism.

The treatment of physiologic pes planus with orthotic devices is controversial.[36] Insole arch supports diminish some of the muscular activity that maintains the arch and tend to weaken the muscles.[35] Two studies suggest an association between wearing shoes at an early age and flat feet.[37,38] This stresses the importance of allowing the feet to grow and develop without constraint. Parents should be reassured about their concerns regarding the child's appearance and gait. This condition tends to improve between 2 and 6 years of age.[39] To promote optimal growth without dysfunctional mechanics, the osteopathic practitioner should consider the global posture of the child. Check for rearfoot valgus by assessing the position and freedom of the calcaneus and talus. Check also for internal rotation dysfunction of any of the tarsal bones. Encourage the child, through their parents, to maintain a healthy lifestyle, to go barefoot as much as possible and not to become overweight. Physical activities that strengthen foot inversion, such as walking on the lateral borders of the feet or picking objects with the toes, should be recommended.

Calcaneovalgus

Positional calcaneovalgus, the result of intrauterine malposition, is a flexible dorsiflexion of the ankle with a mild subtalar joint eversion. It is frequently associated with external tibial torsion and has the appearance of flat feet. Treatment follows the principles of functional procedures to address the subtalar dysfunction.

Sprains and strains

Sprains and strains are common in the pediatric population. Young athletes are particularly vulnerable. Activities that involve jumping and landing, as in skateboarding, often result in such injuries. These

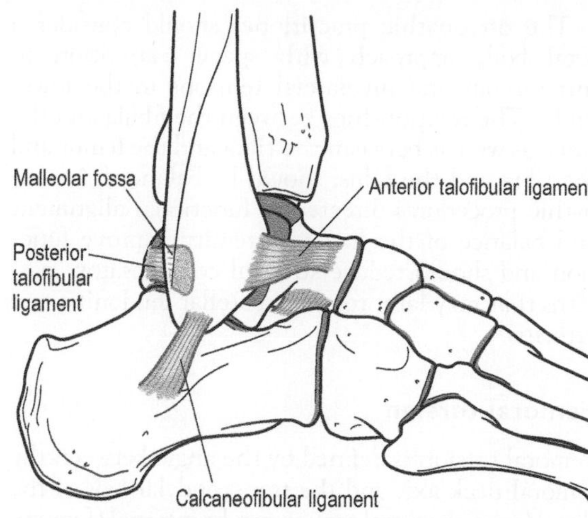

Figure 7.2.5. *Lateral view of the ankle joint.*

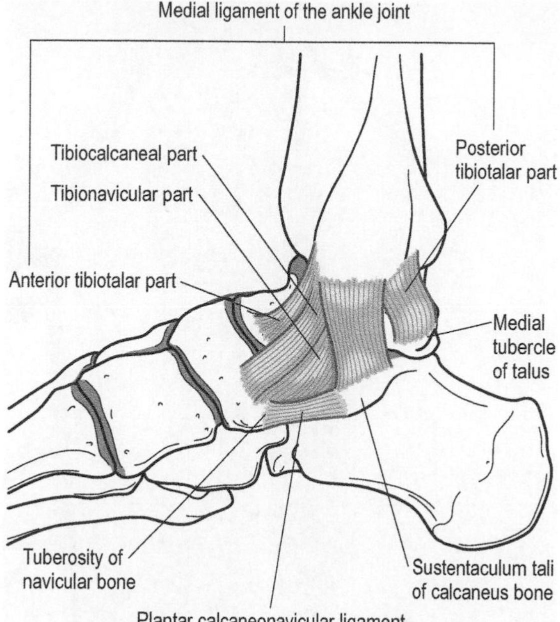

Figure 7.2.6. *Medial view of the ankle joint.*

injuries are, however, not limited to young athletes. Young children can sustain sprains and strains with activities of daily living, such as ascending or descending stairs. These injuries may be overlooked because of the child's tendency to get up and resume activity unless severely injured; however, if not properly addressed, such injuries can be the source of functional asymmetry and somatic dysfunction, often with sequelae in other anatomic areas at a later date. Following a foot or ankle sprain that causes excessive or prolonged midfoot pronation, abnormal patellofemoral mechanics may result.[40]

Traumatic twisting of the forefoot, most often inversion, commonly causes ankle injuries, often resulting in, but not limited to, sprains or strains involving the tibia, fibula and talus. It should be remembered that these stresses may also result in specific dysfunctions between the fibula and talus, the talus and calcaneus, the talus and navicular bone, and the calcaneus and cuboid, as well as dysfunctions between any of the other adjacent tarsal and metatarsal bones (Figs 7.2.5, 7.2.6).

On physical examination, the acutely injured ankle presents with pain and swelling and, with more severe injuries, ecchymosis. Ecchymosis indicates possible ligamentous tears or bony fracture necessitating radiographic evaluation. Further, if the subject is not willing to bear weight on the injured ankle, or if significant edema is present, radiographic evaluation is also appropriate to evaluate the extent of injury.[41]

Once bony fracture has been ruled out, soft tissue injuries may be treated with osteopathic manipulation by employing indirect principles. Under these circumstances, the patient should experience no aggravation of discomfort during the treatment procedure and will often feel a significant reduction of pain and swelling following the intervention. Post-treatment reduced weight bearing and avoidance of stressful activities should be recommended. Immobilization of the injured area with strapping methods should be considered for adolescents and individuals likely to be involved in weight-bearing activities. When there is no more pain for a week, a rehabilitation program can be organized to work the injured ankle in full range of motion with progressive resistance exercises. Exercises with a balance board, to strengthen proprioception, function and coordination, are also indicated. The patient places the foot on the board and first does flexion–extension movements, followed by rotation of the ankle around the ball (Fig. 7.2.7).

DYSFUNCTIONS OF THE LEGS

Tibial torsion

A thorough history and physical examination should be performed to rule out diagnoses such as cerebral palsy, which can present with rotational misalignment of the legs. Internal tibial torsion is said to be

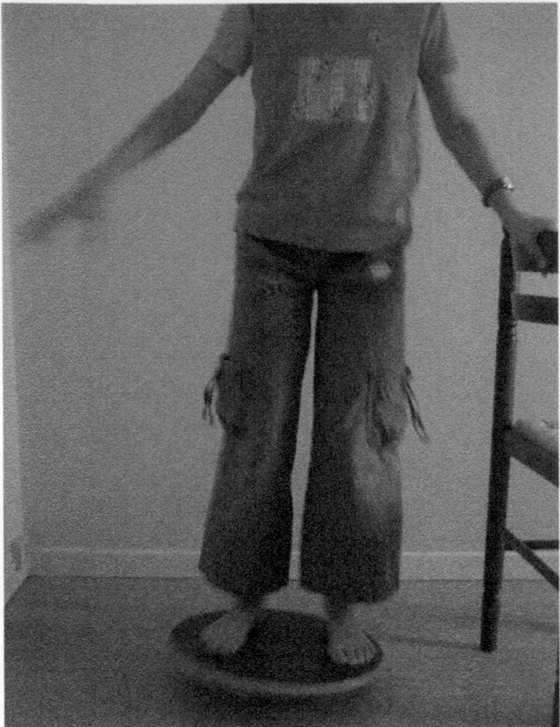

Figure 7.2.7. *Rehabilitation includes exercises with a balance board.*

the result of intrauterine positioning or from the child's habit of sitting on their feet. This is often noticed by the parents between 1 and 2 years of age and is a common cause of intoeing in children under 3 years of age. Internal tibial torsion is more often bilateral; when unilateral, the deformity most commonly affects the left side.[24] Parents complain that their child is clumsy, trips and falls easily, although intoeing in athletes has been suggested as beneficial in activities like sprinting.[42] About 90–95% of all torsional deformities resolve spontaneously by maturity.[43] When it does not resolve, however, dysfunctional rotation results in improper alignment of the lower limb and is associated with arthrosis of the hip, knee and ankle.[44]

External tibial torsion is usually diagnosed later and demonstrates a tendency to increase with age. It is associated with conditions of the extensor apparatus as unstable patellofemoral joints and Osgood–Schlatter disease.[45,46]

Examination of rotation of the tibia is best done with the child in the prone position with their knee flexed to 90°. This allows measurement of the foot–thigh angle, the angle formed between the long axes of the femur and the foot.

The osteopathic practitioner should consider a total body approach with specifi c attention to intraosseous and myofascial tensions in the lower limbs. The relationships between the fibula and the tibia, as well as between the tibia and the femur and the tibia and the talus, should be balanced. Osteopathic procedures directed at functional alignment and balance of the lower extremity improve function and should reduce stressful compensatory patterns that may later result in patellar tendonitis and arthritis.

Femoral torsion

Femoral torsion is defined by the angle between the femoral neck axis and the transcondylar axis of the distal femur. Femoral torsion can be internal (femoral anteversion) or external (femoral retroversion) and results in the knees pointing toward or away from each other, respectively. A normal femur is anteverted, i.e. the femoral head and neck are rotated anteriorly with respect to the femoral condyles. Babies have 30° of femoral anteversion. This decreases by about 1.5° per year to reach 10° in adult life.[33] Femoral anteversion is also a very common cause of intoeing in children under 3 years of age, the child being obliged to internally rotate the femurs in order to re-center the femoral heads in the acetabula. Observation of the child's gait allows one to differentiate between intoeing that is the result of internal tibial torsion as compared to femoral anteversion where the patellae are positioned more medially on the knees. The child trips and falls frequently and does not like to sit with their legs crossed, preferring to sit in a 'W' position (Fig. 7.2.8). Parents note that the child's shoes are very quickly worn out in an asymmetric pattern. Studies in adults in whom the condition remained uncorrected found a correlation between femoral anteversion and arthritis of the knee.[47]

Normally, hip range of motion shows greater amplitude in medial rotation than in lateral rotation. Abnormal femoral anteversion can be predicted (±2 SD from the mean) if the difference between medial and lateral rotation is 45° or more.[48]

The osteopathic practitioner should consider a total body approach and release intraosseous and myofascial tension in the lower limbs. The pelvis should be diagnosed and treated if necessary, as well as the coxofemoral joint. Somatic dysfunction of the innominate, particularly during periods of growth, is signifi cant because of the infl uence it can have on the position of the femur.

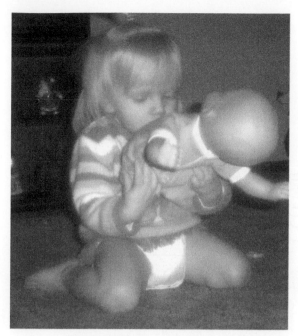

Figure 7.2.8. *Sitting in a 'W' position.*

Genu varum and genu valgum

Genu varum and genu valgum – also known as bowlegs and knock-knees, respectively – are common angular deformities of the lower extremities in children. All babies are born bowlegged. Between the ages of 2 and 3 years the bowlegging gradually decreases, and by 3 years the average child is maximally knock-kneed. The knock-kneeing straightens minimally over the next several years and, by age 7 years, most children have reached the typical adult configuration, which is slightly knock-kneed.

Persistent genu varum is better tolerated functionally than valgus, which causes stress to the medial aspect of the knee joint with the subsequent development of pain. The wider the varus or the valgus, the greater the shear stress (lateral–medial forces) on the joint.

An angular deformity is not physiologic when it is asymmetric or painful and radiographs might be necessary. Bilateral varus is associated with craniosacral flexion of the sacrum, and bilateral valgus with a sacrum in craniosacral extension. Unilateral varus problems are very often associated with flexion–external rotation patterns on the same side at the level of the pelvis, the temporal bone or the occipital bone. Similarly, unilateral valgus problems are associated with extension–internal rotation patterns of these same areas.

Using indirect procedures from a total body perspective, treatment is directed at specifically diagnosed dysfunctional mechanics. The distance between the knees (with the ankles together) of children who have varus, or between the ankles (with the knees together) of children who have valgus, can be measured to follow the response to treatment.

The knee can also present minor strains. A commonly found pattern occurs when an increased medial femoral torsion is combined with excessive lateral torsion of the tibia. This is found more often as the result of physical activities, such as in skiing, when the ski is stuck in the snow, slightly abducted, and the rest of the body moves forward. The relationship between the tibia and the femur should be balanced to address these strains.

Patellar disorders

Congenital dislocation of the patella is rare and may be isolated or associated with other limb malformations.[49] Patellar instability is not a congenital condition, although anatomic configurations such as patella alta, trochlear dysplasia and ligamentous laxity are thought to participate in the instability. MRI permits visualization of the nonosseous components of the patellofemoral articulation in the child. The cartilaginous composition of the articulation provides less restraint to lateral movement of the patella that allows instability.[40] The trilaminar soft-tissue structures[50] surrounding the patella present interconnections with the fibers of the iliotibial tract, lateral hamstrings and lateral quadriceps retinaculum. Tightness in these structures has been suggested as causing excessive posterior and lateral pull, contributing to patellar instability, especially if the medial patellofemoral ligament is injured and cannot stabilize the knee.[40] These structures are linked to the pelvic bone, and recurrent dislocation of the patella can be associated with pelvic dysfunctions that interfere with the balance transmission of weight-bearing forces.

Osgood–Schlatter disease occurs mainly in athletic adolescent boys. It is suggested that a well-developed and inelastic quadriceps creates a traction apophysitis on the tibia, with the development of loose ossicles and elongation of the patellar ligament leading to patella alta.[51] Patients with Osgood–Schlatter disease also present with increased external tibial torsion that, in association with other factors, has been suggested to predispose to the onset of the disease.[46]

The osteopathic practitioner will consider a total body approach and release the pelvis, the hips, the knees and the patellofemoral articulations (Fig. 7.2.9). Myofascial release should be considered for the thigh and patella. Gentle and pain-free stretching exercises should be done at home on a regular basis and should address tension in the quadriceps, the upper and lower iliotibial tract, the hamstrings, the hip flexors, the hip abductors, the gastrocnemius and the soleus. A long-term maintenance program

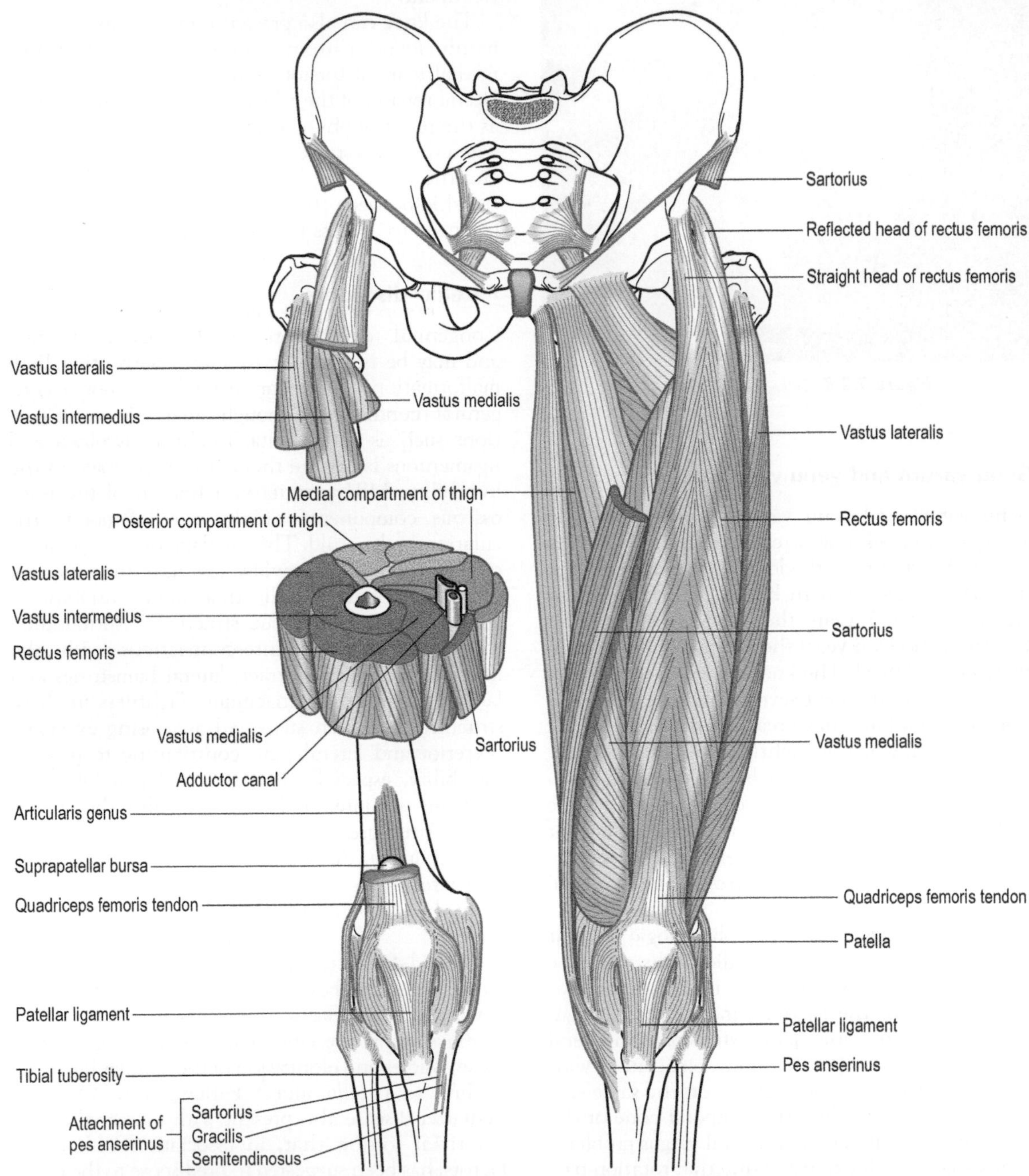

Figure 7.2.9. *Muscles of the thigh functionally and dysfunctionally uniting the pelvis and knee.*

should include strengthening in terminal knee extension in association with isometric exercises of the above muscles. Patellar knee sleeves are sometimes useful. They might have proprioceptive effects offering support. Patients feel less pain and the support provides some kind of reassurance.

DYSFUNCTIONS OF THE HIPS

Different terms describe hip dysfunctions. 'Developmental displacement of the hip' (DDH) is proposed in replacement for 'congenital dislocation of the hip' to stress the fact that the condition can occur prenatally or postnatally.[52] The different variants of the abnormalities of the hip joint include shallowness of the acetabulum and capsular laxity with resultant instability and propensity for dislocation. DDH refers to a deficient development of the acetabulum that could lead to subluxation and dislocation.

The femoral head remains well covered by the acetabulum in the early fetal period (between 6 and 20 weeks) and dislocation does not occur at this early time.[53] However, at birth, the human acetabulum is shallower than at any other time during development and is consequently vulnerable for hip instability.[54] Mechanical factors seem to play a role in neonatal hip instability. Moderate loading of the hips at 45° of flexion maintained for 3 hours has been shown to distend the articular capsule and to produce deformation and dislocation of the joint resembling that found in DDH.[55] Modifications in the pressure on the cartilaginous acetabulum are thought to interfere with normal bone growth.[56]

Uterine constraint is proposed by numerous authors as an explanation for the association between DDH and other deformations. Foot deformity,[57] congenital torticollis, congenital postural scoliosis[56,58] and plagiocephaly[59] are frequently associated with DDH. The sleeping position of the infant, with a preference to lie on one side (the 'side-lying syndrome'), has also been proposed as a contributing factor to DDH.[60]

Leg postures, associating extension and lateral rotation, critically predispose the infant to hip dislocation during fetal life and at birth. Interestingly, the newborn psoas muscle is totally relaxed in full abduction, flexion and lateral rotation. This muscle is always a lateral rotator of the hip, but exerts a much greater effect when the femur is abducted.[61] Extending the hip results in a levering action that is potentially critical if associated with other contributing factors such as acetabular or femoral anteversion and dysplasia.[62] Caution should, therefore, be exerted when moving the leg into combined extension and lateral rotation.

DDH occurs in 1 : 1000 live births and is more frequently encountered on the left side. Being female, first-born, having been carried or delivered in the breech position[57,63,64] and having a family history of acetabular dysplasia or ligamentous laxity are the main risk factors.[60]

Dislocation of the hip requires orthopedic attention. Clinical examination reveals asymmetries in the number of skin folds on the thigh and the inability to completely abduct the thigh when the knee and hip are flexed. The malposition of the femoral head may cause the leg on that side to look shorter than the other.

Barlow and Ortolani positive tests confirm the diagnosis and are performed with the child supine on a flat pad, placing the fingers on the baby's greater trochanters and the thumbs on the inside of the lower portion of the thighs and knees. The hips and knees are flexed to 90°. The Barlow test consists of adducting the legs and pushing down gently on the knees in an attempt to disengage the femoral head from the acetabulum. A 'clunk' will be felt as the femoral head dislocates. The Ortolani test relocates a dislocated hip and is performed by slowly abducting the thighs while maintaining axial pressure. The fingers on the greater trochanter exert a movement in the opposite direction to assist the return of the femoral head to the acetabulum. The examiner will again feel, and hear, a 'clunk.' Diagnostic ultrasonography may be carried out after 4–6 weeks and radiographs after 4–6 months; before these ages there is insufficient ossification for the tests to be diagnostic.

Different methods of treatment are proposed for DDH, with good results. Abduction devices (Pavlik harness) and traction followed by plaster immobilization are always done with special care because of the risk of aseptic necrosis of the femoral head. A program of home abduction–adduction exercises administered by the parents has been successful in infants with limited abduction and acetabular dysplasia without dislocation.[57]

Developmental dysplasia of the hip – insufficient depth of the acetabulum to accommodate the femoral head – in the infant can be associated with pelvic imbalance, such as intraosseous dysfunction of the innominates and sacrum, coxofemoral dysfunctions and eventually with craniosacral dysfunctions. The innominate bone needs to be in a neutral position in order to provide a satisfactory acetabular placement.

An internally rotated innominate results in a higher position of the acetabulum, leading to an apparently shorter leg on that side. This can be confused with the apparent inequity of leg length found in association with hip dislocation.

Osteopathic procedures attempt to balance the craniosacral mechanism of these children. The relationship between the sacrum and the occiput, the temporal bones and the innominates should be balanced.

Special care is given to myofascial structures responsible for pelvic tensions or pelvic asymmetry. Myofascial procedures should be applied to the periarticular muscles of the hip, in particular the iliopsoas, the adductors and the abductors, to release contracture of the joint and improve restrictions of motion in adduction or abduction.

The treatment of dysplasia is intended to stabilize the femoral head in the acetabulum and to allow the growth of a symmetric pelvis with a balanced sacrum, innominates and hips. Dysfunctional interosseous relationships between the sacrum and the innominates, and between the innominates and the femurs, should be identified and treated. Any dysfunctional intraosseous relationship between the ilium, ischium and pubes should be also balanced, and, if present, intraosseous dysfunction of the sacrum treated.

Clinical examination of these children should be repeated during the 1st year, with an annual follow-up, until full skeletal maturity. Dysplasia may result in early development of osteoarthritis of the hip.[65–68] Treatment should be directed at promotion of function and prevention of future degenerative changes.

GAIT DISORDERS

Toewalking

By the age of 4 years children should be walking with a heel–toe gait. After this age, toewalking is abnormal and can be due to an underlying neurologic disorder. A tight Achilles tendon may be present, but in other cases nothing will be found. Look for any extension dysfunction of the craniosacral mechanism. Balance the sacrum and the craniocervical junction. Release the posterior myofascial components of the spine and inferior limbs. Teach the child to walk heel–toe.

The child with a limp

Because serious medical and orthopedic conditions may be responsible for limping, any such underlying pathology should be ruled out before using manipulation as a primary treatment. For example, a limp or a waddling gait between the ages of 2 and 6 years might be associated with a congenital coxa vara, where the angle between the femoral neck and the femoral shaft is less than normal (<130°). Coxa valga is an increase in that angle (>135°) and, in this case, the child may present with increased internal rotation and adduction of the hips.

Observation of the child while walking allows one to determine what area is dysfunctional. It is better to have the child bare legged to best visualize the different components of the lower extremity. Observe the foot angle, the direction in which the child's feet point when they walk. Observe for tibial and femoral torsions and the movements of the hips. Determine which part is not following the global movement of the limb or if one side does not contact the floor in the same fashion.

The postural balance should be evaluated and any dysfunctional asymmetries treated. An asymmetry of leg length might be present as the cumulative result of several dysfunctions. For example, an innominate in external rotation on the right side, combined with an innominate in internal rotation on the left side, will give the appearance of a longer leg on the right side. Evaluate the range of motion of the different joints of the lower limbs and, utilizing appropriate manipulative procedures, treat any dysfunction identified.

REFERENCES

1. Kaplan B, Rabinerson D, Avrech OM, Carmi N, Steinberg DM, Merlob P. Fracture of the clavicle in the newborn following normal labor and delivery. Int J Gynaecol Obstet 1998;63(1):15–20.
2. Lam MH, Wong GY, Lao TT. Reappraisal of neonatal clavicular fracture: relationship between infant size and neonatal morbidity. Obstet Gynecol 2002;100(1):115–9.
3. McBride MT, Hennrikus WL, Mologne TS. Newborn clavicle fractures. Orthopedics 1998;21(3):317–9; discussion 319–20.
4. Oppenheim WL, Davis A, Growdon WA, Dorey FJ, Davlin LB. Clavicle fractures in the newborn. Clin Orthop Relat Res 1990;250:176–80.
5. Uhing MR. Management of birth injuries. Pediatr Clin North Am 2004;51(4):1169–86, xii.
6. Gilbert WM, Nesbitt TS, Danielsen B. Associated factors in 1611 cases of brachial plexus injury. Obstet Gynecol 1999; 93(4):536–40.
7. Gardella C, Taylor M, Benedetti T, Hitti J, Critchlow C. The effect of sequential use of vacuum and forceps for assisted vaginal delivery on neonatal and maternal outcomes. Am J Obstet Gynecol 2001;185(4):896–902.
8. Chauhan SP, Rose CH, Gherman RB, Magann EF, Holland MW, Morrison JC. Brachial plexus injury: a 23-year experience from a tertiary center. Am J Obstet Gynecol 2005; 192(6):1795–800; discussion 1800–2.

9. Alfonso I, Papazian O, Shuhaiber H, Yaylali I, Grossman JA. Intrauterine shoulder weakness and obstetric brachial plexus palsy. Pediatr Neurol 2004;31(3):225–7.
10. Hughes CA, Harley EH, Milmoe G, Bala R, Martorella A. Birth trauma in the head and neck. Arch Otolaryngol Head Neck Surg 1999;125(2):193–9.
11. Sunderland S. Mechanisms of cervical nerve root avulsion in injuries of the neck and shoulder. J Neurosurg 1974;41(6): 705–14.
12. Nehme A, Kany J, Sales-De-Gauzy J, Charlet JP, Dautel G, Cahuzac JP. Obstetrical brachial plexus palsy. Prediction of outcome in upper root injuries. J Hand Surg [Br] 2002; 27(1):9–12.
13. Shenaq SM, Bullocks JM, Dhillon G, Lee RT, Laurent JP. Management of infant brachial plexus injuries. Clin Plast Surg 2005;32(1):79–98, ix.
14. Scott JE. Supramolecular organization of extracellular matrix glycosaminoglycans, in vitro and in the tissues. FASEB J 1992;6(9):2639–45.
15. Silver FH, DeVore D, Siperko LM. Invited Review: Role of mechanophysiology in aging of ECM: effects of changes in mechanochemical transduction. J Appl Physiol 2003;95(5): 2134–41.
16. Gilbert A. Paralysie obstétricale du membre supérieur. Encycl Méd Chir (Editions Scientifiques et Médicales, Elsevier SAS, Paris), Pédiatrie 2000;4–002-R-05.
17. Mehta SH, Bujold E, Blackwell SC, Sorokin Y, Sokol RJ. Is abnormal labor associated with shoulder dystocia in nulliparous women? Am J Obstet Gynecol 2004;190(6):1604–7; discussion 1607–9.
18. Gherman RB. Shoulder dystocia: prevention and management. Obstet Gynecol Clin North Am 2005;32(2):297–305, x.
19. Gurewitsch ED, Kim EJ, Yang JH, Outland KE, McDonald MK, Allen RH. Comparing McRoberts' and Rubin's maneuvers for initial management of shoulder dystocia: an objective evaluation. Am J Obstet Gynecol 2005;192(1): 153–60.
20. Pearl ML, Edgerton BW. Glenoid deformity secondary to brachial plexus birth palsy. J Bone Joint Surg 1998;80A(5): 659–67.
21. Waters PM, Smith GR, Jaramillo D. Glenohumeral deformity secondary to brachial plexus birth palsy. J Bone Joint Surg 1998;80(5):668–77.
22. Moukoko D, Ezaki M, Wilkes D, Carter P. Posterior shoulder dislocation in infants with neonatal brachial plexus palsy. J Bone Joint Surg 2004;86A(4):787–93.
23. Bretland PM. Pulled elbow in childhood. Br J Radiol 1994; 67(804):1176–85.
24. Lincoln TL, Suen PW. Common rotational variations in children. J Am Acad Orthop Surg 2003;11(5):312–20.
25. Rushforth GF. The natural history of hooked forefoot. J Bone Joint Surg 1978;60B(4):530–2.
26. Dietz FR. Intoeing – fact, fiction and opinion. Am Fam Physician 1994;50(6):1249–59, 1262–4.
27. Widhe T. Foot deformities at birth: a longitudinal prospective study over a 16 year period. J Pediatr Orthop 1997; 17(1):20–4.
28. Connors JF, Wernick E, Lowy LJ, Falcone J, Volpe RG. Guidelines for evaluation and management of five common podopediatric conditions. J Am Podiatr Med Assoc 1998; 88(5):206–22.
29. Gore AI, Spencer JP. The newborn foot. Am Fam Physician 2004;69(4):865–72.
30. Waisbrod H. Congenital club foot. An anatomical study. J Bone Joint Surg 1973;55B(4):796–801.
31. Fukuhara K, Schollmeier G, Uhthoff HK. The pathogenesis of club foot. A histomorphometric and immunohistochemical study of fetuses. J Bone Joint Surg 1994;76B(3): 450–7.
32. Roye BD, Hyman J, Roye DP Jr. Congenital idiopathic talipes equinovarus. Pediatr Rev 2004;25(4):124–30.
33. Scherl SA. Common lower extremity problems in children. Pediatr Rev 2004;25(2):52–62.
34. Ponseti IV. The Ponseti technique for correction of congenital clubfoot. J Bone Joint Surg 2002;84A(10):1889–90; author reply 1890–1.
35. Garcia-Rodriguez A, Martin-Jimenez F, Carnero-Varo M, Gomez-Gracia E, Gomez-Aracena J, Fernandez-Crehuet J. Flexible flat feet in children: a real problem? Pediatrics 1999;103(6):e84.
36. Staheli LT. Planovalgus foot deformity. Current status. J Am Podiatr Med Assoc 1999;89(2):94–9.
37. Rao UB, Joseph B. The influence of footwear on the prevalence of flat foot. A survey of 2300 children. J Bone Joint Surg 1992;74B(4):525–7.
38. Sachithanandam V, Joseph B. The influence of footwear on the prevalence of flat foot. A survey of 1846 skeletally mature persons. J Bone Joint Surg 1995;77B(2):254–7.
39. Volpon JB. Footprint analysis during the growth period. J Pediatr Orthop 1994;14(1):83–5.
40. Hinton RY, Sharma KM. Acute and recurrent patellar instability in the young athlete. Orthop Clin North Am 2003;34(3):385–96.
41. Sujitkumar P, Hadfield JM, Yates DW. Sprain or fracture? An analysis of 2000 ankle injuries. Arch Emerg Med 1986; 3:101–6.
42. Fuchs R, Staheli LT. Sprinting and intoeing. J Pediatr Orthop 1996;16(4):489–91.
43. Bruce RW Jr. Torsional and angular deformities. Pediatr Clin North Am 1996;43(4):867–81.
44. Eckhoff DG. Effect of limb malrotation on malalignment and osteoarthritis. Orthop Clin North Am 1994;25(3): 405–14.
45. Turner MS, Smillie IS. The effect of tibial torsion of the pathology of the knee. J Bone Joint Surg 1981;63B(3): 396–8.
46. Gigante A, Bevilacqua C, Bonetti MG, Greco F. Increased external tibial torsion in Osgood–Schlatter disease. Acta Orthop Scand 2003;74(4):431–6.
47. Eckhoff DG, Kramer RC, Alongi CA, VanGerven DP. Femoral anteversion and arthritis of the knee. J Pediatr Orthop 1994;14(5):608–10.
48. Kozic S, Gulan G, Matovinovic D, Nemec B, Sestan B, Ravlic-Gulan J. Femoral anteversion related to side differences in hip rotation. Passive rotation in 1140 children aged 8–9 years. Acta Orthop Scand 1997;68(6):533–6.
49. Ghanem I, Wattincourt L, Seringe R. Congenital dislocation of the patella. Part I: pathologic anatomy. J Pediatr Orthop 2000;20(6):812–6.
50. Dye SF, Campagna-Pinto D, Dye CC, Shifflett S, Eiman T. Soft-tissue anatomy anterior to the human patella. J Bone Joint Surg 2003;85A(6):1012–7.
51. Jakob RP, von Gumppenberg S, Engelhardt P. Does Osgood–Schlatter disease influence the position of the patella? J Bone Joint Surg 1981;63B(4):579–82.
52. Klisic PJ. Congenital dislocation of the hip – a misleading term: brief report. J Bone Joint Surg 1989;71B(1):136.
53. Lee J, Jarvis J, Uhthoff HK, Avruch L. The fetal acetabulum. A histomorphometric study of acetabular anteversion and femoral head coverage. Clin Orthop Relat Res 1992;281: 48–55.

54. Ralis Z, McKibbin B. Changes in shape of the human hip joint during its development and their relation to its stability. J Bone Joint Surg 1973;55B(4):780–5.
55. Hjelmstedt A, Asplund S. Congenital dislocation of the hip: a biomechanical study in autopsy specimens. J Pediatr Orthop 1983;3(4):491–7.
56. Chapple CC, Davidson DT. A study of the relationship between fetal position and certain congenital deformities. J Pediatr 1941;18:483–93.
57. Heikkila E, Ryoppy S, Louhimo I. The management of primary acetabular dysplasia. Its association with habitual side-lying. J Bone Joint Surg 1985;67(1):25–8.
58. Dunn PM. Congenital postural deformities. Br Med Bull 1976;32(1):71–6.
59. Hooper G. Congenital dislocation of the hip in infantile idiopathic scoliosis. J Bone Joint Surg 1980;62B(4): 447–9.
60. Wynne-Davies R. Acetabular dysplasia and familial joint laxity: two etiological factors in congenital dislocation of the hip. A review of 589 patients and their families. J Bone Joint Surg 1970;52(4):704–16.
61. McKibbin B. The action of the iliopsoas muscle in the newborn. J Bone Joint Surg 1968;50B(1):161–5.
62. McKibbin B. Anatomical factors in the stability of the hip joint in the newborn. J Bone Joint Surg 1970;52B(1):148–59.
63. James JI. Congenital dislocation of the hip. J Bone Joint Surg 1972;54B(1):1–3.
64. Hsieh YY, Tsai FJ, Lin CC, Chang FC, Tsai CH. Breech deformation complex in neonates. J Reprod Med 2000; 45(11):933–5.
65. Lloyd-Roberts GC. Osteoarthritis of the hip: a study of the clinical pathology. J Bone Joint Surg 1955;37B:8–47.
66. Klaue K, Durnin CW, Ganz R. The acetabular rim syndrome. A clinical presentation of dysplasia of the hip. J Bone Joint Surg 1991;73B(3):423–9.
67. Chitnavis J, Sinsheimer JS, Suchard MA, Clipsham K, Carr AJ. End-stage coxarthrosis and gonarthrosis. Aetiology. Rheumatology (Oxford) 2000;39(6):612–9.
68. Birrell F, Silman A, Croft P, Cooper C, Hosie G, Macfarlane G; PCR Hip Study Group. Syndrome of symptomatic adult acetabular dysplasia (SAAD syndrome). Ann Rheum Dis 2003;62(4):356–8.

7.3 EARS, NOSE AND THROAT

OTITIS MEDIA

Otitis media (OM) is among the most common of illnesses affecting preschool children.[1] Almost every child experiences OM at least once before their third birthday[2] and 20% of children experience recurrent OM.[3] Its prevalence has increased considerably recently, resulting in an enormous economic burden to society.[4] Clinical classifications include acute otitis media (AOM) and chronic otitis media with effusion (COME).

AOM is a viral or bacterial infection, commonly secondary to an upper respiratory infection and usually occurring in young children from the age 3 months to 3 years. It presents with a sudden inflammation in the middle ear, fever, pain and irritability. An incomplete resolution of AOM or an obstruction of the pharyngotympanic tube (PT), also called the Eustachian or auditory tube, may lead to an effusion in the middle ear containing common pathogenic bacteria. Repeated episodes of acute symptoms are considered to be recurrent AOM.

COME is a chronic inflammation of the middle ear mucosa, with the retention of fluid within the middle ear space that lasts more than 3 months. It is a condition wherein irreversible changes have occurred, affecting the tympanic membrane, the PT or the middle ear.

The multitude of studies attempting to identify the causative factors of OM have provided multiple, and often opposite, results. This is probably because the etiology of individual cases of OM is often multifactorial, including genetic, environmental, nutritional and behavioral factors. Thus, the number of variables necessary for consideration makes such studies extremely difficult. The following have, however, been identified as risk factors for the onset of OM: genetic predisposition,[5,6] low birth weight,[7] male gender,[8] number of siblings,[9] day-care attendance,[10] not being breastfed,[1] use of a pacifier,[11,12] season of the year,[10,13] passive exposure to smoking[14] and low socioeconomic status.[15] On the other hand, breastfeeding, even for periods as short as 3 months, has been shown to reduce the incidence of OM in childhood.[16]

Anatomic factors should also be considered. The ear, particularly the middle ear, and adjacent structures provide a site where genetic, environmental, nutritional and behavioral factors can interact, resulting in the development of OM. The three parts of the ear – external, middle and internal (Fig. 7.3.1) – are related anatomically and functionally to the temporal bone. The external ear consists of the auricle (pinna) and external acoustic meatus. The auricle on the lateral aspect of the head, at the level of the temporal bone, reflects the global position of the temporal bone. A protruding auricle, for example, are often associated with external rotation of the homolateral temporal bone. The auricle functions to collect sound waves. The external acoustic meatus

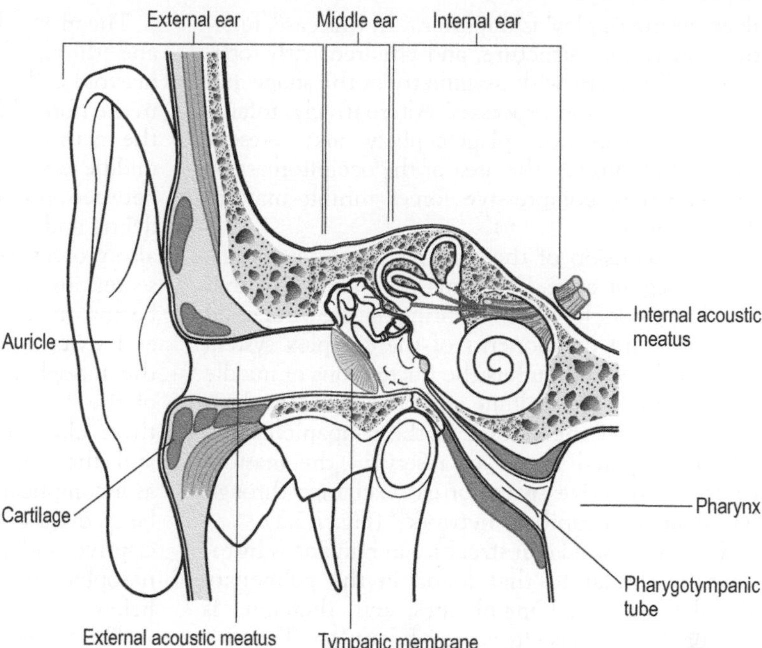

Figure 7.3.1. *Ear.*

terminates in the tympanic membrane. Its lateral part is membranous, continuous with the auricle. The medial part is surrounded by the squamous portion of the temporal bone above and the tympanic portion in front and below.

The middle ear or tympanic cavity, an air-filled space, is located between the tympanic membrane laterally and the lateral wall of the internal ear medially. It contains three bones, or ossicles – the malleus, incus and stapes – that transmit vibrations from the tympanic membrane to the cochlea of the internal ear. The tympanic cavity is open posteriorly to the mastoid antrum, an air sinus located in the petrous portion of the temporal bone, and to the interconnected mastoid air cells. Anteriorly, the tympanic cavity communicates with the nasopharynx through the PT. A mucosa covers the complete cavity, including its contents, the three ossicles and the two muscles (tensor tympani and stapedius), and forms the inner layer of the tympanic membrane. This mucosa is in continuity with that of the pharynx. The mastoid cavity, mastoid antrum and auditory ossicles are nearly completely developed at birth.

The internal ear consists of several bony cavities, the vestibule, the semicircular canals and the cochlea that form the bony labyrinth. It contains the membranous labyrinth with the organ of hearing (the cochlear duct) and the organs of balance (the semicircular ducts). The membranous labyrinth floats in the perilymph, the fluid filling the bony labyrinth. The structures that form the internal ear are also nearly completely developed at birth.

Most of the above structures of the ear can be found nesting within the petrous portion of the temporal bone. In diseases of the ear such as OM, as well as in balance and hearing disorders, this anatomic relationship confers great significance on the temporal bone and its function and dysfunction.

The temporal bone is formed by the squamous, petromastoid, tympanic and styloid parts. The petromastoid part develops in the cartilaginous otic capsule of the cranial base. The squamous and the tympanic portions are ossified from mesenchyme. The tympanic portion (the tympanic ring) unites with the squama just before birth.[17] Total fusion of the temporal bone, except the distal part of the styloid, is complete by the end of the 1st year. Nevertheless, the mastoid portion is completely flat at birth. The mastoid process, a postnatal petrous development, begins to develop with the growth of the mastoid air cells and because of the traction from the tendon of the sternocleidomastoid (SCM) muscle. The development of the mastoid process is dependent on the child's ability to lift their head (extend their cervical spine) and to rotate their cervical spine symmetrically. For this reason the prone position, recommended in the statement 'back to sleep, prone to play' is important. In this case, function determines structure, and children with torticollis will present with asymmetry in the shape and size of the mastoid processes. Alternatively, infants with non-synostotic plagiocephaly may present with a flattening in the area of the occipitomastoid suture, where compressive forces inhibit mastoid development.

The expansion of the mastoid process is of particular signifi ance. The mastoid air cells that develop inside the mastoid during the growth period are important components of the complex system that regulates and buffers the fluctuations of middle ear pressure.[18] The volume of the mastoid air cells is about 20 times the volume of the tympanic cavity. Often compared to an air reservoir, the mastoid cavity is an active space for gas exchange through its submucosal capillary network[19] (Fig. 7.3.2).

The submastoid cell structure in humans is histologically similar to that found in the pulmonary alveolar and nasal membranes, and, therefore, is suitable for gaseous effusion and diffusion. The production of gas within the tympanomastoid cavity keeps the internal pressure at the same level, or higher, than atmospheric pressure.[20] Swallowing allows gas to be expelled through the PT into the pharynx. This positive pressure gradient prevents bacteria from entering the tympanomastoid cavity.[20] The depth of the mastoid air cell system has been found to be shorter in children with secretory OM compared with healthy individuals.[21] Decreased mastoid pneumatization has been proposed as a prognostic indicator for chronic inflammation of the middle ear, as has poor outcome with OM when the mastoid is poorly pneumatized.[22]

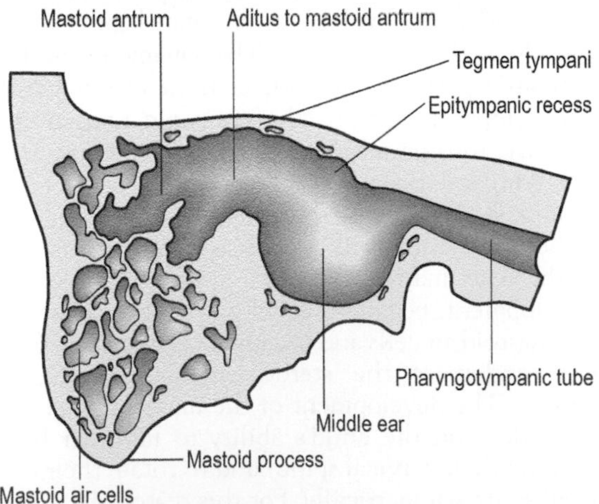

Figure 7.3.2. *Mastoid antrum.*

The mastoid cells connect to the tympanic cavity and through the PT to the nasopharynx. Both mastoid cells and PT are of paramount importance in the normal function of the ear and, consequently, the pathogenesis of OM. The PT connects the middle ear to the nasopharynx, balances pressure between the middle ear and ambient air, clears debris and secretions toward the nasopharynx and also protects the middle ear against nasopharyngeal secretions and noxious agents from the airways. It begins on the anterior wall of the tympanic cavity and extends forward, medially and downward to the nasopharynx posterior to the inferior meatus of the nasal cavity (Figs 7.3.3, 7.3.4). Because of these close relationships between the middle ear and the nasopharynx, OM, frequently described as a complication of rhinitis, may be considered to be a disease of the upper respiratory tract. Descriptive and functional anatomy of the nose and nasopharynx is discussed in 'Rhinitis' and 'Sinusitis' below.

The PT is shaped like two cones joined together at their apices. The posterolateral cone, shorter, approximately one-third of the PT, is osseous (protympanum), located inside the petrous temporal bone. It ends at the junction of the petrous and squamous parts of the temporal bone, immediately posterior to the foramen spinosum. The remaining two-thirds of the PT are fibrocartilaginous, partially fi xed to the cranial base, in a furrow following the sphenopetrosal synchondrosis, between the petrous portion of the temporal bone and the posterior border of the greater wing of the sphenoid. The upper border of the cartilaginous PT is arched laterally and looks like a hook on transverse section. A fi brous membrane completes the tube. The tubal isthmus, where the PT diameter is smallest, joins the two cones of the PT. The cartilaginous portion has a greater vertical inclination than the osseous portion.

The length of the PT in the adult is approximately 35–45 mm. The PT in the newborn is approximately half its adult length and reaches approximately 98% of its adult length by 7 years of age. The ratio of the length of the cartilaginous and junctional portions of the PT to the length of the bony portion is 8:1 in infants and 4:1 in adults.[23] The PT in infants is not only shorter, it is also more horizontal, and, therefore, the clearance function is less effective. Additionally, when the bony portion of the PT of children with secretory OM is compared to that of healthy children, it is found to be even shorter.[21]

The PT connecting the middle ear and nasopharynx has been compared to the bronchial tree

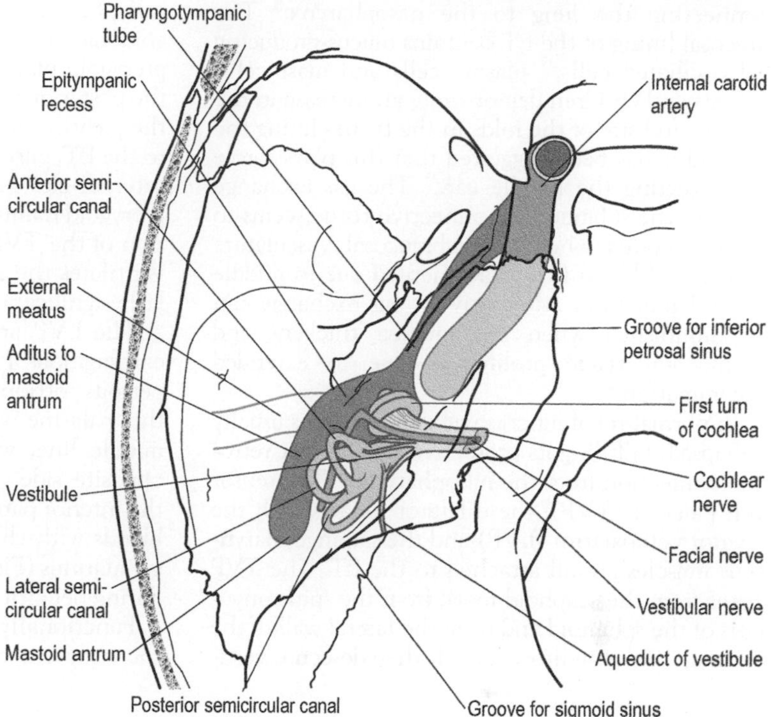

Figure 7.3.3. *Pharyngotympanic tube.*

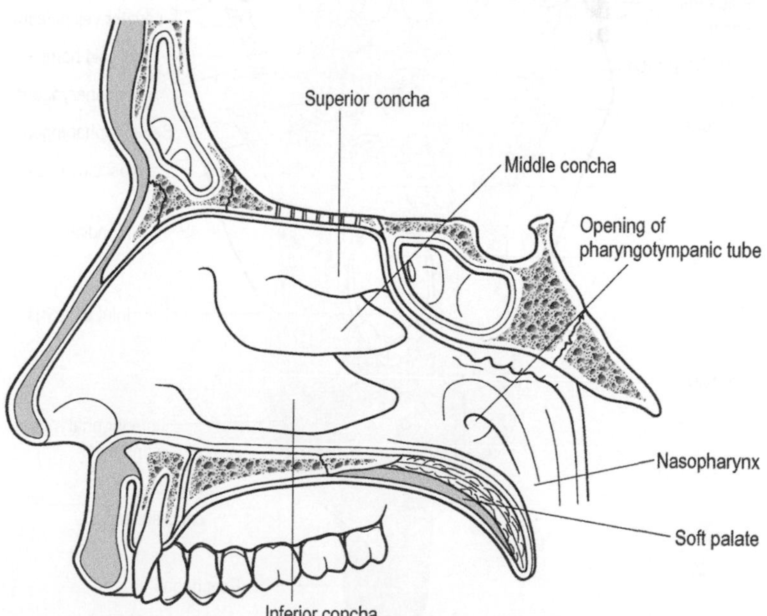

Figure 7.3.4. *Opening of the pharyngotympanic tube in the nasopharynx.*

connecting the lung to the nasopharynx.[8] The mucosal lining of the PT contains mucus-producing cells, ciliated cells,[24] plasma cells and mast cells. Infants and children demonstrate an increase in the density and size of the folds in the tissues lining the PT and it has been suggested that this plays a role in protecting the middle ear.[25] The gas exchange through the submucosal connective tissue seems to be accelerated when the submucosal vasculature dilates and blood flow is augmented due to middle ear inflammation. Alternatively, gas exchange can be diminished when the mucosa thickens and submucosal tissue proliferates due to extended inflammation.[26]

In normal tubal function at rest, the PT is usually collapsed, fulfilling its protective role against retrograde infection from the nasopharynx.[27] The tensor veli palatini (TVP), the dilatator tubae (DT), the levator veli palatini (LVP) and the salpingopharyngeus muscles are all attached to the PT. The TVP arises from the scaphoid fossa, from the spina angularis of the sphenoid and from the lateral wall of the cartilage of the auditory tube. It then descends vertically, becomes tendinous and inserts onto the pterygoid hamulus, the lower extremity of the medial pterygoid plate of the sphenoid, and medially onto the posterior border of the hard palate to form part of the palatine aponeurosis. The DT is attached above to the PT, particularly to its membranous portion. It intermingles below with the TVP and rounds the pterygoid hamulus. Most authors agree that contraction of the TVP opens the PT lumen and therefore ventilates the middle ear;[24,28] this action is particularly significant for the fibers of the DT.[29]

The LVP arises from the medial lamina of the cartilaginous PT and from under the apex of the petrous portion of the temporal bone. It extends into the palatine velum, its fibers broadening to the middle line, where they blend with those of the opposite side. The salpingopharyngeus arises from the inferior part of the PT, is directed downward and blends with the posterior fasciculus of the pharyngopalatinus (Fig. 7.3.5). It contributes to PT opening during deglutition.

Functionally, the PT allows air to enter or exit the tympanic cavity during activities that normally

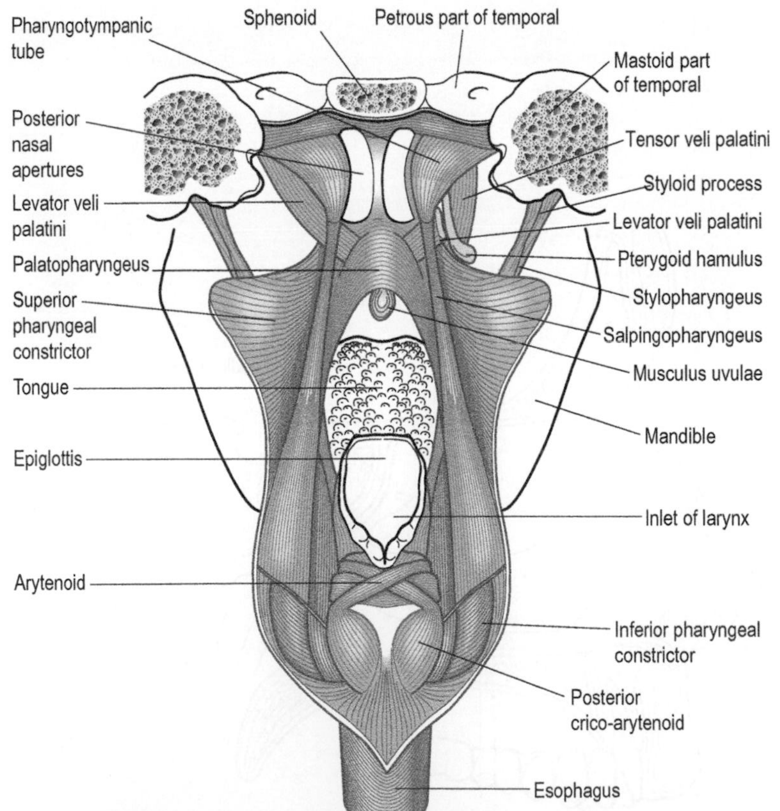

Figure 7.3.5. *Muscles of the palate.*

open it – for example, swallowing, crying or yawning. This balances the pressure gradient between the atmosphere and the tympanic cavity. When the mechanism of swallowing is dysfunctional, opening of the PT is not efficient. Sustained collapse follows with the development of negative middle ear pressure and retraction of the tympanic membrane. The subsequent potential for aspiration of nasopharyngeal secretions into the middle ear may result in OM. Furthermore, dysfunctional swallowing may also cause gastroesophageal refl ux, another risk factor for OM. In addition, if present, the frequent use of a pacifier may encourage infantile deglutition, i.e. forward tongue thrust when swallowing. Although the use of a pacifier does not increase the incidence of respiratory infections, there is evidence that constant use affects the occurrence of AOM, possibly because of alteration in the pressure equilibrating function of the PT.[12]

Dysfunction of the PT may result in negative middle ear pressure that, in turn, impairs auditory sound conduction to the cochlea of the internal ear affecting hearing. PT dysfunction can also affect hearing through its impact on the tensor tympani muscle. The tensor tympani muscle is continuous with the TVP. It arises from the cartilaginous portion of the PT and the adjoining sphenoid, and inserts on the manubrium of the malleus.[24,29] Tensor tympani contraction draws the malleus medially, increasing tympanic membrane tension while pushing the incus and stapes medially against the fenestra vestibuli. This results in an increased intravestibular pressure that, under normal circumstances, serves to dampen violent noises. Consequently, dysfunction of the PT may be associated with both negative middle ear pressure and spasm of the tensor tympani with resultant disturbance of hearing.

Anatomic developmental delays such as immaturities of the PT and surrounding structures or of the neuromuscular system may result in dysfunctional opening of the PT in infants and children.[30] Most of the time, the dysfunctional opening of the PT improves with age as the base of the neurocranium and the viscerocranium develop. This too, however, can contribute to the complex interaction of phenomena that predispose the child to develop OM.

The base of the skull (Figs 7.3.6, 7.3.7) goes through signifi cant developmental changes during the fi rst years of life. Two critical phenomena participate in this development. First, the diverse stimulation produced by normal orofacial functions, such as suckling and swallowing, spurs the growth of structures, particularly the pterygoid processes in which the involved muscles insert. Secondly, but concomitant with the above, the progressive flexion of the cranial base, associated with the anteroposterior growth of the skull, contributes to positional changes of both the pterygoid processes, which become longer and more vertical, and the petrous portions of the temporal bones, which become externally rotated. Additionally, several changes occur in the viscerocranium, such as the increase in

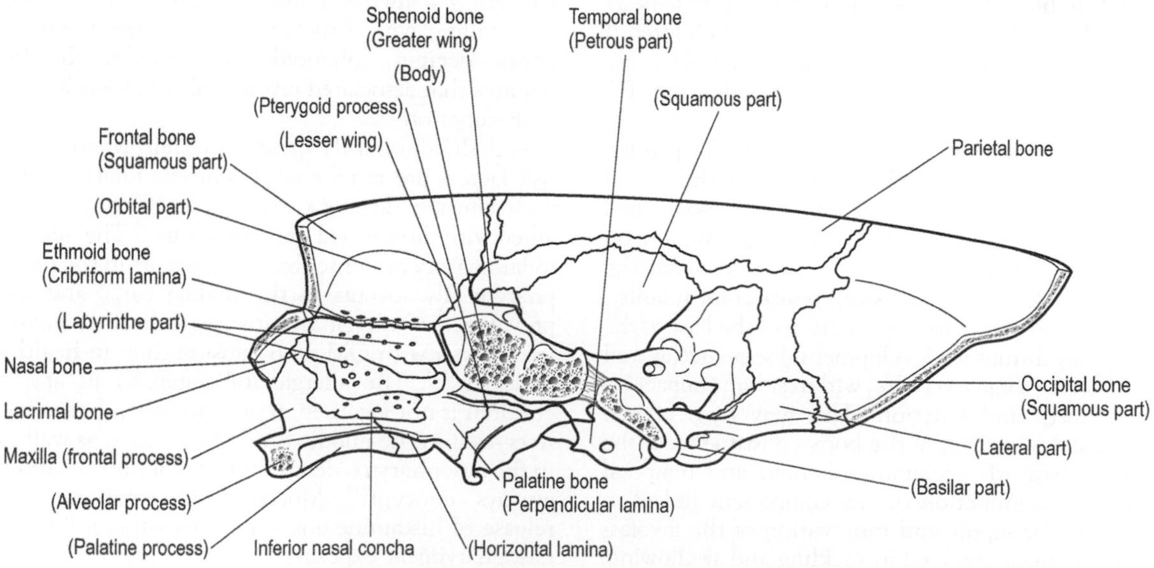

Figure 7.3.6. *Sagittal section of the cranial base at birth.*

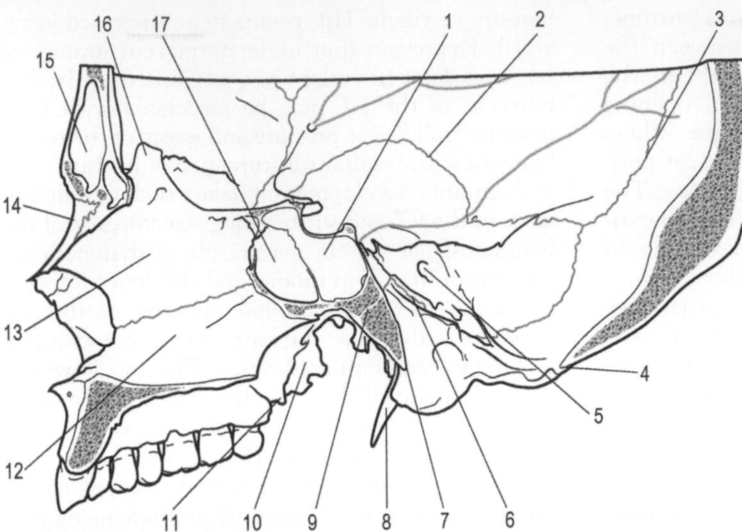

Figure 7.3.7. *Sagittal section of the cranial base in the adult. 1. Right sphenoidal sinus; 2. squamosal suture; 3. lambdoid suture; 4. posterior margin of foramen magnum; 5. internal acoustic meatus; 6. petro-occipital suture; 7. anterior margin of foramen magnum; 8. styloid process; 9. line of sphenobasilar junction; 10. lateral pterygoid plate; 11. pterygoid hamulus; 12. vomer; 13. perpendicular plate of ethmoid; 14. nasal bone; 15. frontal sinus; 16. crista galli; 17. left sphenoidal sinus.*

height of the vomer that accompanies the expansion of the nasal cavity. These developmental changes are concomitant with the development of the PT and its associated muscles. Therefore, any structural imbalance that develops in association with the development of the base of the skull or viscerocranium may adversely affect the ventilation and drainage of the ear.

A dysfunctional tongue posture may affect the tongue's pumping function on the palatine aponeurosis and, therefore, the associated PT ventilation that occurs during swallowing. Tongue posture adapts to oral development and PT function appears to be diminished in long-faced adenoidal children.[31] Additionally, children with significant overbites are found to be more predisposed to develop PT dysfunction.[32]

Body position also seems to influence PT opening. Evidence shows a correlation between the lateral recumbent position, where one ear is positioned downwards, and a lower PT opening function on that side.[20] This reinforces the need to avoid the repeated use of the same sleep position for infants.

Any cranial somatic dysfunction of the base of the skull may disrupt its developmental sequence as well as affecting tongue posture, with resultant impact on PT growth and function. This may be a cranial somatic dysfunction of the bony constituents of the cranial base, the occiput, sphenoid and temporal bones, or dysfunction of any component linked to the vascular supply and innervation of the myofascial structures involved in suckling and swallowing. The TVP and the tensor tympani are innervated by branches from the otic ganglion, located immediately below the foramen ovale, on the medial surface of the mandibular nerve (CN V_3). The glossopharyngeal nerve (CN IX) innervates the stylopharyngeus, and the accessory nerve (CN XI) innervates the palatal muscles through the pharyngeal plexus. They both exit the skull through the jugular foramen. The hypoglossal nerve (CN XII) innervates the intrinsic and extrinsic tongue muscles. It exits the skull through the anterior intraoccipital synchondrosis, the site of the hypoglossal canal of the occipital bone when ossification occurs. Consequently, efficient PT function requires equilibrium among surrounding bony structures, such as the temporal bones, occiput, sphenoid and mandible. It also requires that associated myofascial structures be free of dysfunction.

A dysfunctional PT creates a terrain where other risk factors are reinforced. Recurrent bilateral OM with effusion develops when poor PT function is allied with diminished immune status.[33] The allergic inflammatory response that often occurs in the nasopharynx also occurs in the middle ear,[34] and the prevalence of allergic rhinitis is significantly higher in children with OM with effusion than in healthy children.[35,36] The allergic inflammation in atopic children is not localized in one area only, but manifests itself in the middle ear on both sides, as well as in the nasopharynx, demonstrating totally the united airways concept.[37] Mucosal inflammation with release of histamine and other mediators following nasopharyngeal exposure to an allergen may, consequently, be responsible for PT obstruction and dysfunction. Chronic allergic inflammation of the upper airway may lead to lymphoid hypertrophy with increased size of adenoidal and tonsillar tissue.[38] In such a case, with edema and inflammation of the posterior nasopharynx, the enlarged adenoids may obstruct the pharyngeal ostium of the PT. Tubal tonsil hypertrophy is a possible etiology for OM, when recurrence appears after adenoidectomy.[39]

The PT mucociliary apparatus contains components that have an important role in eliminating middle ear debris by moving it toward the nasopharyngeal orifice. Additionally, specialized epithelial cells express and secrete surface-active materials that appear to facilitate the muscular action of the PT opening and to protect the middle ear against infections.[3] Conversely, many viruses impair the mucociliary function of the PT epithelium and perturb the nasopharyngeal bacterial flora, increasing the adherence of bacteria to the epithelial cells.[40] Bacteria and respiratory viruses (e.g. the respiratory syncytial virus or influenza viruses) are common causes of middle ear infection.[40–42] Because of the connection between the upper and lower airways, the pathophysiologic site of origin is frequently the nasal pathway. Babies born in the fall begin their lives during the peak seasons for viral exposure and the development of respiratory infections, a risk factor for OM.[13] Additionally, impaired or decreased nasal mucociliary activity may also cause PT mucociliary dysfunction.[43] Thus osteopathic procedures that facilitate the clearance of secretions and the mucociliary action of the PT and upper airways are indicated. Blood flow to the region should also be improved.

Gastroesophageal reflux may also predispose to bacterial infection.[44] Possibly because of reflux, infants fed in the supine position demonstrate abnormal postfeeding tympanographic results compared to infants fed in the semi-upright position.[45]

Signs of AOM include fever, insomnia and the presence of pus in the middle ear with a tympanic membrane that appears bulging and erythematous when observed by otoscopic examination. Ear infections may be painful, causing irritability, rubbing of the affected ear, loss of balance and impaired hearing with lack of response to moderate sounds. Although it is generally thought that OM causes permanent hearing loss, this has not been demonstrated.[46] Transient mild to moderate hearing loss associated with OM has, however, been shown to cause delays in communicative development.[47]

Physical examination and treatment

Osteopathic considerations for the treatment of OM are directed at augmenting the body's defenses against infection and its recuperative power after infection is present. Mainstream medical interventions are often fraught with controversy. Because the infectious agents responsible for OM are both viral and bacterial, antibiotic therapy, although appropriate for bacterial infection, is not universally effective. Guidelines for determining when to employ antibiotics and other modalities are available.[2,4,48,49] The use of tympanostomy tubes is controversial.[50,51] Consequently, non-toxic interventions like osteopathic treatment, which appear to reduce the need for antibiotics, have been shown to be of potential benefit as adjuvant therapy for children with recurrent AOM.[52]

Diagnosis should begin with observation. Start with an overall evaluation of the child's posture. Look at the pectoral girdle, often protracted in patients with ENT infections. Observe the cervicothoracic junction, the cervical spine and its relationship to the skull for lack of mobility and vertical compression. These patients may demonstrate a shrugged shoulder posture, with the appearance of a shortened neck.

Observe the auricles of the ear bilaterally for deformity, asymmetry of position and relative external or internal rotation. The appearance of the ear follows the temporal bone which, in turn, affects the function of the PT. Examine the parietomastoid and occipitomastoid sutures bilaterally. Look for flattening or compression of the area. Because ear position reflects temporal bone position, asymmetry of the ears is often associated with asymmetry of cranial shape. Non-synostotic plagiocephaly has been shown to be associated with an increased incidence of OM. Enquire if the child repeatedly pulls at one ear. This will often occur on the side of compression of the parietomastoid and occipitomastoid suture.

Study the face. Open mouth facies are indicative of mouth breathing and nasal obstruction, predisposing to OM. Diagnosis and treatment of dysfunction in this area is discussed in Part 7.4, 'Mouth breathing'.

Next, perform a palpatory examination. Begin by evaluating the upper thoracic spine, ribs and pectoral girdle for somatic dysfunction. The viscerosomatic reflexes from the upper respiratory tract, including the ear, are to be found at level of T1–T4. Somatic dysfunction in this area results in increased sympathetic tone with vasoconstriction affecting the ears, nose and throat through somatovisceral reflexes. Mechanical dysfunction of the upper thoracic spine (T1 and T2), associated ribs, sternum and clavicles impairs lymphatic drainage from the head and neck. Further evaluate the remainder of the thoracic cage and thoracoabdominal diaphragm which, when dysfunctional, can also impair lymphatic circulation. Utilizing indirect principles, treat any dysfunction identified in the above areas.

Examine the cervical region for somatic dysfunction. Pay particular attention to the occipitoatlantal and atlantoaxial articulations, to the myofascial structures for their relation to lymphatic nodes and vasculature, and to the SCM muscles that, when dysfunctional, impact the function of the temporal bone. Treat any identified dysfunction.

Evaluate the skull. Begin by assessing the cranial base, paying attention to the sphenobasilar synchondrosis and temporal bones. The articulations of the temporal bones should be examined. The occipitomastoid sutures are important for their impact on the contents of the jugular foramen: cranial nerves IX, X and XI. The petrobasilar suture and sphenopetrosal synchondrosis are often dysfunctional in the infant's skull. Dysfunction of these articulations may affect the petrous portion of the temporal bone containing the osseous part of the PT. Furthermore, the cartilaginous portion of the PT is located beneath the sphenopetrosal synchondrosis and free motion of the petrous portion of the temporal bone, in external and internal rotation, facilitates the clearance of secretion from the PT. Next, evaluate the temporal bones for intraosseous dysfunctions between the petrous, squamous and tympanic portions. Palpate for the cranial rhythmic impulse (CRI) at the level of the mastoid. Intraosseous mastoid cranial respiration may promote mastoid cell function. Examine the relationship between the mandible and the temporal bones. There is usually tenderness in the area. Any temporomandibular dysfunction can affect the mobility of the temporal bones and the myofascial structures of the anterior neck below. The PT is commonly cleared by the actions of swallowing and yawning. These actions can be impaired by dysfunction of the mandible and its relationship to the tongue and soft palate. Treat identified dysfunction.

Specific attention should be paid to the efficient clearance of secretions from the PT and mastoid cavities. This activity may be stimulated by the mastoid pump procedure and the Galbreath technique.

When possible, the rate and amplitude of the CRI should be monitored during the above procedures. Following the CRI during the mastoid pump enhances the efficacy of the procedure. The specific treatment of cranial dysfunctional patterns will augment the amplitude of the CRI, improving fluid mobility and affecting low frequency oscillations in autonomic nervous system (ANS) physiology.

Advice to caregivers

Counsel the caregivers to maintain a healthy lifestyle for the child. Maintain a regular sleep–wake cycle. Provide a balanced diet with adequate hydration and avoiding refined carbohydrate as much as possible. Bottle feed and nurse in a semi-upright position and never put the infant to bed with a bottle. As much as possible, limit pacifier use to moments when the infant falls asleep and try to eliminate its use after the age of 6 months. Avoid exposure to passive smoke. When bathing the infant, limit the amount of water entering their ears.

Caregivers should be instructed to lay the child on their side, with the problem ear up. They should then massage the mandibular region, applying gentle skin traction from the area anterior to the ear in the direction of the chin. This tends to open the PT and the position employs gravity to facilitate drainage. They can also gently caress around the ear, particularly over the mastoid region. These actions allow the caregiver to actively participate in the child's recovery. They sensitize the caregiver to the health status of the child and promote relaxation for the child. Encourage the caregiver to play with the child in a fashion that promotes mimicry of the production of sounds in the throat and the clicking of the tongue by pulling it quickly from the hard palate. All activities encouraging action of the myofascial structures connected to the PT will tend to open it and facilitate its drainage.

RHINITIS

Rhinitis is the inflammation of the nasal mucous membranes. Acute rhinitis may be the consequence of a viral infection, whereas allergic rhinitis is caused by an immune-mediated response to any one or more of a myriad of allergens. Other classifications include atrophic rhinitis and vasomotor rhinitis. Although these conditions are the result of differing etiologies, they are all affected by the presence of somatic dysfunction. It is an established osteopathic dictum that the body possesses the inherent ability to heal itself. The presence of somatic dysfunction can predispose the individual to develop rhinitis or interfere with the body's recuperative mechanisms. Knowledge of the anatomy and physiology of the nasal cavities and the mucosa lining their walls is absolutely necessary to understand the etiologies of nasal dysfunction and how osteopathic principles may be applied to promote health in this area.

The nose is divided by the nasal septum into two cavities, or fossae. The two nasal cavities open anteriorly by way of the anterior naris, or nostril. They are continuous posteriorly by way of the posterior nasal apertures, or choanae, into the nasopharynx.

The nasal septum represents the medial wall of each nasal cavity. It is formed by the perpendicular plate of the ethmoid, the vomer and the septal cartilage (Fig. 7.3.8).

The roof of the nasal cavities is formed anteriorly by the nasal spine of the frontal bone and the two nasal bones. The cribriform plate of the ethmoid, with numerous perforations for the olfactory nerves, is located behind the nasal bones. More posteriorly, the anterior aspect of the body of the sphenoid causes the roof of the nasal cavities to slope downward. The sphenoidal sinuses open into the nasal cavities from above, on each side of the nasal septum (Fig. 7.3.9).

The floor of the nasal cavities is the upper surface of the osseous palate. The maxillary palatine processes form the anterior two-thirds, while the palatine horizontal plates form the posterior one-third (Fig. 7.3.10).

The lateral walls of the nasal cavities demonstrate numerous structures. They are formed anteriorly by the maxilla, posteriorly by the palatine bone and superiorly by the ethmoid labyrinth and lacrimal bone. The inferior, middle and superior nasal conchae (turbinates), the most central portion of this lateral wall, by virtue of their curled shape add a great amount of surface area to the nasal cavities. The space below each turbinate is referred to as a meatus (Fig. 7.3.11).

The nasal vestibules, just inside the nares, are the anterior-most aspect of the nasal cavities. The nares and vestibules are bounded laterally by the alar and lateral cartilages, and medially by the cartilaginous septum and the connective tissue septum, the columella (Fig. 7.3.12). The vestibule is lined with skin that contains sebaceous and sweat glands and coarse hairs (vibrissae) that assist in air filtration.

The nasal cavities are completely covered with a lining that varies histologically in different areas. At the anterior part of the nasal cavities, in the vestibules, the lining is continuous with the facial skin. Above, at the level of the upper border of the alar cartilages, the limen nasi defines the beginning of a lining formed by a non-keratinizing stratified squamous transitional epithelium that evolves further into a pseudostratified ciliated epithelium, the respiratory mucosa. This mucosa covers the remaining surface of the nasal cavities, except for the olfactory area that is covered with olfactory epithelium. This mucosa is also present in many other parts of the upper respiratory tract.

Several additional cavities communicate with the nasal cavities and demonstrate a continuum of the nasal respiratory mucosa. Each of the nasal cavities communicates directly with the nasopharynx

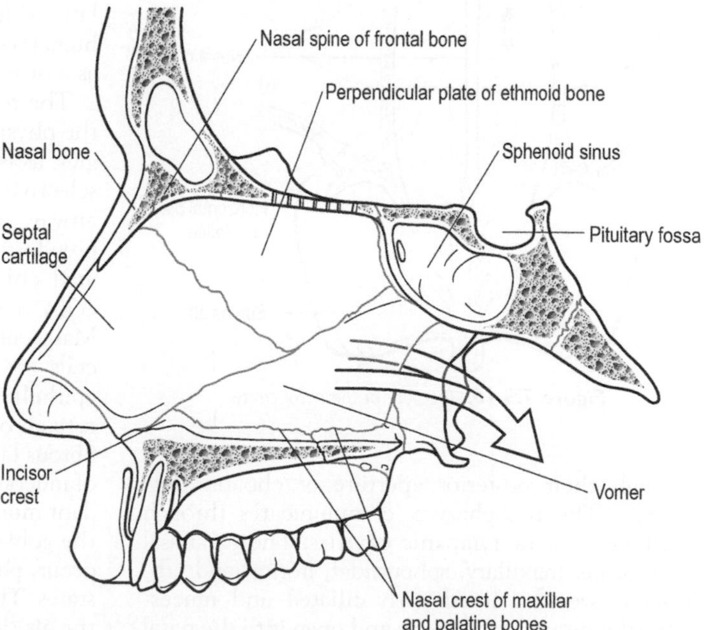

Figure 7.3.8. *The nasal septum, medial wall of the nasal cavity.*

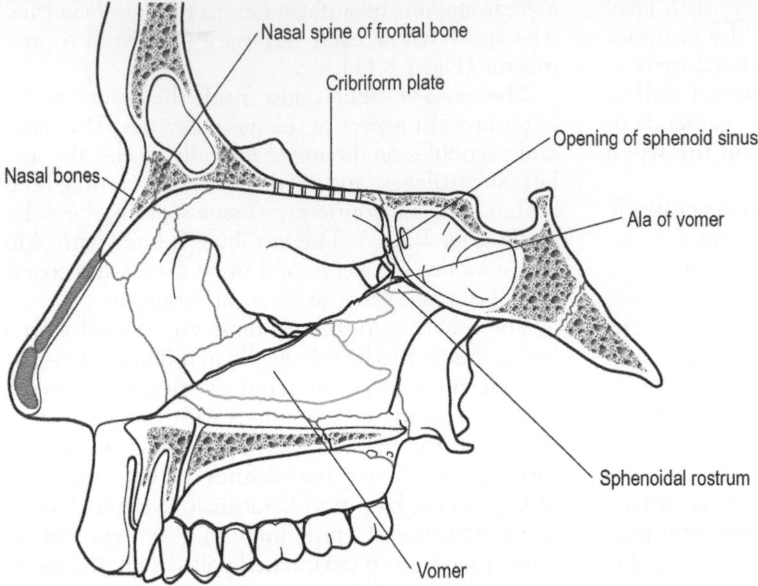

Figure 7.3.9. *The roof of the nasal cavity.*

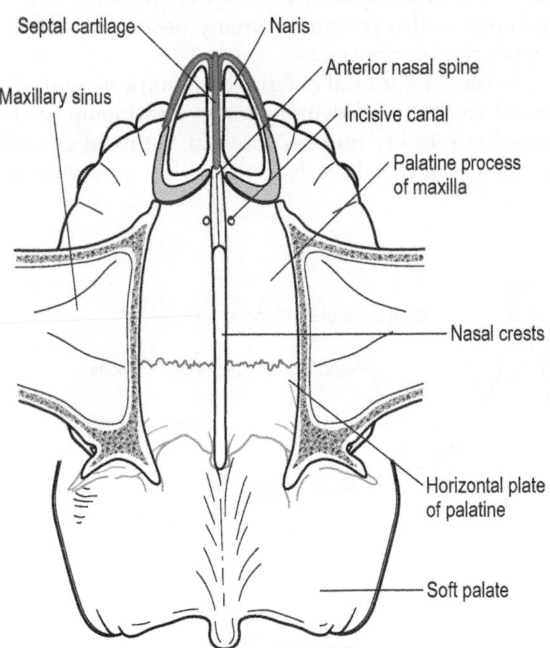

Figure 7.3.10. *The floor of the nasal cavity.*

through their posterior aperture or choana (Fig. 7.3.13). The nasopharynx communicates through the PTs with the tympanic cavities. The paranasal sinuses, i.e. maxillary, sphenoidal, frontal and ethmoidal, are also lined with ciliated and mucus-secreting respiratory mucosa and open into the nasal cavities. The nasopharyngeal mucosa is continuous above with the conjunctiva of the eyes through the nasolacrimal ducts.

Below, the nasopharynx continues to become the oropharynx, the laryngopharynx and the esophagus. The mucous membrane of the pharynx is continuous with that lining the mouth and larynx, as well as, through the trachea and bronchi, into the lungs. This continuum is a perfect example of the interrelationship between the different structures of the human body and exemplifies the concept of the body as a unit.

The respiratory mucosa plays a significant part in the physiology of the nose, as well as in its pathologies, as is the case in rhinitis. The mucosa acts as a selective barrier, essential for the defense of the airways against inhaled pathogens. The respiratory pseudostratified ciliated epithelium is formed by ciliated columnar or cuboidal epithelia with goblets cells, non-ciliated columnar cells and basal cells. Mast cells and migrating lymphocytes, mainly T cells, are also present. Under the basal lamina of this epithelium, the submucosa is adherent to the periosteum of the adjacent cranial bones and includes a fibrous layer with diffuse lymphoid tissue and a layer of mucous, seromucous and serous glands. An abundant mucous film is produced by these glands and by the goblets cells. Additional plasma exudation may occur, particularly in the presence of inflammatory states. This film gathers the particles and debris from the air that is inspired to sweep them away. Almost

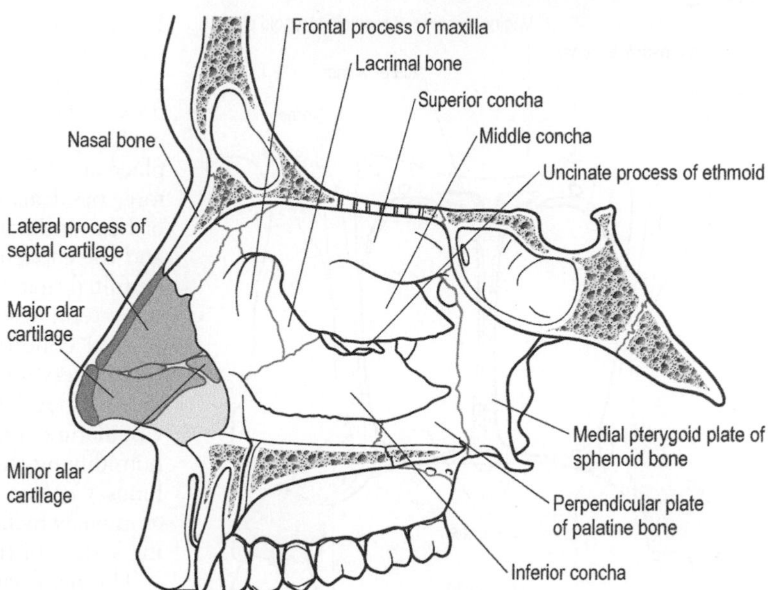

Figure 7.3.11. *The lateral wall of the nasal cavity.*

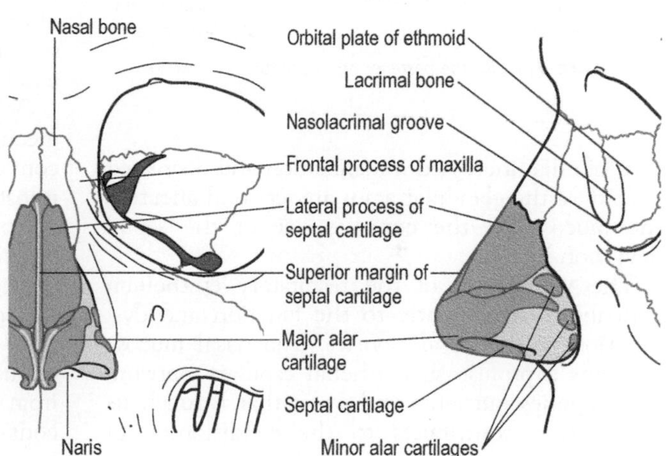

Figure 7.3.12. *The external nose.*

all particles greater than 5 μm and about 50% of those between 2 and 5 μm are collected. They end up either in the nasopharynx and oropharynx to be periodically swallowed, or in the anterior nasal vestibules.

Mucociliary clearance depends on the beating function of the respiratory cilia. They beat about 1000 times per minute.[53] The frequency of the mucociliary transport rate is subject to various influences, such as mucus viscoelastic properties, airway epithelia alkalization that appears to be a stimulator or airway epithelia acidification that decreases the rate.[54] Healthy function of the respiratory cilia results in constant motion of the mucous film. The nasal ciliary beating propels the mucus secretions posteriorly in the direction of the nasopharynx. Conversely, dysfunction of the drainage of the nasal respiratory epithelium leads to stasis and the accumulation of secretions within the nasal cavities. Cranial somatic dysfunction – particularly of the frontal bones, sphenoid, ethmoid, maxillae and vomer, with resultant loss of their inherent motility – is a possible cause of mucociliary stasis. Septal deviations are known to influence the dynamics of the nasal cavity and are often associated with a 'stuffy' nose. Histologic studies confirm this observation.

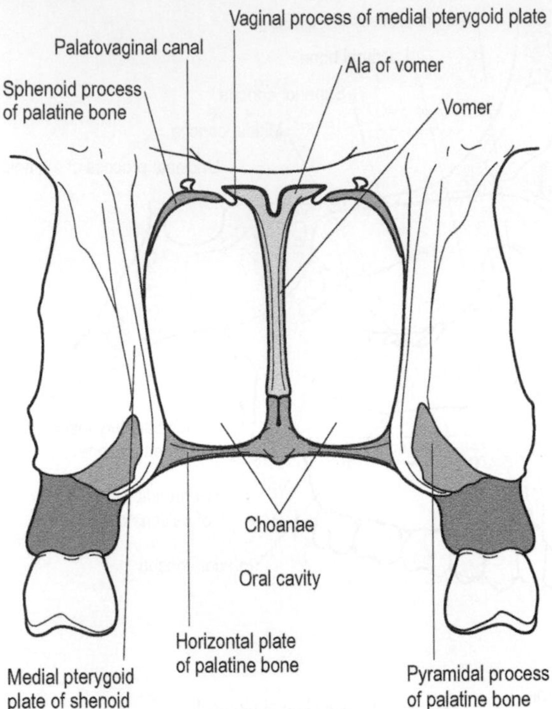

Figure 7.3.13. *The posterior nasal apertures or choana.*

Loss of cilia, increased inflammation and decreased density of the glandular acini are reported affecting the mucosa on the concave side of the septal deviation.[55]

The vasculature of the respiratory epithelium contributes significantly to the function and dysfunction of the nasal cavities. The nasal mucosa contains a profuse subepithelial capillary network that supplies nutrients and water that through its evaporation contributes to the conditioning of inspired air. The vascular supply also includes a number of different capacitance vessels, i.e. the veins, venules and cavernous sinusoids that modulate blood flow. Constriction and relaxation of these sinusoid vessels produce shrinkage or swelling of the mucosal surfaces that consequently regulates airflow and alters nasal patency. Most of the venous cavernous sinusoids are located on the inferior conchae, major sites for nasal congestion.

Air conditioning is a major function of the nose. On inspiration, the air contacts the nasal mucosa and is brought to the appropriately conditioned temperature and humidity. By virtue of their contour, the conchae, located on the lateral walls of the nasal cavities, provide an increased surface area for the flowing air to be in contact with the nasal mucosa. During expiration, some of the heat may be returned to the mucosa. When an individual is in a setting of 23°C, the nasal cavities warm the inspired air to 33°C.[56] The air is also humidified and this allows gas exchange within the alveoli of the lungs that takes place at 37°C and 100% relative humidity.[57] Therefore, nasal air conditioning requires large amounts of heat and water for conditioning the inspired air and the capacitance vessels seem perfectly designed to fulfill that need. They might also operate as a short-term reservoir, either for heat or for water. Special conditions (e.g. hyperventilation) call for these reserves in order to provide cooling and evaporation.[58] Under normal circumstances and normal vasculature, a healthy nose succeeds in warming and humidifying the inspired air in order to protect the lungs. Conversely, paucity in blood supply or moistening may reduce the efficiency of the air conditioning system of the nasal cavity.[56]

The nasal vasculature also contains an extensive system of arteriovenous anastomoses. This allows for the rapid passage of blood through the mucosa without reducing the nasal patency. Great amounts of arterial blood may flow through these anastomoses, providing heat exchange similar to hot water in a radiator.[53]

Brain cooling appears to be the result of several mechanisms including a possible nasal and paranasal convection process. This latter process involves the transfer of cool venous blood from the respiratory mucosa to venous structures of the brain, such as the superior sagittal sinus between the parietal bones or the cavernous sinuses on each side of the body of the sphenoid, where arterial thermoregulation may then occur. On both sides, the cavernous sinus drains venous blood from the skin of the face and from the nose and mouth areas, and is in intimate contact with the internal carotid artery.[59] The direction of flow in these sinuses is reversible.[17] Countercurrent mechanisms are suggested, where the arteriovenous anastomoses, present in the nasal vasculature, may also participate, allowing enhanced thermoregulation and brain cooling in hot conditions.[60] Changes in craniofacial morphology have been observed as adaptations to weather conditions. Wider nasal cavities and larger paranasal sinuses are considered to be adaptive mechanisms that, under hot conditions, offer more evaporating surface and consequently greater cooling capacity, thus protecting the brain.[61] Orofacial dysfunction may alter nasal breathing and consequently the above functions.

Body position also affects the nasal vasculature. The supine position increases vascular congestion, thus decreasing nasal patency and the ability of the nose to condition cold, dry air. Conversely, the upright position decreases vascular congestion.[62] Consequently, it is appropriate to enquire if the patient experiences excessive increased nasal congestion when they lie down as it may result in snoring and sleep disorders.

Furthermore, the nasal vascular supply is under the influence of hormones, psychological stress and diverse substances (e.g. gases or inflammatory molecules) that once in contact with the nasal mucosa seem to produce vascular congestion with edema and plasma exudation. It should be noted that children and teenagers often report nasal vascular congestion as nasal obstruction.

An alternation of breathing between the two nares is known as the nasal cycle. It has been observed as early as 3 years of age, with the duration of a cycle ranging from 40 to 215 minutes.[63] Alternation of the side of nasal breathing has been associated with the central mechanism regulating the dominance of the cerebral hemispheres. Increased sympathetic activity in the nasal mucosa appears to be linked to greater sympathetic tone in the ipsilateral hemisphere and thus with decreased blood flow and mental activity in that hemisphere.[64]

Changes in the tone of the nasal vascular supply are regulated by the ANS. Parasympathetic nerves are vasodilator, sympathetic nerves are vasoconstrictor. Therefore, predominance of parasympathetic activity causes a vasodilatation and nasal congestion, whereas increased sympathetic activity produces a vasoconstriction that decreases nasal airflow resistance.

The preganglionic fibers of the cranial portion of the sympathetic nervous system originate from axons of somata in the lateral gray column of the upper thoracic spinal segments. The fibers enter the superior cervical ganglion adjacent to the second and third cervical vertebrae where they synapse. The postganglionic fibers ascend, following the course of the internal carotid artery, forming the internal carotid plexus.

The greater petrosal nerve, a branch of the facial nerve (CN VII), contains the preganglionic parasympathetic fibers traveling to the pterygopalatine (sphenopalatine) ganglion. Located deeply in the pterygopalatine fossa, between the pterygoid process and maxilla, anterior to the pterygoid canal, the pterygopalatine ganglion is one of the major peripheral parasympathetic ganglia. At the level of the foramen lacerum, the greater petrosal nerve is joined by the deep petrosal nerve from the internal carotid plexus (sympathetic) to form the nerve of the pterygoid canal (Vidian nerve). These fibers synapse in the pterygopalatine ganglion; the postganglionic parasympathetic fibers are secretomotor and supply the glands of the nasal mucosa.

Additionally, the nasal cavities are densely innervated by the sensory nervous system. Nerves are present in respiratory mucosa, particularly in the walls of the venous vessels and the gland acini. Glands are innervated by both parasympathetic and sensory nerve fibers. Sensory nerves are stimulated by mechanical, thermal or chemical stimulation and afferent fibers run in the trigeminal nerve. Sensory nerve stimulation instigates different reflexes, such as the sneeze reflex.[65] Nasal thermal stimulation, as occurs with inhalation of cold dry, dry or moist air, produces a nasopulmonary bronchoconstrictor reflex in normal healthy individuals, inducing changes in airway resistance.[66] Activation of temperature-sensitive nerve endings in the nasal mucosa generates this response and the decrease of airflow through the nose and trachea protect the lungs from insufficiently conditioned air.[66]

The ANS controls several aspects of nasal function, i.e. nasal secretions, mucociliary function, blood flow, microvascular permeability, release of inflammatory cells and nasal patency. The modulation and balance of nasal functions necessitate an interaction between the sympathetic and parasympathetic systems, as well as a well-tuned sensory nervous system. Dysfunction may lead to pathologic nasal syndromes. Because of the relationships between the sympathetic nervous system and the upper thoracic spinal segments, the second and third cervical vertebrae, and between the parasympathetic nervous system and the sphenoid, maxilla or palatine bones, somatic dysfunction of any of these vertebral and cranial areas can result in dysfunction of the ANS with impact on nasal function. Furthermore, because of the role of the trigeminal nerve, particularly the first and second divisions, in the sensory function of the nose, the temporal bone should be added to that list. Osteopathic procedures may be applied to balance the ANS and promote healthy nasal functions.

Unpaired and paired structures form the nasal cavities, as in the remainder of the skull. As such, during the PRM inspiratory phase, the midline unpaired structures of the nasal cavities (i.e. the sphenoid, ethmoid, vomer and septal cartilage) demonstrate cranial flexion and the paired structures (i.e. maxillae, palatine, nasal and lacrimal bones and conchae) externally rotate. In the reciprocal PRM expiratory phase, the midline structures move in the direction of cranial extension and the paired structures internally rotate. Therefore, in health, the nasal cavities follow each cycle of the PRM, with a resultant widening of the cavities during flexion–external rotation of the inspiratory phase and narrowing during extension–internal rotation of the expiratory phase. Cranial somatic dysfunction very frequently follows asymmetric patterns. Thus, the nasal cavity will be wider on one side than on the other. This can be observed by nasoscopic examination, as well as by simply looking at the patient to note asymmetry in the facial features. It may also be observed by comparing the relative size of the nares. One side is usually more open than the other. The open side is the side of the external rotation, whereas the other side is associated with internal rotation. The patient often reports more nasal congestion on the smaller side and in cases of small children the mothers comment on the increase of nasal secretion on that side.

The alternation of cranial flexion and extension, with all cranial structures free to follow this movement, is necessary to ensure effective tissue perfusion of the nasal mucosa. It also promotes venous and lymphatic drainage of the nose, as well as the removal of secretions from the nasal cavities and sinuses. Under these circumstances, mucosal inflammation and hyperreactivity associated with rhinitis may be reduced.

In neurogenic inflammation of the upper airway mucosa, such as in chronic rhinosinusitis, sensory nerves are excited and mediators are released, including histamine, prostaglandins and various neuropeptides such as substance P.[67] They may then cause vasodilatation, vascular congestion, extravasation of plasma with edema, and recruitment and activation of inflammatory cells. Secretion from the submucosal glands may also be increased. These exaggerated sensory and parasympathetic defensive reflexes form the pathophysiologic basis of rhinitis.

Acute rhinitis, one of the symptoms of the common cold, is the result of a viral infection. Numerous viruses cause infections in the respiratory tract and any region of the tract may be inflamed – the nose, the paranasal sinuses, the throat, the larynx, the trachea and the bronchi. Acute rhinitis represents one of the most frequent upper respiratory infections.

Allergic rhinitis is considered to be the most common allergic airway disease, with about 10% of the population experiencing this condition.[53] Allergic rhinitis is common in children and most of the time this condition first develops during childhood or adolescence.[68] Typical behaviors are usually observed such as grimacing and picking of the nose. Older children are likely to blow their noses more often than younger children who present with constant clearing of the throat because of postnasal drip, frequent sniffing or snorting.[69]

Rhinorrhea, nasal obstruction, sneezing, itching of the eyes, nose and palate, and watery eyes are typical symptoms associated with allergic rhinitis. The disease results from exposure to various allergens including foods, pollens, molds, dust mites and animal dander. Two groups are described: seasonal allergic rhinitis, often the result of pollen exposure, and perennial allergic rhinitis, lasting for at least 9 months of the year.

Allergic individuals demonstrate a decreased capacity to warm and humidify inhaled air.[57] They also are prone to develop other diseases of the upper and lower respiratory tract such as sinusitis, otitis media with effusion and asthma that may complicate allergic rhinitis.[70] Although the reason why individuals develop allergic rhinitis is uncertain, a genetic predisposition to develop the allergic response has been suggested.[69] It is thought that these individuals probably have a greater sensitivity to allergens and are predisposed to develop mucosal inflammation and hyperreactivity.

A 'microflora hypothesis' has also been suggested. It is thought that the disturbance of the normal microbiota in the gastrointestinal tract, in part due to the use of antibiotics and dietary changes in industrialized countries over the past two decades, is a factor that may lead to modified airway tolerance to allergens and atopic disorders.[71] Genetics and microbiotic disruption would then be considered as predisposing factors, increasing an individual's susceptibility to develop airway hypersensitivity and allergy.

The nasal dysfunction associated with allergic rhinitis results in various symptoms. Nasal congestion with increased airflow resistance, particularly in the supine position, causes sleep-disordered breathing. It is a risk factor for snoring, affecting teenage males more frequently than females.[72] It is also linked to various systemic symptoms such as headaches, irritability and fatigue that diminish functional capacity. Thus, allergies are one of the main reasons for missed school days in the US.[73] School performance may be decreased because of inattention and decreased concentration.[74] Physical and emotional impairments associated with the allergic condition make it a whole body dysfunction.[75]

Because allergic rhinitis can affect the patient's quality of life to such an extent, and because of its economic impact, prevention and treatment are essential.[73] Osteopathic procedures may be seen as a valuable complement to traditional medical treatment.

Physical examination and treatment

The examination for somatic dysfunction is begun by observing the global postural pattern and/or how the cervical and thoracic regions are, or are not, integrated into this pattern. The child should be observed from behind, from the side and from the front.

From behind, observe upper body postural mechanics. Look for cervical and thoracic sidebending, occipitocervical rotation and slumping of the pectoral girdle.

From the side, observe cervical and thoracic anteroposterior mechanics. There is often upper thoracic flexion with increased cervical lordosis. In this position, the head will very commonly be thrust forward with significant tension placed on the anterior cervical soft tissues. Observe specifi cally the submandibular myofascial structures and the position of the hyoid bone. The child with rhinitis may have to compensate by mouth breathing. As such, they may demonstrate the associated mouth breathing posture to a variable degree, depending on the chronicity of the condition. A double-chin appearance and the demonstration of a slack-jawed posture are indicative of chronic mouth breathing.

From the front, observe and confirm the sidebending and rotation observed from behind. Again look for the presence of mouth breathing and the associated orofacial characteristics. Children who mouth breath demonstrate a lack of tonicity of their facial tissues. The lower lip is typically everted and the tongue slightly protruded. Observe the relationship between the tongue and the teeth. Persistent protrusion of the tongue results in anterior displacement of the upper incisors with an eventual overbite. The child with allergic rhinitis will demonstrate puffiness of the facial soft tissues, particularly noticeable around the eyes, as well as darkening of the tissues beneath the eyes. The nasion is often recessed in the face. Because of the chronic lack of nasal breathing, the bony structures of the nasal cavities are small, resulting in narrowed nasal apertures. Children with persistent nasal congestion demonstrate an observable transverse crease in the skin across the lower third of the nose, at the junction between the nasal bones and cartilages. This develops as the result of repeatedly rubbing and pushing the tip of the nose vertically or laterally with their fi ngers or hand in response to nasal itching – the 'allergic salute'.

Following observation, the palpatory examination is best performed with the child supine. Begin by palpating the upper thoracic region for structure and employ the tests of listening to assess function, paying particular attention to the motion of the vertebrae and ribs. Examine the clavicles in similar fashion. Next, evaluate the cervical spine, with attention to the structural and functional relationships between the occiput, C1, C2, C3 and C4. Palpate the soft tissues in this area for the presence of edema. In acute upper respiratory conditions, the trigeminally mediated upper cervical reflex (occiput, C1) will result in acute tissue texture changes. Assess the anterior cervical soft tissues and midline structures with attention to the hyoid bone. Identify somatic dysfunction and treat it using the principles of indirect technique.

Examine the cranial base. Note the pattern demonstrated between the sphenoid and occiput. SBS compression and inferior vertical strain are often encountered in association with nasal dysfunction. Note the relationship between the occiput and temporal bone. Visualize how this relationship impacts the jugular foramina and consequently CN X. The functional status of the sphenoid bone exerts significant infl uence on the frontal bone and the facial bones below, and should be assessed. Also assess the frontal bone. Any dysfunctional motion restriction will result in diminished movement, and consequently diminished drainage, of the nasal cavities. In particular, dysfunctional frontal internal rotation causes the ethmoidal notch to be narrowed, restricting the movement of the ethmoid below. When evaluating the relationships between the sphenoid, frontal bone and the facial bones with the tests of listening, first assess the global motion of the region and then proceed to assess the individual bones and their interosseous relationships. During this assessment, localized motion restriction may be perceived that requires further identification through visualization. The following sutures are potential sites of interosseous dysfunctions: frontoethmoidal, frontomaxillary, frontonasal and sphenoethmoidal.

The relationships between the vomer and the sphenoid, ethmoid, maxillae and palatine bones, as well as the articulation between the two maxillae, should be evaluated. The nasal cartilages should be assessed in their relationship with the nasal bones and perpendicular plate of the ethmoid.

Following indirect principles, treat any dysfunctions found. Address the upper thoracic and cervical regions for their effect on the ANS. Treat cranial dysfunctions for their effect on the autonomic and sensory nervous systems, venous and lymphatic drainage, and to promote the production and drainage of nasal secretions.

Treatment of nasal structures will affect the total body through the cranial mechanism. The nasal septum consists of the vomer and the perpendicular plate of the ethmoid. Posteriorly, it is continuous with the sphenoidal sagittal septum that divides the body of the sphenoid into two sinus cavities. Posteriorly and superiorly, it is continuous with the falx cerebri and falx cerebelli. These structures combined constitute a vertical septum that separates the paired structures of the head and unites the viscerocranium and the neurocranium and, through the core link, the body below.

The nasal mucosa contains a rich supply of nerve endings and a dense network of microvasculature. For these reasons, it is highly sensitive. This should be kept in mind during the physical examination and treatment. It makes tests of listening and methods of treatment employing indirect principles the techniques of choice. Further, to follow the PRM, its rhythm and potency within nasal tissue, and to employ treatment when appropriate to enhance its potency, may help to modulate the autonomic dysfunction present in rhinitis, as well as help to reduce stasis and edema on a macro level in the mucosa and a micro level in the neuronal synapses.

Advice to caregivers

Recurrent and chronic rhinitis is commonly triggered or aggravated by environmental circumstances. As such, the caregiver should be provided with information as to potentially irritating conditions and substances that will allow them to identify and remove these triggers from the child's environment. Allergens should be sought out, identified and, if possible, removed. The most common allergens include pollens, foods, molds, dusts and animal dander. A detailed list of these substances may be found by doing an Internet search.

Conversely, dietary considerations and respiratory exercises may be employed to improve the function of the immune system. It has been suggested that disruption of the normal microbiota in the gastrointestinal tract contributes to decreased airway tolerance to allergens.[71] Refined foods should be avoided as much as possible, while a diet rich in fresh fruit and vegetables and antioxidants such as vitamins C and E should be recommended. A diet high in probiotics that promote the growth of beneficial bacteria (Bifidobacterium, Lactobacillus, Bacteroides) is recommended. This includes prebiotic carbohydrates such as inulin and oligofructose, plant carbohydrates that are not digestible in the small intestine but rather are fermented by bacteria in the colon.[76] Lactose intolerance should be considered.

Respiratory exercises are intended to enhance nasal breathing, promote mucus drainage and reduce vascular stasis in the nasal mucosa. They should be initiated in such a way that they can be successfully performed and yet avoid frustrating the child. Nasal congestion impairs nasal respiration and if the child is simply told to breathe through their nose, the difficulty of the experience usually limits the success of the exercise. The child will feel frustrated at best, and at worst may experience anxiety and a sense of suffocation. And they will stop doing the exercises.

Begin by explaining to the child the importance of nasal breathing. Explain that breathing through their nose cleans the air they breathe and gives them more oxygen in their blood, and that this will, in turn, enhance their performance in school and in sports.

Next, have the child breathe through their nose and become aware of the sensation of nasal airflow. Have them palpate the lateral aspects of the nasal cartilages as they breathe. Teach them to actively flare the nose by contracting the dilatator nostril muscles as they inhale. Palpating the nose during this process reinforces their awareness of nasal flaring. After 2 or 3 minutes of active nasal breathing the child should observe the difference in the sensation of nasal airflow. They may now be instructed to repeat the above process at home, exercising for 5 minutes at least three times daily. The child should also be taught to breathe using their thoracoabdominal diaphragm.

Successfully implementing these exercises not only allows the child to improve nasal respiratory function, it further teaches them a sense of control over their own respiration. This will reduce and eventually eliminate the sense of suffocation the child experiences when they attempt to breathe through congested nasal passages because, even thought they may experience nasal congestion, they will have been empowered to alleviate it.

SINUSITIS

It is estimated that children get an average of six to eight colds annually, and that 5–10% of all upper respiratory tract infections are complicated by sinusitis.[77] The application of osteopathic principles in the treatment and prevention of sinusitis in children should be utilized, as it is particularly efficient. It is based on an understanding of the anatomic and functional aspects of the nasal cavities and sinuses as part of the upper respiratory tract. A description of the nasal cavities, mucosa and its main characteristics has already been provided in 'Rhinitis' above. We shall, therefore, only consider the description of the paranasal sinuses and the pathophysiology that explains their dysfunction.

Many speculative theories exist concerning the function of paranasal sinuses. Some 2000 years ago, Galen hypothesized that they were 'porous bones' reducing the skull's weight. Since then, other theories have described the paranasal sinuses as shock absorbers, resonance chambers, air conditioning areas or the result of the evolutionary process and parts of the facial development.

There are four paranasal air sinuses associated with each nasal cavity: the ethmoidal, frontal, sphenoidal and maxillary sinuses, all of which open into the lateral walls of the nasal cavities by small apertures that differ from one individual to another. The lateral wall of the nasal cavity is formed anteriorly by the frontal process of the maxilla and the lacrimal bone; centrally by the ethmoid, maxilla and inferior nasal concha; and posteriorly by the vertical plate of the palatine bone and the medial pterygoid plate of the sphenoid. Three meatuses are located in this wall. They consist of three irregular passages directed anteroposteriorly – the superior, middle and inferior meatuses of the nose. The superior meatus is the smallest. Located between the superior and middle nasal conchae, it occupies the middle third of the lateral wall of the nasal cavity. The middle meatus is between the middle and inferior conchae. The inferior meatus is the largest of the three. It lies in the space between the inferior concha and the floor of the nasal cavity. Only the nasolacrimal duct drains into the inferior meatus in the anterior part of the nasal cavity.

The ethmoidal sinuses, on each side, are formed by 3–15 air cells, filling the ethmoidal labyrinth. They are divided into three groups: anterior, middle and posterior. The anterior and middle ethmoidal cells drain into the middle meatus, whereas the posterior ethmoidal cells drain into the superior meatus. The frontal sinuses are the highest. Each frontal sinus develops from an anterior ethmoidal cell that extends posteriorly along the medial part of the orbital roof and laterally above the internal part of the eyebrow at about 5 or 6 years of age. On each side, through the frontonasal duct and the ethmoidal labyrinth, the frontal sinus drains into the middle meatus. The maxillary sinuses are the largest. They form large pyramidal cavities within the bodies of the maxillae and drain into the middle meatus on each side. The sphenoidal sinuses are within the body of the sphenoid, their apertures being on the upper portion of the anterior walls of the sphenoidal body. The sphenoid sinuses drain into the superior meatus, near the roof of the nasal cavities (Figs 7.3.14, 7.3.15).

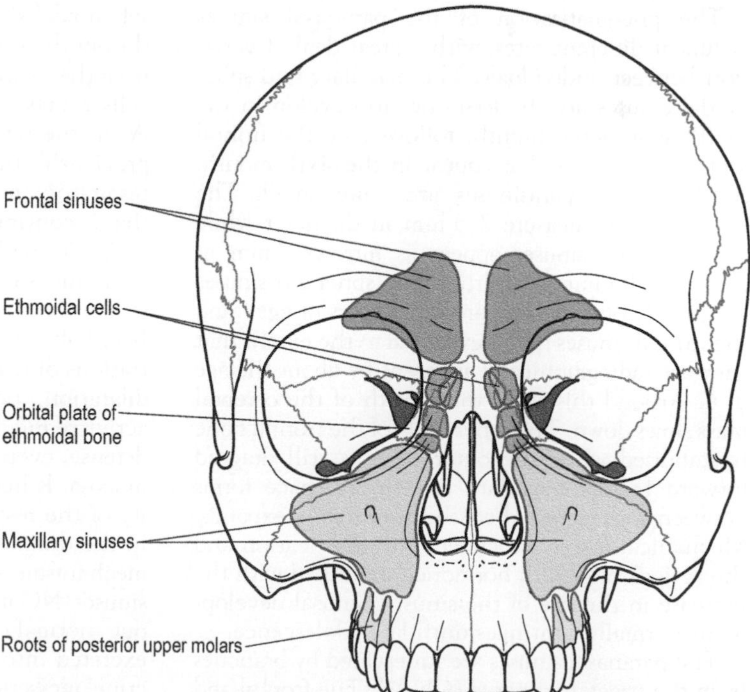

Figure 7.3.14. *Paranasal air sinuses.*

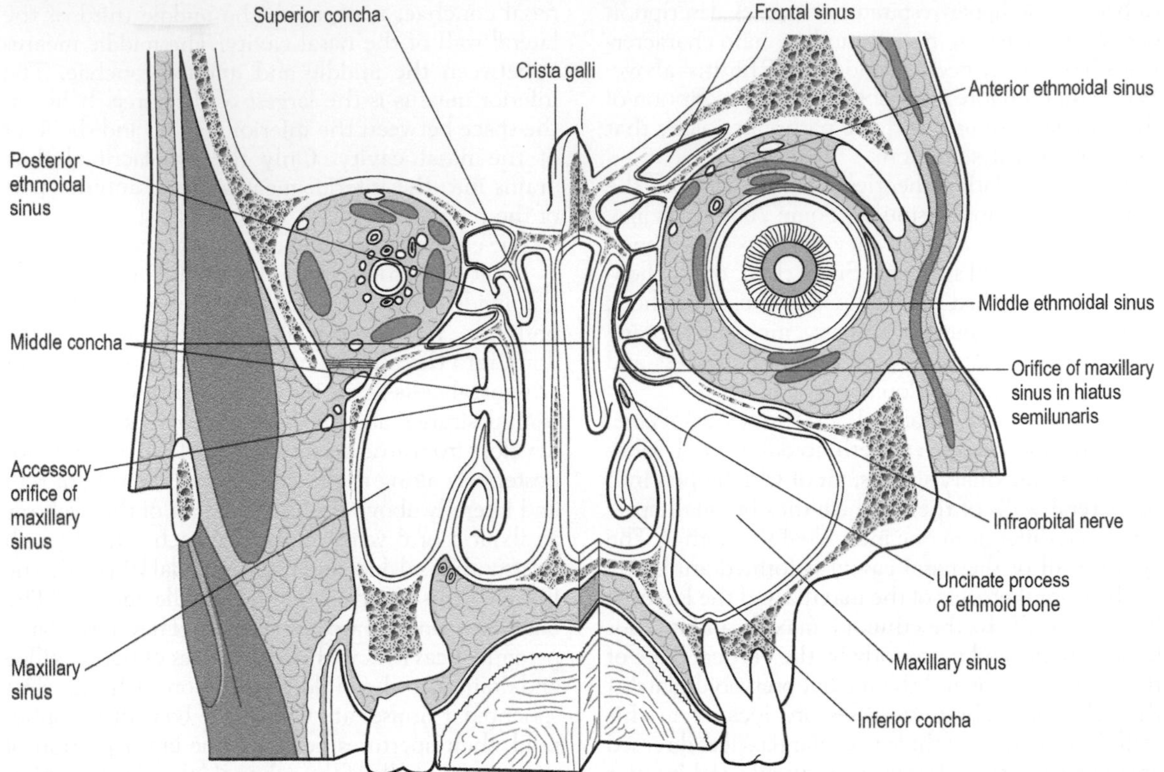

Figure 7.3.15. *Coronal section through the nasal cavity, from the posterior aspect. The plane of the section is more anterior on the right side.*

The pneumatization of the paranasal sinuses occurs at different rates, with a great deal of variation between individuals. The maxillary and sphenoidal sinuses are the first ones to develop in the fourth gestational month, followed by the frontal and ethmoid cells that appear in the sixth month. At birth, the parasinuses are quite small. The ethmoid cells measure 2–5 mm in diameter while the maxillary sinuses appear as furrows 7 mm in length and 4 mm in width.[78] The sphenoid sinuses are usually pneumatized around 5 years of age[79] and the frontal sinuses have developed to the extent that they are radiographically apparent by about the age of 6. Around this time, the growth of the cerebral mass slows down. The inner table of the frontal bone is stabilized while the outer table is still dragged forward by nasomaxillary growth. A space forms between both plates, where the frontal sinus expands. Mechanical forces associated with mastication and the actions of growth hormones are linked with the increase in the size of the sinus.[80] Sinusal development normally continues until late adolescence.

The paranasal sinuses are innervated by branches from the trigeminal nerve (CN V). The frontal and sphenoidal sinuses are innervated by branches from the ophthalmic nerve (CN V_1), the maxillary sinuses from the maxillary nerve (CN V_2), and the ethmoid cells from both the ophthalmic and maxillary nerves. As in the remainder of the nasal cavity, described previously, the paranasal sinuses are lined with a respiratory mucosa, ciliated and mucus-secreting, that is continuous with that of the respiratory tract.

Additionally, the paranasal sinuses seem to be an anatomic source for the excretion of nasal nitric oxide (NO). Mammals lacking paranasal sinuses (e.g. baboons) demonstrate lower exhaled concentrations of this molecule.[81] NO is involved in vasodilatation, neural transmission and immunologic activity, and appears also to participate in local host defense, even before allergens reach the respiratory mucosa. It may also regulate the mucociliary motility of the respiratory mucosa, thereby participating in the drainage of nasal secretions and the defense mechanisms of the mucosa. From the paranasal sinuses, NO may also play distal functions. Throughout normal nasal breathing, NO is constantly excreted into the upper airway, acting as an 'aerocrine' messenger.[82] It follows the airflow to the lungs where it modulates pulmonary function through regulation of blood flow and oxygen uptake.[83] Nasal breathing, therefore, becomes crucial for these vital functions. When compared to oral breathing in healthy individuals, nasal breathing results in an improvement of arterial oxygenation[84] with a reduction of pulmonary vascular resistance. In this manner, NO would be an airborne messenger. It is of prime importance to improve nasal respiration in infants and children as soon as possible. Nasal breathing promotes healthier conditions in association with inspiration. Additionally, it stimulates the development of the maxillofacial skeleton and, therefore, of the nasal cavities.[85]

The paranasal sinuses are a common site for infection in children and adolescents. The most common sinusitis is maxillary, followed by ethmoidal and then frontal sinusitis. The tendency to develop sinusitis can be explained in part by anatomy. Proper ventilation is critical for preservation of sinus integrity. The maxillary sinuses are ventilated, but the ostium of each sinus is positioned high on the lateral wall of the nasal cavity. This encumbers gravitational drainage and probably predisposes patients to infections of the maxillary sinus. The frontal sinus is ventilated and because of the location of its ostium at its base, this sinus benefits the most from gravity. Sphenoidal sinusitis rarely occurs as an isolated infection, being found more often as a part of complete sinusal involvement.

Viral infections of the upper respiratory tract commonly result in an inflammation of the sinuses and nasal mucosa to produce the rhinosinusitis.[86] Bacterial infections with purulent nasal drainage are most often located in the paranasal sinuses.[79] Viral rhinosinusitis precedes about 80% of bacterial sinus infections while the remaining 20% most often follow allergic rhinitis.[77] Persistence of nasal symptoms, such as discharge or congestion, cough and headaches, particularly when awakening, for more than 30 days is defined as chronic sinusitis.

The sinus ostium is a common structure shared by all of the paranasal sinuses. Its function has been compared to that of the pharyngotympanic tube. They both permit drainage. The ostia of the sinuses allow drainage of the paranasal sinuses whereas the PTs drain the tympanic cavities.[87] Therefore, following the same principles as those used to treat otitis media, osteopathic procedures may be applied to affect the bones of the paranasal sinuses to improve their compliance and promote sinus drainage. Inter- and intraosseous techniques for the frontal bones, ethmoid, sphenoid and maxillae are very efficient in the treatment of sinusitis.

The normal size of the sinus ostia is approximately 2.4 mm.[88] The ostia are lined with mucosa and inflammation and swelling of that mucosa may decrease or occlude ostial patency and consequently the drainage of the paranasal sinuses. Obstruction of a paranasal sinus ostium will initially produce an increase of the pressure within the sinus. This is followed by intrasinusal gas absorption that consequently results in negative pressure within the sinus. This condition predisposes aspiration of bacteria-laden secretions into the ethmoid or maxillary sinuses from the nasal cavity, particularly when an individual sniffs or blows their nose.[87] Obstructed drainage generates stasis of mucus in the paranasal sinuses that, in turn, becomes an ideal culture medium for bacteria. More inflammation follows, with a self-perpetuating condition that leads to chronicity.

Additionally, somatic dysfunction may contribute to impaired nasal secretion. Parasympathetic stimulation results in vasodilatation and increased activity of the seromucous glands and goblet cells, with symptoms such as rhinorrhea and nasal congestion. On the other hand, increased sympathetic activity produces vasoconstriction and dryness of the nasal mucosa.[89] Cranial somatic dysfunction of the maxilla, palatine bone and sphenoid can affect the pterygopalatine ganglion and both parasympathetic and sympathetic supply of the nose and paranasal sinuses (see 'Rhinitis' above). Dysfunction of the cranial base and craniocervical junction will reflexly affect the trigeminal nerve and, through it, sympathetic and parasympathetic reflexes. Somatic dysfunction in the cervical and upper thoracic spine can affect sympathetic activity, as well as lymphatic drainage of the facial area. Once again, normal motion of skeletal structures, functional ciliary motion and autonomic regulation are required for a healthy upper respiratory system.

It should be stressed that cranial somatic dysfunction, although it may originate very early in life, may not manifest until years later. Nasal septal asymmetry may affect as many as 1% of newborns as the result of compression of the tip of the baby's nose during vaginal delivery.[90] Nasal suction bulbs or nasogastric tubes may also be traumatic to the nose. A nasal septal deviation may affect the middle concha and predispose to the obstruction of the osteomeatal area.[87] Cranial base dysfunction and vertebral somatic dysfunction may result from difficult labor. Obviously, for all these reasons, a whole body osteopathic evaluation and treatment of the newborn should be performed, including attention to the facial bones, particularly those of the nose. Left untreated, facial somatic dysfunction may restrict full development of the paranasal sinuses. Furthermore, nasal obstruction will lead to mouth breathing and sleep-disordered breathing.[85] Sore throat and sinusitis may follow. Nasal obstruction is frequently associated with chronic maxillary sinusitis, adenotonsillar hypertrophy and otitis media as well as dental malocclusion and facial maldevelopment.[31]

Later in childhood and adolescence, somatic dysfunction can occur as the result of traumatic forces from physical bumps, falls, athletic strains and the like. The resultant dysfunction, depending on the direction of the traumatic force, may be established in the pattern of the individual's underlying postural balance or completely independent of it. Somatic dysfunctions of the facial bones and upper thoracic region are of particular consequence in the development and maintenance of sinus dysfunction.

The cranial respiration of the PRM differs from the thoracoabdominal respiration. However, they may entrain each other. This happens during states of relaxation, where the rate of the pulmonary respiration decreases to that approximating the rate of the PRM. Thereby, the two respirations combine their action to affect the entire body. This principle is particularly significant in the upper airway to promote movement of the nasal secretions, the gaseous contents of the paranasal sinuses, blood and lymph.

The normal cranial motion associated with the PRM consists of an inspiratory phase (flexion–external rotation) during which the paranasal sinuses as paired structures expand laterally and decrease in height. Conversely, during the expiratory phase of the PRM (extension–internal rotation), the sinuses decrease their lateral dimension and increase their height.

During cranial inspiration, the maxilla and the zygomatic bone move in external rotation, but at the same time a slight twisting occurs between them that contributes to the drainage of the maxillary sinus. The movements of all bones in association with the biphasic PRM may be described as the result of the combined movements in the three cardinal planes. The twisting between the zygomatic bone and the maxilla occurs predominantly in the sagittal plane. During external rotation, the zygoma demonstrates a component of anterior rotation, while the maxilla simultaneously demonstrates posterior rotation. The reverse occurs during internal rotation. This motion may be compared to the wringing out of a wet rag.

The zygomatic bones are an interface between the greater wing of the sphenoid, the maxilla, the frontal and the temporal bones. Their position is strategic and they play a key role in the balance of the face. The vomer is located between the sphenoidal body and the hard palate. Its inferior border articulates anteriorly with the intermaxillary suture between the palatine processes of the maxillae and posteriorly with the interpalatine suture between the horizontal plates of the palatine bones. The vomer rotates posteriorly during cranial flexion or inhalation, when the body of the sphenoid rotates anteriorly. Conversely, the vomer rotates anteriorly during cranial extension or expiration, when the body of the sphenoid rotates posteriorly. Accordingly, Sutherland stated: 'During inhalation the zygomatic bones and the vomer function somewhat like a plumber's plunger on the sphenoidal sinus and the maxillary sinuses.'[91] Every component of the facial skeleton is involved as part of the global functional pattern and should be assessed. Again according to Sutherland, even the smallest structures should be considered: 'See the turbinates on the side of the nose as they are in the living body, curling and uncurling during inhalation and exhalation.'[92]

The treatment of sinusitis is intended to promote the PRM. The osseous structures as well as the potency of the PRM should be considered.

Physical examination and treatment

Manipulative treatment of the somatic dysfunction associated with sinusitis should be employed in conjunction with standard medical treatments. The sooner it is initiated, the more rapid and successful the response. Failure to treat chronic sinusitis effectively will result in altered growth patterns of the viscerocranium. Nasal breathing will be impaired with concomitant malposition of the tongue and resultant dental malalignment.

Osteopathic examination and treatment of sinusitis are very similar to that of rhinitis. Examination is directed at the identification of somatic dysfunction that affects normal mucociliary clearance and impairs blood and lymphatic circulation, as well as ANS function. For this and the associated treatment discussion, the reader is directed to 'Rhinitis' above.

Manipulative treatment for sinusitis should focus on the reduction of mucosal edema, which will increase osteal patency. Procedures should be employed to drain the sinuses and provide symptomatic relief. Treatment should also include procedures that address sympathetic and parasympathetic somatovisceral reflex activity affecting the sinuses.

The sympathetic supply of the paranasal sinuses emanates from the upper thoracic spine. When examining the child with sinusitis, it is all too easy to become focused on dysfunction of the viscerocranium and forget this significant area. Additionally, when working with children it is less intrusive to begin in an area away from the face. Perform tests of listening to evaluate the motion of the upper thoracic vertebrae and associated ribs. Because of its relationship with the trigeminal nerve, the occipitocervical region should also be assessed.

The rhythmic motion of the cranial bones under the influence of the PRM significantly facilitates sinus drainage. It is, therefore, appropriate to examine the global cranial pattern, looking specifically for dysfunction that reduces the motion of the sphenoid, ethmoid, vomer, palatine and zygomatic bones, maxillae and conchae.

Observe the face of the child, looking for puffiness in the nasal area. Look for asymmetry of the nares and asymmetric nasal respiration. Compare the degree of nasal alar flare with inspiration. In addition, inspect the nasal cavity, noting secretions, edema and erythema of the mucosa. Observe the child for open mouth posture that may be indicative of enlarged adenoids. Listen to the child's speech for hyponasality.

Utilizing tests of listening, evaluate the sphenoid and frontal bones. Proceed to assess the facial bones, paying particular attention to the ethmoid, maxillae and zygomatic bones. The function of the vomer, palatine bones and conchae should also be considered.

The zygomatic bones are easily accessible and their manipulation readily results in drainage of the maxillary sinuses. This procedure (see Chapter 6) is straightforward and easily mastered by the novice. Manipulation of the zygoma, in turn, affects the ipsilateral maxilla and greater wing of the sphenoid.

The motion of the sphenoid should be assessed. It exerts significant influence on the facial bones and on proper drainage of the sphenoid sinuses whose ostia are located in the upper portion of the anterior walls of the sphenoidal body. The ethmoid bone is a common site of dysfunction in children and adolescents, and should be assessed in its relationships with the frontal bones, sphenoid and maxillae. Proper motion of the ethmoid bone is necessary to facilitate the emptying of secretions from the ethmoid air cells.

Intra- and interosseous motion of the maxilla should be assessed because it is necessary for the effective drainage of the maxillary sinus. Additionally, in conjunction with the pterygoid process of the sphenoid and the palatine bone, it forms the pterygopalatine fossa where the pterygopalatine (sphenopalatine) ganglion is located. Any dysfunction of these bones may affect the ganglion and its effects on mucosal secretions.

The vomer's contribution is very important to the mechanism of the pumping action of the paranasal sinuses. Its assessment is often performed with one finger placed intraorally. When treating very young children, this procedure should be done only when absolutely necessary and then only with the greatest delicacy. The examiner should never attempt intraoral palpation of the vomer if the child is not completely cooperative. An alternative procedure is to employ visualization of the vomer while palpating the anterior edge of the nasal septal cartilage.

Treat any dysfunctional areas identified. Treatment is normally performed in continuity with assessment. Because indirect treatment procedures are used preferentially for children and adolescents, the effective treatment of a given area results in further relaxation of the patient, thereby facilitating the treatment of the next area to be evaluated and treated. Furthermore, when performing indirect techniques, tissue responses are continuously monitored, so that in acute conditions the patient's tolerance to the procedure is also continuously assessed. The tissues dictate the treatment; they guide your actions and determine the dosage.

The upper thoracic region should be treated for its sympathetic somatovisceral effects, to facilitate lymphatic drainage of the head and neck, and for functional reasons because it is the foundation on which the above structures rest. The occipitocervical junction should be treated for its reflex impact on the trigeminal nerve and its relationship to the cranial base. The sphenoid, frontal and facial bones should be treated for their direct effect on the paranasal sinuses.

Paranasal sinuses are intraosseous cavities and their drainage is dependent on the inherent motility of their respective bones: frontal, sphenoid, ethmoid and maxillae. As such, intraosseous dysfunctions of any of these bones can impact the associated sinus. Specifically pumping the individual bones may be employed to facilitate drainage of their sinuses. Positioning the patient contributes to the drainage of the paranasal sinuses by using gravity. Drainage of the sinuses is best performed as follows:

- drainage of the frontal sinus in the seated position
- drainage of the sphenoidal sinus in the seated position with the head of the patient bent forward
- drainage of the maxillary sinus in the supine position with the patient's head rotated to the

opposite side so that the sinus to be drained is up.

When treating the vomer, if the child resists the digital intraoral approach, the child's pacifier, if they have one, may be utilized. By allowing the child to actively suck on the pacifier the resultant alternation of intraoral pressure and tongue movement, pressing the pacifier on the roof of the child's mouth, may be employed to manipulate the vomer, while the practitioner works on the adjacent sphenoid and ethmoid bones.

Advice to caregivers

The caregiver should be encouraged to maintain a healthy lifestyle for the child, including a balanced diet with adequate hydration and the avoidance, as much as possible, of refined carbohydrate.

Respiratory exercises including nasal respiration and diaphragmatic breathing may be taught. Vocal activities such as humming can be beneficially employed to increase sinus ventilation.[93]

PHARYNGITIS AND TONSILLITIS

The pharynx is a musculomembranous half-cylinder that connects the nasal and oral cavities with the larynx and esophagus. It extends from the base of the skull to the level of the sixth cervical vertebra where it joins the esophagus. The pharynx is divided into three portions: the nasopharynx located above the hard palate, the oropharynx that extends from the hard palate to the base of the epiglottis and the laryngopharynx from the base of the tongue to the larynx. The oropharynx can be further subdivided into the retropalatal or velopharynx from the hard palate to the caudal margin of the soft palate and retroglossal from the most inferior tip of the soft palate to the base of the epiglottis (Fig. 7.3.16).

The pharyngeal wall consists of an internal mucous layer, an intermediate fibrous layer and an external layer of skeletal muscle. In the superior part of the pharynx, the pharyngobasilar fascia is the thickest portion of the intermediate fibrous layer of the pharyngeal wall and is firmly attached to the base of the skull. The attachment forms an irregular U-shaped line. The anterior part inserts on the posterior margin of the medial plate of the sphenoidal pterygoid process. It then curves under the cartilaginous part of the PTs where it inserts onto the petrous part of the temporal bone and continues to the pharyngeal tubercle of the occipital basilar part to meet the attachment from the other side (Fig. 7.3.17).

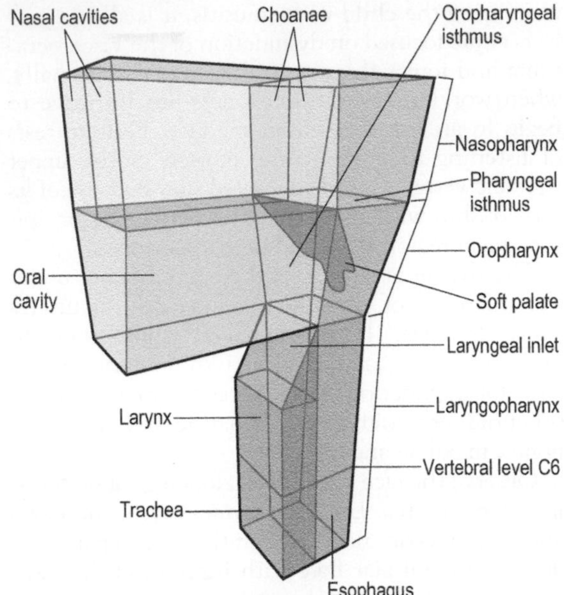

Figure 7.3.16. *Pharynx.*

The anterior part of the pharyngeal wall is not continuous; rather, it has multiple attachments to the medial pterygoid plate, the pterygomandibular raphe, the mandible, the tongue, the hyoid bone, and the thyroid and cricoid cartilages.

Six muscles contribute to constitute the pharyngeal wall. The bilateral superior, middle and inferior constrictor muscles constrict the pharyngeal cavity and, on each side, three longitudinal muscles – the stylopharyngeus, salpingopharyngeus and palatopharyngeus – elevate the pharyngeal wall and participate in swallowing (Figs 7.3.18, 7.3.19). The fibers of the three constrictor muscles fan out posteriorly into the median pharyngeal raphe, a fibrous band that is attached above to the pharyngeal tubercle of the occipital basilar part. The pharyngeal raphe descends to the level of the sixth cervical vertebra where it blends into the posterior wall of the esophagus. A thin retropharyngeal space filled by loose areolar tissue connects the pharynx with the cervical portion of the vertebral column and the prevertebral fascia covering the longus colli and longus capitis muscles.

The pharynx is the common route for air and food, and seven cavities communicate with it: the two nasal cavities, the mouth, the larynx, the two tympanic cavities and the esophagus (Fig. 7.3.20). The nasal cavities open posteriorly into the nasopharynx through the choanae. The oral cavity also opens posteriorly through the oropharyngeal isthmus

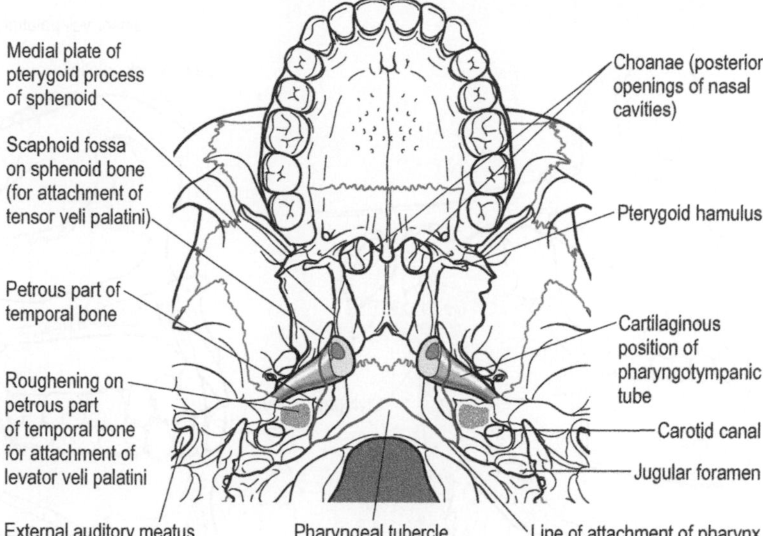

Figure 7.3.17. *Pharyngeal attachments to the base of the skull.*

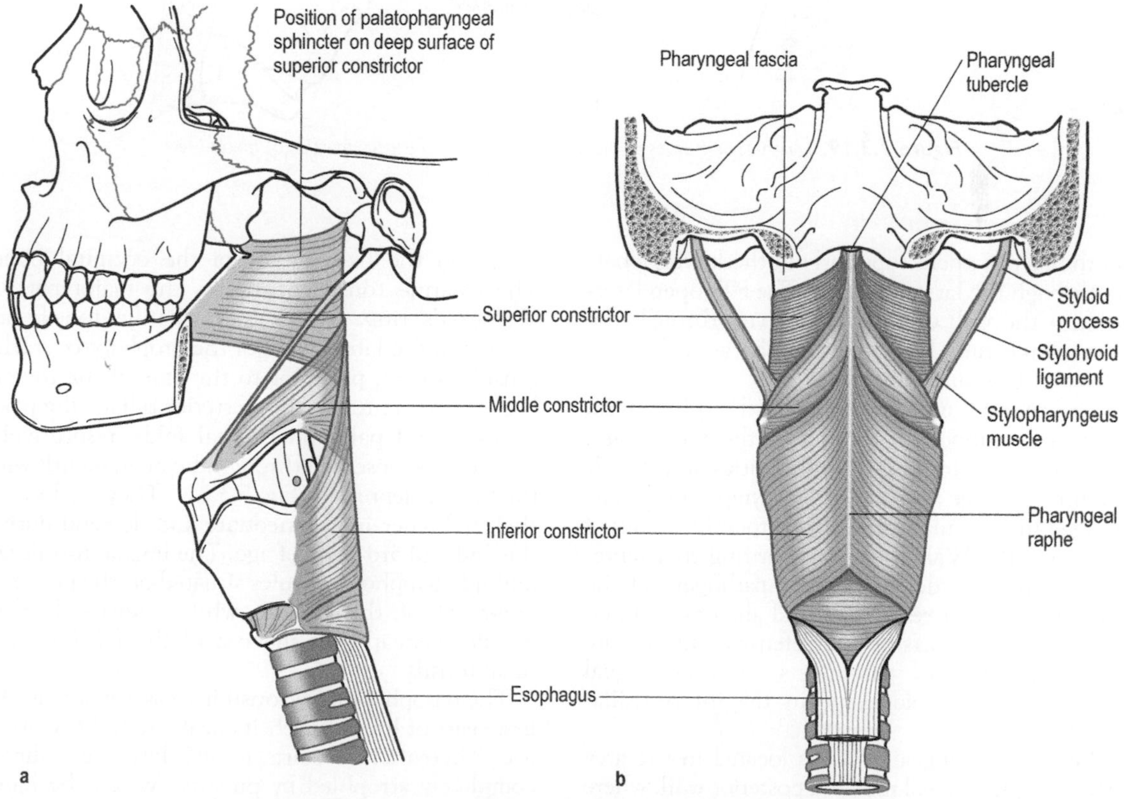

Figure 7.3.18 *Constrictor muscles of the pharynx: (a) lateral view; (b) posterior view.*

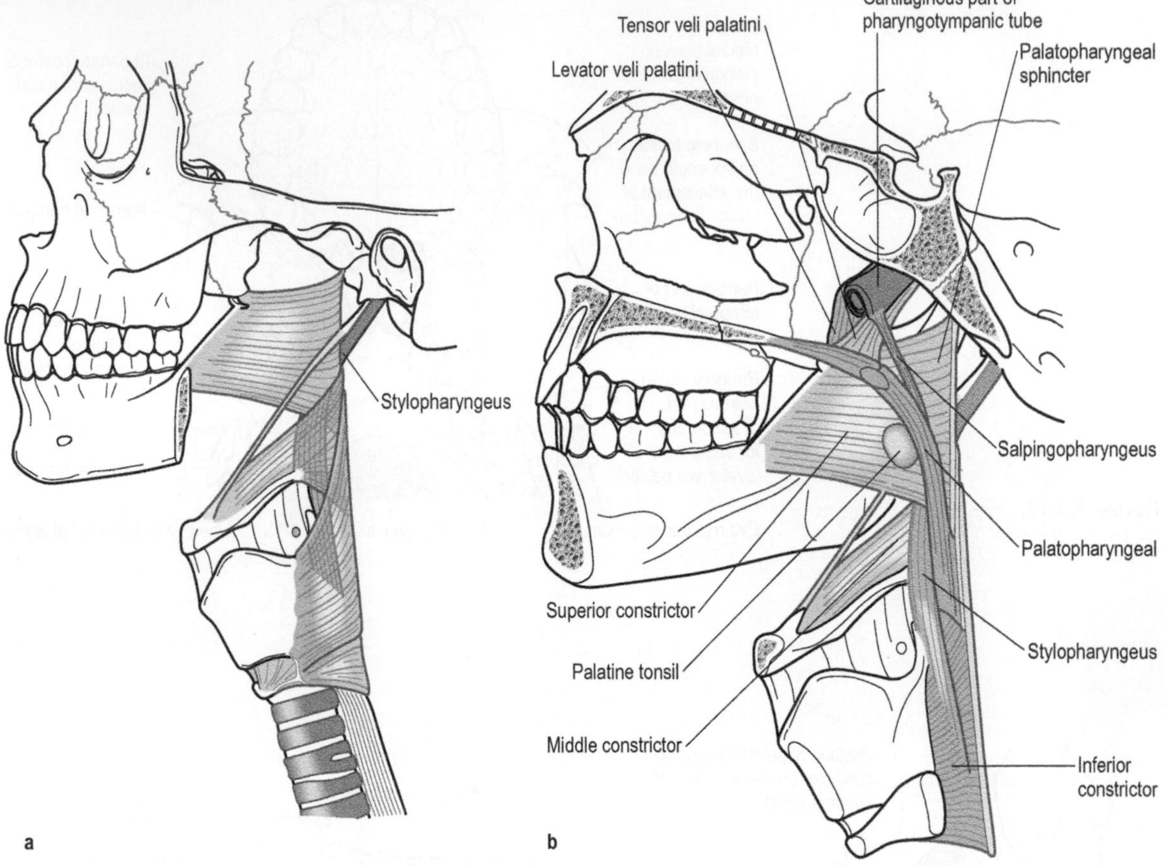

Figure 7.3.19. *Longitudinal muscles of the pharynx: (a) stylopharyngeus muscle; (b) medial view.*

and the larynx opens superiorly in the laryngopharynx through the laryngeal inlet. The PTs open laterally into the wall of the nasopharynx through the pharyngeal ostium located in the pharyngeal recess, or fossa of Rosenmüller.

The internal mucous layer of the pharyngeal cavity is continuous with that of the mouth and larynx and that lining the nasal cavities and PTs. It contains a large collection of lymphoid tissue, arranged in a circular orientation around the wall of the throat, the Waldeyer's tonsillar ring that represents the primary defense against pathogens at the entry of the upper respiratory and alimentary tract. The constituent parts of this defensive annulus are the nasopharyngeal, palatine, tubal and lingual tonsils, plus lymphoid tissue in the intertonsillar intervals.

The nasopharyngeal tonsil is located in the area of the nasopharyngeal roof and posterior wall, where the mucosa covers the inferior part of the sphenoidal body and the basilar part of the occipital bone. The palatine tonsil constitutes the major part of Waldeyer's ring. The paired palatine tonsils are located in the lateral wall of the oropharynx, in the tonsillar fossae, posterior to the base of the tongue between the anterior and posterior pillars, the palatoglossal and palatopharyngeal folds, respectively. They can be observed through the open mouth with the tongue depressed (Fig. 7.3.21). They are located slightly higher in the neonate and descend during the 2nd and 3rd years of age. The lingual tonsils are multiple lymphoid nodules situated on the posterior one-third of the tongue while additional small nodules beneath the mucosa of the PT form the tubal tonsils.

The nasopharyngeal tonsil increases in size in the first years of life to reach its peak around 6 years of age. Thereafter, it starts to involute until almost completely atrophied by puberty. When the nasopharyngeal tonsil is enlarged it is referred to as

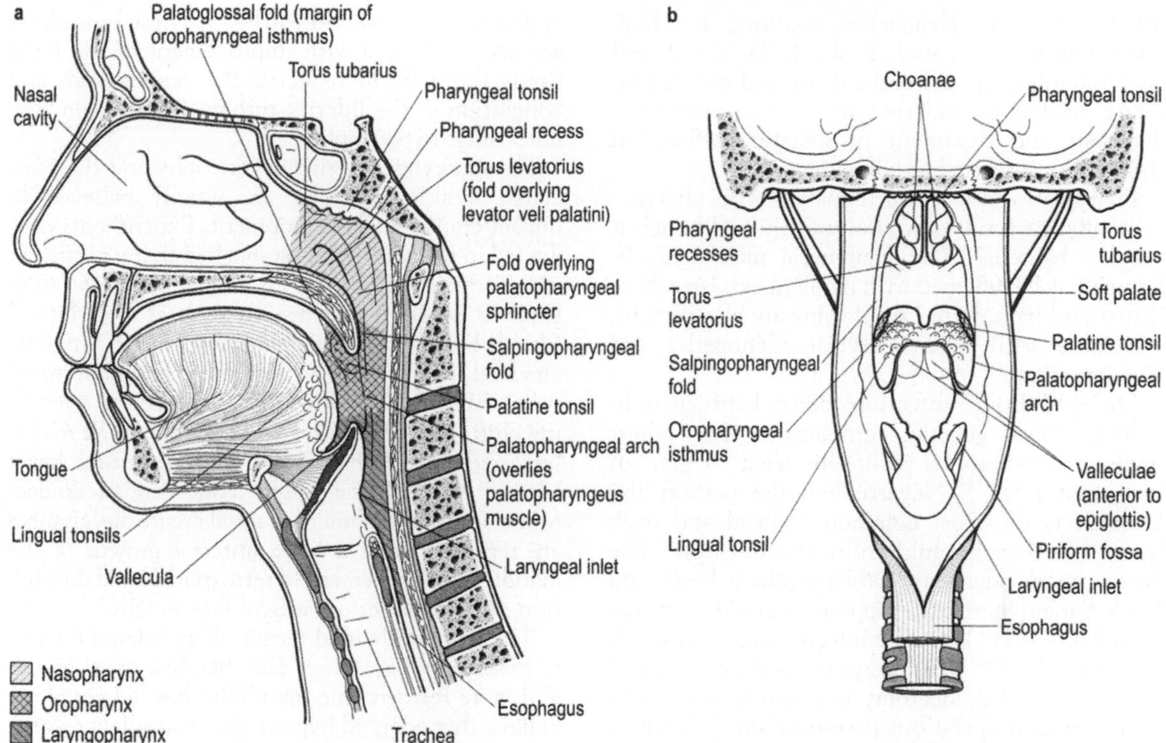

Figure 7.3.20. *Sagittal section of the oral and pharyngeal regions in the adult: (a) lateral view; (b) posterior view with the pharyngeal wall opened.*

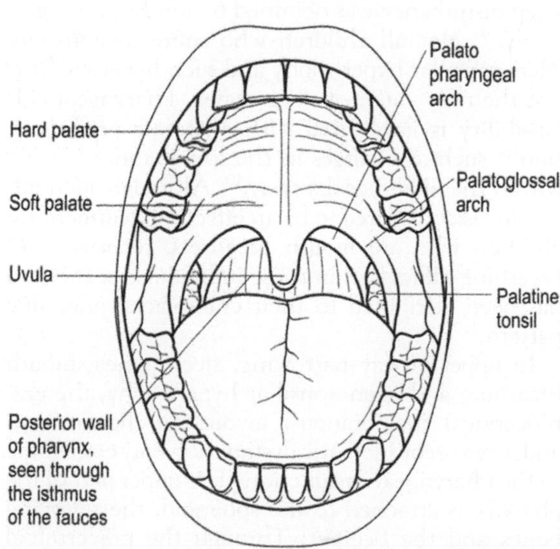

Figure 7.3.21. *The palatine tonsils located in the lateral wall of the oropharynx are observed through the open mouth, with the tongue depressed.*

adenoid or adenoids; 'tonsils' is usually the common name for the palatine tonsils.

Waldeyer's tonsillar ring is located at a strategic point where numerous antigens, both food-supported and airborne, first come into contact with the body. Thus, it plays an important role in the immune system as a site of antigen recognition and synthesis of antibodies, including IgE.[94] The nasopharyngeal and palatine tonsils are major sources of T lymphocytes that participate in cell-mediated immunity and B lymphocytes that produce immunoglobulins.[95] The nasopharyngeal tonsil also seems to participate in immune peripheral tolerance to harmless foreign antigens commonly inhaled or present in digested nutrients.[96]

Bacterial, or less frequently viral, infections are most often responsible for tonsillitis, where the tonsils may be acutely inflamed. Bacterial infections are often streptococcal, usually from group A streptococci, the most virulent species in humans. Differential diagnosis between viral and bacterial infection, based on physical examination alone, is difficult. Tonsillitis is characterized by sore throat and pain, particularly during swallowing, which may involve the ears. Headaches, vomiting and high fever may be associated. It should be noted that bacterial infections are correctly treated with appropriate antibiotics and that in these instances the diagnosis and treatment of somatic dysfunction should be considered as adjunctive.

Pharyngitis, an acute inflammation of the pharynx, is usually the result of a viral infection, although it may be bacterial. The pharyngeal mucous membranes may be inflamed with purulent exudates. Sore throat and pain during swallowing are also present, associated with fever, cervical adenopathy and leukocytosis.

Susceptibility to infections differs between individuals. Host genetic components that adjust immune responses to pathogens seem to play an important role.[97,98] Nevertheless, the peritonsillar location is the most common of head and neck space infections in children in 49% of cases.[99] The American Academy of Otolaryngology–Head and Neck Surgery currently proposes adenoidectomy as a guideline after '3 or more infections of tonsils and/or adenoids per year despite adequate medical therapy'.[100] Adenoidectomy is currently one of the most common operations performed on children in the United States.[39,101]

Besides bacterial and viral infections, allergies such as allergic rhinitis are considered to be common risk factors for adenoid hypertrophy.[102] The continuity between the internal mucous layer of the pharyngeal cavity, the nasal cavities, the mouth, the larynx, the tympanic cavities and the esophagus explains the interrelationship and diversity of clinical presentations in allergic conditions.

Increased immune activity results in hypertrophy of Waldeyer's tonsillar ring, in particular at the level of the nasopharyngeal tonsil. Chronic nasal airway obstruction may follow a condition quite common in childhood that leads to a persistent mouth-open posture and mouth breathing. Adenotonsillar hypertrophy has also been associated with a myriad of symptoms such as obstructive sleep disorder syndrome, nocturnal snoring, rhinosinusitis, hyponasal speech and impairment of the ability to smell.[103] Furthermore, hypertrophy of the nasopharyngeal tonsil or adenoids predisposes the individual to recurrent otitis media or otitis media with effusion, in part because of the diminution of the patency of the orifices of the PT, located just laterally to the nasopharyngeal tonsil.

Tonsillectomy and adenoidectomy in children is reported to improve symptoms associated with obstructive sleep apnea syndrome, such as snoring and restless sleep, as well as behavioral, emotional and neurocognitive difficulties.[104] These procedures are also associated with improvement of the nasal cavity geometry by reducing the venous stasis and congestion of the inferior turbinate present in adenotonsillar hypertrophy.[105]

Nasopharyngeal tonsil hypertrophy and the associated mouth breathing are usually believed to impact craniofacial development. Experiments conducted in primates have established that a persistent mouth-open posture and associated oral respiration leads to dental malocclusions such as cross-bite.[106] Mouth-breather children may present with a narrow, elevated palate and a decreased nasopharyngeal space. In such cases, they may demonstrate a receding chin (retrognathia) with crowding of the maxillary and mandibular teeth, and increased lower anterior vertical face height. Following adenoidectomies and establishment of nasal breathing, changes are reported, with a more anterior growth of the mandible, improvement of retrognathia and diminution of lower anterior vertical face height.[107]

The commonly used terminology 'adenoid' facies to describe longer lower face heights, open mouth and more retrognathic mandibles has led people to believe that adenoid hypertrophy was solely responsible for mouth breathing and associated disorders. This is an overly simplified conclusion. Once again, a multifactorial approach to diagnosis and, consequently, treatment may be necessary.

A study of children 12 years after adenotonsillectomy showed that upper airway narrowing during sleep was still present, although some resolution of sleep disturbance was obtained 6 months postoperatively.[108] Not all children who snore demonstrate adenotonsillar hypertrophy and such hypertrophy is not the only cause of sleep apnea. Pharyngeal collapsibility is implicated with anatomic predisposition[109] such as changes in the longitudinal tension within the pharyngeal airway.[109] Although adenoidectomy is considered to be an effective treatment for children who are mouth breathers, recurrence of breathing difficulties in these individuals occurs and has been attributed to their craniofacial anatomic pattern.[110]

In upper airway narrowing, sleep apnea, mouth breathing and adenotonsillar hypertrophy, the craniocervical membranous, myofascial, ligamentous and interosseous somatic dysfunction may contribute to the pharyngeal dysfunction. The upper part of the pharynx is attached to the sphenoid, the temporal bones and the occiput. Through the prevertebral fascia the pharynx is linked to the cervical spine and movements of the cervical spine are associated with changes of pharyngeal size: cervical flexion decreases oropharyngeal size; cervical extension does the opposite.[111–113]

Any dysfunction of the cervical spine or of any of the structures on which the pharynx is inserted can impair normal pharyngeal function. Movement is necessary to mobilize body fluids, particularly lymph, and somatic dysfunction affecting the structures surrounding lymph nodes and vessels is associated with impaired motion and can thus interfere with lymph flow. Lymphatic vessels from the pharynx drain into the deep cervical lymph nodes through the retropharyngeal, paratracheal and infrahyoid nodes. The retropharyngeal nodes consist of a median and two lateral groups located in front of the lateral masses of the atlas. They are positioned between the pharyngeal and prevertebral fasciae and drain the nasopharynx and PT, as well as the two upper cervical joints.

The deep cervical lymph nodes are beneath the SCM muscle. Among them, a large node surrounded with several small ones forms the jugulodigastric group that receives drainage from most of the lymphatic vessels from the tonsil. The tonsils differ from the lymph nodes in that they do not receive afferent lymphatic vessels. Small lymphatic vessels organize as efferents from the tonsils that traverse the superior constrictor muscle before draining to the jugulodigastric nodes. Located against the posterior belly of the digastric muscle, these nodes swell during tonsillitis and may be palpable in front of the anterior border of the digastric muscle, below the mandibular angle.

The vessels that supply the pharyngeal wall come from the external carotid artery. The tonsillar branch of the facial artery (external maxillary) is the main blood supply to the palatine tonsil. The veins of the pharynx drain through the pterygoid plexus in the infratemporal fossa and into the facial and internal jugular veins.

Physical examination and treatment

Because the pharynx is so intimately linked to the cervical spine and the cranial base, as well as associated muscles and fasciae, optimal pharyngeal function necessitates that these areas are unimpaired. The upper thoracic spine is the anatomic origin of the sympathetic supply to the pharynx and, consequently, along with associated ribs, should also be considered when addressing pharyngeal dysfunction and disease. Finally, the functional freedom of the clavicles, thoracic inlet and cervical spine, together with associated soft tissues above, is necessary to facilitate lymphatic drainage of the pharynx.

Having performed a total body structural examination to identify the global postural pattern and its relationship to the pharyngeal complaint, with the child in a supine position, it is appropriate to begin the local examination by evaluating the cervical and upper thoracic regions. First, palpate for tissue texture abnormalities in the paravertebral muscles and superficial soft tissues, looking for areas of muscular tension and subcutaneous edema. Similarly, palpate the anterior and lateral aspects of the neck. Observe and palpate the location of the hyoid bone and larynx that should be in the midline. Palpation of the anterior neck structures should be done with great delicacy to prevent irritating already inflamed tissues and because this is an area of increased sensitivity, particularly in infants who were born with a nuchal cord. Assess the anterior and lateral cervical musculature, paying specific attention to the SCM muscle because of its relationship to the deep cervical lymph nodes. Follow the SCM inferiorly to its attachment on the clavicles and assess clavicular motion.

Evaluate the cervical vertebrae, noting the alignment of the spinous processes. Clinical experience has shown a strong association between pharyngitis and cervical articular somatic dysfunction that, when treated, appears to prevent recurrent pharyngitis. Next, evaluate the upper thoracic vertebrae and associated ribs.

Assess the functional status of the cranial base, noting the relationships between the occiput, temporal bones and sphenoid. The pharynx is suspended beneath the skull and tone of the pharyngeal musculature is impacted by cranial dysfunction. For proper function, the pharyngeal muscles require precise interrelationships between their origins and insertions. Dysfunctional mechanics that affect these relationships will impair function of the pharynx and associated Waldeyer's tonsillar ring.

The pharyngeal tonsil is located directly beneath the cranial base, at the level of the sphenobasilar junction. As such, freedom of motion of the cranial base may facilitate lymphatic drainage of the adenoids.

Mandibular function should also be examined. Dysfunction of the mandible may impact anterior cervical myofascial function, contribute to impaired lymphatic drainage of the jugulodigastric node and participate in chronic mouth breathing.

Apply indirect principles to treat any identified articular dysfunction of the spine, ribs and clavicles. Myofascial release techniques may be employed to address pharyngeal, anterior cervical and spinal muscular dysfunctions. Normalizing the cranial and thoracoabdominal diaphragms and the thoracic inlet may be employed to promote lymphatic and venous circulation. Following the inherent motility of the PRM may enhance all of these interventions. This slow, gentle rhythm is soothing to the child and is integral in the maintenance of homeostasis.[114]

REFERENCES

1. Lanphear BP, Byrd RS, Auinger P, Hall CB. Increasing prevalence of recurrent otitis media among children in the United States. Pediatrics 1997;99(3):E1.
2. Rovers MM, Schilder AG, Zielhuis GA, Rosenfeld RM. Otitis media. Lancet 2004;363(9407):465–73.
3. Paananen R, Sormunen R, Glumoff V, van Eijk M, Hallman M. Surfactant proteins A and D in Eustachian tube epithelium. Am J Physiol Lung Cell Mol Physiol 2001;281(3): L660–7.
4. American Academy of Pediatrics Subcommittee on Management of Acute Otitis Media. Diagnosis and management of acute otitis media. Pediatrics 2004;113(5):1451–65.
5. Ehrlich GD, Post JC. Susceptibility to otitis media: strong evidence that genetics plays a role. JAMA 1999;282(22): 2167–9.
6. Casselbrant ML, Mandel EM, Rockette HE et al. The genetic component of middle ear disease in the first 5 years of life. Arch Otolaryngol Head Neck Surg 2004;130(3): 273–8.
7. Kvaerner KJ, Nafstad P, Jaakkola JJ. Upper respiratory morbidity in preschool children: a cross-sectional study. Arch Otolaryngol Head Neck Surg 2000;126(10):1201–6.
8. Fireman P. Otitis media and eustachian tube dysfunction: connection to allergic rhinitis. J Allergy Clin Immunol 1997;99(2):S787–97.
9. Rovers MM, Zielhuis GA, Straatman H, Ingels K, van der Wilt GJ, van den Broek P. Prognostic factors for persistent otitis media with effusion in infants. Arch Otolaryngol Head Neck Surg 1999;125(11):1203–7.
10. Daly KA, Brown JE, Lindgren BR, Meland MH, Le CT, Giebink GS. Epidemiology of otitis media onset by six months of age. Pediatrics 1999;103(6 Pt 1):1158–66.
11. Niemela M, Uhari M, Mottonen M. A pacifier increases the risk of recurrent acute otitis media in children in day care centers. Pediatrics 1995;96(5 Pt 1):884–8.
12. Niemela M, Pihakari O, Pokka T, Uhari M. Pacifier as a risk factor for acute otitis media: a randomized, controlled trial of parental counseling. Pediatrics 2000;106(3):483–8.
13. Alho OP, Oja H, Koivu M, Sorri M. Risk factors for chronic otitis media with effusion in infancy. Each acute otitis media episode induces a high but transient risk. Arch Otolaryngol Head Neck Surg 1995;121(8):839–43.
14. Bennett KE, Haggard MP. Accumulation of factors influencing children's middle ear disease: risk factor modelling on a large population cohort. J Epidemiol Community Health 1998;52(12):786–93.
15. Paradise JL, Rockette HE, Colborn DK et al. Otitis media in 2253 Pittsburgh-area infants: prevalence and risk factors during the first two years of life. Pediatrics 1997;99(3): 318–33.
16. Duffy LC, Faden H, Wasielewski R, Wolf J, Krystofik D. Exclusive breastfeeding protects against bacterial colonization and day care exposure to otitis media. Pediatrics 1997;100(4):E7.
17. Williams PL (ed). Gray's anatomy, 38th edn. Edinburgh: Churchill Livingstone; 1995.
18. Koc A, Ekinci G, Bilgili AM, Akpinar IN, Yakut H, Han T. Evaluation of the mastoid air cell system by high resolution computed tomography: three-dimensional multiplanar volume rendering technique. J Laryngol Otol 2003;117(8): 595–8.
19. Park MS, Yoo SH, Lee DH. Measurement of surface area in human mastoid air cell system. J Laryngol Otol 2000;114(2): 93–6.
20. Okubo J, Watanabe I. Aeration of the tympanomastoid cavity and the Eustachian tube. Acta Otolaryngol Suppl 1990;471:13–24.
21. Kemaloglu YK, Goksu N, Ozbilen S, Akyildiz N. Otitis media with effusion and craniofacial analysis – II: 'Mastoid–middle ear–Eustachian tube system' in children with secretory otitis media. Int J Pediatr Otorhinolaryngol 1995;32: 69–76.
22. Sade J, Fuchs C. Secretory otitis media in adults: II. The role of mastoid pneumatization as a prognostic factor. Ann Otol Rhinol Laryngol 1997;106(1):37–40.
23. Ishijima K, Sando I, Balaban C, Suzuki C, Takasaki K. Length of the Eustachian tube and its postnatal development: computer-aided three-dimensional reconstruction and measurement study. Ann Otol Rhinol Laryngol 2000; 109(6):542–8.
24. Prades JM, Dumollard JM, Calloc'h F, Merzougui N, Veyret C, Martin C. Descriptive anatomy of the human auditory tube. Surg Radiol Anat 1998;20(5):335–40.
25. Sudo M, Sando I. Developmental changes in folding of the human Eustachian tube. Acta Otolaryngol 1996;116(2): 307–11.
26. Ikarashi F, Takahashi S, Yamamoto Y. Carbon dioxide exchange via the mucosa in healthy middle ear. Arch Otolaryngol Head Neck Surg 1999;125(9):975–8.
27. Bluestone CD. Pathogenesis of otitis media: role of Eustachian tube. Pediatr Infect Dis J 1996;15(4):281–91.
28. Huang MH, Lee ST, Rajendran K. A fresh cadaveric study of the paratubal muscles: implications for Eustachian tube function in cleft palate. Plast Reconstr Surg 1997;100(4): 833–42.
29. Barsoumian R, Kuehn DP, Moon JB, Canady JW. An anatomic study of the tensor veli palatini and dilatator tubae muscles in relation to Eustachian tube and velar function. Cleft Palate Craniofac J 1998;35(2):101–10.
30. Bylander A, Tjernstrom O. Changes in Eustachian tube function with age in children with normal ears. A longitudinal study. Acta Otolaryngol 1983;96(5–6):467–77.
31. Mew JR, Meredith GW. Middle ear effusion: an orthodontic perspective. J Laryngol Otol 1992;106(1):7–13.
32. McDonnell JP, Needleman HL, Charchut S et al. The relationship between dental overbite and Eustachian tube dysfunction. Laryngoscope 2001;111(2):310–6.
33. Straetemans M, van Heerbeek N, Sanders EA et al. Immune status and Eustachian tube function in recurrence of otitis media with effusion. Arch Otolaryngol Head Neck Surg 2005;131(9):771–6.
34. Nguyen LH, Manoukian JJ, Tewfik TL et al. Evidence of allergic inflammation in the middle ear and nasopharynx in atopic children with otitis media with effusion. J Otolaryngol 2004;33(6):345–51.
35. Fireman P. Otitis media and eustachian tube dysfunction: connection to allergic rhinitis. J Allergy Clin Immunol 1997;99(2):S787–97.
36. Miceli Sopo S, Zorzi G, Calvani M Jr. Should we screen every child with otitis media with effusion for allergic rhinitis? Arch Dis Child 2004;89(3):287–8.

37. Nguyen LH, Manoukian JJ, Sobol SE et al. Similar allergic inflammation in the middle ear and the upper airway: evidence linking otitis media with effusion to the united airways concept. J Allergy Clin Immunol 2004;114(5): 1110–5.
38. Lack G. Pediatric allergic rhinitis and comorbid disorders. J Allergy Clin Immunol 2001;108(1 Suppl):S9–15.
39. Emerick KS, Cunningham MJ. Tubal tonsil hypertrophy: a cause of recurrent symptoms after adenoidectomy. Arch Otolaryngol Head Neck Surg 2006;132(2):153–6.
40. Heikkinen T, Chonmaitree T. Importance of respiratory viruses in acute otitis media. Clin Microbiol Rev 2003; 16(2):230–41.
41. Andrade MA, Hoberman A, Glustein J, Paradise JL, Wald ER. Acute otitis media in children with bronchiolitis. Pediatrics 1998;101(4 Pt 1):617–9.
42. Fleming DM, Pannell RS, Elliot AJ, Cross KW. Respiratory illness associated with influenza and respiratory syncytial virus infection. Arch Dis Child 2005;90(7):741–6.
43. Cingi C, Altin F, Cakli H, Entok E, Gurbuz K, Cingi E. Scintigraphic evaluation of nasal mucociliary activity in unilateral chronic otitis media. J Laryngol Otol 2005; 119(6):443–7.
44. Tasker A, Dettmar PW, Panetti M, Koufman JA, Birchall JP, Pearson JP. Reflux of gastric juice and glue ear in children. Lancet 2002;359(9305):493.
45. Tully SB, Bar-Haim Y, Bradley RL. Abnormal tympanography after supine bottle feeding. J Pediatr 1995;126(6): S105–11.
46. Roberts JE, Rosenfeld RM, Zeisel SA. Otitis media and speech and language: a meta-analysis of prospective studies. Pediatrics 2004;113(3 Pt 1):e238–48.
47. Roberts JE, Burchinal MR, Medley LP et al. Otitis media, hearing sensitivity, and maternal responsiveness in relation to language during infancy. J Pediatr 1995;126(3): 481–9.
48. Neff MJ; American Academy of Pediatrics; American Academy of Family Physicians. AAP, AAFP release guideline on diagnosis and management of acute otitis media. Am Fam Physician 2004;69(11):2713–5.
49. Cober MP, Johnson CE. Otitis media: review of the 2004 treatment guidelines. Ann Pharmacother 2005;39(11): 1879–87.
50. Johnston LC, Feldman HM, Paradise JL et al. Tympanic membrane abnormalities and hearing levels at the ages of 5 and 6 years in relation to persistent otitis media and tympanostomy tube insertion in the first 3 years of life: a prospective study incorporating a randomized clinical trial. Pediatrics 2004;114(1):e58–67.
51. Vayalumkal J, Kellner JD. Tympanocentesis for the management of acute otitis media in children: a survey of Canadian pediatricians and family physicians. Arch Pediatr Adolesc Med 2004;158(10):962–5.
52. Mills MV, Henley CE, Barnes LL, Carreiro JE, Degenhardt BF. The use of osteopathic manipulative treatment as adjuvant therapy in children with recurrent acute otitis media. Arch Pediatr Adolesc Med 2003;157(9): 861–6.
53. Dahl R, Mygind N. Anatomy, physiology and function of the nasal cavities in health and disease. Adv Drug Deliv Rev 1998;29(1–2):3–12.
54. Sutto Z, Conner GE, Salathe M. Regulation of human airway ciliary beat frequency by intracellular pH. J Physiol 2004;560(Pt 2):519–32.
55. Jang YJ, Myong NH, Park KH, Koo TW, Kim HG. Mucociliary transport and histologic characteristics of the mucosa of deviated nasal septum. Arch Otolaryngol Head Neck Surg 2002;128(4):421–4.
56. Wolf M, Naftali S, Schroter RC, Elad D. Air-conditioning characteristics of the human nose. J Laryngol Otol 2004; 118(2):87–92.
57. Rouadi P, Baroody FM, Abbott D, Naureckas E, Solway J, Naclerio RM. A technique to measure the ability of the human nose to warm and humidify air. J Appl Physiol 1999;87(1):400–6.
58. Widdicombe J. The airway vasculature. Exp Physiol 1993; 78(4):433–52.
59. Cabanac M. Selective brain cooling in humans: 'fancy' or fact? FASEB J 1993;7(12):1143–6; discussion 1146–7.
60. Widdicombe J. Microvascular anatomy of the nose. Allergy 1997;52(40 Suppl):7–11.
61. Irmak MK, Korkmaz A, Erogul O. Selective brain cooling seems to be a mechanism leading to human craniofacial diversity observed in different geographical regions. Med Hypotheses 2004;63(6):974–9.
62. Assanasen P, Baroody FM, Naureckas E, Solway J, Naclerio RM. Supine position decreases the ability of the nose to warm and humidify air. J Appl Physiol 2001;91(6):2459–65.
63. Werntz DA, Bickford RG, Bloom FE, Shannahoff-Khalsa DS. Alternating cerebral hemispheric activity and the lateralization of autonomic nervous function. Hum Neurobiol 1983;2:39–43.
64. Werntz DA, Bickford RG, Shannahoff-Khalsa D. Selective hemispheric stimulation by unilateral forced nostril breathing. Hum Neurobiol 1987;6(3):165–71.
65. Baraniuk JN, Kaliner M. Neuropeptides and nasal secretion. Am J Physiol 1991;261(4 Pt 1):L223–35.
66. Fontanari P, Burnet H, Zattara-Hartmann MC, Jammes Y. Changes in airway resistance induced by nasal inhalation of cold dry, dry, or moist air in normal individuals. J Appl Physiol 1996;81(4):1739–43.
67. Lacroix JS. Chronic rhinosinusitis and neuropeptides. Swiss Med Wkly 2003;133(41–42):560–2.
68. Fischer A, Wussow A, Cryer A, Schmeck B, Noga O, Zweng M, Peiser C, Dimb QT, Heppt W, Groneberg DA. Neuronal plasticity in persistant perennial allergic rhinitis. J Occup Environ Med 2005;47(1):20–5.
69. Skoner DP. Allergic rhinitis: definition, epidemiology, pathophysiology, detection, and diagnosis. J Allergy Clin Immunol 2001;108(1 Suppl):S2–8.
70. Skoner DP. Complications of allergic rhinitis. J Allergy Clin Immunol 2000;105(6 Pt 2):S605–9.
71. Noverr MC, Huffnagle GB. The 'microflora hypothesis' of allergic diseases. Clin Exp Allergy 2005;35(12):1511–20.
72. Ng DK, Chan CH, Kwok KL, Cheung JM. Allergic rhinitis as a risk factor for habitual snoring in children. Chest 2005;127(6):2285–6; author reply 2286.
73. Schoenwetter WF, Dupclay L Jr, Appajosyula S, Botteman MF, Pashos CL. Economic impact and quality-of-life burden of allergic rhinitis. Curr Med Res Opin 2004;20(3):305–17.
74. Blaiss MS; Allergic Rhinitis in Schoolchildren Consensus Group. Allergic rhinitis and impairment issues in schoolchildren: a consensus report. Curr Med Res Opin 2004; 20(12):1937–52.
75. Juniper EF, Guyatt GH, Dolovich J. Assessment of quality of life in adolescents with allergic rhinoconjunctivitis: development and testing of a questionnaire for clinical trials. J Allergy Clin Immunol 1994;93(2):413–23.

76. Cherbut C. Inulin and oligofructose in the dietary fibre concept. Br J Nutr 2002;87(Suppl 2):S159–62.
77. Fireman P. Diagnosis of sinusitis in children: emphasis on the history and physical examination. J Allergy Clin Immunol 1992;90:433–6.
78. Gruber DP, Brockmeyer D. Pediatric skull base surgery. 1. Embryology and developmental anatomy. Pediatr Neurosurg 2003;38(1):2–8.
79. American Academy of Pediatrics Subcommittee on Management of Sinusitis and Committee on Quality Improvement. Clinical practice guideline: management of sinusitis. Pediatrics 2001;108(3):798–808.
80. McLaughlin RB Jr, Rehl RM, Lanza DC. Clinically relevant frontal sinus anatomy and physiology. Otolaryngol Clin North Am 2001;34(1):1–22.
81. Lewandowski K, Busch T, Lohbrunner H et al. Low nitric oxide concentrations in exhaled gas and nasal airways of mammals without paranasal sinuses. J Appl Physiol 1998;85(2):405–10.
82. Lundberg JO, Weitzberg E. Nasal nitric oxide in man. Thorax 1999;54(10):947–52.
83. Settergren G, Angdin M, Astudillo R et al. Decreased pulmonary vascular resistance during nasal breathing: modulation by endogenous nitric oxide from the paranasal sinuses. Acta Physiol Scand 1998;163(3):235–9.
84. Swift AC, Campbell IT, McKown TM. Oronasal obstruction, lung volumes, and arterial oxygenation. Lancet 1988;1(8577):73–5.
85. Rappai M, Collop N, Kemp S, deShazo R. The nose and sleep-disordered breathing: what we know and what we do not know. Chest 2003;124(6):2309–23.
86. Smart BA, Slavin RG. Rhinosinusitis and pediatric asthma. Immunol Allergy Clin North Am 2005;25(1):67–82.
87. Wald ER. Chronic sinusitis in children. J Pediatr 1995; 127(3):339–47.
88. Aust R, Drettner B. The functional size of the human maxillary ostium in vivo. Acta Otolaryngol 1975;78:432–5.
89. Maltinski G. Nasal disorders and sinusitis. Prim Care 1998;25(3):663–83.
90. Olnes SQ, Schwartz RH, Bahadori RS. Consultation with the specialist: diagnosis and management of the newborn and young infant who have nasal obstruction. Pediatr Rev 2000;21(12):416–20.
91. Sutherland WG. Teachings in the science of osteopathy. Fort Worth, TX: Sutherland Cranial Teaching Foundation; 1991:84.
92. Sutherland WG. Teachings in the science of osteopathy. Fort Worth, TX: Sutherland Cranial Teaching Foundation; 1991:105.
93. Weitzberg E, Lundberg JO. Humming greatly increases nasal nitric oxide. Am J Respir Crit Care Med 2002; 166(2):144–5.
94. Ganzer U, Bachert C. Localization of IgE synthesis in immediate-type allergy of the upper respiratory tract. ORL J Otorhinolaryngol Relat Spec 1988;50(4):257–64.
95. Bourges D, Wang CH, Chevaleyre C, Salmon H. T and IgA B lymphocytes of the pharyngeal and palatine tonsils: differential expression of adhesion molecules and chemokines. Scand J Immunol 2004;60(4):338–50.
96. Pajusto M, Tarkkanen J, Mattila PS. Human primary adenotonsillar naive phenotype CD45RA CD4 T lymphocytes undergo apoptosis upon stimulation with a high concentration of CD3 antibody. Scand J Immunol 2005;62(6): 546–51.
97. Kotb M, Norrby-Teglund A, McGeer A, Green K, Low DE. Association of human leukocyte antigen with outcomes of infectious diseases: the streptococcal experience. Scand J Infect Dis 2003;35(9):665–9.
98. Goldmann O, Chhatwal GS, Medina E. Role of host genetic factors in susceptibility to group A streptococcal infections. Indian J Med Res 2004;119(Suppl):141–3.
99. Ungkanont K, Yellon RF, Weissman JL et al. Head and neck space infections in infants and children. Otolaryngol Head Neck Surg 1995;112:375.
100. American Academy of Otolaryngology–Head and Neck Surgery. 2000 Clinical indicators compendium. Alexandria, VA; 2000:19. [Bulletin June 2000, Vol 19, No. 6]
101. Paradise JL, Bluestone CD, Colborn DK, Bernard BS, Rockette HE, Kurs-Lasky M. Tonsillectomy and adenotonsillectomy for recurrent throat infection in moderately affected children. Pediatrics 2002;110(1 Pt 1):7–15.
102. Huang SW, Giannoni C. The risk of adenoid hypertrophy in children with allergic rhinitis. Ann Allergy Asthma Immunol 2001;87(4):350–5.
103. Paradise JL, Bernard BS, Colborn DK, Janosky JE. Assessment of adenoidal obstruction in children: clinical signs versus roentgenographic findings. Pediatrics 1998;101(6): 979–86.
104. Goldstein NA, Post JC, Rosenfeld RM, Campbell TF. Impact of tonsillectomy and adenoidectomy on child behavior. Arch Otolaryngol Head Neck Surg 2000;126(4): 494–8.
105. Kim YK, Kang JH, Yoon KS. Acoustic rhinometric evaluation of nasal cavity and nasopharynx after adenoidectomy and tonsillectomy. Int J Pediatr Otorhinolaryngol 1998; 44(3):215–20.
106. Harvold EP, Tomer BS, Vargervik K, Chierici G. Primate experiments on oral respiration. Am J Orthod 1981;79(4): 359–72.
107. Kerr WJ, McWilliam JS, Linder-Aronson S. Mandibular form and position related to changed mode of breathing – a fiveyear longitudinal study. Angle Orthod 1989;59(2): 91–6.
108. Tasker C, Crosby JH, Stradling JR. Evidence for persistence of upper airway narrowing during sleep, 12 years after adenotonsillectomy. Arch Dis Child 2002;86(1):34–7.
109. Schwartz AR, Eisele DW, Smith PL. Pharyngeal airway obstruction in obstructive sleep apnea: pathophysiology and clinical implications. Otolaryngol Clin North Am 1998; 31(6):911–8.
110. Finkelstein Y, Wexler D, Berger G, Nachmany A, Shapiro-Feinberg M, Ophir D. Anatomical basis of sleep-related breathing abnormalities in children with nasal obstruction. Arch Otolaryngol Head Neck Surg 2000; 126(5):593–600.
111. Reed WR, Roberts JL, Thach BT. Factors influencing regional patency and configuration of the human infant upper airway. J Appl Physiol 1985;58(2):635–44.
112. Thut DC, Schwartz AR, Roach D, Wise RA, Permutt S, Smith PL. Tracheal and neck position influence upper airway airflow dynamics by altering airway length. J Appl Physiol 1993;75(5):2084–90.
113. Isono S, Tanaka A, Tagaito Y, Ishikawa T, Nishino T. Influences of head positions and bite opening on collapsibility of the passive pharynx. J Appl Physiol 2004;97(1): 339–46.
114. Hyndman BW. The role of rhythms in homeostasis. Kybernetik 1974;15:227–36.

7.4 RESPIRATORY DYSFUNCTIONS

MOUTH BREATHING

Humans may breathe through their noses, mouths or intermittently through both. It is commonly held that, between birth and at least 2 months of age, infants breathe exclusively through their noses. This belief has, however, been challenged and some authors propose that infants are 'preferential nasal breathers' rather than 'obligate nasal breathers'.[1] In older children and adults, under normal conditions and at rest, the nasal respiratory route is used, and oronasal breathing occurs typically when a higher degree of ventilation is necessary, as during exercise.

In order to breathe through the nose, the nasal airway (nostril, nasal cavity and nasopharynx) should be patent. Nasal obstruction consists of partial or complete blockage of one or more of these components of the air passages. In the newborn, the posterior nasal aperture may be blocked by choanal atresia. Because of the infant's preferential nasal breathing route, such total nasal obstruction is a medical emergency.[2]

In the young infant, and later in life, several other factors can cause nasal airway obstruction. 'Stuffy nose' or rhinitis is a common cause of nasal obstruction in young infants that results in mouth breathing (see p. 224). Viral upper respiratory tract infections, foreign body, deviated nasal septum, hypertrophy of the inferior turbinates and nasal polyps are other factors that can also predispose to mouth breathing and produce an open mouth posture. Nasal endoscopy may be necessary to assess children with severe nasal obstruction that may require surgical repair.[3]

Tonsillar hypertrophy is believed by many to be the main cause of nasal obstruction in children. The pharyngeal tonsil, or adenoids, is a large collection of lymphoid tissue located beneath the roof of the nasopharynx, at the level of the SBS. Enlargement of the pharyngeal tonsil commonly occurs as the result of frequent bacterial or viral infections and can obstruct the nasopharyngeal route so that mouth breathing is the only possible alternative. 'Tonsils' is the common name for the palatine tonsils, which are lymphoid tissue located laterally on the oropharyngeal walls, just posterior to the base of the tongue.

Children with enlarged adenoids are described as having 'adenoidal facies' (long faces). They share common features with other mouth breathers, having low body weight and short stature, circles around their eyes, receding chins, small mouths, dry, large lower lips and short upper lips that are held apart from one another. They also tend to have multiple allergies and to demonstrate a specific postural configuration, the most commonly described feature of which is the anteriorly displaced or extended position of the head.[4]

Efficient respiration is the result of multiple intricate neurophysiologic processes and several anatomic structures contribute to this complex system. The extended, or forward, head posture may follow nasal obstruction as a solution to compromised nasal breathing. Experimental studies have shown that cervical extension increases maximum oropharyngeal airway size.[5] Therefore, children with nasal obstruction will spontaneously tend to assume the extended or forward head posture.

An extended head position is associated with an anterior displacement of the condyles of the occiput on the superior articular surfaces of the atlas, while the squamous portion of the occiput is lowered. The distance between the occiput and dorsal arch of the first cervical vertebra has been shown to be decreased in mouth breathers.[6] The condyles of the occiput are convex and the superior articular surfaces of the atlas are concave. Extension of the head for the shift from nasal to mouth breathing results in anterior and ascending displacement of the occipital condyles on the superior articular surfaces of the atlas. This causes the horizontal line of sight of the orbits to be angled upward, with resultant shift of the visual field and the need for postural compensation. One way to accomplish this, which is commonly observed in mouth breathers, is to increase the thoracic kyphosis. Another way – possible with young children when the synchondroses of the cranial base are still patent – is to increase the amount of flexion in the cranial base. Such an increase of cranial base flexion is present in mouth-breathing children.[7] Interestingly, an increase in cranial base flexion in primates has been shown to result in a decrease of the anteroposterior length of the nasopharynx and shortening of the anteroposterior length of the mandibular ramus.[8] The decrease of the anteroposterior length of the nasopharynx reinforces the tendency for mouth breathing, while the shortening of the anteroposterior length of the mandibular ramus correlates with the receding of the chin (retrognathia) that is observed in children who are mouth breathers.

Adenoidectomy is considered to be an effective treatment for children with enlarged adenoids who are mouth breathers. However, recurrence of breathing difficulties in these children has been observed and is attributed to their craniofacial anatomic pattern.[7] An extended craniocervical junction, or any dysfunctional pattern in the surrounding myofascial structures, may, therefore, be considered a primary dysfunction that could, in turn, predispose the child to chronic mouth breathing. This is confirmed by clinical observations that some children present with chronic mouth breathing secondary to nasal airway obstruction, while others tend to be mouth breathers without any obvious obstruction of the nasal airway.

Mouth breathing has also been correlated with an inferoposterior displacement of the hyoid bone and an anteroinferior positioning of the tongue.[4,7,9] The hyoid bone, a 'U-shaped' bone with an anterior convexity, is not directly articulated with any other skeletal structures. Through its myofascial attachments it acts as an interface between the tongue, the pharynx, the larynx and the skull and thorax. Therefore its position is influenced by dysfunction of any of these related structures and it can, in turn, exert influence on them. In mouth breathers, both the hyoid bone and the tongue are displaced to a position lower than normal.

Chronic mouth breathers often demonstrate premature molar eruption. Mouth breathing also influences the growth of the mandible, resulting in anterior mandibular rotation[9] and increase of the gonial angle between the ramus and the body of the mandible.[7] Consequently, the vertical height of the lower face of mouth breathers is usually increased, with a resultant open bite that is an augmentation of the vertical dimension separating the jaws.[9]

Nose breathing performs several functions of importance, such as warming and humidification of the inspired air, facilitation of arterial oxygenation[10] and regulation of pulmonary function.[11] Nasal obstruction is linked to obstructive sleep apnea in children as well as in adults. Therefore, nasal obstruction is a significant dysfunction and osteopathic procedures can often be applied to improve the patency of the nasal airway. Preventive treatment should be carried out for infants and toddlers to ensure normal development of the cranial base and craniocervical junction.

Physical examination and treatment

Mouth breathing is present with and without nasal obstruction and the child should be evaluated to determine if nasal obstruction is present. In severe cases, nasal endoscopy and medical treatment may be necessary. Hyponasal speech usually indicates an obstructed airway. A simple way to check for nasal patency is to ask the child to breathe, at least 10 times, through their nose while keeping their mouth closed. The child should be able to perform this test without becoming short of breath. Difficulty in achieving the test may be associated with rhinitis or chronic sinusitis. Successfully completing the test indicates that the prognosis for a positive response to manipulative treatment is good.

An alternative method to assess nasal patency is to hold a mirror under the nostrils of the subject. Normally patent nasal respiration will fog the mirror. If nasal obstruction is not demonstrated, the child should be examined to define somatic dysfunction possibly responsible for mouth breathing. Identified somatic dysfunction should be treated and then procedures to establish nasal breathing should be taught to the child.

The objective of treatment is to obtain optimal posture, improve function of the cervical and thoracic spine, balance the cranial base and its relationships with the hyoid bone and mandible, and facilitate nasal passage patency. As the pharyngeal tonsil is located immediately below the cranial base, at the level of the sphenobasilar junction, augmentation of the motion of the cranial base may increase tonsilar lymphatic drainage.

When treating the child it is best to begin by addressing their global standing posture. Observe the relationship between the head and the remainder of the body. Look for any asymmetries of cervical rotation and sidebending. Look for an exaggerated position of cervical extension or flexion and for increased thoracic kyphosis and lumbar lordosis.

Next, with the child in the supine position, palpate for tissue texture change in the suboccipital area and in the cervical and thoracic spine below. Palpate the soft tissue in the submandibular area; look for any lack of tonicity of the genioglossus muscles. Palpate for texture change in the tissues surrounding the mouth and the nose.

Assess the motion of the suboccipital area, cervical and thoracic spine. The cranial base, sphenobasilar synchondrosis and sphenoid should be evaluated next. The motions of the frontal bone, ethmoid and facial bones, particularly the maxillae, are considered next. Identify any membranous myofascial dysfunction that might also be present and treat accordingly, following indirect principles.

Teaching the child activities for the rehabilitation of normal breathing habits should complete the treatment. The child should be trained to breathe through their nose. They should be taught to control the nasalis muscle that compresses the nasal aperture with its transverse part and laterally opens the nostril with its alar part. With their index finger and thumb bilaterally contacting their nose, lateral to the nasal ala, they can be taught to feel the expansion of the nares when breathing. Next, they can be encouraged to open their nostrils more dynamically during inhalation while palpating the resultant nasal expansion. Encouraging them to smell pleasant odors such as flowers or favorite foods may further increase awareness of nasal function. Small children may be taught to intermittently flare and relax their nostrils by telling them to move their noses as a rabbit does, while keeping their mouths closed, but not so tight as to purse their lips by constricting the orbicularis oris muscle.

SLEEP APNEA

The upper airway is a very complex area that participates in several physiologic functions as diverse as deglutition, vocalization and respiration. Multiple anatomic structures take part in the mechanics of respiration. Consequently, more than one specific site of the upper airway can be blocked in obstructive disorders such as sleep-disordered breathing (SDB) where the different parts of the pharynx, the base of the tongue and the esophagus may be involved.[12] In SDB, several factors may be present along with the obstructive phenomenon. These include abnormalities or diseases of the paranasal sinuses, tonsilses, soft palate and tongue, as well as obesity.[13–15] A review of the development and relationships between the multiple constituents of the upper respiratory system is helpful in understanding the dysfunctional patterns of the region.

The respiratory system consists of the larynx, trachea, bronchi, lungs and pleura. The larynx is situated between the trachea and the root of the tongue. It forms the lower part of the anterior wall of the pharynx and is the organ of voice. In the infant, during the first 2 months of life, the larynx is located in a high position and, throughout both deglutition and respiration, contact is maintained between the epiglottis and the soft palate.[16] By approximately 6 months of age, however, this contact is maintained only during deglutition and separation occurs during respiration. The larynx progressively descends from a high position in the neck at the level of C1–C3 during the first 2½–3 years of life to a lower position in the adult, where it is located between the upper border of C4 and the upper border of C7.[16]

During the first 2 years of life the descent of the larynx is associated with important changes in the relationships of the structures that constitute the pharynx. In the newborn and the very young infant, the tongue is located totally within the oral cavity. As the larynx descends, the posterior part of the tongue is drawn posteriorly and inferiorly to participate in the constitution of the superior part of the anterior wall of the pharynx, i.e. the oropharynx.

The pharynx is shaped like a funnel, having a length of about 12.5 cm. The upper wide end of the pharynx is tipped forward and consists of the oral and nasal cavities, whereas the lower part, at about the level of C6, is continuous with the esophagus. Superiorly, it is attached above to the base of the skull on the posterior borders of the medial plates of the pterygoid processes of the sphenoid bone, on the petrous parts of the temporal bones and on the pharyngeal tubercle of the occipital bone. Laterally, the pharynx is connected to the styloid processes of the temporal bones and posteriorly to the cervical spine and the prevertebral fascia that envelops the longus colli and longus capitis muscles. The anterior portions of the pharynx are attached to the medial pterygoid plates of the sphenoid bone, the pterygomandibular raphes, the mandible, the tongue, the hyoid bone, and the thyroid and cricoid cartilages.

The pharyngeal wall consists of two groups of muscles, the constrictor muscles and the longitudinal muscles, grouped according to the arrangement of the muscle fibers. The three constrictor muscles – the inferior, middle and superior – function to constrict the pharyngeal cavity. The longitudinal muscles are the paired stylopharyngeus muscles that connect the pharynx with the styloid processes of the temporal bones, the salpingopharyngeus muscles that connect the pharynx with the cartilaginous part of the pharyngotympanic tubes and the palatopharyngeus muscles that connect the pharynx with the soft palate. The three longitudinal muscles elevate the pharyngeal wall. The pharyngeal muscles are innervated by the vagus nerve (CN X), except for the stylopharyngeus muscles that are innervated by the glossopharyngeal nerve (CN IX). The pharynx consists of three parts: the nasopharynx into which the choanae of the nasal cavity open, the oropharynx that constitutes the posterior portion of the oral cavity and the laryngopharynx into which the superior portion of the larynx opens. The soft palate is located between the nasopharynx and the oropharynx.

The soft palate is a determining factor in the establishment of the breathing route. It is compared to a curtain hanging from the posterior border of the hard palate, i.e. the posterior borders of the two palatine bones. The soft palate extends downwards and backwards between the mouth and pharynx. It consists of muscular fibers, aponeurosis, vasculature, nerves, adenoid tissue and mucous glands enclosed in a fold of mucous membrane. Its posterior surface is convex and is continuous with the floor of the nasal cavities. Its anterior surface is concave and is continuous with the roof of the mouth (Fig. 7.4.1).

The position of the soft palate determines the route of breathing. It acts as a valve hanging over the oropharyngeal isthmus. In its more horizontal position it separates the nasopharynx from the oropharynx, its posterior tip being closer to the posterior wall of the pharynx, facilitating the oral route of breathing. When it is depressed against the base of the tongue, the oropharyngeal isthmus is closed and the nasal breathing route is made possible. When respiration is through both mouth and nose, the position of the soft palate is shown to be between the tongue and the posterior pharyngeal wall.[13]

The soft palate is under the control of five pairs of muscles. The levator veli palatini (LVP) and tensor veli palatini (TVP) arise from the base of the skull. The LVP originates from the apex of the petrous part of the temporal bone and from the cartilage of the PT and spreads in the palatine velum

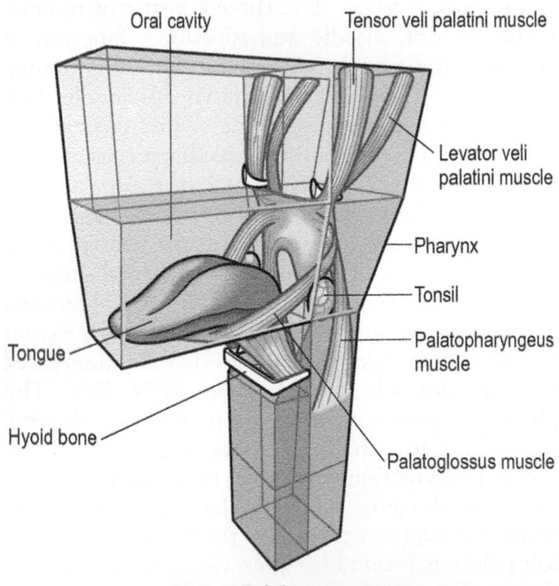

Figure 7.4.1. *Soft palate.*

to blend with the muscle of the opposite side. The TVP arises from the scaphoid fossa of the medial pterygoid plate, from the spina angularis of the sphenoid and from the lateral wall of the cartilage of the PT. It descends vertically and then turns around the pterygoid hamulus to insert into the palatine aponeurosis. The musculus uvulae is related to the uvula. The palatopharyngeus arises from the pharynx and the palatoglossus from the tongue. All the soft palate muscles are innervated by the vagus nerve (CN X) except the TVP that is innervated by the mandibular nerve (CN V_3).

The TVP muscles tense the soft palate; the LVP muscles elevate the soft palate and, therefore, close the nasopharynx. The palatopharyngeus muscles depress the soft palate and participate in the closing of the oropharyngeal isthmus. The palatoglossus muscles depress the soft palate caudally and ventrally and elevate the root of the tongue. The function of the soft palate is supposed to be actively determined, with dominant activity of the palatoglossus muscle when a subject is breathing quietly, and more activity from the LVP muscle during forced expiration.[13] Some activities such as breathing exercises or singing require both the nasal and oral breathing routes and the position of the soft palate consequently adapts to the situation.

Normal breathing relies on a patent nasal and pharyngeal airway. This patency depends on neural regulatory mechanisms as well as normal anatomic structures. The neural regulation is in part under the control of reflexes mediated through the trigeminal nerve (CN V) or the vagus nerve (CN X). The role of the vagus nerve is of paramount importance in the preservation of pharyngeal airway patency and any dysfunction of the upper cervical spine, in particular at the level of the jugular foramen, should be considered when airway patency is functionally compromised.

Considering the anatomic structures, the soft palate has been found to be the most common site of obstruction in infants presenting with significant obstructive sleep apnea (OSA).[17] Furthermore, an increase of cranial base flexion has also been demonstrated in mouth breathing or SDB children.[7] One can assume that, because of the insertion of the soft palate muscles, a dysfunction of the cranial base would lead to modified soft palate mechanics. The soft palate occupies a strategic position, an intersection between the muscles arising from the base of the skull and the muscles connected to the tongue and the pharynx. Considering these relationships, it is logical that any disturbance in the anatomic features influencing the soft palate, the tongue and the pharynx may also play a role in the development of SDB.

Adenotonsillar hypertrophy is described as being the most common cause of OSA in children; its importance correlates with the dimension of the adenoids.[18] OSA, the result of airflow obstruction, occurs in older children as well as in infants, where symptoms may include apneic spells.[17] Pharyngeal collapse is involved and it is proposed that airway muscle dysfunction[19] or anatomic alterations predispose to that collapse.[20] Loss of longitudinal tension within the pharyngeal airway is suggested as being responsible for the collapsibility.[20] Subtle abnormalities in upper airway neuromuscular function or structure are proposed additions to the etiology of adenotonsillar hypertrophy.[21,22] The craniocervical junction is under great stress in the infant and dysfunction of the pharynx, which is attached to the base of the skull and to the cervical spine and prevertebral fascia, may be associated with any somatic dysfunction of the craniocervical junction and cranial base.

The position of the cervical spine is correlated with pharyngeal changes: cervical flexion reduces oropharyngeal size; cervical extension increases it.[5,23,24] Studies have demonstrated that patients with obstructive SDB present a narrower or more obstructed oropharynx and laryngopharynx than controls, particularly during sleep.[15] Besides the effect of cervical posture, alteration of reflexes due to sleepiness may play a role. When present, nasal obstruction also disturbs nasopharynx reflexes, mediated through the trigeminal or vagus nerves, which may result in decreased patency of the oropharynx.[25]

Multiple sites are considered as potential causes for SDB. In view of the intricate anatomic relationships of the soft palate, the pharyngeal wall, the tongue and the mandible, any dysfunction of one affects the associated structures and their positions. Biomechanical interactions between the tongue and lateral pharyngeal walls have been described[26] and displacement of the mandible also affects oropharyngeal size.[5] Mouth opening reduces oropharyngeal size.[27] The modified mandible position affects the function of the genioglossus, one of the tongue muscles that protrude the anterior part of the tongue out of the mouth. This, in turn, increases upper airway collapsibility, the position of the tongue being a strong determinant of the patency of the oropharynx. This explains why mouth breathers present with snoring and SDB.[7]

Alterations in the electromyographic activity of the geniohyoid and genioglossus muscles follow experimental nasal obstruction in monkeys with affected mandibular growth as a result. Similar mechanisms are believed to exist in humans[27] where mouth breathing in children, associated with SDB, may cause developmental facial abnormalities.[25] Maxillary and mandibular protrusions are smaller in children with OSA and the position of the hyoid bone is lower.[28] Mouth breathing generates the development of a craniofacial type that includes an increased value of the anterior facial height and an open bite.[29] The increased respiratory effort that these children must exert is responsible for functional impairment and eventually structural changes in their craniofacial anatomy. OSA is also associated with poor sleep quality, failure to thrive, impaired daytime psychomotor performance, irreversible developmental delay[17] and enuresis.[30] Osteopathic procedures should consequently be employed at the earliest possible time to avoid the establishment of dysfunctional patterns and their sequelae.

Physical examination and treatment

Begin by assessing for, and treating, any dysfunctional imbalances in the global postural pattern, particularly the craniocervical junction and upper aspects of the thoracic region including clavicle, sternum, upper thoracic vertebrae and associated ribs. Next, attention should be paid to the mechanics of the hyoid bone, including the infra- and suprahyoid muscles because of their relationship with the pharynx and tongue.

The synchondroses of the cranial base, the occipitomastoid sutures and the relationship between the sphenoid and temporal bones should be considered next. Any dysfunction of the temporal bones should be addressed in the treatment of SDB because of the connection between the longitudinal muscles of the pharynx and the styloid processes of the temporal bones. Evaluate the temporomandibular joint, the mandible and surrounding myofascial elements.

The inferior part of the pharynx is continuous with the esophagus that connects the pharynx to the stomach. Possible stomach as well as tracheal visceral dysfunctions may affect the pharynx, either through mechanical imbalance or through disturbed vagal reflex; therefore, they should be treated if present.

Teaching the child activities that strengthen and tone the soft palate and tongue can complete the treatment. Vocal exercises employed in singing are beneficial. The tongue, particularly the genioglossus muscles, can be strengthened by having the child alternately attempt to touch the tip of their tongue up to the tip of their nose and down to their chin.

BRONCHIOLITIS

Bronchiolitis is an acute viral infection of the lower respiratory tract that affects infants and young children. In Europe, Australasia and North America, an average of 3% of all children born every year present with bronchiolitis.[31] Respiratory syncitial virus (RSV) and influenza A virus are the most important viral causes of lower respiratory tract infection in young children. Infections with influenza viruses B and coronavirus may also be common.[32] Influenza viruses are highly contagious and are responsible for epidemics presenting various degrees of severity, although only a small proportion of children infected with the virus develop severe disease. Risk factors are childcare attendance, exposure to environmental pollutants, school-aged siblings, congenital abnormalities of the airways and neuromuscular disease.[33]

RSV is so named because, in tissue culture, it grows as a giant syncytia, a mass of protoplasm containing several nuclei. Multiple genotypes of RSV cocirculate every year,[34] along with an important variability in influenza virus occurrence from year to year.[32] The infecting virus first establishes in the upper respiratory tract and then spreads to the medium and small bronchi and bronchioles, resulting in inflammation of the epithelium with edema and bronchial obstruction that manifests principally during expiration. Air is trapped within the alveoli and hyperinflation of the lungs follows. Respiratory distress appears with tachypnea and tachycardia. Expiration is difficult and prolonged, and when the infant presents with severe tachypnea, breath is rapid and short, with poor air exchange. Wheezing, crepitus and fever may be present.

RSV is an important childhood pathogen in infants younger than 24 months of age.[35] Once infected, an infant does not develop complete immunity and recurrence of infection is common. Pneumonia and bacterial superinfections of the respiratory tract are frequent complications.[32] RSV may be severe in infants under 3 months of age and is an important cause of hospitalization for acute lower respiratory tract infection in infants and young children.[36]

Bronchiolitis, particularly when due to RSV, may be a precursor of the later development of asthma. Allergic rhinitis also exacerbates bronchial inflammation and may be a risk factor for the development of asthma.[37] Young children who have more than three episodes of infectious bronchiolitis, and those with a family history of asthma who have more than two episodes of infectious bronchiolitis, may also be predisposed to asthma. Widespread respiratory viruses like RSV are also possible factors in the cause of acute otitis media in young children.[38,39] Consequently, preventive considerations should be applied.

The primary defense against common pathogens of acute lower respiratory infections is Waldeyer's (circumpharyngeal) tonsillar ring, a collection of lymphoid tissue in the mucosa of the nasopharynx. It consists of the pharyngeal tonsil, the palatine tonsils and the lingual tonsil that are the multiple lymphoid nodules located on the posterior part of the tongue, plus small other nodules in the PT and lymphoid tissue in the intertonsillar intervals. The nasopharyngeal tonsil increases in size in the first years of life, are largest at 6 years and atrophies by the time of puberty.

The efferent lymphatics of these mucosa-associated lymphoid tissues start in plexuses surrounding every lymphoid follicle and drain through the retropharyngeal lymph nodes or directly into the upper deep cervical nodes. The retropharyngeal nodes consist of three groups, two of which are located on either side, anterior to the lateral masses of C1, following the lateral borders of the longi capitis.

Somatic dysfunction of the cervical spine, the frontal bone, the maxillae, the ethmoid bone, the nasal bones and the zygomatic bones can alter the function of the upper respiratory tract as a primary defense against common pathogens. Dysfunction of the thoracic cage and diaphragm can impair efficient return of lymph to the general circulation and the ciliary clearance current of mucus in the bronchial tree. Thus, somatic dysfunction can contribute to the creation of a fertile environment wherein pathogens can thrive. It has been shown that osteopathic manipulative treatment (OMT), particularly the lymphatic pump, results in decreased morbidity and mortality in patients with influenza.[40,41]

The ANS is of prime importance in the regulation of bronchial secretion and its dysfunction may facilitate bronchiolitis. The sympathetic postganglionic fibers between T2 and T4 stimulate bronchial and bronchiolar dilatation and decrease fluidity of the secretions. The pulmonary branches of the vagus nerve are motor to the muscles fibers of the bronchi and bronchioles and are consequently bronchoconstrictor. Thus, somatic dysfunction of the upper thoracic, upper cervical and cranial regions can affect the lower respiratory tract through somatovisceral reflex action.

Physical examination and treatment

The objective of osteopathic treatment in the acutely ill, non-emergent child with bronchiolitis is to stimulate the expectoration of mucus, reduce air trapping and promote homeostasis by balancing the ANS and enhancing the venous and lymphatic drainage of the lungs. Furthermore, it is important to reduce somatic dysfunction that can predispose the child to the recurrence of the illness.

Observe the chest and the way the child is breathing, paying particular attention to the mobility of the ribs and sternum. Children with respiratory obstruction may demonstrate suprasternal, infrasternal, subcostal and intercostal retraction when breathing. On percussion, the chest is hyperresonnant. Prolonged expiration, wheezing, and fine moist crackles may be observed at auscultation. It is important to auscult the lungs before and after the osteopathic treatment.

Using indirect principles, restore thoracic spine and rib motion. Thoracic pumping may be used to loosen mucus, stimulate expectoration and decrease bronchial obstruction. The thoracic diaphragm and thoracic inlet should be evaluated and treated as findings dictate. Rib raising and sternal molding may be applied to further mobilize the thoracic cage, increase ventilation, loosen mucus and stimulate expectoration.

Sympathetic activity should be balanced by treating any dysfunction of the upper thoracic spine (T2–T4). Parasympathetic tone can be normalized with treatment of the suboccipital area. Using indirect principles, treat any cervical somatic dysfunction that is present. Improve lymphatic drainage from the upper deep cervical lymph nodes with soft tissue techniques applied to the cervical myofascial structures.

Observe the child's face. The frontal bone, the maxillae, the ethmoid bone, the nasal bones and the zygomatic bones form the upper respiratory tract. Look for asymmetries of these structures and for any tissue texture change. Palpation and motion testing will confirm these observations and treatment should be applied accordingly. It is imperative that the child is breathing through their nose, so any dysfunction that impairs nasal respiration should be addressed.

Following manipulative treatment it is important to re-evaluate the child. Re-evaluate the musculoskeletal areas treated and auscult the lungs again to check clearance of the secretions and progress of airflow.

It is important to maintain hydration of the respiratory tract. The caregivers should be advised to encourage consumption of fluids and to maintain sufficient humidification of the child's environment.

ASTHMA

Asthma is the most frequently encountered chronic disease in childhood. Allergic disorders and asthma in childhood have increased in prevalence in many countries over the past 20–30 years.[42,43] Asthma is characterized by chronic inflammation leading to airway hyperreactivity and recurrent reversible airflow obstruction.

A multifaceted interaction of genetic and environmental factors appears to cause asthma. A genetic predisposition seems to exist[42,44,45] and the risk is greater if both parents present with the disease.[46] In the predisposed host, immune responses to different exposures such as allergens and air pollutants may trigger pathogenic inflammation.[47]

Children from lower socioeconomic groups more often present with asthma, rhinitis and allergic sensitization, especially to food allergens.[48] Different factors may explain this susceptibility, the quality of food being one of them. Evaluation of different diets demonstrates the asthma preventive effect of dietary management for children with a family history of asthma. Of demonstrable benefit are diets with increased anti-inflammatory 'n-3' polyunsaturated fatty acids (omega-3 polyunsaturated fatty acids), alone[49] and in combination with house dust mite allergen prevention.[50] There is also some evidence that dietary omega-3 polyunsaturated fatty acid supplementation during pregnancy and early childhood may potentially reduce infant atopy and asthma.[51,52]

The controversial 'hygiene hypothesis' was developed in the late 1980s to explain the high prevalence of allergic diseases and asthma in industrialized countries.[53] The attention to hygiene in these countries is associated with reductions in microbial exposures and decreased incidence of infectious diseases. Microbial encounters in infancy and early childhood stimulate the development of the immune system and the 'hygiene hypothesis' states that atopic disorders are the consequences of the lack of early life infections.[54] Alternatively, the use of antibiotics in the 1st year of life may increase the risk of asthma.[55]

Opposite to the hygiene hypothesis, however, there is evidence that the pathogenesis of asthma may include early exposure to viruses and bacteria.[56,57] A high frequency of respiratory tract infections in the 1st year of life is a predictor of asthma between the ages of 6 and 8 years.[46,58] Elevated IgE levels at 6 months are also a predictor.[46] Alternatively, the association of atopy with asthma is controversial and the onset of eczema during the 1st year of life is not always found to be associated with the later development of asthma in childhood.[46]

A clinical association between rhinosinusitis and asthma is strongly suggested. Furthermore, effective treatment of rhinosinusitis has a positive effect on concomitant asthma.[59] Elements that contribute to the concept of 'united airway' disease include the dissemination of postnasal drip of inflammatory cells into the lungs. A vascular circulatory route with the migration of inflammatory cells to the lungs is another suggested pathway to explain the connection.

Another possible link between the upper and lower airways is through the nervous system, with naso-pharyngo-bronchial reflexes involving the trigeminal and the vagus nerves.[60] Upper airway inflammation may have an effect on receptors in the nose and pharynx. Afferent (sensory) fibers from these receptors participate in the constitution of the trigeminal nerve that connects with the dorsal vagal nucleus in the brainstem through the reticular formation. The vagus sends parasympathetic efferent fibers to the bronchi to preserve bronchial muscle tone and modulate bronchospastic responses. In asthmatic children, bronchoconstriction and mucus secretion is increased due to augmented parasympathetic nerve activity.[61] A neurogenic inflammation activated by inflammatory mediators and environmental irritants along the neural reflex pathway may be the cause of a neuronal dysfunction.[62]

The osteopathic principle of holistic integration of the different parts of the body applies perfectly to this hypothesis where an initial body reaction is followed by distant manifestations. The theory of 'one airway – one response' states that the common histopathology in both upper and lower airways results in a global allergic inflammation of the whole airway.

The total body allergic response is also illustrated through interactions between the respiratory system, the skin and the gastrointestinal tract. The lung and the gut are part of a unified mucosal system. The circulation of cells of the blood, from the bone marrow and the mucosal lymphoid tissue explain a possible interaction between these different areas and allergens.[63] The intestine is one of the most significant immune organs of the body. The composition of its microflora differs between infants with and without atopy, and the differences are verifiable before the occurrence of some clinical manifestation such as asthma.[64]

Alternatively, there is a link between the mode of obstetrical delivery and the maturation of the humoral immune system. Infants delivered by cesarean section demonstrate a delay in intestinal colonization.[65] The initial stimulation by the gut microflora may possibly be more significant than that of a sporadic infection and there is evidence of a relationship between cesarean section delivery and increased occurrence of atopic asthma.[66]

There is another connection between the lung and the guts with asthmatic patients. About 50–80% of adults and children with asthma present with gastroesophageal reflux – reflux of gastric contents into the esophagus – which may not be clinically obvious.[67] Intracellular acidification diminishes the ciliary beat frequency of the epithelial cells of the human tracheobronchial apparatus.[68] This point is significant in asthma, as well as in other respiratory dysfunction, as a factor contributing to decreased mucociliary clearance.

The lungs and esophagus are both innervated by the vagus and upper thoracic distribution of the sympathetic nervous system. Autonomic dysfunction may explain symptoms related to both gastroesophageal reflux and asthma.[69] Under normal conditions, the parasympathetic nervous system through the vagus sustains bronchial muscle tone while sympathetic fibers evoke bronchodilatation. Sympathetic nerve fibers also innervate the bronchial and gut-associated lymphoid tissue that seems to be essential in neuroimmune interactions.[70]

The parasympathetic visceral sensory system collects internal information that, in turn, influences emotions as much as emotional states impact autonomic function.[71] The influence of stress is potentially negative on neuroimmunoregulation.[70] In asthmatic patients, there is evidence that stress experienced prenatally or in the 1st years of life may participate in the development of asthma.[72,73] Increased psychological stress may impact respiratory illnesses in children and contribute to immune deregulation. There is evidence that stress facilitates susceptibility to infections[74] and may be associated with the development of asthma. Very often, asthmatic children present with anxious facial expression.

Most of the time, an asthmatic reaction is triggered by exposure to numerous environmental agents. Asthmatic children have hyperresponsive or hyperreactive airways. Various stimuli such as dust mites, pollutants and tobacco smoke produce an exaggerated bronchoconstrictor response with sensations of shortness of breath and chest tightness. There is evidence that the pathogenic development occurs early in the lungs, producing architecturally altered lungs later in life.[47] Treatment, therefore, should be initiated as soon as possible.

Asthma presents in different forms. The patient may demonstrate prodromal symptoms such as itching over the upper part of the chest and associated dry cough. This can be followed by episodes of dyspnea, tachypnea and tightness in the chest with wheezing and coughing that result from exposure to allergens, air pollution[75] or exercise. In asthmatic patients, a bronchoconstrictor response follows nasal inhalation of cold air.[76] Other patients present with chronic coughing and wheezing, associated with shortness of breath and decrease of vital capacity. Anxiety may occur related to the sensations of shortness of breath and chest tightness.

Physical examination and treatment

Osteopathic considerations for the treatment of asthma, although directed as a whole body intervention, are specifically focused on somatic dysfunctions of the thoracoabdominal diaphragm, thoracic cage, upper thoracic spine, cervical spine, sacrum, cranium and face. The goals of treatment are to encourage expectoration of mucus, reduce the mechanical impact of somatic dysfunction, enhance the recuperative effect of balanced sympathetic and parasympathetic tone, and facilitate the arterial, venous and lymphatic components of tissue perfusion. Because signs and symptoms are often observed first by the parents, these children may present to the osteopathic practitioner before the diagnosis of asthma has been formally made. It must be stressed that asthma is a potentially life-threatening condition, and although the treatment of somatic dysfunction can greatly benefit the patient,[77,78] the need for other methods of medical management should never be dismissed. The earlier somatic dysfunction is effectively addressed, the better the possible outcome. Manipulative treatment should begin with the area most easily accessible without distressing the child. The sequence of treatment is determined by the patient's acceptance of the intervention. Older children are commonly tolerant and treatment may be begun on the treatment table. For younger children, it is often easier to begin with the evaluation and treatment of the upper thoracic cage because this can be done with the child seated, even in the caregiver's lap. After a trusting physician–patient relationship has been established, the child may then be transferred to the treatment table for further treatment.

With the child seated or supine, observe the upper thoracic cage, looking for decreased compliance to respiratory excursion, i.e. tension of the scalene, trapezius and sternocleidomastoid muscles in the region of the supraclavicular triangle. Evaluate sternoclavicular motion and flexibility of the sternum for dysfunction. Articular motion of this region becomes mechanically discrete as the skeletal structures become more developed around 7 years of age. Palpate the thoracic spine and ribs for somatic dysfunction, paying attention to the area from T2 to T4 because of viscerosomatic input and somatovisceral impact with the lungs in this region. Utilizing indirect principles, treat identified somatic dysfunctions.

Following this, with the child, if possible, in the supine position, evaluate the lower thoracic cage and thoracoabdominal diaphragm. Observe the mechanical pattern of respiration. Asthmatic children tend to demonstrate forced expiration. Palpate for lower thoracic cage compliance, comparing the inspiratory and expiratory phases of respiration. Greater resistance will typically be appreciated during the expiratory phase and the child will often manifest shallow, rapid respiration. Palpating the lower thoracic cage bilaterally, evaluate for general tension and asymmetry in the excursion of the thoracoabdominal diaphragm. Assess the lumbar spine for dysfunction that can impact the diaphragm through the diaphragmatic crura. Examine the sacrum and pelvis to identify dysfunctional mechanics that can affect the asthmatic through the core link. Treat identified somatic dysfunction with indirect procedures. Entraining the movement of the manipulative treatment with the patient's breathing allows the practitioner to follow and gradually augment the amplitude of respiratory excursion.

Next, evaluate the cervical spine and myofascial structures of the neck. After general screening for dysfunction, attention should be directed at the upper cervical spine because of the viscerosomatic and somatovisceral vagal influence of the area. Treat identified dysfunction.

Examination can now proceed to the cranial base. Using your preferred hand placement, evaluate the motion of the SBS. Anecdotally, children with asthma and eczema seem to present frequently with SBS compression and decreased amplitude of the CRI. Assess the relationship between the occiput and temporal bones for compromise of the jugular foramen with its potential to interfere with vagal function. Evaluate the temporal bones where part of the tentorium cerebelli attaches. Dysfunction at this level affects the respiratory breathing pattern. An external rotation of one temporal bone tends to limit the freedom of expiration. Examine the relationship between the sphenoid, frontal and facial bones. The bones of the face – ethmoid, lacrimal, maxillary and nasal bones, which contribute to the structure of the nasal airway – are suspended beneath the frontal bones. Additionally, the ethmoid bone articulates posteriorly with the sphenoid. It is not uncommon to encounter compression between the frontal bones and the bones of the face. Treat specifically identified dysfunctional patterns. It is important that the nasal airway is unobstructed because of the effect of nasal respiration on inspired air and thoracopulmonary function. The interrelationship between rhinosinusitis and asthma further stresses the importance of appropriate function of the facial bones in asthmatic children. Treatment of the cranial mechanism with attention to the inherent rhythm augments the CRI with a resultant total body effect.

Following manipulative treatment, various activities can be prescribed to facilitate the results of the intervention. For small children the caregiver should be encouraged to regularly gently stroke the thoracic paravertebral region, particularly T1–T5, bilaterally.

The child can be encouraged to perform expiratory activities like blowing soap bubbles. Older children can be taught breathing exercises to improve lung function to increase vital capacity, facilitate the clearing of airway secretions and enhance the quality of life. Begin by encouraging the child to breathe slowly and deeply, employing the thoracoabdominal diaphragm and with the least possible utilization of the accessory muscles of respiration – scalene, sternocleidomastoid, trapezius and abdominal wall muscles. They should learn to breathe on demand with particular attention to control of expiration. Further, they should be taught to hold their breath in the most relaxed possible way. This allows them to experience apnea without anxiety. As they become experienced in these activities, they can be encouraged to practice this method of respiratory relaxation at the first perception of an asthma attack. Because controlled breathing is an integral part of singing, they may benefit from participation in a choral group.

Teach them to maintain good posture. A simple procedure is to have the child walk with a book balanced on the top of their head. Finally, children and adolescents with asthma should participate in regular physical activity.[79,80]

Diet considerations should be initiated. Daily intake of fresh fruit and vegetables should be recommended. Processed sugars and foods that increase gastric acidity should be limited. Dairy products (e.g. ice cream) which increase mucus production should be consumed moderately and preferably before 5 p.m. to facilitate gastric emptying before bedtime and avoid gastroesophageal reflux.

REFERENCES

1. Rodenstein DO, Perlmutter N, Stanescu DC. Infants are not obligatory nasal breathers. Am Rev Respir Dis 1985;131(3):343–7.
2. Olnes SQ, Schwartz RH, Bahadori RS. Consultation with the specialist: diagnosis and management of the newborn and young infant who have nasal obstruction. Pediatr Rev 2000;21(12):416–20.
3. Kubba H, Bingham BJ. Endoscopy in the assessment of children with nasal obstruction. J Laryngol Otol 2001;115(5):380–4.
4. Behlfelt K, Linder-Aronson S, Neander P. Posture of the head, the hyoid bone, and the tongue in children with and without enlarged tonsils. Eur J Orthod 1990;12(4):458–67.
5. Isono S, Tanaka A, Tagaito Y, Ishikawa T, Nishino T. Influences of head positions and bite opening on collapsibility of the passive pharynx. J Appl Physiol 2004;97(1):339–46.
6. Kumar R, Sidhu SS, Kharbanda OP, Tandon DA. Hyoid bone and atlas vertebra in established mouth breathers: a cephalometric study. J Clin Pediatr Dent 1995;19(3):191–4.
7. Finkelstein Y, Wexler D, Berger G, Nachmany A, Shapiro-Feinberg M, Ophir D. Anatomical basis of sleep-related breathing abnormalities in children with nasal obstruction. Arch Otolaryngol Head Neck Surg 2000;126(5):593–600.
8. McCarthy RC, Lieberman DE. Posterior maxillary (PM) plane and anterior cranial architecture in primates. Anat Rec 2001;264(3):247–60.
9. Principato JJ. Upper airway obstruction and craniofacial morphology. Otolaryngol Head Neck Surg 1991;104(6):881–90.
10. Swift AC, Campbell IT, McKown TM. Oronasal obstruction, lung volumes, and arterial oxygenation. Lancet 1988;1(8577):73–5.
11. Settergren G, Angdin M, Astudillo R et al. Decreased pulmonary vascular resistance during nasal breathing: modulation by endogenous nitric oxide from the paranasal sinuses. Acta Physiol Scand 1998;163(3):235–9.
12. Boudewyns AN, Van de Heyning PH, De Backer WA. Site of upper airway obstruction in obstructive apnoea and influence of sleep stage. Eur Respir J 1997;10(11):2566–72.
13. Rodenstein DO, Stanescu DC. Soft palate and oronasal breathing in humans. Appl Physiol 1984;57(3):651–7.
14. Schwab RJ. Upper airway imaging. Clin Chest Med 1998;19(1):33–54.
15. Nishimura T, Suzuki K. Anatomy of oral respiration: morphology of the oral cavity and pharynx. Acta Otolaryngol Suppl 2003;550:25–8.
16. Laitman JT, Crelin ES. Developmental change in the upper respiratory system of human infants. Perinatol Neonatol 1980;4:15–22.
17. Don GW, Kirjavainen T, Broome C, Seton C, Waters KA. Site and mechanics of spontaneous, sleep-associated obstructive apnea in infants. J Appl Physiol 2000;89(6):2453–62.
18. Jain A, Sahni JK. J. Polysomnographic studies in children undergoing adenoidectomy and/or tonsillectomy. Laryngol Otol 2002;116(9):711–5.
19. Cohen G, Henderson-Smart DJ. Upper airway stability and apnea during nasal occlusion in newborn infants. J Appl Physiol 1986;60(5):1511–7.
20. Schwartz AR, Eisele DW, Smith PL. Pharyngeal airway obstruction in obstructive sleep apnea: pathophysiology and clinical implications. Otolaryngol Clin North Am 1998;31(6):911–8.

21. Marcus CL, McColley SA, Carroll JL, Loughlin GM, Smith PL, Schwartz AR. Upper airway collapsibility in children with obstructive sleep apnea syndrome. J Appl Physiol 1994; 77(2):918–24.
22. Tasker C, Crosby JH, Stradling JR. Evidence for persistence of upper airway narrowing during sleep, 12 years after adeno-tonsillectomy. Arch Dis Child 2002;86(1):34–7.
23. Reed WR, Roberts JL, Thach BT. Factors infl uencing regional patency and confi guration of the human infant upper airway. J Appl Physiol 1985;58(2):635–44.
24. Thut DC, Schwartz AR, Roach D, Wise RA, Permutt S, Smith PL. Tracheal and neck position influence upper airway airflow dynamics by altering airway length. J Appl Physiol 1993;75(5):2084–90.
25. Rappai M, Collop N, Kemp S, deShazo R. The nose and sleep-disordered breathing: what we know and what we do not know. Chest 2003;124(6):2309–23.
26. Trudo FJ, Gefter WB, Welch KC, Gupta KB, Maislin G, Schwab RJ. State-related changes in upper airway caliber and surrounding soft-tissue structures in normal subjects. Am J Respir Crit Care Med 1998;158(4):1259–70.
27. Chen W, Kushida CA. Nasal obstruction in sleep-disordered breathing. Otolaryngol Clin North Am 2003;36(3):437–60.
28. Shintani T, Asakura K, Kataura A. Adenotonsillar hypertrophy and skeletal morphology of children with obstructive sleep apnea syndrome. Acta Otolaryngol Suppl 1996;523: 222–4.
29. Zucconi M, Caprioglio A, Calori G et al. Craniofacial modifi cations in children with habitual snoring and obstructive sleep apnoea: a case-control study. Eur Respir J 1999;13(2): 411–7.
30. Brooks LJ, Topol HI. Enuresis in children with sleep apnea. J Pediatr 2003;142(5):515–8.
31. Sharland M, Bedford-Russell A. Preventing respiratory syncitial virus bronchiolitis. BMJ 2001;322(7278):62–63.
32. Lina B, Valette M, Foray S et al. Surveillance of community-acquired viral infections due to respiratory viruses in Rhone-Alpes (France) during winter 1994 to 1995. J Clin Microbiol 1996;34(12):3007–11.
33. Centers for Disease Control and Prevention (CDC). Respiratory syncytial virus activity – United States, 2003–2004. MMWR Morb Mortal Wkly Rep 2004;53(49):1159–60.
34. Sato M, Saito R, Sakai T et al. Molecular epidemiology of respiratory syncytial virus infections among children with acute respiratory symptoms in a community over three seasons. J Clin Microbiol 2005;43(1):36–40.
35. Rakes GP, Arruda E, Ingram JM et al. Rhinovirus and respiratory syncytial virus in wheezing children requiring emergency care. IgE and eosinophil analyses. Am J Respir Crit Care Med 1999;159(3):785–90.
36. Hussey GD, Apolles P, Arendse Z et al. Respiratory syncytial virus infection in children hospitalised with acute lower respiratory tract infection. S Afr Med J 2000;90(5):509–12.
37. Braunstahl GJ. The unifi ed immune system: respiratory tract–nasobronchial interaction mechanisms in allergic airway disease. J Allergy Clin Immunol 2005;115(1):142–8.
38. Pitkaranta A, Virolainen A, Jero J, Arruda E, Hayden FG. Detection of rhinovirus, respiratory syncytial virus, and coronavirus infections in acute otitis media by reverse transcriptase polymerase chain reaction. Pediatrics 1998;102(2 Pt 1):291–5.
39. Rovers MM, Schilder AG, Zielhuis GA, Rosenfeld RM. Otitis media. Lancet 2004;363(9407):465–73.
40. Smith RK. One hundred thousand cases of influenza with a death rate of one-fortieth of that reported under conventional medical treatment. JAOA 1920;19:172–5.
41. Magoun HI Jr. More about the use of OMT during influenza epidemics. J Am Osteopath Assoc 2004;104(10):406–7.
42. Steinke JW, Borish L. Genetics of allergic disease. Med Clin North Am 2006;90(1):1–15.
43. Burr ML, Wat D, Evans C, Dunstan FD, Doull IJ. British Thoracic Society Research Committee. Asthma prevalence in 1973, 1988 and 2003. Thorax 2006;61(4):296–9.
44. Puthothu B, Krueger M, Heinze J, Forster J, Heinzmann A. Impact of IL8 and IL8-receptor alpha polymorphisms on the genetics of bronchial asthma and severe RSV infections. Clin Mol Allergy 2006;4:2.
45. Apter AJ, Szefler SJ. Advances in adult and pediatric asthma. J Allergy Clin Immunol 2006;117(3):512–8.
46. Klinnert MD, Nelson HS, Price MR, Adinoff AD, Leung DY, Mrazek DA. Onset and persistence of childhood asthma: predictors from infancy. Pediatrics 2001;108(4):E69.
47. Liu AH. Consider the child: how early should we treat? J Allergy Clin Immunol 2004;113(1 Suppl):S19–24.
48. Almqvist C, Pershagen G, Wickman M. Low socioeconomic status as a risk factor for asthma, rhinitis and sensitization at 4 years in a birth cohort. Clin Exp Allergy 2005;35(5):612–8.
49. Nagakura T, Matsuda S, Shichijyo K, Sugimoto H, Hata K. Dietary supplementation with fish oil rich in omega-3 polyunsaturated fatty acids in children with bronchial asthma. Eur Respir J 2000;16(5):861–5.
50. Peat JK, Mihrshahi S, Kemp AS et al. Three-year outcomes of dietary fatty acid modification and house dust mite reduction in the Childhood Asthma Prevention Study. J Allergy Clin Immunol 2004;114(4):807–13.
51. Devereux G, Seaton A. Diet as a risk factor for atopy and asthma. J Allergy Clin Immunol 2005;115(6):1109–17; quiz 1118.
52. Dunstan JA, Mori TA, Barden A et al. Fish oil supplementation in pregnancy modifies neonatal allergen-specific immune responses and clinical outcomes in infants at high risk of atopy: a randomized, controlled trial. Allergy Clin Immunol 2003;112:1178–84.
53. Kim DS, Drake-Lee AB. Infection, allergy and the hygiene hypothesis: historical perspective. J Laryngol Otol 2003; 117(12):946–50.
54. Christen U, von Herrath MG. Infections and autoimmunity – good or bad? J Immunol 2005;174(12):7481–6.
55. Cohet C, Cheng S, MacDonald C et al. Infections, medication use, and the prevalence of symptoms of asthma, rhinitis, and eczema in childhood. J Epidemiol Community Health 2004;58(10):852–7.
56. Weinberger M. Clinical patterns and natural history of asthma. J Pediatr 2003;142(2 Suppl):S15–9; discussion S19–20.
57. Pelaia G, Vatrella A, Gallelli L et al. Respiratory infections and asthma. Respir Med 2006;100(5):775–84.
58. de Marco R, Pattaro C, Locatelli F, Svanes C; ECRHS Study Group. Infl uence of early life exposures on incidence and remission of asthma throughout life. J Allergy Clin Immunol 2004;113(5):845–52.
59. Smart BA, Slavin RG. Rhinosinusitis and pediatric asthma. Immunol Allergy Clin North Am 2005;25(1):67–82.
60. Togias A. Systemic effects of local allergic disease. J Allergy Clin Immunol 2004;113:S8–14.
61. Coulson FR, Fryer AD. Muscarinic acetylcholine receptors and airway diseases. Pharmacol Ther 2003;98(1):59–69.
62. Undem BJ, Carr MJ. The role of nerves in asthma. Curr Allergy Asthma Rep 2002;2(2):159–65.
63. Braunstahl GJ. The unifi ed immune system: respiratory tract–nasobronchial interaction mechanisms in allergic airway disease. J Allergy Clin Immunol 2005;115(1):142–8.

64. Bjorksten B, Sepp E, Julge K, Voor T, Mikelsaar M. Allergy development and the intestinal microflora during the first year of life. J Allergy Clin Immunol 2001;108(4): 516–20.
65. Gronlund MM, Arvilommi H, Kero P, Lehtonen OP, Isolauri E. Importance of intestinal colonisation in the maturation of humoral immunity in early infancy: a prospective follow up study of healthy infants aged 0–6 months. Arch Dis Child Fetal Neonatal Ed 2000;83(3):F186–92.
66. Kero J, Gissler M, Gronlund MM et al. Mode of delivery and asthma – is there a connection? Pediatr Res 2002;52(1): 6–11.
67. Harding SM. Gastroesophageal reflux: a potential asthma trigger. Immunol Allergy Clin North Am 2005;25(1):131–48.
68. Sutto Z, Conner GE, Salathe M. Regulation of human airway ciliary beat frequency by intracellular pH. J Physiol 2004; 560(Pt 2):519–32.
69. Canning BJ, Mazzone SB. Reflex mechanisms in gastroesophageal reflux disease and asthma. Am J Med 2003;115(Suppl 3A):45S–48S.
70. Elenkov IJ, Wilder RL, Chrousos GP, Vizi ES. The sympathetic nerve – an integrative interface between two supersystems: the brain and the immune system. Pharmacol Rev 2000;52(4):595–638.
71. Saper CB. The central autonomic nervous system: conscious visceral perception and autonomic pattern generation. Annu Rev Neurosci 2002;25:433–69.
72. Wright RJ. Stress and atopic disorders. J Allergy Clin Immunol 2005;116(6):1301–6.
73. Chen E, Fisher EB, Bacharier LB, Strunk RC. Socioeconomic status, stress, and immune markers in adolescents with asthma. Psychosom Med 2003;65(6):984–92.
74. Meyer RJ, Haggerty RJ. Streptococcal infections in families. Factors altering individual susceptibility. Pediatrics 1962; 29:539–49.
75. McCunney RJ. Asthma, genes, and air pollution. J Occup Environ Med 2005;47(12):1285–91.
76. Fontanari P, Burnet H, Zattara-Hartmann MC, Jammes Y. Changes in airway resistance induced by nasal inhalation of cold dry, dry, or moist air in normal individuals. J Appl Physiol 1996;81(4):1739–43.
77. Bockenhauer SE, Julliard KN, Lo KS, Huang E, Sheth AM. Quantifiable effects of osteopathic manipulative techniques on patients with chronic asthma. J Am Osteopath Assoc 2002;102(7):371–5; discussion 375.
78. Guiney PA, Chou R, Vianna A, Lovenheim J. Effects of osteopathic manipulative treatment on pediatric patients with asthma: a randomized controlled trial. J Am Osteopath Assoc 2005;105(1):7–12.
79. Counil FP, Varray A, Matecki S et al. Training of aerobic and anaerobic fitness in children with asthma. J Pediatr 2003;142(2):179–84.
80. Lucas SR, Platts-Mills TA. Physical activity and exercise in asthma: relevance to etiology and treatment. J Allergy Clin Immunol 2005;115(5):928–34.

7.5 DISORDERS OF THE EYES

LACRIMAL DUCT OBSTRUCTION

Approximately 20% of infants demonstrate symptoms of imperfect lacrimal drainage during their first months of life. Most of the time spontaneous resolution takes place and by their 1st birthday only about 0.7% of infants still present with the condition.[1] Congenital nasolacrimal duct obstruction (dacryostenosis) may result from an abnormality in the lacrimal drainage system or from an infection.

The diagnosis of congenital nasolacrimal duct obstruction is clinical. It is based on a history of epiphora (tearing), mucopurulent discharge, or both, in the presence of non-inflamed conjunctiva, usually affecting only one eye and occurring in the first few weeks of life. The condition may be continuous or intermittent and crusting on the lid margins is common. Parents will often report that the eyelids are stuck together on the child's awakening or that the child has a persistently watering or sticky eye. Digital pressure applied medial to the eye over the lacrimal sac will produce increased discharge from the excretory puncta.

There is much debate regarding a standard medical approach for the management of congenital nasolacrimal duct obstruction.[2] The availability of multiple therapeutic approaches for any given condition indicates that none of them works particularly well in all cases. The list of procedures that are employed as standard to correct symptomatic nasolacrimal duct obstruction includes probing and irrigation, intubation with a silicone tube, balloon dilatation of the nasolacrimal duct and infracture of the inferior turbinate.[3] Osteopathic manipulation offers an alternative approach and, since it is benign, it should be attempted before more aggressive procedures are employed. The earlier the infant or child is treated, the better the chance of rapid resolution of the obstruction. Additionally, a good mental image of the anatomy of the nasolacrimal duct and lacrimal drainage system, on the part of the practitioner, will provide the basis necessary to improve the efficacy of manipulation.

The lacrimal apparatus consists of several parts that develop simultaneously. The lacrimal gland secretes the tears and the excretory ducts (lacrimal canaliculi) deliver the fluid to the surface of the eye, while the lacrimal sac and the nasolacrimal duct collect and transport the fluid into the nasal cavity.

The lacrimal gland consists of two portions: the superior orbital part and the inferior lacrimal part. The superior orbital part is located in the lacrimal fossa, in the superolateral part of the orbit, on the medial side of the zygomatic process of the frontal bone. Shaped like an almond, it is connected to the periosteum of the orbit and rests on the levator palpebrae superioris and the lateral rectus. The inferior lacrimal gland is separated from the superior by a fibrous septum and projects into the lateral part of the upper eyelid. Although the lacrimal gland reaches full development at about 3–4 years of age, the production of tears in infants is similar to that in adults.[4]

On each eyelid, the lacrimal canaliculus originates at a lacrimal punctum, a minuscule orifice on the medial margins of the lids. The superior canaliculus is the smaller and shorter. First it goes up, then turns at an acute angle to meet the lacrimal sac, while the inferior canaliculus descends, then turns upward toward the lacrimal sac (Fig. 7.5.1). At their angles the canaliculi are dilated and form ampullae. Their mucous lining is covered by stratified squamous epithelium, positioned on a basement membrane. The external wall consists of a layer of skeletal muscle fibers, continuous with the lacrimal part of the orbicularis oculi.

The lacrimal sac is the upper dilated end of the nasolacrimal duct. It is located in a fossa formed by the lacrimal bone, the frontal process of the maxilla and the lacrimal fascia. It measures from 12 to 15 mm in length and extends to form the nasolacrimal duct. Its superficial surface is sheltered by the lacrimal fascia (an extension of the orbital periosteum) and by the medial palpebral ligament. Its deep surface is crossed by the lacrimal part of the orbicularis oculi, which is attached to the posterior lacrimal crest on the lacrimal bone. The lacrimal sac is lined by a mucosal membrane continuous with the conjunctiva through the lacrimal canals and with the nasal cavity through the nasolacrimal duct.

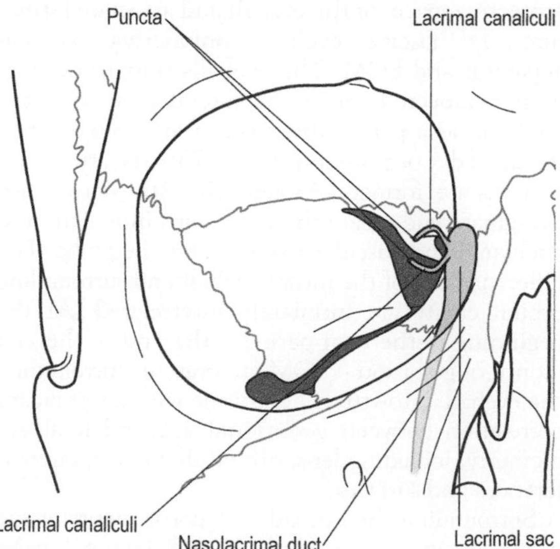

Figure 7.5.1. *The lacrimal sac.*

The relationship with the orbicularis oculi is of particular interest. This muscle surrounds the circumference of the orbit, with osseous attachments on the frontal bone, the frontal process of the maxilla and the lacrimal bone. When it contracts, as during 'blinking', compression of the lacrimal sac occurs through the lacrimal part of the muscle, pushing fluid into the nasolacrimal duct to drain into the inferior meatus of the nasal cavity. During muscular relaxation, fluids are drawn into the canaliculi and the expanded lacrimal sac.[5]

The nasolacrimal duct extends from the lacrimal sac caudally to open in the inferior nasal meatus. Both ends of the duct are wider than its middle portion, where it is enclosed in an osseous canal formed by the maxilla, the lacrimal bone and the inferior nasal concha. It is directed downward, backward and slightly laterally.

The nasolacrimal duct is formed embryologically from ectodermal cells enclosed between the maxillary and lateral nasal processes. During the 3rd month of gestation a canal appears in the center of this epithelial cord. It will develop progressively in a cephalocaudal direction from the 6th month of gestation until birth. In the third trimester of gestation the lower portion of the duct opens into the inferior meatus of the nasal cavity to constitute the nasolacrimal duct, while the epithelium from the nasal cavity invests the duct in a caudocephalad direction. A mucosal fold – the valve of Hasner – is located just above the nasal opening of the nasolacrimal duct. Total canalization of the epithelial cord may fail to occur with the persistence of membranous tissue that should normally disappear at birth or in the first days of life. In congenital nasolacrimal duct obstruction, the lower part of the duct may be closed at birth by fusion of the mucosa covering the nasal folds. The resultant obstruction is usually observed in infants at about the 10th or 12th day of life.

Nasolacrimal duct obstruction is frequently associated with dysfunction of the bones forming the osseous canal in which the nasolacrimal duct is located, i.e. the maxilla, the lacrimal bone and the inferior nasal concha. It frequently follows compression of the frontal bone and may also be associated with an inferior vertical strain of the SBS. Consequently, the relationships between the frontal bone, maxilla and lacrimal bone are affected, potentially modifying the patency of the nasolacrimal duct. This type of compression occurs frequently during pregnancy, difficult labor or delivery and appears to be a prediposing factor. Furthermore, dysfunction of the frontal bone, maxilla and lacrimal bone changes the relationship between the points of attachment of the orbicularis oculi, predisposing to muscular dysfunction.

Physical examination and treatment

When treating nasolacrimal duct obstruction, the delicacy of the intervention necessitates that the infant moves as little as possible. This may be accomplished by arranging to see the infant at a time that coincides with their nap time. The best approach is to have the caregiver arrive with the infant about 30 minutes before the scheduled appointment. Place the infant and caregiver in a quiet examining room and allow the infant to have their bottle or to nurse. Allow sufficient time thereafter for the infant to go to sleep, preferably in a supine position on the examining table.

Once the infant is asleep, quietly commence treatment. First observe the frontal bones. Often the frontal bone on the side of the lacrimal duct obstruction will be found to be lower than the other side. Look next at the area of the nasion, nasal bones and frontal processes of the maxillae, noting asymmetry and compression of these structures. The forces commonly involved in lacrimal duct obstruction are most often vertical compression between the frontal and nasal bones, sometimes with sidebending and rotation of the facial block beneath the frontal bone, with the obstruction on the side of the facial concavity.

Confirm the observations with tests of listening, paying close attention to the frontal bones, nasal bones, maxillae and lacrimal bones. Keep a mental picture of the minute details of the area to help this process. Define areas of restricted motility and employing the inherent forces of the PRM and its rhythm, utilize the most delicate indirect treatment procedure. The treatment procedure should be so gentle as not to awaken the infant.

Advice to caregivers

Encourage the caregiver to regularly clean the secretions from the eye to avoid the development of an infection. To promote drainage into the nasolacrimal duct, the caregiver can milk the lacrimal sac by intermittently applying gentle digital pressure medial to the punctum of the eye in a superior to inferior direction.

Actively playing with the child to encourage facial expression stimulates the function of the orbicularis oculi. If the child is old enough, have them blink tightly and make faces. Contracting the orbicularis oculi promotes drainage by placing pressure on the lacrimal sac.

STRABISMUS

Strabismus – the deviation of the alignment of one eye in relation to the other – is a condition frequently encountered in infants and children. It is a very complex subject and its complete discussion is beyond the focus of this text. However, the treatment of somatic dysfunction can prove very beneficial in certain presentations of the condition. Strabismus must be taken seriously and significant underlying pathologies, such as congenital cataract and retinoblastoma, ruled out. It is imperative that, on presentation, every case of strabismus, no matter what the age of the patient, has a thorough ocular examination, including cornea, lens, retina and optic nerve, as well as the neurologic status of the eye and extraocular muscles (EOM). Treatment of strabismus should be initiated at the earliest possible time to avoid loss of the ocular stimulation that normally contributes to the maturation of the visual system.

The eyeball – the organ of sight – is contained in the skeletal cavity of the orbit, which provides a protective space for the eyeball and associated structures, i.e. fasciae, eyelids, conjunctiva, lacrimal apparatus and EOM. The eyeballs start to develop from neuroectoderm of the lateral aspects of the forebrain as a pair of diverticulae at approximately the 22nd day of gestation. At the 25th day, two optic vesicles are formed. Around the 4th week, they invaginate and create the optic cups in which mesenchymal and vascular tissues enter the globe. The different parts of the future eyeball and surrounding orbital cavity are intimately interrelated. At the beginning of the fetal period – the end of the 2nd month of gestation – EOM are present, surrounding the eyeball. Growth will continue with a significant correlation between gestational age and fetal eye biometry, including lens, orbital diameters, circumferences and surfaces.[6]

Surrounding the eyeball, the constituents of the orbital cavity consist of the frontal, lacrimal, palatine and zygomatic bones, ethmoid, maxilla and sphenoid. They develop in membrane and are quite responsive to the growth stimulation of the eyeball. Thus, the orbital cavity is growing as a result of the increase of the volume of the eyeball and the activity of the EOM, with more and more elaborate eye movements. From this time up to 5 years of age, the eyeballs will continue to grow, acting continuously as a growth stimulator for the skeletal cavity of the orbit. At birth, the orbit height is already 55% of its adult height. At 3 years of age it is 79%, while at 7 years of age it is about 94%, nearly its adult size.[7]

Evidence of the importance of this stimulating factor is demonstrated by conditions like microphthalmia, where the development of the eyeball does not occur correctly, or when an individual is enucleated in early childhood. Underdevelopment of the orbital cavity is typically associated with these conditions. An anophthalmic bony orbit may be 14.5% smaller when compared to the other orbit.[8] The concept that function affects structure, one of the basic osteopathic principles, is perfectly illustrated in this instance.

At the same time, structure affects function. In this case, the structures forming the orbital cavity may affect the ocular function of sight, associated vascular and neurologic aspects, and extra- and intraocular muscular activity. Therefore, it is appropriate to consider the protective case for the eye, i.e. the orbital cavity, and to see how its osseous components play a part in the etiology of ocular dysfunction.

The orbits are located in the upper and anterior part of the viscerocranium. They are shaped like pyramids, with their apices and long axes directed backward and medially. Each orbit consists of a roof, a floor, a medial and a lateral wall, a base and an apex. The roof is concave, directed downward and slightly forward. The orbital plate of the frontal bone forms most of the roof, while the lesser wing of the sphenoid forms its posterior part. Therefore, there is a suture on the roof of the orbital cavity between the frontal bone and the lesser wing of the sphenoid. The lacrimal fossa for the lacrimal gland is located laterally on the orbital surface of the frontal plate. Medially, below and behind the end of the supraorbital margin of the frontal bone, is the trochlear fovea for the attachment of the cartilaginous pulley of the superior oblique muscle. This feature is of particular interest in understanding ocular dysfunction, since the frontal bone is frequently under stress from fetal positioning, difficult labor or trauma sustained by young children, such as a fall on the head. Although most of this anatomy is not directly palpable, the supraorbital margin of the frontal bone is completely accessible and its position should always be evaluated in strabismus.

The floor of the orbit is directed upward and laterally. It consists mostly of the orbital surface of the maxilla; behind that and medially, the orbital process of the palatine; and in front and laterally, the orbital process of the zygomatic bone (Fig. 7.5.2). The maxilla articulates with both the palatine and the zygomatic bones. The lacrimal notch is located anteriorly, on the medial border of the maxilla, and provides the superior opening of the nasolacrimal canal. On this border the maxilla articulates with the lacrimal bone and the ethmoid's orbital plate behind. A depression situated just lateral to the lacrimal notch is the location of the origin of the inferior oblique muscle. The posterior border of the maxilla forms most of the anterior edge of the inferior orbital fissure, discussed further below.

The medial wall of the orbit is formed anteriorly by the frontal process of the maxilla, the lacrimal bone, the orbital plate of the ethmoid and a tiny part of the body of the sphenoid in front of the optic foramen. The lacrimal groove for the lacrimal sac is located anteriorly. It is limited behind by the posterior lacrimal crest, from which the lacrimal part of the orbicularis oculi arises. Three vertical sutures – the lacrimomaxillary, lacrimoethmoidal

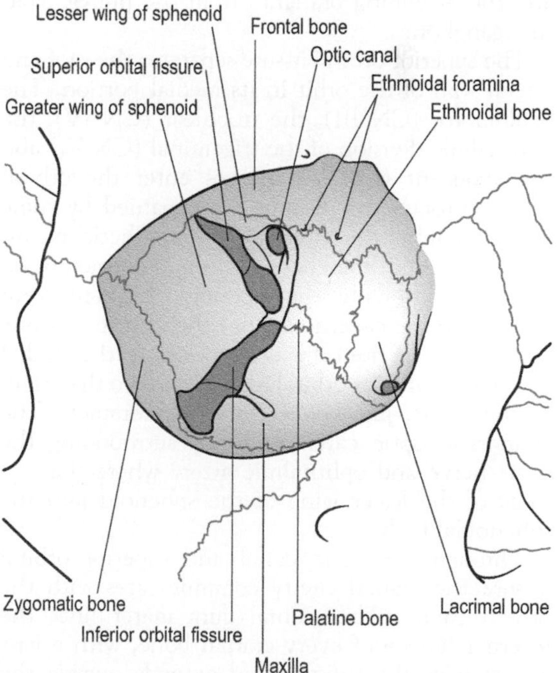

Figure 7.5.2. *The bony orbit.*

and sphenoethmoidal – are present, while the frontomaxillary, frontolacrimal, and frontoethmoidal sutures are situated between the superior border of the medial wall and the orbital roof.

The lateral wall of the orbit is directed medially and forward. It consists of the orbital process of the zygomatic and the orbital surface of the greater wing of the sphenoid. The sphenozygomatic suture unites them. This is another site of particular interest since the zygomatic bone is easily palpable. Through palpation of the zygoma one can visualize, indirectly assess and treat the less accessible greater wing of the sphenoid. The sphenozygomatic suture ends below at the anterior end of the inferior orbital fissure. The upper end of the sphenozygomatic suture meets with two other sutures, creating a sutural crossroads for consideration in the treatment of any ocular dysfunction. Anteriorly, the frontozygomatic suture can be observed, and posteriorly the suture between the frontal bone and the greater wing of the sphenoid. Just under the frontozygomatic suture, on the orbital process of the zygomatic bone, is a tubercle for the attachment of the levator palpebrae superioris' aponeurosis.

The inferior orbital fissure lies between the lateral wall and floor of the orbit, posterior to the zygomaticomaxillary suture. It communicates with the pterygopalatine and infratemporal fossae, and transmits the infraorbital vessels, the maxillary nerve (CN V_2) and the ascending branches from the pterygopalatine ganglion.

The superior orbital fissure separates the roof and lateral wall of the orbit in its medial portion. The oculomotor (CN III), the trochlear (CN IV), the ophthalmic division of the trigeminal (CN V_1) and the abducent (CN VI) nerves enter the orbital cavity through this fissure, accompanied by some filaments from the cavernous sympathetic plexus and the orbital branches of the middle meningeal artery. Additionally, the superior ophthalmic vein drains into the cavernous sinus through this fissure.

The apex of the orbit corresponds to the medial end of the superior orbital fissure, close to the origin of the EOM, just below the optic foramen. The cylindrical optic canal forms by surrounding the optic nerve and ophthalmic artery where the two roots of the lesser wing of the sphenoid join the sphenoidal body.

Through the optic canal and superior orbital fissure, the cranial cavity communicates with the orbital cavity. The cranial dura mater lines the internal surface of every cranial bone, with a firm adhesion at the sutures, and extends outside the cranial cavity through foramina and fissures, forming tubular sheaths for the cranial nerves as they leave the neurocranium. Thus, the endosteal layer of the cranial dura mater is continuous through the superior orbital fissure with the orbital periosteum. In addition, a tubular dural sheath from the meningeal layer of the dura surrounds the optic nerve as it passes through the optic canal. This dural layer blends with the ocular sclera and adheres intimately to the common annular tendon of the four recti muscles. There is an anatomic continuity between the dura and the lining and structures of the orbital cavity, such as the eyeball and the EOM.

The seven extraocular, or extrinsic, muscles include the levator palpebrae superioris, superior rectus, inferior rectus, medial rectus, lateral rectus, superior oblique and inferior oblique muscles (Fig. 7.5.3). They control the movements of the upper lid and eyeball. All the EOM are tied together in a complex fashion by fascial sheaths. There are also intrinsic muscles within the eyeball that are responsible of the shape of the lens and size of the pupil.

The levator palpebrae superioris arises from the lesser wing of the sphenoid, above and in front of the optic foramen, from which it is separated by the origin of the rectus superior. From a narrow tendon it soon broadens into a flat, triangular shape that ends anteriorly in a wide aponeurosis. The superficial fibers are prolonged forward, piercing the orbicularis oculi muscle, to insert on the deep surface of the skin of the upper eyelid. The deepest fibers blend with an expansion from the sheath of the rectus superior. Some fibers also attach to the upper margin of the superior tarsus and are referred to as the superior tarsal muscle.

A thickening of the sheath of the levator palpebrae superioris is referred to as the superior transverse ligament of Whitnall. It extends laterally and medially to insert in the orbital walls just behind the superior orbital rim. Medially, it attaches to the trochlea of the superior oblique muscle and to the frontal bone. Laterally, it is fixed to the capsule of the lacrimal gland and to the frontal bone.

When the levator palpebrae superioris contracts, it raises the upper eyelid. It is innervated by a superior branch of the oculomotor nerve (CN III). Interestingly, the superior tarsal muscle is innervated by postganglionic sympathetic fibers from the superior cervical ganglion. Therefore, a complete ptosis reflects the loss of oculomotor function, whereas a partial ptosis is associated with loss of sympathetic supply.[5]

The four rectus muscles arise from a fibrous ring – the common tendinous annulus of Zinn – that extends across the superior orbital fissure and

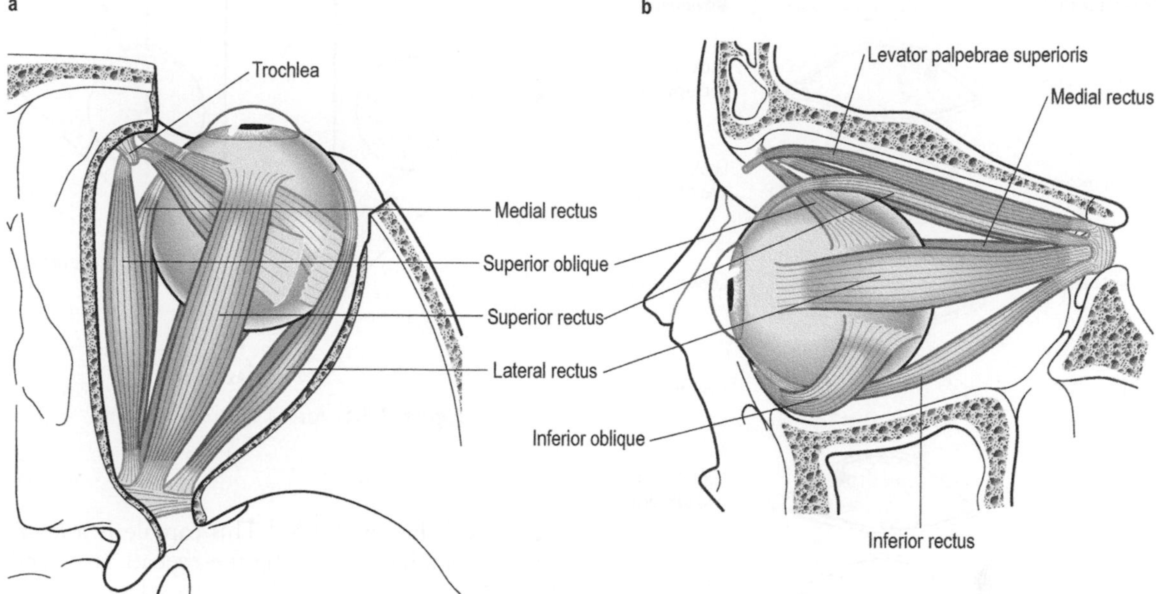

Figure 7.5.3. *Muscles of the eyeball: (a) superior view; (b) lateral view.*

surrounds the upper, medial and lower margins of the optic foramen, where it adheres strongly to the tubular dural sheath surrounding the optic nerve. The common tendinous annulus consists of two parts. Superiorly, the tendon of Lockwood gives origin to the superior rectus muscle, part of the medial rectus and the upper fibers of the lateral rectus; inferiorly, the tendon of Zinn gives origin to the inferior, medial and lateral rectus muscles. At their origin, the rectus muscles are tightly set in Zinn's annulus and start to separate at about 8 mm anterior to the optic canal.[9] The medial rectus is the broadest while the lateral rectus is the longest. The four rectus muscles go forward and insert through tendinous expansions into the sclera, the superior and inferior recti passing anterolaterally.

The superior oblique muscle originates from the body of the sphenoid, above and medial to the margin of the optic foramen and origin of the superior rectus. It passes forward, ending in a round tendon, which goes through a fibrocartilaginous ring or trochlea attached to the frontal bone. From that point, the tendon turns backward, laterally and downward beneath the superior rectus to insert into the sclera, behind the equator of the eyeball in its superolateral posterior quadrant.

The inferior oblique muscle originates from the orbital surface of the maxilla, just posterior to the orbital rim and lateral to the lacrimal groove. It traverses the floor of the orbit in a lateral, backward and upward direction, and inserts into the inferolateral posterior quadrant of the eyeball.

The EOM produce mobility of the eyeball with extreme amplitude in all directions (Fig. 7.5.4). This is because the type of attachment they demonstrate to the periorbita – an interlocking of tendinous and muscular fibers – provides them with a strong anchor.[10] The contraction of the EOM rotates the eyeball according to their insertions and the orientation of their fibers. However, in all cases it should be remembered that these muscles function together and not as isolated entities. The ocular movements of individual muscles can be simplified as follows:[5]

- The superior and inferior recti adduct the eyeball, in association with elevation and intorsion from the superior rectus and depression and extorsion from the inferior rectus.
- The medial rectus adducts the eyeball while abduction is the result of contraction of the lateral rectus.
- The superior oblique is considered to act from the trochlea.
- Both the superior and inferior oblique abduct the eye, with a component of depression and intorsion from the superior oblique and elevation and extorsion from the inferior oblique.

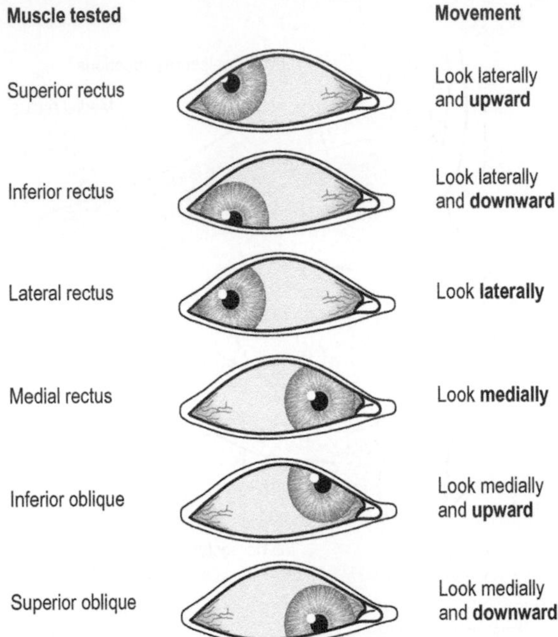

Figure 7.5.4. *Action of muscles of the eyeball.*

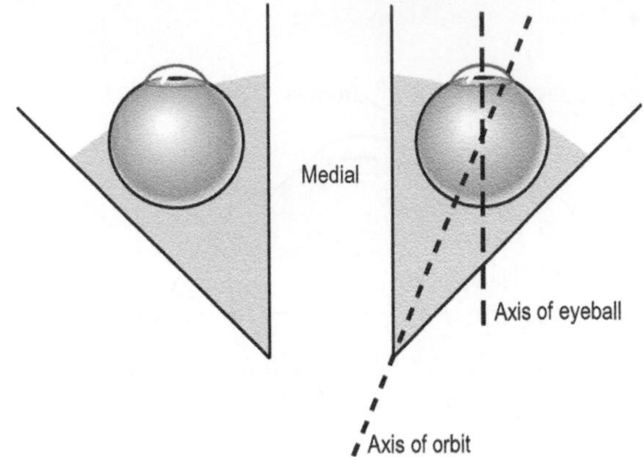

Figure 7.5.5. *Axes of the eyeball and orbit.*

It should be noted that while the longitudinal axis of the orbit deviates laterally in a posterior to anterior direction, the axis of the eyeball approximates the sagittal plane (Fig. 7.5.5). Therefore, muscular activity between medial and lateral muscles is not equal. At birth, infants tend to demonstrate intermittent ocular misalignments. This is associated with lack of maturity in visual function. It should disappear by 4 months of age when orthotropic ocular alignment and sensory binocularity should be present.[11] Transitory esotropic misalignments are usually considered to be typical in infants. However, if the condition is permanent with a fixed restriction of any of the EOM movements, or if it persists after 6 months of age, further evaluation is necessary.[12] In any case, osteopathic examination and treatment are indicated to balance the bony components of the orbit and their relationship with other parts of the skull. Dysfunction can also manifest through myofascial and membranous components. Entrapment neuropathy can result. Evaluation and treatment of these components are indicated to promote the best possible muscular activity and ocular function.

Although the study of EOM function is complex, it is imperative that it includes the orbital connective tissues that sheath the muscles. These tissues have long been recognized, the capsule of Tenon being described in 1806.[13] This capsule is a fascial sheath completely covering the eyeball. It extends from the optic nerve to the corneoscleral junction and separates the eyeball from the orbital fat. It is perforated by the tendons of the EOM on which it reflects to form tubular sheaths. Tenon described this capsule as a 'muscle pulley'.[13] After much controversy, this theory is again accepted, and further studies have established that each rectus and inferior oblique muscle passes through a pulley formed by a ring or sheath of collagen, elastin and smooth muscle that is located close to the equator of the eyeball, in Tenon's capsule.[14] In this manner, the rectus and the inferior oblique muscles have their paths constrained by pulleys that serve as functional origins for the muscles, in a fashion similar to that of the trochlea for the superior oblique muscle.[15] Thus, the position of a pulley insertion relative to the eyeball affects the forces of the EOM, and a translation of the eyeball of 1.5 mm modifies the pulling direction of the rectus muscle by 6°.[16] These pulleys are under active muscular control, allowing for constant ocular adjustments.[14] Conversely, their instability and modification of location are associated with ocular dysfunction.[16]

The EOM connective tissue sleeves that act as pulleys are firmly attached to each other and, through extensions, to the orbital walls. Those from the lateral and medial rectus are anchored to the orbital tubercle of the zygomatic bone and posterior to the lacrimal crest of the lacrimal bone, respectively. They are referred to as check ligaments. This point is of great significance. The zygomatic bone should not be overshadowed as a site of insertion for the EOM sheaths by the sphenoid on which the common tendinous annulus of Zinn inserts. In subjects with strabismus or other ocular misalignments, the consideration of the orbital bones on which the EOM insert should include the zygomatic bone. Its location makes it vulnerable to being struck during the course of normal childhood activities. This may, in turn, affect the diameter of the orbit and the functional balance of the EOM, particularly the lateral rectus. Another site of importance is the trochlea for the superior oblique muscle on the frontal bone. Frontal dysfunctions are often found in infants, with one side lower than the other resulting in frontal trochlear asymmetry. This may be seen with a superior–medial deviation of the eye encountered with dysfunction of the superior oblique muscle. Dysfunction of the maxilla can also influence visual activity through its effect on the insertion of the inferior oblique muscle. Through these complex interactions the orbit functions as a unit and each part, when dysfunctional, is a potential site for muscular instability and resultant ocular dysfunction.

The somatic components of ocular dysfunction also involve oculomotor supply. The oculomotor nerve (CN III) exits the brain medially to the cerebral peduncles. It traverses the dura at the top of the clivus, enters the cavernous sinus and courses forward in the lateral wall of the cavernous sinus where it receives sympathetic fibers from the internal carotid plexus and connects with the ophthalmic division of the trigeminal nerve (CN V_1). It then divides into two branches that enter the orbit through the superior orbital fi ssure The general somatic efferent fi bers of the oculomotor nerve innervate nearly all of the EOM. The superior division innervates the superior rectus and the levator palpebrae muscles, whereas the inferior division innervates the medial and inferior rectus and inferior oblique muscles. The general visceral efferent fi bers of CN III are part of the parasympathetic ANS and supply the sphincter of the iris that regulates the size and shape of the pupil and the ciliary muscle that modulates the shape of the lens.

The trochlear nerve (CN IV) is the only cranial nerve to emerge from the dorsal surface of the brainstem. It curves around the midbrain, pierces the dura between the lesser and greater circumferences of the tentorium cerebelli, enters the lateral border of the cavernous sinus, receives sympathetic fi bers from the internal carotid plexus and traverses the superior orbital fissure to the orbit. It carries somatic efferent fibers to the superior oblique muscle.

The abducent nerve (CN VI) emerges from the brainstem between the pons and medulla oblongata. It pierces the dura covering the clivus and passes over the ridge of the petrous apex of the temporal bone through an osteofi brous canal underneath Gruber's petrosphenoidal ligament. It then enters the cavernous sinus where it receives sympathetic fibers from the internal carotid plexus and the orbit through the medial end of the superior orbital fissure and within the annulus of Zinn. CN VI carries somatic efferent fibers to the lateral rectus muscle.

Additionally, the EOM contain proprioceptive receptors that provide input as to the position and movement of the eye in the orbit.[17] This contributes to the control of eye's movements and facilitates central control of the direction of gaze and the relationship of the child to their environment. These afferent fi bers appear to travel with the motor CN III, IV and VI before joining the ophthalmic branch of CN V to enter the CNS. Afferent input from these receptors not only affects static eye position but can also modify linear visual tracking, saccadic eye movement and the vestibulo-ocular reflex.[18]

Each of these nerves is subject to intracranial entrapment from osseous compression, membranous tension, ligamentous pull or the pressure of edema from venous congestion.[19] The anterior attachments of the tentorium cerebelli are a site with particularly great potential to cause such neurologic dysfunction. The ganglion of the trigeminal nerve may become entrapped by the tentorium in the trigeminal cave formed at the apex of the petrous part of the temporal bone. Bilaterally, the anterior fibers of the tentorium twine on each side as the fibers of the lesser circumference attach to the anterior clinoid processes and the fibers of the greater circumference attach to the posterior clinoid processes. Between these two attachments, the fibers of the tentorium cerebelli are oriented horizontally and contribute to the formation of the roof of the cavernous sinus. CN III and IV pierce the dura at this level to enter the cavernous sinus. Any dural membranous strains in these areas can result in entrapment neuropathy and each bone on which the tentorium cerebelli attaches should be considered as potentially critical in the development of ocular dysfunction. The petrosphenoidal ligament is another significant site under which CN VI may be compressed. Furthermore, as the nerve bends sharply in its course over the petrous ridge, it is, therefore, vulnerable to the changes in position of the petrous portion of the temporal bone.

Adequate arterial supply and drainage are necessary for healthy nervous function. Edema and stasis encumber this function, as is the case with a jugular foramen dysfunction and impediment of the drainage from the cavernous sinus, resulting in venous congestion. This, in turn, will affect the cranial nerves passing through the cavernous sinuses to the orbits. The same rationale applies to the superior orbital fissure Intraosseous dysfunction in infants between the greater and lesser wings of the sphenoid, or narrowing of the fissure because of greater wing dysfunction with surrounding structures, such as the temporal bone, impairs venous drainage or impulse conduction of the nerves passing through the fissure.[19] Additionally, lymphatic stases outside the skull can also entrap nerves at their foramina of exit.[19]

Multiple theories exist concerning the cause of non-paralytic or concomitant strabismus, including sensorimotor, anatomic and mechanical or muscular origins.[10] Prematurity[20] and difficult labor are considered to be risk factors. A supranuclear developmental abnormality in the CNS is thought to be the cause of strabismus occurring in the first 6 months of life. Impaired vision and amblyopia may also cause strabismus.

It is abnormal for an infant or child to have strabismus and, if present, a thorough ocular and neurologic examination by a specialist should be performed. Osteopathic procedures may, however, be applied to provide balance to the musculoskeletal and nervous systems. Such balance improves the self-healing capacities of the body and contributes to the success of other treatments. Osteopathic treatment should be initiated at the earliest possible time because the prognosis of strabismus is correlated to the time when the strabismus first appears and the time when treatment is initiated. Additionally, early treatment may positively impact the vestibulo-ocular reflexes and thereby the child's posture.

Physical examination and treatment

Young children and infants are most likely to present for the treatment of strabismus. As such the following treatment description must be appropriately adapted to fit the age of the patient. The following is not intended to treat organic pathologies of the eye; it is directed at problems of functional balance.

The examination and treatment for the eye should address different levels of anatomic dysfunction. These include osseous, myofascial, neurologic and vascular dysfunction and the intrinsic structure of the eye. Observation and palpation are directed at determining on which of these levels treatment should focus. Observe the relationship between the eye and the functional pattern of the skull. If the functional pattern of eye position and movement is consistent with the dysfunctional pattern of the skull, the focus of treatment should be on the cranial dysfunction. If eye position and movement is not consistent with the pattern of the skull, treatment should focus directly on the eye, EOM and associated fascial structures.

Start with observation of the bony orbit, relative to how it fits the global pattern of the skull. Look at the shape of the face and skull of the child to determine if a global pattern of cranial flexion–external rotation, extension–internal rotation, sidebending–rotation or torsion is present. Observe the orbital diameter, the distance between the superior medial and inferior lateral angles of the orbit. It is increased with cranial flexion–external rotation, resulting in an orbital cavity that is wider. Cranial extension–internal rotation decreases the orbital diameter, with a resultant orbital cavity that is narrower. Look for asymmetry between the visible constituents of the bony orbits, specifically the frontal bones, zygomae and maxillae.

Look at the eyes and observe for difference in size and shape. Cranial flexion–external rotation is associated with a prominent eyeball and an almond-shaped eye. In cranial extension–internal rotation, the eyeball is less prominent, with a smaller, rounder shaped eye. Epicanthus – a vertical fold of skin covering the medial portion of the eye – may give the impression of esotropia. Active motion testing will, however, demonstrate normal function of the eye.

Next, observe the spontaneous movements and neutral resting position of the eyes. Note the direction of gaze, the presence of esotropia or exotropia. The easiest way to evaluate the ocular movement of younger children is to hold a toy or some interesting object in front of the child to catch their attention. Move the object horizontally, vertically and in both diagonals, and observe the movement of the child's eyes as they follow the moving object. Note any asymmetric movement of the cervical spine that can be employed to compensate for the absence of ocular movement. This may be a sign of amblyopia that requires further evaluation. If possible, assess both eyes together and each eye separately by covering one eye with the child's or caregiver's hand and pretending to play 'peek-a-boo'. Comparatively note the speed and ease with which the eyes move to follow the object. Convergence may be determined by observing as the toy is brought closer to the infant's face. This procedure tests the actions of the EOM and normal responses are illustrated in Figure 7.5.4.

Determine if a correlation exists between the dysfunction of the EOM and the pattern of cranial dysfunction. The two most commonly encountered types of strabismus that are amenable to cranial manipulation are the consequence of dysfunction involving the superior oblique muscle and the lateral rectus. A superior–medial–oblique deviation of the eye resulting from dysfunction of the superior oblique muscle may be associated with ipsilateral dysfunction of the frontal bone affecting its relationship to the muscle at the trochlea. Medial deviation of the eye resulting from dysfunction of the lateral rectus may be associated with ipsilateral temporal bone or sphenoid dysfunction that affects CN VI as it passes beneath the petrosphenoidal ligament.

Palpate for function to confirm the above observations. Tests of listening should be performed with specific attention to the anatomic structures associated with the eyes in order to define the dysfunctional area responsible for ocular deviation. Areas of specific interest include the bones on which the EOM are attached: the sphenoid, frontal, maxillae and zygomae. Assess the anatomic areas of neurovascular passage to the orbital cavity. These include the superior orbital fissure between the greater and lesser wing of the sphenoid and the cavernous sinus for their contents. Also evaluate the apex of the petrous portion of the temporal bone and the sphenoid for their relationship to the petrosphenoidal ligament. In actual practice, these assessments and the treatment of identified dysfunction flow seamlessly into one another.

Diagnostic palpation of the sphenoid, and to a lesser degree of the frontal bone, is complex because the movements of the EOM are transmitted to these bones. These additional movements on top of the biphasic PRM create multifaceted palpatory sensations that can be confusing to the inexperienced examiner. Consequently, it is desirable to evaluate the child when they are quiet with minimal eye movement. This occurs most readily when the child is sleeping. If the examiner is skilled with indirect procedures, the act of palpation will often soothe the child enough to bring them to a quiet state.

Complete examination of the sphenoid is somewhat difficult because of the limited surface area of the bone that is available for direct palpation. The areas of contact over the lateral-most aspects of the membranous greater wings, because of their flexibility, transmit an incomplete representation of the movement of the body of the sphenoid. For this reason, the lightest touch must be employed when evaluating the sphenoid and even then information about the body must be obtained indirectly. To assess the sphenoid body and associated lesser wings more effectively, visualize the relationship between the frontal bone and the sphenoid behind. The body and lesser wings of the sphenoid are in continuity with the orbital plates of the frontal bone. When palpating, one hand can be placed transversely on the frontal bone with the thumb and middle finger contacting the greater wings on either side. The movement of the lesser wings and body of the sphenoid is transmitted through the orbital plates of the frontal bone. This provides a method of augmenting the palpatory sensations from the body of the sphenoid through the frontal bone.

Similarly, the sensation of movement of the greater wings of the sphenoid may be enhanced through the zygomatic bones and their relationship with the greater wings at the sphenozygomatic sutures. These visualization procedures may be employed during both tests of listening and treatment, and require that the bones being palpated in association with the sphenoid are themselves free of somatic dysfunction.

In infants and younger children, intraosseous dysfunctions of the frontal bone and sphenoid should be considered. Listen to the movement between the two halves of the frontal bone. Palpate for deformation affecting the trochlea of the superior oblique muscle. Visualize and listen to the synchondroses between the greater wings and the body of the sphenoid.

Listen to the relationship between the greater and lesser wings at the superior orbital fissure, visualizing the neurovascular content, and try to promote the inherent forces of the PRM in the area. Similarly, assess the cavernous sinus because of its relation with the nerves and venous drainage of the eyes. Visualize the dura that constitutes the walls of the cavernous sinus and its relationship to the remainder of the reciprocal tension membranes.

Finally, if the child permits, and while utilizing the gentlest of indirect methods, palpate the globes of the eyes. Evaluate the tone and quality of the myofascial structures surrounding the eyeballs. Identify the functional point of balance between the EOM.

Treat any dysfunction as identified above, using indirect principles. Only after any osseous, membranous and fascial dysfunctions have been treated, and the EOM have been balanced, employ myofascial rehabilitation. In the patient with ocular deviation, the EOM provide dysfunctional proprioception to the CNS. The child should learn to experience the sensations of the normal range of ocular movements. Older children can be taught to move their eye while the practitioner gently applies digital contact intended to guide the eye through the normal range of ocular movements. In this exercise, particular attention should be directed at establishing awareness of the sensation of eye movements in the directions that they are deficient. The process of myofascial rehabilitation is accomplished with greater ease once pre-existing osseous, membranous and fascial dysfunctions have been treated.

ASTIGMATISM, MYOPIA, HYPEROPIA

A description of the anatomy of the bony orbit and the EOM has already been provided in 'Strabismus' above. We shall, therefore, only consider the description of the eyeball and somatic dysfunction as they relate to the pathophysiology of astigmatism, myopia and hyperopia.

The eyeball occupies the anterior part of the cavity of the orbit. It is surrounded by the EOM and embedded in the fat of the orbit. Two spheres of different diameters form the eyeball. The anterior cornea is smaller, transparent, bulging outward and represents approximately one-sixth of the eyeball. Posteriorly, a larger opaque sphere constitutes the rest of the eyeball.

Anatomically, the eyeball may be described as being formed by three tunics or walls that are, from front to back, the fibrous tunic, the vascular pigmented tunic and the nervous tunic, and by internal components or refracting media, the aqueous humor, the vitreous body and the crystalline lens.

The outside fibrous tunic of the eyeball is formed by the sclera and cornea. In the front, the sclera is continuous with the cornea at the sclerocorneal junction. The sclera is a dense and firm membrane that preserves the shape of the eyeball. It is covered with a fascial membrane, the capsule of Tenon, posteriorly from the optic nerve to the corneoscleral junction anteriorly. This fascial membrane reflects onto each of the EOM tendons as they perforate Tenon's capsule to attach on the sclera. Posteriorly, the sclera is pierced by the nervous filaments of the optic nerve (CN II), forming the lamina cribrosa sclerae. The sclera is continuous with the fibrous sheath of CN II and, therefore, with the meningeal layer of the dura mater. Several small apertures exist around the lamina cribrosa sclerae for the ciliary vessels and nerves. The central artery and vein of the retina pass through CN II.

The cornea projecting in front of the sclera is almost circular, with its width slightly greater than its height. Its anterior convexity demonstrates varying degrees of curvature throughout life and between individuals. A rapid change in the corneal curvature occurs during the first 2–4 weeks of life. This rate of change then decreases considerably after the 8th week.[21] The corneal curvature usually stabilizes at approximately the end of the 1st year of life.[5] Its coating of tears constitutes the most important site of refraction of the eyeball.

The middle tunic of the eyeball is a vascular pigmented layer consisting of the choroid posteriorly and the ciliary body and iris anteriorly. The choroid is a thin, highly vascular membrane that constitutes approximately the posterior five-sixths of the globe. Its outer surface adheres firmly to the sclera while its inner surface is attached to the retina. This layer provides a significant percentage of the vascular supply to the retina.

The ciliary body consists of the ciliary processes and the ciliary muscle. The ciliary processes are circularly arranged as a ruche behind the iris surrounding the lens. They are continuous at their periphery with the layers of the choroid and anteriorly with the periphery of the iris. Posteriorly, they are connected with the zonule that is the suspensory ligament of the lens. The ciliary muscle plays an important role in accommodation. It adjusts the shape of the lens in order to change the focus of the eye. When the ciliary muscle contracts, it draws forward the ciliary body, thus reducing tension in the fibers of the suspensory ligament. This results in a relaxation of the lens' capsule with resultant increased convexity of the lens. The parasympathetic stimulation of fibers from CN III produces contraction of the ciliary muscle.

The iris is a thin, circular, contractile disk, located between the cornea and lens, and continuous peripherally with the ciliary body. The iris differs in color among individuals, and at birth is light blue because of a lack of pigment. Iris pigmentation is well developed at 6 months of age. The iris divides the space between the cornea and lens into an anterior and a posterior chamber that communicates through the center of the iris, the pupil. Pupillary dilatation or constriction results from the contraction of the dilatator or sphincter pupillae. Responses to light and accommodation produce the two dominant pupilloconstrictor reflexes. Axons from preganglionic parasympathetic fibers course with CN III to the ciliary ganglion, located behind the eyeball. From there, postganglionic fibers supply the smooth muscle of the iris; this may result in pupillary constriction. Inhibition of the tonic activity of the oculomotor system in the midbrain Edinger–Westphal nucleus leads to pupillary dilatation. Extreme pupillary dilatation is referred to as mydriasis, extreme constriction as miosis.

The nervous tunic, i.e. the retina or inner layer of the walls of the eyeball, is truly a sensory extension of the brain. During embryogenesis, the optic vesicles develop from the lateral aspects of the forebrain. When they invaginate, forming two optic cups, the inner walls of the cups become the retinal sensory mesh and send axons back to the optic stalk. On activation of the receptors of this sensory stratum, brain activity starts the visual sensory processing. Light and images of external objects are received on the retinal receptors, stimulating a chemical reaction and action potentials transmitted through the optic nerve to the visual cortex within the occipital lobe.

The vascular supply of the retina comes partly from the choroid that is in contact with the external layer of the retina. Internally, the retina lies in contact with the vitreous body. The thickness of the retina varies, its thickest portion being located in the back of the eye, near the central retinal area or macula lutea. The fovea centralis, the center of the macula lutea, is a point of maximum vision and could be considered as the posterior point of the eyeball's axis. It is approximately 3–4 mm lateral and 1 mm inferior to the center of the optic disc, a point where the retina is insensitive to light, referred to as the blind spot. The macula continues to develop until 16–18 weeks after birth. Fully developed visual acuity is normally established by 2 years of age.[22]

Light passes through various refracting media in the eye, the aqueous humor, the lens and the vitreous body. The aqueous humor fills the anterior and posterior chambers of the eyeball. It is secreted into the posterior chamber by the ciliary processes. It flows into the anterior chamber through the pupil and is absorbed into the scleral venous sinus between the iris and cornea. The lens is situated directly behind the iris and in front of the vitreous body. It is a transparent, biconvex structure surrounded by a capsule and is connected to the ciliary muscle through the suspensory ligament. It measures approximately 6 mm in diameter at birth and from the first years of life offers excellent refractive power. As the child grows, more layers are added on the lens periphery, and around 14 years of age it reaches its adult size. From then on, progressively, it will loose its hydration and thereby its flexibility and refractive power. Accommodation, normally occurring when tension of the lens' capsule decreases, becomes more difficult. This leads, for most individuals in their fifties, to the need for glasses to compensate. The postrenal (vitreous) chamber forms about four-fifths of the eyeball and is filled with the vitreous body (vitreous humor) that is situated between the retina and the lens. It is transparent, of a gel-like consistency, and is composed of about 99% water.

When light enters the eye, the cornea and crystalline lens normally focus the rays of light through accommodation specifically on the retina. When properly functioning, this is referred to as the emmetropic state and requires that normal ocular growth occurred resulting in normal eye biometry.

The central point of the anterior curvature of the eyeball is referred to as the anterior pole; the central point of the posterior curvature is the posterior pole. A line joining the two poles is referred to as the optic axis. The optic axes of the two eyeballs are almost parallel, approximating in the sagittal plane, while the longitudinal axes of the orbits are directed forward and laterally (Fig. 7.5.5). Therefore, for each eye, these two axes are aligned in different directions. The optic nerves enter the orbit with the ophthalmic artery, through the optic canal, and follow the direction of the axes of the orbits. This explains why the optic disc is medial to the fovea centralis in the center of the macula lutea. The transverse and anteroposterior diameters of the eyeball are slightly greater (24 mm) than its vertical diameter (23.5 mm). At birth the anteroposterior diameter is about 17.5 mm and at puberty is between 20 and 21 mm.

Ocular growth and refraction are dynamic processes evolving during infancy and childhood, well through adult life. Color vision develops rapidly after birth and in most individuals some color vision is usually present at 3 months of age.[23] Although difficult to evaluate in infants, normal visual acuity is thought to be present by 2 years of age.[22] Even though complete anatomic and functional maturity of the visual system is reached around 10 years of age, many important milestones occur during the first 2 years of life. For these reasons, when examining and treating infants and children, an osteopathic practitioner should pay close attention to any somatic dysfunction that may potentially alter the normal shift of the refractive state of the eye to emmetropia. The sites of dysfunction with potential for alteration of the visual system are the different bony components of the orbit, the eyeball, EOM and surrounding fascial and dural sheaths. Because the vestibulo-ocular reflexes link the individual's posture with ocular function, the axial skeleton and postural balance of the child should also be addressed.

Any disturbance in the visual components may alter vision, usually asymmetrically. If this occurs during the developmental process, the resulting absence of stimulation in the visual part of the cortex will cause partial loss of sight, or amblyopia. This could be associated with an important difference of visual acuity between both eyes. Normally orthotropic ocular alignment and sensory binocularity should be present by 4 months of age.[11] If there are signs of misalignment and lack of sensory binocularity, further evaluation should be carried out.

Emmetropization allows a distant object to be projected as a focused image on the retina without accommodative effort.[24] This is possible when the optical power and the axial length of the eye are balanced. Normally, in the emmetropic eye with relaxed accommodation, objects are focused on the retina. If the point of focus falls behind the retina, increased accommodation is necessary to bring the point of focus on the retina. This occurs with hyperopia and has been associated with decrease of the axial length of the eyeball. Conversely, in myopia, the point of focus falls in front of the retina and this is associated with increase of the axial length of the eyeball (Fig. 7.5.6). Some compensation usually occurs in these conditions, since eyes with decreased axial length are associated with a more rounded cornea, whereas increased axial length is associated with flattening of the cornea.

Typically, infants demonstrate hyperopic eyes that tend to improve with ocular growth and, by the age of 5–8 years, they are emmetropic. By age 6 years, only a few children are myopic, but between the ages of 6 and 7 years, myopic children have the fastest progression of all age groups.[25] Myopia is a common condition affecting approximately 4.4% of Caucasian children, 13.2% of Hispanics and demonstrates the highest prevalence in Asians (18.5%).[26] This condition and its progression are influenced by

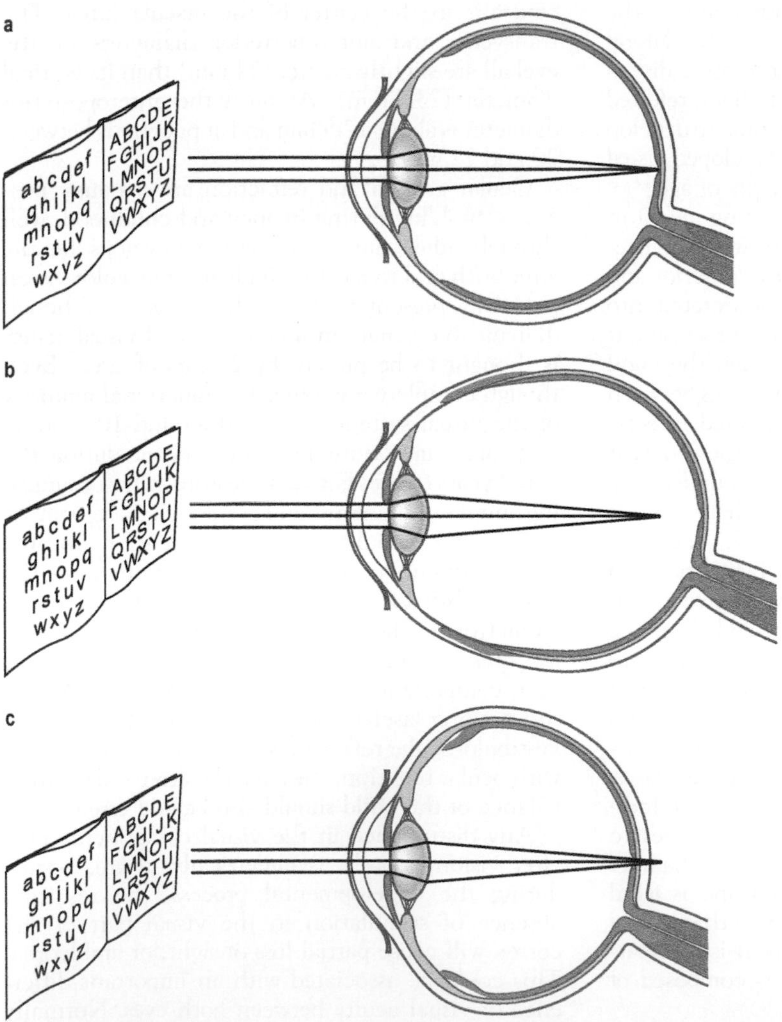

Figure 7.5.6. *Accommodation: (a) in the emmetropic eye, objects are focused on the retina; (b) in myopia, associated with increase of the axial length of the eyeball, the point of focus falls in front of the retina; (c) in hyperopia, associated with decrease of the axial length of the eyeball, the point of focus falls behind the retina.*

various factors such as demography and the environment[27].

The etiology of myopia seems to be multifactorial, with a genetic component since myopic individuals are more likely to have myopic parents.[29] A greater reading exposure in childhood has often been suggested as a contributing factor and is especially associated with myopia in Asian children, more often encountered around 7–9 years.[30]

Intrinsic ocular factors are also associated with myopias. Greater dimensions are present in myopic eyes than in emmetropic eyes when the vitreous chambers are measured along the axial direction, i.e. the optical and visual axes.[31,32] Heavier newborns with large heads have longer optical axial lengths, deeper vitreous chambers and flatter corneas. However, refraction is maintained and satisfactory, suggesting the presence of accommodative mechanisms in the cornea that compensate for the longer axial length.[24] Myopia usually develops because of a lack of coordination between postnatal growth and the refractive power of the eyeball components. There is some probability that the CNS influences the development of myopia.[28]

Unequal curvature(s) along the meridians of the refractive surfaces of the eye – cornea, anterior or posterior surfaces of the lens – result in astigmatism. Thus, when light enters the eye, instead of having the cornea and the crystalline lens focusing the rays of light at a single point on the retina, they are spread out as a line in one direction or another. The orientation of the axis of corneal astigmatism is affected by the mode of delivery. Infants delivered vaginally when compared to those delivered by cesarean section demonstrate a higher frequency of with-the-rule astigmatism, with the greater curvature of that astigmatism tending to be in the vertical meridian.[33] These astigmatic corneas usually flatten significantly by the age of 6 months.

Because astigmatism, myopia and hyperopia are associated with anatomic variations in the biometry of the eye, any form of treatment that may affect the refractive power and shape of the eye is desirable. This is particularly important in children less than 1 year of age, when the eye is still growing and the ocular reflexes are not totally developed. Prevention of the ocular complications of myopia, such as retinal detachment and glaucoma, may be facilitated by relaxation of tension in surrounding ocular structures. Addressing somatic dysfunction of the upper thoracic and cervical vertebrae may further assist relaxation of ocular tension. For these reasons, osteopathic procedures may be applied directly to the eyeball itself or the structures surrounding the eyeball including the orbit and its myofascial contents. Procedures may also be employed to affect the control of refractive mechanisms through the impact that the ANS has on the intrinsic ocular muscles.

Physical examination and treatment

The osteopathic structural examination of the eye and orbit for the patient with astigmatism, myopia and hyperopia is essentially the same as that described above for strabismus. The patient should be thoroughly evaluated for dysfunction affecting the component bones of the orbit, the EOM and associated fascial sheaths. In addition, because these ocular conditions involve changes in the shape of the eyeball, the physical evaluation of the individual with myopia or hyperopia should specifically include the search for any somatic dysfunction that affects the axial length of the eyeball. For the patient with astigmatism, somatic dysfunction responsible for changes in orbital shape and tension of myofascial structures that affect the curvatures along the meridians of the refractive surfaces of the eye should be identified.

Cranial flexion–external rotation is associated with a decrease of the orbital depth, whereas extension–internal rotation is associated with increased orbital depth. For these reasons, potentially contributory craniosacral somatic dysfunction should be sought out and treated. This includes dysfunction involving the SBS and bony components of the orbit as well as all components of the craniosacral mechanism, including, but not limited to, the sacrum and pelvis. A posture in which the child projects their head forward may be the result of poor sight. On the other hand, dysfunction affecting the posture, because of its effect on the cervical myofascial structures, particularly those attaching to the base of the skull, will tend to impair the inherent motility of the skull and potentially the components of the orbit. A craniosacral somatic dysfunction of the sacrum in flexion will produce a decrease of spinal AP curves and a tendency toward cranial flexion. This can, in turn, favor decreased orbital depth that is particularly significant in infants and young children at a time when ocular growth is occurring. As such, a complete postural assessment is appropriate when examining a child with ocular dysfunction.

It is also appropriate in these individuals to begin working on the global postural pattern because vestibulo-ocular reflexes link posture with ocular function. Using an indirect approach, begin with the treatment of postural dysfunction.

Because of their action on the PRM, the use of indirect techniques will relax the patient. The treatment of ocular dysfunction requires the most delicate touch and as the patient relaxes it becomes easier to treat the eyes.

After addressing the global postural pattern, proceed to the examination of the neurocranium and viscerocranium. Assess the SBS with tests of listening, then progress to observe the size and shape of the orbit. Look at the relationship of the eyeball to the orbit. Prominence of the eyeball is associated with a wider orbit and a pattern of cranial flexion–external rotation, whereas a recessed eye is associated with a narrower orbit and cranial extension–internal rotation. Also observe the patient in profile bilaterally, comparing the amount of corneal curvature.

Determine if the dysfunctional mechanics identified at the SBS is consistent with the pattern of orbit and eyeball. If so, treat the SBS; if not, look for dysfunction in the orbit. (*Note*: In infants the state of development of the frontal bone with small brow ridges causes the eyeballs to appear as if they are bulging.)

Next, assess the different bones that constitute the orbit, particularly the frontal bone, zygomae, maxillae and sphenoid. The effect of cranial dysfunction on the depth and shape of the orbit is significant in astigmatism, myopia and hyperopia. The apex of the orbit is situated at the medial end of the superior orbital fissure between the lesser and greater wings of the sphenoid, near the origin of the EOM and inferior to the optic foramen. Thus, the length and direction of the orbital axes are influenced by the sphenoid. Dysfunctions of the sphenoid that can affect the orbit include dysfunction of the SBS, dysfunction between the sphenoid and the bones articulating with its wings and intraosseous dysfunction. With cranial flexion the apex of the orbit moves forward, thus decreasing the AP orbital diameter, whereas in extension the apex is displaced posteriorly, increasing the AP orbital diameter. With SBS torsion or sidebending–rotation, on the side of associated external rotation, the AP orbital diameter is decreased and on the side of associated internal rotation it is increased. Intraosseous dysfunctions of the sphenoid have variable effects on the orbit and eyeball. They must be identified and treated as early as possible, sphenoid ossification being essentially complete by 1 year of age. Dysfunction of the frontal bones, zygomae and maxillae, either individually or in conjunction with the sphenoid, can affect the shape of the orbit and, when present, should be treated using indirect principles.

An extension of the dura surrounds the optic nerve and is attached to the optic canal. Intraosseous dysfunction of the sphenoid can affect the cylindrical optic canal that is formed where the two roots of the lesser wing of the sphenoid join the sphenoidal body. The dura also extends through the superior orbital fissure and blends with the orbital periosteum. Consequently, membranous strain can affect the sphenoid and through the sphenoid the shape of the orbit. Dural membranous dysfunction should thus be sought out and treated at the youngest possible age.

To ensure autonomic balance for the orbital contents, the rhythmic motility of the orbit and neurocranium is necessary. Change of the AP diameter of the orbit is associated with altered tension of the intraorbital soft tissues with resultant stasis, edema and compression. This, in turn, will affect the function of nervous structures, in this case CN III and the ciliary ganglion. Treatment of regional dysfunction, ensuring the rhythmic flexion–extension of the PRM in the orbit, fissures and foramina, provides a pumping action mobilizing the extracellular fluids surrounding the nerves and facilitating their function.

The sympathetic supply to the orbit originates in the upper thoracic spine and, through the upper cervical ganglia, reaches the ciliary ganglia via the carotid plexus. Somatic dysfunction affecting these structures in the upper thoracic and cervical spine and the cranial base should be sought out and treated to ensure optimal sympathetic function.

REFERENCES

1. MacEwen CJ, Young JD. Epiphora during the first year of life. Eye 1991;5(Pt 5):596–600.
2. Honavar SG, Prakash VE, Rao GN. Outcome of probing for congenital nasolacrimal duct obstruction in older children. Am J Ophthalmol 2000;130(1):42–8.
3. Coats DK. A simple model for practicing surgery on the nasolacrimal drainage system. J AAPOS 2004;8(5):509–10.
4. Isenberg SJ, Apt L, McCarty J, Cooper LL, Lim L, Del Signore M. Development of tearing in preterm and term neonates. Arch Ophthalmol 1998;116:773–6.
5. Williams PL (ed). Gray's anatomy, 38th edn. Edinburgh: Churchill Livingstone; 1995.
6. Dilmen G, Koktener A, Turhan NO, Tez S. Growth of the fetal lens and orbit. Int J Gynaecol Obstet 2002;76(3): 267–71.
7. Scott JH. The growth of human face. Proc Roy Soc Med 1954;47(2):91–100.
8. Hintschich C, Zonneveld F, Baldeschi L, Bunce C, Koornneef L. Bony orbital development after early enucleation in humans. Br J Ophthalmol 2001;85(2):205–8.
9. Ettl A, Zwrtek K, Daxer A, Salomonowitz E. Anatomy of the orbital apex and cavernous sinus on high-resolution magnetic resonance images. Surv Ophthalmol 2000;44(4): 303–23.
10. Sevel D. The origins and insertions of the extraocular muscles: development, histologic features, and clinical significance. Trans Am Ophthalmol Soc 1986;84:488–526.

11. Thorn F, Gwiazda J, Cruz AA, Bauer JA, Held R. The development of eye alignment, convergence, and sensory binocularity in young infants. Invest Ophthalmol Vis Sci 1994; 35(2):544–53.
12. Algranati PS. Effect of developmental status on the approach to physical examination. Pediatr Clin North Am 1998; 45(1):1–23.
13. Roth A, Muhlendyck H, De Gottrau P. La fonction de la capsule de Tenon revisitée. J Fr Ophtalmol 2002;25(9): 968–76.
14. Demer JL, Oh SY, Poukens V. Evidence for active control of rectus extraocular muscle pulleys. Invest Ophthalmol Vis Sci 2000;41(6):1280–90.
15. Demer JL. Pivotal role of orbital connective tissues in binocular alignment and strabismus: the Friedenwald lecture. Invest Ophthalmol Vis Sci 2004;45(3):729–38; 728.
16. Oh SY, Clark RA, Velez F, Rosenbaum AL, Demer JL. Incomitant strabismus associated with instability of rectus pulleys. Invest Ophthalmol Vis Sci 2002;43(7):2169–78.
17. Donaldson IM. The functions of the proprioceptors of the eye muscles. Philos Trans R Soc Lond B Biol Sci 2000; 355(1404):1685–754.
18. Weir CR, Knox PC, Dutton GN. Does extraocular muscle proprioception influence oculomotor control? Br J Ophthalmol 2000;84(9):1071–4.
19. Magoun HI Sr. Entrapment neuropathy of the central nervous system. II. Cranial nerves I–IV, VI–VIII, XII. J Am Osteopath Assoc 1968;67(7):779–87.
20. Robaei D, Rose KA, Kifley A, Cosstick M, Ip JM, Mitchell P. Factors associated with childhood strabismus: findings from a population-based study. Ophthalmology 2006;113(7): 1146–53.
21. Inagaki Y. The rapid change of corneal curvature in the neonatal period and infancy. Arch Ophthalmol 1986;104(7): 1026–7.
22. Edward DP, Kaufman LM. Anatomy, development, and physiology of the visual system. Pediatr Clin North Am 2003; 50(1):1–23.
23. Brown AM. Development of visual sensitivity to light and color vision in human infants: a critical review. Vision Res 1990;30(8):1159–88.
24. Saw SM, Tong L, Chia KS et al. The relation between birth size and the results of refractive error and biometry measurements in children. Br J Ophthalmol 2004;88(4): 538–42.
25. Hyman L, Gwiazda J, Hussein M et al. Relationship of age, sex, and ethnicity with myopia progression and axial elongation in the correction of myopia evaluation trial. Arch Ophthalmol 2005;123(7):977–87.
26. Kleinstein RN, Jones LA, Hullett S et al; Collaborative Longitudinal Evaluation of Ethnicity and Refractive Error Study Group. Refractive error and ethnicity in children. Arch Ophthalmol 2003;121(8):1141–7.
27. Saw SM. A synopsis of the prevalence rates and environmental risk factors for myopia. Clin Exp Optom 2003;86(5): 289–94.
28. Saw SM, Tan SB, Fung D et al. IQ and the association with myopia in children. Invest Ophthalmol Vis Sci 2004;45(9): 2943–8.
29. Wong TY, Foster PJ, Hee J et al. Prevalence and risk factors for refractive errors in adult Chinese in Singapore. Invest Ophthalmol Vis Sci 2000;41(9):2486–94.
30. Saw SM, Chua WH, Hong CY et al. Nearwork in early-onset myopia. Invest Ophthalmol Vis Sci 2002;43(2): 332–9.
31. Gwiazda J, Marsh-Tootle WL, Hyman L, Hussein M, Norton TT; COMET Study Group. Baseline refractive and ocular component measures of children enrolled in the correction of myopia evaluation trial (COMET). Invest Ophthalmol Vis Sci 2002;43(2):314–21.
32. Atchison DA, Jones CE, Schmid KL et al. Eye shape in emmetropia and myopia. Invest Ophthalmol Vis Sci 2004; 45(10):3380–6.
33. Isenberg SJ, Del Signore M, Chen A, Wei J, Christenson PD. Corneal topography of neonates and infants. Arch Ophthalmol 2004;122(12):1767–71.

7.6 DIGESTIVE TRACT DYSFUNCTIONS

SUCKING AND SWALLOWING DYSFUNCTIONS

Sucking and swallowing are complex activities that are partially conscious and partially unconscious. They require the participation of many structures, including a significant percentage of the cranial nerves, and should be considered in the context of a sensory–motor complex that begins to develop well before birth.

Swallowing appears in utero after 11 weeks[1] with movements of the fetal tongue visible after 14 weeks. At that time, fetuses suck their thumbs reflexively in response to oral stimulation from the digital extremities.[2] Protrusion of the upper lip appears after the 17th week of gestation and protrusion of the lower lip at the 20th week. The real activity of sucking is seen at the 24th week. After that time, sucking and swallowing become more and more developed and appear as coordinated movements around 33 weeks.[1] At term, the fetus swallows about 500–900 ml of amniotic fluid per day. This daily exercise stimulates the maturation of oral structures, including the tongue, lips, soft palate and pharynx, and, therefore, prepares the fetus to perform the orofacial functions that will be vital at birth.

Sucking is one of the primitive reflexes that are totally present at birth in term infants. In the first days of life, oral feeding is almost entirely reflex, apparently without suprabulbar activity for rooting, latching, sucking and swallowing.[3] These reflexes are functionally important in infants to ensure successful ingestion. The primitive sucking reflex lasts for about a year, and then becomes more difficult to obtain because of central nervous system maturation and the development of voluntary motor activity.

The tongue is one of the major participants in the process of sucking. It is a muscular structure with intrinsic and extrinsic muscles. The intrinsic muscles allow the precise movements necessary for sucking, swallowing and speech. They are the superior longitudinal, inferior longitudinal, transverse and vertical muscles. The extrinsic muscles originate from other parts of the skull and hyoid bone, and consist of four paired muscles:

- the genioglossus muscles originate from the mandible, attach to the hyoid bone and blend with the intrinsic muscles of the tongue
- the hyoglossus muscles originate from the hyoid bone and insert into the tongue
- the styloglossus muscles originate from the styloid processes of the temporal bones and insert into the lateral part of the tongue
- the palatoglossus muscles originate from the soft palate aponeurosis and insert into the lateral part of the tongue.

A midline fibrous sagittal septum divides the tongue into two halves and attaches to the body of the hyoid bone. Additionally, on the undersurface of the tongue, the frenulum linguae – a vertical fold of mucous membrane – connects the tongue to the floor of the mouth. As such, although anchored at its root, the tongue is mobile, allowing the different functions of sucking, suckling, latching, swallowing and eating, and later speech.

In infants, the tongue is totally contained in the oral cavity, although it is quite wide in proportion to the container and protrudes beyond the alveolar gum pads. However, its development is far from being complete and its position will go through many changes before the end of adolescence. One of the biggest changes occurs in the first years of life, as the child grows, the posterior third of the tongue descends following the larynx.[1]

When evaluating tongue malposition in children, the bony attachments of the tongue muscles should be evaluated for somatic dysfunction. Dysfunction of the mandible, the temporal bones through the styloid processes and the hyoid bone may potentially interfere with the position of the tongue. One of the most common lingual dysfunctions is forward and inferior displacement of the tongue. This predisposes to malocclusion and mouth breathing. Mouth breathing and a low posture of the tongue are also associated with an inferoposterior displacement of the anterior convexity of the hyoid bone.[4–6]

To ensure the lingual mobility necessary in the infant for feeding and the development of proper speech, the frenulum linguae should not be too short. Ankyloglossia, or tongue-tie, is a congenital anomaly characterized by an unusually short frenulum linguae. Breastfeeding is more difficult in the presence of ankyloglossia, and children have more difficulty pronouncing lingual and sibilant sounds such as T, D, Z, S, TH, N and L.[7] Furthermore, the tongue affects the growth and development of the maxillae and mandible and, therefore, the teeth in the alveolar processes, acting as a natural orthodontic appliance 'for better or for worse'.[8] Its position should be unencumbered as early in life as possible in order to play a satisfactory functional role. As such, clipping of the frenulum (frenuloplasty) may be necessary in association with osteopathic procedures to ensure a correct tongue placement.

Sucking has been classified in two categories: nutritive and non-nutritive sucking (NNS).[9] Nutritive sucking results in the delivery of milk and exhibits a slower rate of sucks that are continuous, whereas NNS consists of a series of bursts of rapid sucks, approximately twice the rate of nutritive sucking, followed by rest periods. During breastfeeding, before the initiation of sucking, the tongue protrudes beyond the lower gum and then retracts, repeating this protrusive and retrusive displacement of the tongue to draw the nipple into the mouth. If the newborn recognizes the odor of the breast's nipple, frequent sucking is initiated that, in turn, will stimulate the mechanism of lactation. The mother's milk odor results in increased sucking and stronger pressure than when the infant is fed formula or water.[10] Successful sucking is produced by a peristaltic wave in the medial portion of the tongue moving from the front to the back of the tongue.[11,12] This is the result of successive contraction and relaxation of the genioglossus and transverse muscles of the tongue. At the same time, a repetitive thrust of the mandible participates in the compressive action on the nipple to produce milk. Sucking results from the combined actions of the masseters, orbicularis oris and buccinator muscles, as well as from the muscles of the tongue and the mandible, in particular the lateral pterygoid muscles. This activity of the pterygoid muscles is important. At birth the pterygoid processes of the sphenoid are not fully developed, and because the activity of sucking requires a significant effort from the infant, the stimulation produced contributes to their development.

At approximately the 10th month of life, a new sucking pattern appears. It resembles that of later years, as when sucking from a straw, and demonstrates less movement of the tongue.[13]

Reflexes are of paramount importance in the actions of the oral cavity. They facilitate various vital functions, including suckling and swallowing, but also breathing, eating and drinking. Sucking elicits a swallowing reflex in the infant by stimulating the lips and the oral cavity. This reflex results from sensory input that induces a series of motor responses. It is mediated through neural receptors located on sensory fibers, the afferent pathway of sensory fibers, central synaptic connections and interneurons, and the efferent pathway composed of motoneurons or autonomic postganglionic neurons innervating the effector organ. In a somatic reflex, the effector is the striated muscle innervated by the alpha motoneuron. In an autonomic reflex, the effector includes a peripheral neuron extending its postganglionic axon to visceral structures. In sucking and swallowing, the sensory receptors – the tongue, gums, palate and pharynx – are located in the oral cavity. The sensory input passes through the superior laryngeal nerve, trigeminal nerve (CN V) and glossopharyngeal nerve (CN IX) to the brainstem, in the nucleus tractus solitarius (NTS) and adjacent reticular formation. From there, second order neurons engage brainstem deglutitive pharyngeal and laryngeal motoneurons in the nucleus ambiguus and in the facial, trigeminal and hypoglossal nuclei. The palate and palatopharyngeal muscles respond, separating the mouth from the nasal cavity to prevent passage of food from the oral cavity to the nasal cavity during the swallowing process.[14]

The integrity of the infant's oral cavity is of significance when considering the development of orofacial reflexes. The concept that structure affects function, and vice-versa, is perfectly illustrated in this area. The different structures that constitute the oral cavity evolve as the infant is developing, thus producing changes in function that will, in turn, further affect those structures. Conversely, malposition of any of the structures contributing to the oral cavity, such as lingual malposition, will affect function and consequently viscerocranial development in infants and children.

Breastfeeding differs from bottle feeding. Breastfed infants have better control of the amount of milk obtained than bottle-fed infants. Bottle feeding is greatly influenced by the force of gravity, with higher volumes resulting in faster flow of milk. In order to control this increased fluid flow, the newborn tends to adapt with a lingual and mandibular posture that is less protrusive. This decreases muscular participation and bottle-fed infants demonstrate a reduction of masseter muscle activity.[15] The positive effect of muscular traction on bony development and thus on orofacial development[16] is decreased and may, in turn, contribute to malocclusion.[17] The type of nipple employed during bottle feeding, i.e. its material, density and location of holes, requires different adaptive patterns from the infant. Most of the time, the root of the tongue does not come up to the tip of the nipple, as is the case with breastfeeding, but rather demonstrates a more posterior position.

Sucking is considered to be a determining factor in orofacial morphogenesis. It influences mandibular growth through the traction of myofascial attachments. The upper head of the lateral pterygoid muscle inserts into the developing condyle of the mandible. Active sucking as produced by breastfeeding is considered to be of paramount importance in mandibular development. It contributes to the change from the retrognathic mandibular posture seen in infants to a more centered position at 1 year of age.[18,19] During breastfeeding, the shape of the breast and the sucking pressure of the infant's tongue against their palate has a modeling effect on the palate. The pressure of the tongue on the anterior portion of the palate produces a pattern of cranial flexion–external rotation. The rhythmic sucking pressure on the infant's palate results in a pumping action that may contribute to the balancing of their skull and cranial mechanism. Additionally, breastfeeding seems to have a positive effect on orofacial morphogenesis,[20] and a protective effect for the development of posterior cross-bite in deciduous dentition.[21]

Human milk is a complex fluid that contains more than 200 components and is highly effective for the health and wellbeing of the infant.[22] Breastfeeding provides multiple benefits, such as decreased gastrointestinal and respiratory infections in childhood,[23] in particular otitis media, as well as protection against atopic disease.[24,25] It also seems to reduce pain in infants[26] and to enhance cognitive and visual development, as well as to have a potentially positive impact on the mother's health.[22]

Breastfeeding is thus recommended as the optimal source of nutrition for infants during the first 6 months of life. Although thought of as a natural process, it is not always easy, and some infants demonstrate difficulties. Such is the case for preterm infants, or infants with developmental anomalies such as micrognathia or ankyloglossia. Nursing difficulties may also be related to developmental anomalies of the mother's breast or variations of nipple size or shape that reduce the effectiveness of sucking. When developmental anomalies are not present, but nursing difficulties persist, an evaluation for somatic dysfunction should be performed. The oral structures, including the mandible, should be assessed, and the function of the tongue should be checked. The intrinsic muscles of the tongue are all innervated by the hypoglossal nerve (CN XII), as are all the extrinsic muscles, with the exception of the palatoglossus muscle which is innervated by the vagus nerve (CN X). The hypoglossal nerve leaves the skull through the hypoglossal canal, situated in the anterior intraoccipital synchondrosis, between the basiocciput and the exocciput. The hypoglossal nerve may be subject to compressive forces during a difficult labor, with consequent impact on tongue motor function and resultant suckling difficulties.

Feeding is a highly complex activity in young infants since it requires the integration of sucking, swallowing and breathing. Normally, coordination of the buccopharyngeal functions takes place by 35 weeks postconceptional age,[14] although reflex swallowing occurs when sucking stimulates the lips and the oral cavity. A spoon of food placed on the tongue of term infants will also produce a reflex where the tongue pushes against the spoon.[1] It is only around the 4th or 5th month of age that infants open their mouth when a spoon is brought before them or touches their lips, and approximately 2 weeks later that they use their tongue to move food to the back of the mouth to swallow.[27]

The mechanism of deglutition is divided into oral, pharyngeal and esophageal stages. The oral stage occurs when the milk or food is in the mouth and when the child tastes, plays, experiments with the food and forms a bolus to be pushed into the pharynx and esophagus. At that time, the anterior part of the tongue presses against the hard palate, while in infants the buccinator muscles participate with resultant suction. Next, the tongue propels the bolus in the back of the mouth into the pharynx and the swallowing reflex is elicited. Multiple receptors around the opening of the pharynx are stimulated by the bolus, resulting in sensory impulses conducted to the swallowing center via CN V, IX and X. Consequent motor activity is triggered by CN IX and X.

During this pharyngeal stage, while the tongue propels the bolus posteriorly, the hyoid is displaced anteriorly, the larynx superiorly and anteriorly toward the base of the tongue, and the epiglottis moves to cover the superior opening of the larynx. The displacement of the epiglottis and the approximation of the vocal cords of the larynx combine to prevent the passage of food into the trachea. Thus, the bolus passes into the pharynx, dividing around the epiglottis while the soft palate moves against the posterior pharyngeal wall to close the nasopharyngeal entrance. The stylopharyngeus muscles draw the sides of the pharynx superiorly and laterally. This stretches the opening of the esophagus, and the bolus, always under the influence of gravity and contractions of the pharyngeal constrictors, enters into the esophagus. This third stage of the mechanism of swallowing – the esophageal phase – is totally under the influence of the ANS via the vagus nerves and the cervical and thoracic sympathetic ganglia.

Several differences in the coordination of swallowing are observed between infants and adults. Human infants, like non-human primates, demonstrate the ability to breathe and suckle simultaneously with swallowing phases between respirations (Fig. 7.6.1). They will keep this ability until approximately 2 years of age when the neuromuscular system matures. At that time, the larynx and tongue have completed their descent and the posterior third of the tongue is more vertical, forming the upper anterior wall of the pharynx.[28] The larynx and hyoid bones are involved in the descent, with separation of the epiglottis away from the uvula of the soft palate. The tip of the epiglottis is located at the level of the first cervical vertebra at 4 months of age and at the level of the third vertebra between 12 and 18 months of age.[29]

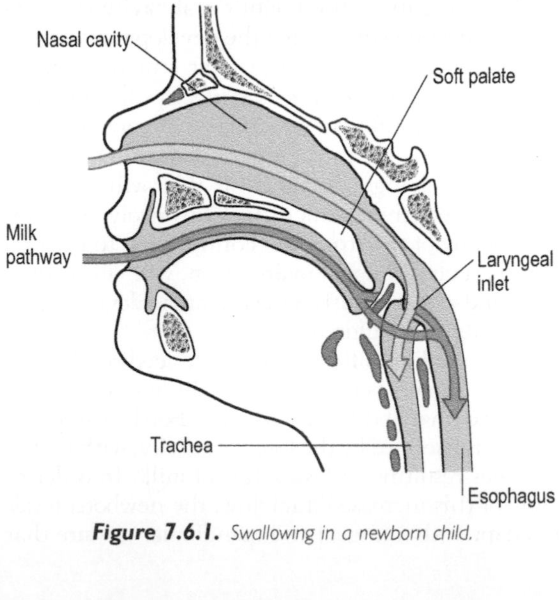

Figure 7.6.1. *Swallowing in a newborn child.*

In infants, swallowing is immature, different from that of the adult and characterized by an important anterior displacement of the posterior pharyngeal wall. During immature swallowing, the tongue protrudes over the lower lip with active contraction of the facial muscles, in particular the orbicularis oris and mentalis muscles. With progression of time, the teeth erupt in surroundings that can have an influence on their development, as much as they can influence the adjacent structures. Therefore, with maturation, the tongue rests lower in the mouth and is located between the teeth. Now, during swallowing, the tip of the tongue is posterior to the incisors, the lips are sealed and facial muscles relaxed. Infantile or immature swallowing should disappear around 2–3 years of age, and the positioning of the tongue against the palate will contribute to the development of a broad palate and a well-developed facies.

The act of swallowing is complex, involving the lips, jaw, tongue, palate, pharynx, larynx and esophagus, and each of these structures may be affected by somatic dysfunction. Conversely, the functions of sucking and swallowing are of paramount importance for the development of structures to which they are related. Oropharyngeal development is influenced by the functional posture of the tongue, lips and jaws.

The pharynx is attached superiorly to the base of the skull, the pterygoid processes of the sphenoid bone, the petrous portions of the temporal bones and the pharyngeal tubercle of the occipital bone. Laterally, the pharynx is connected to the styloid processes of the temporal bones and posteriorly to the cervical spine. Consequently, any dysfunction of the cranial base, cervical spine, hyoid bone and mandible should be considered when evaluating dysfunctional swallowing. Craniocervical dysfunctions are very frequently associated with an anterior displacement of the tongue, predisposing the individual to tongue thrusting. Furthermore, because CN IX and X trigger the motor activity of swallowing, the relationship between the occiput and temporal bones should be assessed for its effect on the jugular foramina.

The process of maturation of swallowing is not always established, leading to swallowing dysfunction or immature swallowing. Many individuals swallow with their tongues barely touching the palate or with their tongues between their teeth, in a dysfunctional manner. Swallowing occurs between 1500 and 2000 times a day, and, when dysfunctional, the thrusting force applied on the incisors with every swallow results in labial tilting. The child or adolescent who swallows immaturely also demonstrates some contraction in the orbicularis oris and mentalis muscles, failure to contact the molars and tongue protrusion when swallowing.[30] Furthermore, they have a narrow, high, palatal arch, and thus do not benefit from the pumping action of the tongue on the palate, and the palatine aponeurosis, which is suggested as being necessary for aeration of the pharyngotympanic tube (Eustachian tube).[31]

Physical examination and treatment

Begin by observing the face, specifically noting the proportion between the upper, middle and lower thirds of the face. The lower two regions are proportionately smaller in newborns than in older children, adolescents and adults. Observe the tonicity of the lips and note whether or not pursing is present. Observe the tonicity of the perioral musculature.

Have the child open the mouth and observe the position of the tongue; note any protrusion and if the tongue is at rest or demonstrates slight muscular activity. Assess the length of the frenulum linguae. It may be too short, inserting near the tip of the tongue, sometimes giving the tongue a heart-shaped appearance due to it.

Observe the movements of the tongue and, if the child is old enough, have them protrude the tongue to note its mobility. Ask them to pretend they are going to touch the tip of their nose with their tongue to observe its undersurface. With severe ankyloglossia, the tongue will tend to curl under during protrusion and will not be able to protrude because the tip is tied down by the short frenulum.

In infants, test the suck response by introducing a cotted finger, with the palmar surface in the direction of the hard palate, into the infant's mouth and allow them to suckle. The infant should respond by latching tightly. Feel coordination and strength of tongue movements.

Note any oral habits, such as tongue sucking, thumb or finger sucking, pacifier sucking or nail biting. When present, observe the position the child assumes when sucking a finger, thumb or pacifier and note in what direction the object being sucked is oriented. These positions will usually be taken to reinforce a dysfunctional pattern. For example, placement of an index finger relatively vertically in the mouth is associated with a narrow, high, palatal arch. Thumb sucking with the index finger curled over the nose is consistent with a cranial pattern in extension because the ethmoid bone is placed in anterior rotation as during extension.

Utilizing tests of listening, assess the cranial base, noting the movement of the occiput and the temporal bones. Intraosseous dysfunction of the occipital bone at the anterior intraoccipital synchondrosis will compress CN XII in the hypoglossal canal, while interosseous dysfunction between the occiput and temporal bones can affect the jugular foramen, entrapping CN IX and X.

Also examine the temporal bones because they affect the position of the mandible and because of the insertion of the styloglossus muscles on the styloid processes. Assess the mandible, temporomandibular joint, hyoid bone and cervical spine. These areas should be balanced to ensure satisfactory function of the associated myofascial structures.

Patient education and advice to caregivers

Patient education should be approached in three steps:

1. Instruct them to consciously keep their tongue in their mouth.
2. They must learn to swallow with their lips closed.
3. While keeping their lips closed, they must learn to swallow with the tip of their tongue resting against the palate behind their upper incisors.

An exercise to accomplish this is to place a small piece of food between the tongue and palate and keep it there while attempting to swallow several times. This may be repeated up to the point where swallowing with the tip of the tongue resting against the palate becomes an automatic reflex.

In young children with minor ankyloglossia, have them perform exercises to mobilize the tongue as much as possible in order to stretch the frenulum. Stress that mispronunciation often associated with baby talk may appear to be cute, but that it is actually dysfunctional and should not be encouraged. Insist, when speaking, that the child repeats incorrectly articulated sounds as correctly as possible to improve tongue mobility. Have them play sound-making games where they repeat certain sounds that cause the tongue to make a clicking noise against the palate.

Be aware that functional asymmetries are often associated with repetitive asymmetric activities, such as unilateral bottle feeding or thumb sucking. Educate the caregiver and patient to lose these habits. The use of a pacifier should be limited as much as possible. Suggest that pacifiers should be used only during the first 10 months of life, when the need for sucking is strongest.[32]

REGURGITATION AND GASTROESOPHAGEAL REFLUX

Gastroesophageal reflux (GER) is the retrograde flow of gastric contents into the esophagus and above. It is rather frequent during infancy and is often considered as 'physiologic' under 2 months of age with a benign prognosis in the majority of cases. However, it is a problem of considerable concern for the parents that ranges from minimal regurgitation with the bringing up of small amounts after feeds, to significant vomiting with failure to thrive. Because the latter may be indicative of a serious condition, it requires further medical evaluation.

GER is one of the most recurrent symptomatic clinical disorders affecting the gastrointestinal tract of infants and children, and regurgitation in infancy is a complaint in 5.8% of children seen in osteopathic practice.[33] Daily regurgitation is present in 50% of infants in the first 3 months of life, with a peak incidence at 4 months.[34] Most of the time, the condition resolves before the end of the 1st year and only 5% of infants still bring up their food between 13 and 14 months of age; however, when the condition is present for at least 90 days before 2 years of age, children are predisposed to demonstrate GER symptoms into middle childhood.[35] There is no association with gender,[35,36] nor with the mode of feeding the infant, breast or bottle; nevertheless, a genetic component seems to be present and a correlation exists between maternal symptoms of GER and the occurrence of regurgitation in infancy and GER in middle childhood.[35] Additionally, there is a stronger prevalence of GER among Caucasian infants.[36,37]

Normal gastroesophageal function is a complex mechanism where the relaxation and contractility of the lower esophageal sphincter are important factors. The esophagus is a tube connecting the pharynx and stomach, with muscular sphincters – the upper and lower esophageal sphincters. The upper portion of the esophagus (the cervical esophagus) consists of skeletal muscle; the remainder (the thoracic esophagus) consists of smooth muscle. After swallowing, the bolus of food passes through the pharynx to enter the esophagus. A primary wave of contraction starts in the pharynx and travels along the whole length of the esophagus, reinforced by secondary waves in the body of the esophagus. These peristaltic waves assist gravity to propel the bolus through the esophagus and into the stomach. Normally, at the gastroesophageal junction (GEJ), the lower esophageal sphincter (LES) relaxes to allow the bolus of liquid or food to pass into the stomach.

In GER, the GEJ is a critical site. The LES is formed by circular smooth muscle surrounding the terminal esophagus. The LES is under tonic contraction that relaxes during swallowing as well as following esophageal distension by a bolus of liquid or food. Additionally, the crura of the diaphragm participate in this sphincteric mechanism. The esophagus traverses the diaphragm through an opening in the right diaphragmatic crus, the esophageal hiatus, which is located between the central tendon and the hiatus aorticus. The two vagus nerves (CN X) also traverse the diaphragm through the esophageal hiatus. At this hiatus, one crus, most often the right crus, surrounds the esophagus forming an external sphincter; however, the fibers from the crus are not directly connected to the esophageal wall. Rather, fibers coming from the transversalis fascia, and thus continuing to form a fascia under the diaphragm, pass into the esophageal hiatus and surround the esophagus to blend into its walls 2–3 cm above the GEJ. Some of the elastic fibers of the fascia extend into the esophageal submucosa.[1] This connection between the diaphragm and esophagus is called the phrenoesophageal ligament. This ligament simultaneously allows GEJ mobility, permitting the displacement associated with respiration and swallowing, while providing restriction of upward movement of the esophagus. Additionally, during pulmonary inspiration, the diaphragmatic esophageal hiatus contracts in response to increased intra-abdominal pressure.[1]

The fascial relationships between the esophagus and the diaphragm must be balanced when addressing dysfunction of the GEJ. The transversalis fascia is a vast layer of fascia lying between the peritoneum and the abdominal walls, in continuation below with the pelvic fasciae, behind with the thoracolumbar fascia and above with the fascial sheet covering the undersurface of the diaphragm. The phrenoesophageal ligament, described above, consists of fibers extending from this layer to form the cone surrounding the GEJ. Furthermore, the stomach is connected to the diaphragm through the gastrophrenic ligament, i.e. the portion of the greater omentum that extends from the greater curvature of the stomach to the inferior surface of the diaphragm. From a functional point of view, the diaphragm must be balanced to allow satisfactory GEJ function.

The smooth muscle of the LES generates a tonic pressure at the GEJ that is the major barrier to reflux of gastric contents into the esophagus. Thus, reflux of acidic fluid backward, out of the stomach and into the esophagus, is normally controlled at the GEJ. At birth, neuromuscular activity and esophageal and LES peristalsis are undeveloped, resulting in frequent retrograde spilling out of gastric contents. The achievement of full development of the LES occurs as the infant matures, with the pressure at the LES reaching adult levels between 3 and 6 months of age. At the same time, the average capacity of the stomach at birth, i.e. around 30 ml, will rise to 100 ml at the end of the first month and will reach 1000 ml in the adolescent.

In order to act as a protective barrier against reflux from the stomach, pressure in the GEJ has to be higher than in the adjacent stomach or esophagus. Inhibitory and excitatory factors influence the tone of the LES. As mentioned above, a bolus of liquid or food initiates the relaxation of the sphincter in response to esophageal distension. This mechanism is under the control of intramural plexuses of the enteric nervous system. The motor fibers start in the dorsal motor nucleus of the vagus and the nucleus ambiguus, and the neural release of nitric oxide and vasoactive intestinal peptide among others by postganglionic fibers triggers the relaxation of the LES. Additionally, neurological activity from the dorsal motor nucleus of the vagus and nucleus ambiguus is also sent to the crura of the diaphragm.[14] Thus, both the esophageal and crural musculature are inhibited.

Embryologically, both the esophagus and stomach develop from the foregut. The dilatation of the foregut for the stomach starts in the sagittal plane at 4 weeks of gestation. Several spatial changes occur before the stomach reaches its final position. Because growth is greater along the dorsal border of the stomach, the greater and lesser curvatures are formed. This is followed by rotation, with the greater curvature moving to the left and the lesser curvature moving to the right. The two vagus nerves follow this rotation. Thus, the right vagus becomes posterior and supplies the dorsal part of the stomach, while the left vagus is anterior and supplies the ventral part of the stomach. Some torsion of the stomach occurs between the lower part of the esophagus and the pyloric canal, which are consequently no longer in the same plane. This has been suggested as a risk factor for GER.[38] This developmental process results in what is felt when the stomach is palpated. The identification of a strong torsional sensation in this region of the gut is an indication for osteopathic treatment that should be directed at the alleviation of the identified torsional dysfunction.

The etiology of GER is multifactorial, with often more than one factor being present in children with this condition. However, a transient LES relaxation (TLESR) as the result of a vasovagal reflex appears to be frequently associated with GER, producing a complete relaxation of the LES without pharyngeal swallowing.[39,40] Other factors for GER include ineffective esophageal motility or delayed gastric emptying.[41] A high fat diet can contribute to an increase in the number of episodes of TLESR.[42] Additionally, in infants, gravitational and positional factors associated with the supine position may exacerbate the reflux. Most infants spend more time in this recommended position since the 'Back to Sleep' campaign to prevent sudden infant death syndrome (SIDS). The return of the gastric acid contents into the esophagus predisposes the infant and the child to esophagitis; for these patients, crying becomes common.[43]

Acid reflux into the esophagus can reach the upper esophagus, the pharynx and larynx, and may possibly be aspirated into the trachea. Chemoreceptors in the mid or upper esophageal mucosa are stimulated, resulting in reflex respiratory inhibition, hypertension and bradycardia. Approximately 1% of infants demonstrate reflux-induced apnea with airway closure or laryngospasm.[44] The severity of these reactions may lead to SIDS.[43] Bronchospasm may also occur and, in turn, accentuate the symptoms of asthma, although GER does not seem to increase the risk of developing asthma.[45] Recurrent bronchitis or pneumonia is frequent and can be caused by repeated pulmonary aspiration of acid reflux. ENT problems such as nasal obstruction are sometimes related to GER, with secondary inflammation and narrowing of the posterior nasal apertures.[46,47] With premature infants, the most common complication of recurrent GER is failure to thrive.

In children and adolescents, GER is frequently associated with abdominal pain in the midepigastrium, eventually substernal heartburn and possible chronic irritative coughing. Furthermore, regurgitation of gastric contents into the oral cavity is responsible for dental erosion and dental caries.[48]

The vagus nerve (CN X) is essential in the control of LES tone. It contains both motor and sensory fibers, with a course and distribution more widespread than any of the other cranial nerves, passing through the neck and thorax to the abdomen. About 80% of vagal fibers are afferent fibers and may be general somatic, general visceral or special afferent. They provide significant sensory input from the viscera. In infants, children and adolescents with GER, there is a definitive dysfunctional viscerosomatic and/or somatovisceral component. This may, in turn, lead to altered behavioral responses. Possible dysfunction affecting CN X in its extensive course may facilitate GER. Critical sites are the jugular foramina and the passages through the diaphragm at the esophageal hiatus. Additionally, the stomach and esophagus may demonstrate visceral dysfunction in relation to somatic dysfunction in the surrounding structures, i.e. diaphragm, fasciae and ligaments.

The osteopathic approach to GER consists, therefore, of addressing any dysfunction that can impede the vagus, balancing the stomach and esophagus together and in their relationships with surrounding structures – the diaphragm, fasciae and ligaments.

Physical examination and treatment

Inspect the abdomen, noting its shape, contour and movement with respiration. The abdomen should be rounded and dome-shaped in infants because of the lack of abdominal muscular tone. Observe for abdominal asymmetry, noting areas of tension under the inferior border of the thoracic cage, in particular under the xiphoid process. Note if the umbilicus is centered or displaced or if it is protruded. In children and adolescents, observe the inside of the mouth for dental caries.

Examine and treat the craniocervical junction, with particular attention to the relationship between the occiput and temporal bones because compression of the jugular foramen can impact the exit of CN X. Check and balance the cervical area (C3, C4, C5) because of the phrenic nerve and its action on the diaphragm. Examine and treat identified somatic dysfunction affecting the thoracolumbar junction because of its potential to affect the crura of the diaphragm.

Evaluate and treat the diaphragm, paying particular attention to the freedom and symmetry of its excursion and its attachment around the xiphoid process as well as its anterior costal attachments. Balance the fasciae at the level of the LES by balancing the area below the xiphoid process with the diaphragm.

Balance the relationship between the stomach and diaphragm. The stomach itself demonstrates curling and uncurling movements, similar to those that created its curvatures. Palpation should reveal a balance between these curling and uncurling movements. A predominance of one phase can be treated using indirect procedures. Balance the torsional relationship between the stomach and the esophagus. Address somatic dysfunction related to both viscerosomatic and somatovisceral reflexes: occiput, C1, C2 for the vagus; upper thoracic for the esophagus; midthoracic for the stomach.[49]

Advice to caregivers

Infants should have small and frequent feeds, and should be fed in a semi-upright position. Feeding should occur under calm circumstances. Instruct children and adolescents to eat slowly and to avoid swallowing air. They should eat and drink small amounts to prevent distension of the stomach. They should also be instructed to avoid the consumption of fatty foods, caffeinated beverages and chocolate. Lifestyle changes such as avoiding eating before bedtime and, if appropriate, weight loss should be encouraged.

COLIC

The term colic is derived from the Greek, *kblikos*, meaning in relation to the colon. In the list of the most frequent gastrointestinal (GI) dysfunctions encountered in infants, colic is second only to regurgitation. It occurs in 10–40% of infants[50–52] and is one of the most common complaints for which parents seek professional advice.

The colicky infant presents with abdominal distension, frequent gas emissions, apparent abdominal pain, irritability and excessive crying. The mechanisms that explain this disorder are not entirely understood. They may be discussed in anatomic or physiologic terms, reflecting dysfunction at one or more levels of the brain–gut axis. Additionally, because the ontogeny of the GI system is under multiple influences – genetic heritage, intrinsic development, endogenous regulatory mechanisms and the environment[53] – the etiology of colic is commonly multifactorial. Thus, various etiologies have been proposed, including GI diseases such as allergy to cow's milk protein, lactose intolerance and intestinal hyperperistalsis, as well as neurodevelopmental dysmaturation or psychological difficulties in the parent–child relationship.

On average, it is estimated that infants cry for 2.2 hours per day during the first 2 months of life, with a peak around 6 weeks of age.[54] Crying time then slowly decreases to less than 1 hour a day by 12 weeks of age. The 'rule of three' proposed by Wessel et al. in 1954 is usually the reference employed to identify colicky children. These children are said to cry for more than 3 hours per day, more than 3 days per week and for longer than 3 weeks.[55] Colic usually starts in the 1st month of life and may persist until 3 or 4 months of age. Crying is commonly concentrated in the late afternoon and evening, occurs in prolonged bouts and is unpredictable and spontaneous. Colicky children are described as crying without identifiable cause, fussing and hard-to-soothe, although being otherwise healthy infants, well fed and showing no signs of failure to thrive. Individual variation may be present in the cries, such as duration or intensity, associated fussing or the resulting parental distress, adding complexity to the definition.[56] Colic cries convey acoustic information that the infant is highly aroused or distressed.[57] During a crying episode, the infant usually positions their legs flexed over their abdomen, in association with a hard distended abdomen, gurgling noises from the abdomen (borborygmi), sometimes gas and regurgitation, as well as facial grimacing and clenched fists. This presentation is indicative of a GI etiology for colic. When evaluating the colicky infant, several aspects of GI development and associated neuro–hormonal factors should be considered.

Bacterial colonization of the sterile GI tract of the neonate starts quickly on delivery. A flora develops, resulting from microbial and host interactions. The main factors that influence this developing microbial population are the maternal intestinal flora, the use of antibiotics by the mother during pregnancy and when nursing, the mode of delivery (vaginal or cesarean) and the mode of feeding (bottle feeding or breastfeeding). The bacterial flora in breastfed infants is composed typically of bifidobacteria, whereas in bottle-fed infants anaerobic bacteria as well as aerobic species are present.[58] It is also recognized that the flora of breastfed infants includes far fewer species that are liable to be pathogenic.[59] The developing bacterial flora usually becomes stable by the end of the first week of life. By 2 years of age the infantile flora resembles that of the normal adult. This process is one of the main components, along with host cells and nutrients, that form the complex ecosystem of the intestine.

The intestinal lumina are lined by a very large surface of mucosa that is the principal interface with the external environment. Besides its function of digestion and absorption of the nutrients contained in food, the intestinal mucosa forms a protective barrier against foreign substances and potentially pathogenic microorganisms from the external environment. The mucosal barrier consists of cellular and stromal components covered by a mucus layer. Within the mucosal barrier various secretions form a viscoelastic gel, creating a site for bacteria–bacteria interactions. Thus, the microbiota play an important role in the development of the endogenous barrier mechanism in the gut and are involved in the maturation of humoral immunity in humans.[60]

The intestine can be considered the primary immune organ, housing more than 70% of all immune cells.[25] The gut-associated lymphoid tissue (GALT) develops through innate and acquired immunity and consists of organized and diffuse lymphoid tissues that constitute the aggregated lymphoid follicles (Peyer's patches) and the mesenteric lymph nodes. This arrangement permits rapid response to any challenge in order to maintain the integrity and protective functions of the immune barrier at the GI mucosal surface. The GALT contains B lymphocytes, implicated in the synthesis of secretory antibodies of the immunoglobulin A (IgA) class, and T lymphocytes. In this ecosystem, the equilibrium of the microbiota is important in the maintenance of homeostasis and intestinal immune responses. It is also of paramount importance in the prevention of food allergies, and it is during the first 2 years of life, when the infantile flora is not well diversified, that food allergies and enteropathies are more apt to be established.

Particular circumstances in infants, such as prematurity, cesarean section delivery and antimicrobial treatment, delay intestinal colonization and its important immunostimulating effect.[60,61] On the other hand, breastfeeding is considered to confer beneficial effects on the microbiota, explaining its protective role against atopic disease, although it does not appear to have a protective effect on the development of colic.[62] Differences in the gut microbiota of breastfed colicky infants have been shown to exist when compared to non-colicky, and Lactobacilli are present less than in controls.[63]

That breastfed infants may suffer from colic might be explained by the fact that breast milk contains intact proteins similar to those of cow's milk and that colic often appears to be related to a food allergy, particularly to cow's milk protein.[64,65] This exposure would trigger the production of specific IgE to milk protein and may be considered a manifestation of an allergic predisposition. This is, however, subject to debate because no data support the hypothesis that infantile colic leads to an increased risk for subsequent allergic disease or atopy,[66] although more irritability during the 7th week and colic-type crying during the 12th week has been observed in children with atopic disease at 2 years of age.[67] Furthermore, lactose intolerance also contributes to infantile colic.[68] Incomplete lactose absorption encourages bacterial growth with resultant flatulence and cramping. As the etiology of infantile colic is multifactorial, cow's milk protein elimination may be an effective treatment for infantile colic,[64] and for colicky breastfed infants a maternal diet free of cow's milk may be considered.[69] Other maternal dietary modifications during breastfeeding should include reduction of cruciferous vegetables, onion and chocolate, foods that are associated with colic symptoms in infants.[70]

Hyperperistalsis is another theory included in the GI disorder etiology to explain abdominal cramping and colic. Intestinal smooth muscle normally generates rhythmic peristaltic activity. Movements of the intestine with the regulation of gut motility are the result of complex neural and muscular interactions that take place at several levels and under the influence of neurotransmitters and hormones.[71] The innervation of the gut consists of intrinsic and extrinsic nerves. Ganglionated and non-ganglionated plexi, part of the enteric nervous system (ENS), form the intrinsic innervation, while the vagus, splanchnic and pelvic nerves form the extrinsic innervation. The intrinsic afferent neurons project within the myenteric and submucous plexuses and information from activated sensory receptors reaches the CNS through vagal and spinal afferent nerves. The gut interacts constantly with the CNS through either somatic or autonomic neurons (brain–gut axis). Consequently, the CNS modulates the gut motor activity through the ANS (sympathetic and parasympathetic), maintaining the normal rhythm of activity in the GI tract as well as adjusting autonomic output to accommodate any external challenge. The release of acetylcholine by the parasympathetic fibers increases gut motility, whereas the release of norepinephrine, somatostatin and neuropeptide Y by sympathetic fibers decreases the motility. Multiple factors, such as emotion, stress, nervousness, fasting or eating, can also influence the activity of the ANS. Additionally, communication occurs between the different parts of the GI tract through myogenic and neurogenic signals along the gut, and through reflex arcs transmitted via autonomic neurons.

Individual differences are present in the functioning of the CNS. Accordingly, an increased sensitivity to stimuli, such as distension of the gut, is demonstrable in patients with functional GI disorders,[72] and excessive crying in colicky infants may be the result of hypersensitivity in the perception of gut stimuli or excessive afferent responses to these stimuli.[73] Genetic susceptibility to functional GI disorders may exist. Supporting this theory, a correlation is found between high responsiveness of the newborn during neurobehavioral assessment in the first days of life and crying behavior at home.[74] Additionally, intestinal hypersensitivity may alter motility of the GI tract by increasing intestinal afferent–efferent reflexes.[75]

Cranial osteopathy offers a therapeutic option for these patients. Osteopathic treatment of colicky infants has been demonstrated to decrease crying and increase sleep time.[76] Somatic dysfunction affects the

ANS. The resulting state of facilitation, in turn, increases the perception of either mechanical or chemical intestinal stimuli, and visceral hypersensitivity or dysfunction follows. Somatic dysfunction can involve any osseous, articular, ligamentous, membranous, fascial, muscular, visceral and vascular component associated with the GI tract. Vagal viscerosensory neurons have their cell bodies in the inferior ganglion located under the jugular foramen. The spinal sensory input takes place through perivascular nerves passing through the prevertebral ganglia to the dorsal horn of the spinal cord, and these neurons have their cell bodies in the dorsal root ganglia. Pain perception is thought to be mediated essentially by the spinal innervation.[77] The craniocervical junction (parasympathetic), the thoracic and thoracolumbar spine (sympathetic) and sacropelvic region (parasympathetic) may be sites of somatic dysfunction resulting in somatovisceral dysfunction. Treating these areas may contribute to balance the gut function of the colicky infant.

Changes in internal sensory states, acting in a bidirectional manner between the viscera and the brain, are obviously related to interoception and visceral hypersensitivity, and are considered as the key pathogenetic factors underlying the emotional state present in subjects with functional GI disorders.[78] Stress, in a broad sense, as with any menace to one's individual homeostasis, may come from the external or internal environment.[78] As such, visceral hypersensitivity, milk allergy or somatic dysfunction may be stressful, and colicky infants are quite often described as demonstrating difficult temperament.

An infant who is crying is expressing distress without indication of its origin. This can be a significant source of stress for parents and caregivers. They respond differently to these cries according to cultural and sociodemographic factors that, in turn, may affect the amount of infant crying. Responses of mothers to infant crying diverge from putting the child to bed, to holding and carrying them, riding around in the car, rocking or swaddling.[79] Globally, first-born babies are usually reported as crying more excessively, and the Western caregiving style is associated with a higher incidence of reported crying.[79,80]

Touching, holding and caressing a child results in positive effects on the emotion regulation and stress reactivity in the infant.[81] Maternal care facilitates the development of central corticotropin-releasing factor (CRF) systems which regulate the expression of behavioral, endocrine and autonomic responses to stress.[82] It is well established that infant–maternal contact is of paramount importance in mediating infant emotional reactivity. Gut–brain peptide cholecystokinin (CCK) and endogenous opioid analgesic agent production are increased following contact.[81] This contributes to the development of attachment through the 'interactive regulation of biological synchronicity between organisms'.[83] Under normal conditions, this relationship between mother and infant contributes to the wellbeing of both.

Conversely, infantile irritability can prove to be a major source of distress to caregivers. In extreme circumstances the irritability of the child can prove so stressful as to create an impulse to shake the child.[73] A potential psychosocial etiology for colic in the 1st year of life is associated with pre-existing maternal anxiety.[62] If the caregiver is stressed, the child will cry more, and the caregiver will be further worried by their incapacity to help the child. Furthermore, a baby is frequently described as crying excessively when the crying distresses the parents. Infants' cries can also be indicative of a behavioral problem resulting from a less than optimal parent–infant interaction. This complex interrelationship between the child and caregiver has led to a behavioral hypothesis for the etiology of colic where interventions such as modifying parental responsiveness, using motion and sound to calm the baby, and reducing stimuli have been suggested.[64] These caregivers do not need to be told that they are bad parents; they need to be supported and managed with understanding. The circumstances must be discussed and the caregiver given the opportunity to vent their anxiety and frustration. Behavioral adaptations, when appropriate, should be encouraged. Maternal smoking may contribute to the disorder.[84]

One hypothesis for colic suggests that it is the result of transient developmental dysmaturation based on the fact that infantile colic often stops after 5 or 6 months.[85] It is important, nonetheless, to treat these children and help the parents, because persistent behavioral difficulties, including crying, sleeping or feeding behavior in infancy, are precursors of hyperactivity or behavioral problems and academic difficulties in childhood.[86]

Physical examination and treatment

It is important to perform a thorough physical examination to rule out other causes for persistent crying to ensure that there is no organic cause for the crying. Once this has been done, osteopathic manipulation may be employed to reduce the somatic afferent load of somatovisceral reflexes into the CNS as well as to alleviate the mechanical impact that somatic dysfunction can have on the GI tract.

Treatment is appropriate not only for infants, but also for children and adolescents, because colic may persist later in life as a functional GI disorder.[87]

The osteopathic component of the examination should begin with observation of the infant's posture. The infant may position themselves with their legs flexed to their chest. If the patient is a child, they might present with an apparent increased lumbar lordosis that occurs when bowel dysfunction creates a distended abdomen with consequent relaxation of the abdominal muscles. Observe the abdomen to see if it is tense with bowel distension from flatulence. Note the power and rhythm of the inherent motility of the PRM in the head and throughout the body, particularly noting the abdomen. Somatic dysfunction should be sought out, especially in the regions of, but not limited to, the posterior neurocranium; the occipitocervical junction and upper cervical spine; the thoracic spine, ribs and upper lumbar spine; the thoracoabdominal diaphragm, the anterior abdominal wall and the sacrum and pelvis.

Treatment should employ indirect principles and manipulation should be directed at somatic dysfunction, when identified, involving the temporo-occipital relationship for its impact on the jugular foramen, and the occipitocervical junction and upper cervical spine for their effect on the vagus and parasympathetic somatovisceral reflexes. Somatic dysfunction of the thoracic spine, ribs and upper lumbar spine may be treated to affect sympathetic somatovisceral reflexes. In acute cases, practice inhibition in the lumbothoracic area. Avoid active massage of the abdomen which can be irritating. Dysfunction of the thoracic spine, ribs and thoracoabdominal diaphragm should be addressed for its impact on the lymphatic and venous drainage of the contents of the abdomen. Diaphragmatic, abdominal wall and pelvic dysfunction should be treated to alleviate the impact of dysfunctional fascial tensions on the GI tract. Dysfunction of the thoracoabdominal diaphragm is related to the function of the mesenteric plexus. Sacropelvic somatic dysfunction may be treated to affect pelvic splanchnic parasympathetic somatovisceral reflexes. Using indirect principles, release the periumbilical area and intestine. In every treatment procedure pay attention to the inherent motility of the PRM as manifest throughout the body. Treating this mechanism affects the ANS and probably facilitates tissue perfusion, reducing congestion.[88]

Patient education and advice to caregivers

The caregiver should be encouraged to create an environment of comfort, calm and relaxation for the infant. Gently caressing the frontal area of the neurocranium will often facilitate this. Obtaining relaxation of the infant will also have a calming effect on the caregiver(s) that will, in turn, further relax the infant. This relaxation will often make it easier to obtain such a state of calm in the future and will also demonstrate to the caregiver(s) that it can be obtained. Avoid, however, active massage of the abdomen which can be irritating.

Dietary considerations may be employed to improve the function of the GI and the immune system. Breastfeeding should, if at all possible, be encouraged. The mother should pay attention to her diet, avoiding cow's milk, cruciferous vegetables, onion and chocolate.

In colicky children, lactose intolerance should be considered. A diet rich in fresh fruit and vegetables and antioxidants such as vitamins C and E should be recommended, while refined foods should be avoided as much as possible.

CONSTIPATION

Constipation is the chief complaint in 3% of all pediatric outpatient visits and defecation disorder is present in 10–25% of children referred to pediatric gastroenterologists.[89] Constipation in children is usually defined as abdominal pain, difficulty or pain when passing stool, with the passage of feces that are either large and too hard or in small pebble-like pieces, with difficulty defecating and a frequency of two times or less per week.

The first intestinal discharge, meconium, is passed in healthy newborns within 24 hours.[90] After that, the mode of feeding determines the frequency and quality of stools. Bottle-fed infants demonstrate less frequent stools than breastfed infants, who have soft yellow stools up to five times a day. However, breastfed infants may go for 3 or more days without defecation. Weaning – the commencement of nourishment with food other than milk – usually occurs between 4 and 6 months of age and results in firmer feces. Although the frequency of bowel evacuation varies from one infant to another, it is generally admitted that a frequency of less than one stool a day before 6 months of age, and three times or less per week after 6 months, may be considered as pathologic. In preschool children, constipation is present when the child has less than two stools per week.

Most of the time, constipation is functional, without any objective evidence of an underlying pathologic condition and a thorough history and physical examination are sufficient to make the diagnosis. It is, however, important to rule out failure to thrive or endocrine, metabolic or structural disease such as Hirschsprung's disease. Children presenting with this latter condition, characterized by the total absence of ganglion cells in Meissner's and Auerbach's plexuses, suffer from constipation with massive colonic dilatation proximal to the segment of affected bowel. The onset, however, occurs at birth with delayed passage of meconium and children suffering from the disease demonstrate poor growth.[91]

Functional constipation has also been described as functional fecal retention, voluntary withholding, psychogenic megacolon or idiopathic constipation. It affects boys more often than girls, contrary to the adolescent and adult populations where women suffer more often from constipation. Another difference between children and the adult population is the presence of fecal incontinence in children, which is not present in adults with functional constipation.[91]

During the first months of life, infants may present with dyschezia, i.e. difficulty in defecation. In this case they experience severe problems when trying to defecate and strain and scream during prolonged endeavors. This behavior may last up to 20 minutes, until they successfully pass stools that are usually soft or liquid. The cause is hypothesized to be the failure to coordinate the augmentation of intra-abdominal pressure with the relaxation of the pelvic muscles.[89] Painful defecation quite often results in chronic fecal retention with fecal impaction (the immovable collection of compressed or hardened feces in the colon or rectum) and resultant fecal soiling (the passage of liquid stool around the impaction). More than 50% of school-aged children suffering constipation have a history of painful defecation before 36 months of age.[92] Toddlers may succeed in avoiding defecation for several days. The evacuation that then occurs is often painful and may be associated with bleeding, thereby strengthening the behavior of fear and retention. Fecal retention, in turn, is associated with subsequent abnormal contraction of the anal sphincters (anismus) and contraction of the pelvic floor during attempted retention. The child develops a retentive posture with contraction of the gluteal muscles. With overstretching of the rectal wall and muscle fatigue in the pelvic floor, incompetent anal function results in spontaneous relaxation of the sphincters, with consequent fecal soiling with soft or liquid stool. Fecal soiling often follows constipation facilitated by rectal distension.[93] Constipated children demonstrate several associated symptoms including irritability, abdominal cramps and decreased appetite. Most of the time, children with constipation have a withholding type of behavior and very often feel ashamed. They demonstrate more behavioral problems than children who are not constipated; however, these accompanying symptoms disappear immediately following the effective treatment of constipation.[94]

The role of psychological and emotional components in the etiology of defecation disorders is subject to debate. It is uncertain which problem comes first: the emotional disorder or the defecation disorder.[94]

Toilet training is normally initiated between the ages of 18 months and 3 years. When conducted in an overly coercive and stressful fashion, the associated stress has been proposed as a cause of fecal retention. However, when hard bowel movements or painful defecation are present in association with stool toilet training refusal, constipation should be considered because the first episode of constipation in children usually occurs before stool toilet training refusal.[95] Familial environmental factors, or added parental anxiety because they want their child to be able to go to school, may add a psychological factor to a physical predisposition to constipation.

A decrease in colonic peristalsis has been proposed as a cause of constipation in childhood. It is well recognized that reduction of physical activity and reduction of fluid intake in adults can be associated with constipation. Because children tend to be normally physically active, inactivity is not a major cause of constipation for this population. However, food allergy, particularly cow's milk allergy with cow's milk protein hypersensitivity, seems to be associated with constipation in children.[96,97]

Constipation may certainly be multifactorial. The behavioral approach does not explain every case of constipation. Furthermore, children with constipation demonstrate a higher incidence of bladder disorders such as urinary incontinence, bladder overactivity, dyscoordinated voiding, large bladder capacity, poorly emptying bladder, recurrent urinary tract infection and vesicoureteral reflux.[98] This constitutes a syndrome, an aggregate of associated symptoms and signs that may be addressed by an osteopathic approach. Most cases of functional constipation respond well to osteopathic manipulative procedures.

Defecation is a complex process that involves a mixture of voluntary and involuntary actions. It is triggered by the excitation of anorectal mechanoreceptors sensitive to distension of the rectum. It is followed by coordinated voluntary activity of the abdominal and pelvic musculature and involuntary relaxation of anal sphincters. As the fecal mass moves, the pelvic floor muscles relax in order to allow alignment of the rectum with the anal canal. Defecation can be inhibited by voluntary contraction of the external anal sphincter and pelvic floor muscles.

Normally, the anal canal is occluded by the internal and external anal sphincters. Additionally, the puborectalis muscle, the medial part of the levator ani muscle, contributes to the loop surrounding the anorectal junction by mixing some of its fibers with the deep part of the external sphincter of the anal sphincters. Additional fibers of the levator ani muscle join the conjoint longitudinal coat that surrounds the anal canal between the internal and external canal. Behind the rectum, the pubococcygeal fibers of the levator ani muscles attach to the anterior surface of the coccyx.

The internal anal sphincter has an autonomic innervation: the sympathetic fibers are from the hypogastric plexus and the plexuses located around the superior rectal artery; the parasympathetic fibers are from the pelvic splanchnic nerves (S2–S4). The external sphincter has a voluntary motor supply that comes from the inferior rectal branch of the pudendal nerve (S2–S3) and the perineal branch of the fourth sacral nerve.

Physical examination and treatment

If the child is old enough to be standing and walking, observe their postural mechanics, noting particularly the degree of abdominal protrusion, thoracolumbar mechanics as they relate to psoas muscle mechanics, the degree of lumbar lordosis as it relates to abdominal protrusion and psoas muscle mechanics.

With the patient supine, observe the abdomen, noting its contour and possible distension. Palpate the abdomen, looking for tension in the abdominal wall and for palpable stool. In many cases of chronic constipation, stool will be palpable throughout the colon. Define stool consistency and assess the quantity of the rectal fecal mass by looking at the height of transabdominally palpable stool above the pelvic brim. Diagnostic digital rectal examination should be performed gently to avoid perpetuation of dyschezia. Maneuvers that result in rectal stimulation produce potentially noxious sensory experiences and should be discouraged.[89]

Specifically look for somatic dysfunction affecting the thoracolumbar junction that can be associated with psoas muscle dysfunction and sympathetic somatovisceral reflexes. Examine the sacrum, coccyx and pelvis for dysfunction that can affect the pelvic floor and also be the source of parasympathetic somatovisceral reflexes.

The general medical treatment approach includes dietary changes with behavioral modification techniques (cognitive and behavioral interventions such as toilet training, which diminishes phobia and provides positive reinforcement through a rewards system). This approach is often combined with prolonged courses of laxatives. Treatment is usually successful, but may take up to 6–12 months.[93] When somatic dysfunction has been identified, the correct osteopathic treatment can result in significantly faster results with a resolution of constipation, often in one or two treatments.

Therefore, treat any somatic dysfunction as identified. Treat somatic dysfunction of the sacrum for its relation with pelvic splanchnic nerves and the pudendal nerve. Release sacroiliac joints and surrounding myofascial structures. It is important to remember that the sacrum is not completely ossified in infants and children and that intraosseous dysfunction may be present between the different sacral segments. In the infant the sacral molding procedure often provides good results. Treat somatic dysfunction of the coccyx, paying attention to its relationship to the insertion of the levator ani muscles. Treat somatic dysfunction of the thoracolumbar area for its somatovisceral effect on the sympathetic output to the intestine. With hypersympathetic drive, the bowel becomes less active and may result in constipation. It is also important to be sure that child's posture is balanced, without dysfunctional tension at the level of the psoas for its relationship with the sympathetic chain near the psoas muscle origin.

Patient education and advice to caregivers

It is important to increase the amount of fluid that the child drinks every day. Infants may be given fruit juices such as prune and pear which contain fructose and sorbitol for their mild laxative effect. If the child is old enough to be eating solid foods, increase bran cereal and fruits and vegetables that are high in fiber. Encourage the consumption of meals at regular times. If the child is relatively sedentary, as tends to occur these days with the playing of computer games, encourage increased physical activity.

Tell the parents to watch for infrequent, difficult or painful defecation that heralds the recurrence of constipation. When identified, they should respond quickly, encouraging the child to go to the bathroom more frequently and modifying the child's diet and physical activities.

REFERENCES

1. Williams PL (ed). Gray's anatomy, 38th edn. Edinburgh: Churchill Livingstone; 1995.

2. Gaspard M. Acquisition et exercice de la fonction masticatrice chez l'enfant et l'adolescent. Première partie. Rev Orthop Dento-Faciale 2001;5(3):349–403.
3. Stevenson RD, Allaire JH. The development of normal feeding and swallowing. Pediatr Clin North Am 1991; 38(6):1439–53.
4. Behlfelt K, Linder-Aronson S, Neander P. Posture of the head, the hyoid bone, and the tongue in children with and without enlarged tonsils. Eur J Orthod 1990;12(4):458–67.
5. Principato JJ. Upper airway obstruction and craniofacial morphology. Otolaryngol Head Neck Surg 1991;104(6): 881–90.
6. Finkelstein Y, Wexler D, Berger G, Nachmany A, Shapiro-Feinberg M, Ophir D. Anatomical basis of sleep-related breathing abnormalities in children with nasal obstruction. Arch Otolaryngol Head Neck Surg 2000;126(5):593–600.
7. Lalakea ML, Messner AH. Ankyloglossia: does it matter? Pediatr Clin North Am 2003;50(2):381–97.
8. Couly G. La langue, appareil naturel d'orthopédie dento-faciale 'pour le meilleur et pour le pire'. Rev Orthop Dento-Faciale 1989;23(1):9–17.
9. Wolff PH. The serial organization of sucking in the young infant. Pediatrics 1968;42(6):943–56.
10. Mizuno K, Ueda A. Antenatal olfactory learning influences infant feeding. Early Hum Dev 2004;76(2):83–90.
11. Bosma JF, Hepburn LG, Josell SD, Baker K. Ultrasound demonstration of tongue motions during suckle feeding. Dev Med Child Neurol 1990;32(3):223–9.
12. Hayashi Y, Hoashi E, Nara T. Ultrasonographic analysis of sucking behavior of newborn infants: the driving force of sucking pressure. Early Hum Dev 1997;49(1):33–8.
13. Iwayama K, Eishima M. Neonatal sucking behaviour and its development until 14 months. Early Hum Dev 1997;47(1): 1–9.
14. Miller MJ, Kiatchoosakun P. Relationship between respiratory control and feeding in the developing infant. Semin Neonatol 2004;9(3):221–7.
15. Inoue N, Sakashita R, Kamegai T. Reduction of masseter muscle activity in bottle-fed babies. Early Hum Dev 1995; 42(3):185–93.
16. Pottenger FM, Krohn B. Influence of breast feeding on facial development. Arch Ped 1950;57:454–61.
17. Raymond JL. Approche fonctionnelle de l'allaitement et malocclusions. Rev Orthop Dento-Faciale 2000;34:379–402.
18. Couly G. Morphogenèse temporo-mandibulaire. Actual Odontostomatol 1979;128:793–811.
19. Couly G. Structure fonctionnelle du condyle mandibulaire humain en croissance. Rev Stomatol 1980;81:152–63.
20. Labbok MH, Hendershot GE. Does breast-feeding protect against malocclusion? An analysis of the 1981 Child Health Supplement to the National Health Interview Survey. Am J Prev Med 1987;3(4):227–32.
21. Viggiano D, Fasano D, Monaco G, Strohmenger L. Breast feeding, bottle feeding, and non-nutritive sucking; effects on occlusion in deciduous dentition. Arch Dis Child 2004; 89(12):1121–3.
22. Zembo CT. Breastfeeding. Obstet Gynecol Clin North Am 2002;29(1):51–76.
23. Duffy LC, Faden H, Wasielewski R, Wolf J, Krystofi k D. Exclusive breastfeeding protects against bacterial colonization and day care exposure to otitis media. Pediatrics 1997; 100(4):E7.
24. Kramer MS, Chalmers B, Hodnett ED et al; PROBIT Study Group (Promotion of Breastfeeding Intervention Trial). Promotion of Breastfeeding Intervention Trial (PROBIT): a randomized trial in the Republic of Belarus. JAMA 2001; 285(4):413–20.
25. Noverr MC, Huffnagle GB. The 'microfl ora hypothesis' of allergic diseases. Clin Exp Allergy 2005;35(12):1511–20.
26. Potter B, Rindfleisch K. Breastfeeding reduces pain in neonates. J Fam Pract 2003;52(5):349, 352.
27. Carruth BR, Skinner JD. Feeding behaviors and other motor development in healthy children (2–24 months). J Am Coll Nutr 2002;21(2):88–96.
28. Laitman JT, Heimbuch RC, Crelin ES. Developmental change in a basicranial line and its relationship to the upper respiratory system in living primates. Am J Anat 1978;152: 467–82.
29. Sasaki CT, Levine PA, Laitman JT, Crelin ES Jr. Postnatal descent of the epiglottis in man. A preliminary report. Arch Otolaryngol 1977;103(3):169–71.
30. Subtelny JD, Subtelny JD. Oral habits – studies in form, function, and therapy. Angle Orthod 1973;43(4):349–83.
31. Mew JR, Meredith GW. Middle ear effusion: an orthodontic perspective. J Laryngol Otol 1992;106(1):7–13.
32. Niemela M, Uhari M, Mottonen M. A pacifier increases the risk of recurrent acute otitis media in children in day care centers. Pediatrics 1995;96(5 Pt 1):884–8.
33. Sergueef N, Nelson KE, Glonek T. Palpatory diagnosis of plagiocephaly. Complement Ther Clin Pract 2006;12(2): 101–10.
34. Nelson SP, Chen EH, Syniar GM, Christoffel KK. Prevalence of symptoms of gastroesophageal reflux during infancy. A pediatric practice-based survey. Pediatric Practice Research Group. Arch Pediatr Adolesc Med 1997;151(6):569–72.
35. Martin AJ, Pratt N, Kennedy JD et al. Natural history and familial relationships of infant spilling to 9 years of age. Pediatrics 2002;109(6):1061–7.
36. Nazer D, Thomas R, Tolia V. Ethnicity and gender related differences in extended intraesophageal pH monitoring parameters in infants: a retrospective study. BMC Pediatr 2005;5:24.
37. Tolia V, Wuerth A, Thomas R. Gastroesophageal refl ux disease: review of presenting symptoms, evaluation, management, and outcome in infants. Dig Dis Sci 2003;48(9): 1723–9.
38. Mansfi eld LE. Embryonic origins of the relation of gastroesophageal refl ux disease and airway disease. Am J Med 2001;111(Suppl 8A):3S–7S.
39. Mittal RK, Holloway RH, Penagini R, Blackshaw LA, Dent J. Transient lower esophageal sphincter relaxation. Gastroenterology 1995;109(2):601–10.
40. Orlando RC. Overview of the mechanisms of gastroesophageal reflux. Am J Med 2001;111(Suppl 8A):174S–177S.
41. Stacher G, Lenglinger J, Bergmann H et al. Gastric emptying: a contributory factor in gastro-oesophageal reflux activity? Gut 2000;47(5):661–6.
42. Osatakul S. The natural course of infantile reflux regurgitation: a non-Western perspective. Pediatrics 2005;115(4): 1110–1; author reply 1111.
43. Fonkalsrud EW, Ament ME. Gastroesophageal refl ux in childhood. Curr Probl Surg 1996;33(1):1–70.
44. Orenstein SR. An overview of reflux-associated disorders in infants: apnea, laryngospasm, and aspiration. Am J Med 2001;111(Suppl 8A):60S–63S.
45. Ruigomez A, Rodriguez LA, Wallander MA, Johansson S, Thomas M, Price D. Gastroesophageal refl ux disease and asthma: a longitudinal study in UK general practice. Chest 2005;128(1):85–93.
46. Olnes SQ, Schwartz RH, Bahadori RS. Consultation with the specialist: diagnosis and management of the newborn and

young infant who have nasal obstruction. Pediatr Rev 2000;21(12):416–20.
47. Bluestone CD. Humans are born too soon: impact on pediatric otolaryngology. Int J Pediatr Otorhinolaryngol 2005; 69(1):1–8.
48. Linnett V, Seow WK. Dental erosion in children: a literature review. Pediatr Dent 2001;23(1):37–43.
49. Van Buskirk RL, Nelson KE. Osteopathic family practice: an application of the primary care model. In: Ward RC (ed). Foundations for osteopathic medicine, 2nd edn. Philadelphia: Lippincott Williams and Wilkins; 2002:289–97.
50. Stagnara J, Blanc JP, Danjou G, Simon-Ghediri MJ, Durr F. Eléments cliniques du diagnostic de coliques du nourrisson. Enquête chez 2773 nourrissons âgés de 15 à 119 jours. Arch Pediatr 1997;4(10):959–66.
51. Lucassen PL, Assendelft WJ, van Eijk JT, Gubbels JW, Douwes AC, van Geldrop WJ. Systematic review of the occurrence of infantile colic in the community. Arch Dis Child 2001;84(5):398–403.
52. Iacono G, Merolla R, D'Amico D et al; Paediatric Study Group on Gastrointestinal Symptoms in Infancy. Gastrointestinal symptoms in infancy: a population-based prospective study. Dig Liver Dis 2005;37(6):432–8.
53. Lebenthal A, Lebenthal E. The ontogeny of the small intestinal epithelium. JPEN J Parenter Enteral Nutr 1999;23(5 Suppl):S3–6.
54. Brazelton TB. Crying in infancy. Pediatrics 1962;29:579–88.
55. Wessel MA, Cobb JC, Jackson EB, Harris GS Jr, Detwiler AC. Paroxysmal fussing in infancy, sometimes called colic. Pediatrics 1954;14(5):421–35.
56. Reijneveld SA, Brugman E, Hirasing RA. Excessive infant crying: the impact of varying defi nitions. Pediatrics 2001; 108(4):893–7.
57. St James-Roberts I. What is distinct about infants' 'colic' cries? Arch Dis Child 1999;80(1):56–61; discussion 62.
58. Fanaro S, Chierici R, Guerrini P, Vigi V. Intestinal microfl ora in early infancy: composition and development. Acta Paediatr Suppl 2003;91(441):48–55.
59. Bourlioux P, Koletzko B, Guarner F, Braesco V. The intestine and its microflora are partners for the protection of the host: report on the Danone Symposium "The Intelligent Intestine', Paris, 14 June 2002. Am J Clin Nutr 2003;78(4): 675–83.
60. Gronlund MM, Arvilommi H, Kero P, Lehtonen OP, Isolauri E. Importance of intestinal colonisation in the maturation of humoral immunity in early infancy: a prospective follow up study of healthy infants aged 0–6 months. Arch Dis Child Fetal Neonatal Ed 2000;83(3):F186–92.
61. Penders J, Thijs C, Vink C et al. Factors infl uencing the composition of the intestinal microbiota in early infancy. Pediatrics 2006;118(2):511–21.
62. Clifford TJ, Campbell MK, Speechley KN, Gorodzinsky F. Infant colic: empirical evidence of the absence of an association with source of early infant nutrition. Arch Pediatr Adolesc Med 2002;156(11):1123–8.
63. Savino F, Cresi F, Pautasso S et al. Intestinal microfl ora in breastfed colicky and non-colicky infants. Acta Paediatr 2004;93(6):825–9.
64. Lucassen PL, Assendelft WJ, Gubbels JW, van Eijk JT, van Geldrop WJ, Neven AK. Effectiveness of treatments for infantile colic: systematic review. BMJ 1998;316(7144): 1563–9.
65. Lindberg T. Infantile colic and small intestinal function: a nutritional problem? Acta Paediatr Suppl 1999;88(430): 58–60.
66. Castro-Rodriguez JA, Stern DA, Halonen M et al. Relation between infantile colic and asthma/atopy: a prospective study in an unselected population. Pediatrics 2001;108(4): 878–82.
67. Kalliomaki M, Laippala P, Korvenranta H, Kero P, Isolauri E. Extent of fussing and colic type crying preceding atopic disease. Arch Dis Child 2001;84(4):349–50.
68. Kanabar D, Randhawa M, Clayton P. Improvement of symptoms in infant colic following reduction of lactose load with lactase. J Hum Nutr Diet 2001;14(5):359–63.
69. Jakobsson I, Lindberg T. Cow's milk as a cause of infantile colic in breast-fed infants. Lancet 1978;2(8087):437–9.
70. Lust KD, Brown JE, Thomas W. Maternal intake of cruciferous vegetables and other foods and colic symptoms in exclusively breast-fed infants. J Am Diet Assoc 1996;96(1): 46–8.
71. Hansen MB. Neurohumoral control of gastrointestinal motility. Physiol Res 2003;52(1):1–30.
72. Kellow JE, Delvaux M, Azpiroz F, Camilleri M, Quigley EM, Thompson DG. Principles of applied neurogastroenterology: physiology/motility-sensation. Gut 1999;45(Suppl 2):II17–24.
73. Barr RG. Changing our understanding of infant colic. Arch Pediatr Adolesc Med 2002;156(12):1172–4.
74. St James-Roberts I, Goodwin J, Peter B, Adams D, Hunt S. Individual differences in responsivity to a neurobehavioural examination predict crying patterns of 1-week-old infants at home. Dev Med Child Neurol 2003;45(6):400–7.
75. Mertz H. Role of the brain and sensory pathways in gastrointestinal sensory disorders in humans. Gut 2002;51(Suppl 1):i29–33.
76. Hayden C, Mullinger B. A preliminary assessment of the impact of cranial osteopathy for the relief of infantile colic. Complement Ther Clin Pract 2006;12(2):83–90.
77. Boeckxstaens GE. Understanding and controlling the enteric nervous system. Best Pract Res Clin Gastroenterol 2002; 16(6):1013–23.
78. Van Oudenhove L, Demyttenaere K, Tack J, Aziz Q. Central nervous system involvement in functional gastrointestinal disorders. Best Pract Res Clin Gastroenterol 2004;18(4): 663–80.
79. van der Wal MF, van den Boom DC, Pauw-Plomp H, de Jonge GA. Mothers' reports of infant crying and soothing in a multicultural population. Arch Dis Child 1998;79(4): 312–7.
80. Michelsson K, Rinne A, Paajanen S. Crying, feeding and sleeping patterns in 1 to 12-month-old infants. Child Care Health Dev 1990;16(2):99–111.
81. Weller A, Feldman R. Emotion regulation and touch in infants: the role of cholecystokinin and opioids. Peptides 2003;24(5):779–88.
82. Francis DD, Caldji C, Champagne F, Plotsky PM, Meaney MJ. The role of corticotropin-releasing factor–norepinephrine systems in mediating the effects of early experience on the development of behavioral and endocrine responses to stress. Biol Psychiatry 1999;46(9):1153–66.
83. Schore AN. Attachment and the regulation of the right brain. Attach Hum Dev 2000;2(1):23–47.
84. Reijneveld SA, Brugman E, Hirasing RA. Infantile colic: maternal smoking as potential risk factor. Arch Dis Child 2000;83(4):302–3.
85. Barr RG. Colic and crying syndromes in infants. Pediatrics 1998;102(5 Suppl E):1282–6.
86. Wolke D, Rizzo P, Woods S. Persistent infant crying and hyperactivity problems in middle childhood. Pediatrics 2002;109(6):1054–60.

87. Gudmand-Hoyer E. The clinical significance of disaccharide maldigestion. Am J Clin Nutr 1994;59(3 Suppl):735S–741S.
88. Nelson KE. The primary respiratory mechanism. AAO Journal 2002;12(4):25–34.
89. Rasquin-Weber A, Hyman PE, Cucchiara S, Fleisher DR, Hyams JS, Milla PJ. Childhood functional gastrointestinal disorders. Gut 1999;45(Suppl 2):II60–8.
90. Clark DA. Times of first void and first stool in 500 newborns. Pediatrics 1977;60(4):457–9.
91. DiLorenzo C, Hyman PE. Gastrointestinal motility in neonatal and pediatric practice. Gastroenterol Clin North Am 1996;25(1):203–24.
92. Partin JC, Hamill SK, Fischel JE, Partin JS. Painful defecation and fecal soiling in children. Pediatrics 1992;89(6 Pt 1): 1007–9.
93. Catto-Smith AG. Constipation and toileting issues in children. Med J Aust 2005;182(5):242–6.
94. Benninga MA, Voskuijl WP, Akkerhuis GW, Taminiau JA, Buller HA. Colonic transit times and behaviour profiles in children with defecation disorders. Arch Dis Child 2004; 89(1):13–6.
95. Blum NJ, Taubman B, Nemeth N. During toilet training, constipation occurs before stool toileting refusal. Pediatrics 2004;113(6):e520–2.
96. Iacono G, Cavataio F, Montalto G et al. Intolerance of cow's milk and chronic constipation in children. N Engl J Med 1998;339(16):1100–4.
97. Carroccio A, Iacono G. Review article. Chronic constipation and food hypersensitivity – an intriguing relationship. Aliment Pharmacol Ther 2006;24(9):1295–304.
98. Chase JW, Homsy Y, Siggaard C, Sit F, Bower WF. Functional constipation in children. J Urol 2004;171(6 Pt 2): 2641–3.

7.7 OROFACIAL DYSFUNCTIONS

ORAL CAVITY AND OROFACIAL FUNCTIONS

In a holistic approach to health care, any one area of the body is linked directly or indirectly to all the other areas of the body. Consequently, observation of the oral cavity not only provides information about the mouth, it also provides knowledge as to many other aspects of the individual. The oral cavity provides access to the posterior nasal cavity, pharynx, esophagus and lower respiratory tract. It contains an ecosystem that reflects the overall health status of the individual. Dental occlusion reflects the functional balance of the musculoskeletal system, both locally and at distant areas of the body. Muscular tone, facial expression and orofacial habits mirror the individual's psychoemotional status. The oral cavity is also an area that allows communication with others through facial expression and speech. It is the major point of entry for nutrition and hydration and a secondary portal for respiration. Optimal function of the area is essential for the very survival of the individual.

Oral cavity

The main osseous structures of the oral cavity are the mandible, maxillae and palatine bones. The latter two bones are part of the viscerocranium and as such their growth and development extend through adolescence. This process is under genetic influence as well as epigenetic factors in which orofacial functions play a significant part. The long period through which development occurs allows extensive opportunities for dysfunction to be established. Thus, a thorough understanding of the structure and function involved in this evolution, combined with attentive observation of the infant and growing child, is imperative to identify somatic dysfunction, the effective treatment of which is necessary to promote health and balance.

The oral cavity, the mouth, is surrounded by the lips and cheeks and consists of two parts: the oral cavity proper and the vestibule. The oral cavity proper is limited anteriorly and laterally by the alveolar arches, teeth and gums, and above by the hard and soft palate; posteriorly, it communicates with the pharynx through the oropharyngeal isthmus. It includes the tongue, which is totally contained in the oral cavity in infants. As the child grows, only the anterior two-thirds remain in the oral cavity while the posterior third descends following the larynx.[1] The vestibule is located between the lips and cheeks externally, and the gums and teeth internally. It connects with the outside through the oral fissure between the lips.

The entire oral cavity is covered by mucosa, starting at the labial margins and consisting of three portions: the lining and the masticatory and specialized mucosae.[1] These portions demonstrate different properties according to their location. The oral mucosa is in continuity with the pharyngeal mucosa at the oropharyngeal isthmus.

Several bones within the viscerocranium define the oral cavity. The maxillae are the first to come to mind; together with the mandible, they are among the largest of the facial bones. Nevertheless, all of the components that constitute the skeletal framework of the oral cavity must be taken into consideration. Myofascial structures attached to this framework affect it and are, in turn, affected by it. Besides the mandible and maxillae, these bony boundaries include the paired palatine and temporal bones, and unpaired sphenoid and hyoid bones.

The maxilla consists of a body with zygomatic, frontal, alveolar and palatine processes. Bilaterally their bodies contain the maxillary sinuses, the largest of the paranasal sinuses. Although these cavities are large in the adolescent, at birth they are small furrows 7 mm in length and 4 mm in width.[2] Consequently, in the infant, the vertical diameter of the maxilla is smaller than the transverse and anteroposterior diameters.

The maxillary body is shaped as a pyramid, having four surfaces: anterior, posterior (infratemporal), superior (orbital) and medial (nasal). The lower part of the anterior surface demonstrates multiple eminences above the roots of the teeth. Several facial muscles insert on the anterior surface of the maxilla and their traction during orofacial activities such as sucking and chewing contributes to the development of the maxilla. The depressor septi nasi muscle arises above the eminences of the incisor teeth. A slip of the orbicularis oris muscle is attached on the alveolar border below this incisive fossa, and the nasalis muscle is attached superiorly. The levator anguli oris muscle arises from the canine fossa, lateral to the incisive fossa. Above the canine fossa is the infraorbital foramen, the anterior end of the infraorbital canal, which transmits the infraorbital vessels and nerve. Above the foramen on the margin of the orbit is attached part of the levator labii superioris. The nasal notch medially limits the anterior surface of the maxilla and nearby the nasalis and depressor septi muscles are attached. Bilaterally the two nasal notches join to form a pointed process, the anterior nasal spine.

Laterally, the convex infratemporal surface of the maxilla forms the inferior part of the infratemporal fossa. The maxillary tuberosity forms the lower part of this surface and on its medial side articulates with the pyramidal process of the palatine bone. Inconstantly, it articulates with the lateral pterygoid plate of the sphenoid and gives origin to a few fibers of the medial pterygoid muscle. Just above this is the pterygopalatine fossa, with a groove for the maxillary nerve.

The maxillary orbital surface forms part of the floor of the orbit. Medially, behind the lacrimal notch, the margin articulates with the lacrimal bone, the ethmoid's orbital plate and the palatine's orbital process. Posteriorly, it constitutes the posterior border of the inferior orbital fissure. Anteriorly it forms part of the orbital margin, which is continuous medially with the frontal process and laterally with the zygomatic process. Anteriorly and medially, the inferior oblique muscle originates just lateral to the lacrimal groove.

On the nasal surface is the maxillary hiatus, the large opening of the maxillary sinus. The superior border of the maxillary nasal surface articulates with the ethmoid and lacrimal bones. The inferior meatus of the nasal cavity is located below the maxillary hiatus and behind a surface for articulation with the perpendicular plate of the palatine bone. A groove crosses this surface, running obliquely downward and forward, and forms, with the palatine bone, the greater palatine canal. Anterior to the maxillary hiatus a deep groove forms part of the nasolacrimal canal.

The zygomatic process of the maxilla is triangular and is situated at the convergence of the anterior, posterior and orbital surfaces. The frontal process forms part of the lateral boundary of the nose projecting posterosuperiorly. It gives attachment to part of the orbicularis oculi and levator labii superioris alaeque nasi. Its medial surface forms part of the lateral wall of the nasal cavity. The upper border articulates with the frontal bone, the anterior border with the nasal bone and the posterior border with the lacrimal bone.

The alveolar process is very thick, being broader behind than it is in front. It contains eight deep cavities for the roots of the teeth. These cavities vary in size and depth: the cavities for the canine teeth are the deepest; the cavities for the molars are the widest. The alveolar processes of the maxillae articulated together form the alveolar arch. The buccinator muscle arises from the lateral surface of the alveolar process, as far forward as the first molar.

The palatine process projects horizontally and medially from the nasal surface of the maxilla. It constitutes an important part of the floor of the nasal cavity and the roof of the mouth. Its inferior surface is concave and forms, with the palatine process of the opposite side, the anterior three-quarters of the osseous plate of the palate. In young skulls, a fine linear suture, the incisive suture, may be observed. It extends from the incisive fossa, behind the incisor teeth, to the space between the lateral incisor and canine teeth. The small part in front of this suture forms the premaxilla (os incisivum) that contains the sockets of the incisor teeth. The two palatine processes join to form the median intermaxillary palatal suture. The margins are sometimes raised and form a prominent palatine torus. The medial border of the superior surface of the palatine process forms a ridge, the nasal crest. With the opposite side, it forms a groove for the vomer. The posterior border is articulated with the horizontal plate of the palatine bone (Figs 7.7.1, 3.5).

The maxilla ossifies in a mesenchymatous sheet. The number of ossification centers is debated and between two and four such centers may appear during the 7th week of fetal life. They form a premaxilla (os incisivum) and a maxilla that start to unite at the beginning of the 3rd month of development. The identification of the junction between these two parts as a suture is also debated,[3] and information is lacking to demonstrate its role as a growth site.[4] A line or cleft, however, may be observed in the anterior part of the palate until the middle decades of life.[1] This site – be it suture, line or cleft – is of consequence in osteopathic practice because it provides a hinge-like location where intraosseous maxillary somatic dysfunction can develop. Such dysfunction is commonly found in infants and children as the result of activities such as thumb sucking and from falls where the area is injured. If not treated, this dysfunction will have a significant impact that can only increase as the structures grow. Orofacial dysfunctions such as malocclusion or speech disorders may follow.

The maxillary sinus, described as a small furrow at birth, reaches its full size after the second dentition. As such, the size of the maxillary body at birth is small, the teeth sockets located almost at the level of the floor of the orbit. The relatively small length of the maxillary vertical dimension, when compared to that of the adult, gives the infant the appearance of having large eyes. Augmentation in volume of the maxillary sinus and development of the alveolar processes will contribute to an increase in the vertical dimension of the maxillary body (Fig. 2.13).

The maxilla articulates with nine bones including the frontal, ethmoid, zygomatic, nasal, lacrimal, inferior nasal concha, palatine, vomer and the opposite maxilla. The articulation with the orbital surface or with the lateral pterygoid plate of the sphenoid is inconstant.

On the other hand, the mandible articulates only with the two temporal bones. It consists of a curved horizontal body and two perpendicular portions, the rami. It is the largest and strongest bone of the face and contains the alveoli for the roots of the lower teeth. Its shape and position determine the positional arrangement of the lower teeth and as such it contributes to the relationship between the occlusal surfaces of the maxillary and mandibular teeth when they are in contact.

The mandibular body has two surfaces and two borders. In the midline of the external surface is a small ridge, the remnant of the line of fusion between the two halves of the mandible at the symphysis menti. This ridge divides inferiorly to surround the mental protuberance. The mentalis muscle and a small portion of the orbicularis oris are inserted below the incisor teeth on either side of the ridge. Laterally, the depressor labii inferioris, depressor anguli oris and platysma muscles are attached.

The internal surface is concave and the paired superior and inferior mental spines are situated on either side of the symphysis menti. The genioglossi muscles have their origins on the superior spines and insert on the lingual fascia beneath the mucous membrane and on the hyoid bone. They depress and protrude the tongue. If their origin on the mandible is dysfunctionally positioned, their leverage will be altered and consequently their effect on the tongue will, in turn, be dysfunctional. The geniohyoid muscles insert on the inferior mental spines, and the

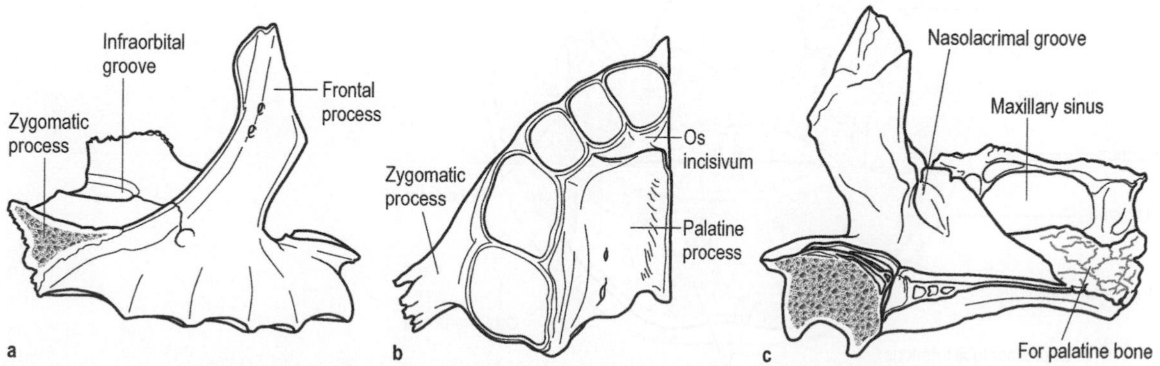

Figure 7.7.1. *Right maxilla at birth: (a) lateral aspect; (b) inferior aspect; (c) medial aspect.*

anterior belly of the digastric insert below the mental spines, on either side of the midline.

On either side, an oblique line, the mylohyoid line, runs from a point inferior to the mental spine upward and backward to the ramus behind the third molar tooth. It gives attachment to the mylohyoid muscle, the lower-most part of the superior constrictor of the pharynx, and the pterygomandibular raphe. The superior constrictor, pterygomandibular raphe and buccinator are intimately joined together to the mandibular periosteum. Furthermore, they form a continuous band that unites the orofacial structures with the cranial base and cervical spine (Fig. 7.7.3). Thus, postural imbalances in the axial skeleton can affect the orofacial structures, potentially leading to orofacial dysfunction and malocclusion.

The upper or alveolar border contains 16 cavities for the roots of the teeth. On either side, the buccinator muscle is attached on the outer lip of the superior border, as far forward as the first molar tooth. The buccinator has its origin posteriorly on the lateral aspect of the maxilla and oblique line of the mandible, the pterygoid hamulus and pterygomandibular raphe (Figs 7.7.2, 7.7.3). It inserts anteriorly on the angle of the mouth, the middle fibers of the muscle crossing in the region of the modiolus, the lower set passing to the upper lip, the upper set to the lower lip.[5] The modiolus located near the corner of the mouth represents a convergence of several muscles of facial expression and, as such, observation of this area is highly indicative of the psychoemotional state of the individual. The fibers of the buccinator muscle are interspersed with more horizontal portions of the orbicularis oris muscle. The buccinator flattens the cheek, retracts the angle of the mouth and plays an important role in mastication in conjunction with the tongue and orbicularis oris muscle to form a belt on each side of the oral cavity, preventing food from accumulating in the oral vestibule.

The quadrilaterally shaped mandibular ramus consists of two surfaces, four borders and two processes. The lateral surface is flat and gives attachment to the masseter muscle. The masseter muscle is attached above on the inferior border of the anterior two-thirds of the zygomatic arch and the medial surface of the zygomatic arch. It inserts inferiorly on the lateral surface of the ramus and the coronoid process of the mandible. It elevates the mandible and its function is of paramount importance in the development, growth and maturation of the mandibular condyles and fossae. A reduction of masseter muscle activity in bottle-fed babies has been observed[6] and, with the loss of chewing behavior, may predispose to chewing/swallowing disorders and malocclusions.[7]

Located on the medial surface of the mandibular ramus, approximately in its center, is the mandibular foramen leading to the mandibular canal. It contains the alveolar nerve and vessels. A sharp spine on the anterior margin of the foramen, the lingula (Spix spine), provides attachment for the sphenomandibular ligament. This site is of particular interest in mandibular kinematics because mandibular motion

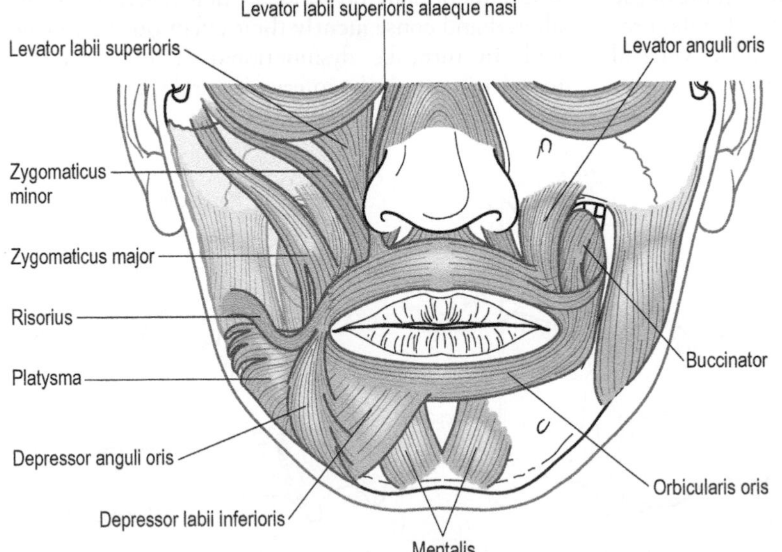

Figure 7.7.2. *Orofacial muscles.*

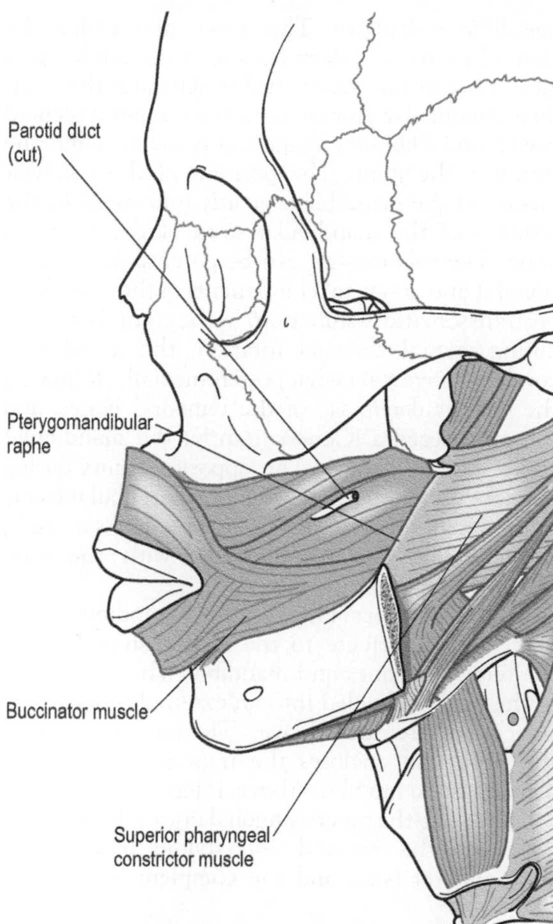

Figure 7.7.3. *Buccinator muscle.*

is centered on a point located near the lingula. The vascular–neural bundle is, therefore, protected from injury caused by normal mandibular motion.[8]

The medial pterygoid muscle inserts below the mandibular foramen, on the medial surface of the mandibular angle. Thus, the mandibular angle is affected by the action of the masseter laterally and medial pterygoid medially. Traction from these muscles dynamically influences the growth of the mandible. This influence has to be balanced unilaterally between the masseter and medial pterygoid, as well as bilaterally.

The coronoid process is a thin, flattened piece that forms the anterior limit of the mandibular incisure. The temporalis and masseter muscles are attached on its lateral surface; the temporalis also covers part of the medial surface and anterior border of the ramus. The temporalis muscle has its origin on the temporal fossa and functions to elevate the mandible and close the jaw. Its posterior, almost horizontally oriented fibers are the primary retractors of the protruded mandible. These muscles determine chewing action and, when dysfunctional, can have significant impact on the mandible.

The condylar process provides an articular surface with the disk of the temporomandibular joint (TMJ). Its long axis is slightly oblique and directed medially and posteriorly. The neck that unites the head or condylar process to the ramus has the pterygoid fovea (anteriorly) for the attachment of the lateral pterygoid muscle. This masticatory muscle has two heads: the inferior head has its origin on the lateral plate of the pterygoid process; the superior head originates on the infratemporal crest and adjacent greater wing of the sphenoid. In addition to its insertion on the mandible, some of its fibers join the articular disk and capsule of the TMJ. It acts to protrude the lower jaw and also contributes to the opening of the mouth. Unilateral pterygoid contraction deviates the chin laterally, enabling grinding motion for chewing. This muscle is important in the development of children's orofacial structures, where unilateral functional patterns will stimulate growth in an asymmetric fashion. Alternatively, structural asymmetries may, in turn, prevent the individual from having symmetric functional patterns.

Ossification of the mandible occurs in the fibrous membrane covering the outer surfaces of Meckel's cartilages. These cartilages develop bilaterally in the first pharyngeal arches. The primitive TMJ starts to organize during the 7th week of development, concomitantly with the emergence of muscular activity in the masticatory apparatus. At birth the mandible consists of two parts separated by a cartilaginous symphysis menti not yet ossified. The body, although rather underdeveloped, is much larger than the rami. It consists of relatively thin cortices with tooth buds almost totally occupying its volume.[9] Each side contains the sockets of the two incisors, the canine and the two deciduous molar teeth. The angle between the body and the ramus is obtuse (175°), and the coronoid process, of rather large size, projects above the level of the condyle. At birth, the TMJ is slack. The mandibular fossa of the temporal bone in which the condylar process of the mandible is located is almost flat, providing little stability.[10] During the first years of life growth will occur through bony deposition and resorption. Bone deposition occurs on the mandibular labial side, whereas resorption occurs on the lingual side, thus allowing for elongation of the mandible and more space for the deciduous dentition.[11] The two halves of the mandible join during the 1st year, although a line of separation may still be seen in the beginning of the 2nd year. Concomitant development of mastication stimulates growth of the alveolar and subdental portions of the mandibular body, allowing in turn more powerful traction from the masticatory muscles. During the first 3 years of life, mandibular bicondylar width grows rapidly, in synchrony with cranial base growth. It is the fastest growth period of the mandible. With the development of permanent dentition, the angle becomes less obtuse – 140° at about the 4th year. Crown formation of the permanent teeth, and their following eruption, is a time of possible occlusal instability, lasting up to 10–12 years of age when the majority of the permanent teeth have erupted. After puberty, the mandibular angle is 120° (Fig. 7.4.4).

Development of the teeth, like the development of the other components of the craniofacial complex – jaws, dental arches, tongue and myofascial structures – is under the infl uence of genetic and environmental factors. This development is largely infl uenced by the surrounding structures of the cranium, particularly the temporal bones with which the mandible articulates, and the sphenoid and hyoid bones that are part of the skeletal framework of the oral cavity.

At the root of the zygomatic process, in the squamous portion of the temporal bone, is the mandibular fossa, with which the condylar process of the mandible articulates. This fossa, also called the glenoid cavity, is a deep hollow in the adult but is almost flat in the infant. A disk separates the mandibular condylar process from the temporal glenoid cavity, and a fibrous capsule and synovial membrane surround the joint. The position of the condylar process of the mandible is greatly influenced by the position of the mandibular fossa of the temporal bone. The relationship can be potentially dysfunctional if one or several components of the TMJ demonstrate somatic dysfunction. In the cranial concept, during cranial external rotation, the mandibular condyles move somewhat posteromedially, following the mandibular fossae of the temporal bones, and the chin recedes. Concomitantly, the mandibular angles move laterally. The opposite occurs during cranial internal rotation when the mandibular fossae of the temporal bones move anteriorly. As a result, the mandible moves anteriorly, with the chin becoming more prominent.

The deep cervical fascia and stylomandibular ligament also contribute to the relationship between the temporal bones and mandible. The deep fascia of the neck is divided into an external or investing layer and a pretracheal layer. The former surrounds the neck and encloses the trapezius and sternocleidomastoid muscles. Above, it fuses with the periosteum along the superior nuchal line of the occipital bone, on the mastoid and styloid processes of the temporal bone and the complete base of the

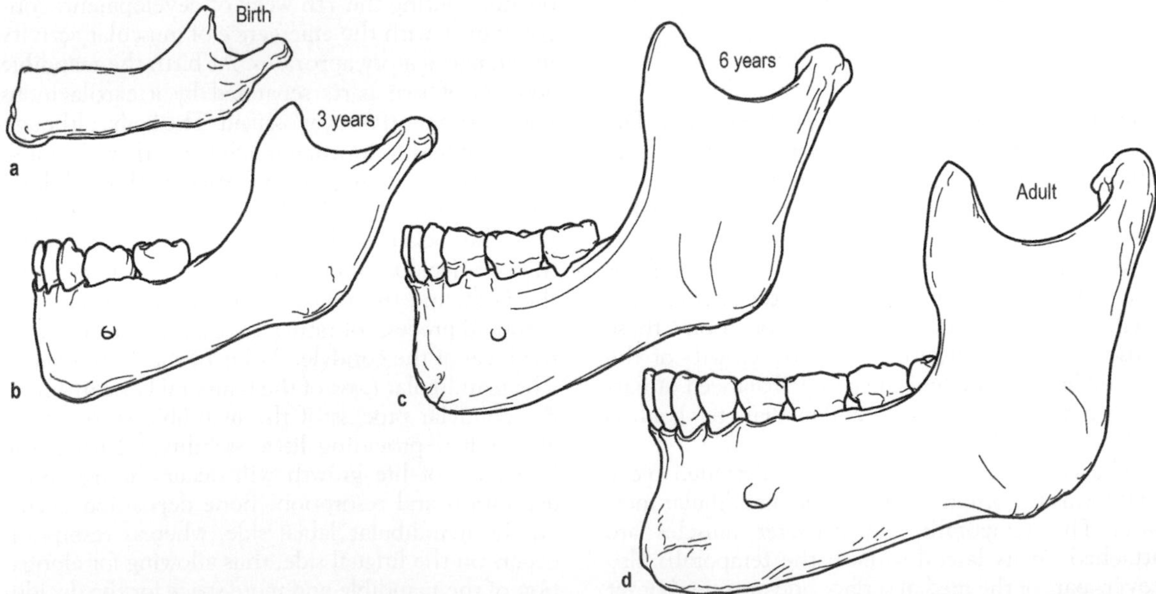

Figure 7.7.4. *(a–d) Development of the mandible.*

mandible.[1] The stylomandibular ligament, a condensation of the deep cervical fascia, extends from the tip of the styloid process of the temporal bone to the posterior border of the angle of the mandible. This fascia links the mandible to the base of the skull. Thus, dysfunction of the cranial base may affect the mandible, and vice versa. It is of great significance in the first years of life, when structures have not yet completed their growth. As such, torticollis or plagiocephaly, if untreated, may predispose to somatic dysfunction of the mandible and viscerocranium, leading to malocclusion.[12]

As it belongs to the cranial base, the sphenoid also influences the mandible through its muscular and ligamentous relations. The sphenomandibular ligament is of particular importance. This fibrous band, a remnant of Meckel's cartilage, runs from the spine of the sphenoid's greater wing to the lingula of the mandible. It constitutes the primary passive support of the mandible, with the area of the lingula acting as an anchor. An artificial axis passing through the two lingulae may be proposed, around which motions of the mandible occur. These motions include depression of the mandible during opening of the mouth and elevation during closure, as well as protraction and retraction. The mandible may be compared to a swing hanging under the sphenoid's greater wings. This comparison is particularly valid in infants and young children, where the TMJ is quite loose and the sphenomandibular ligament well defined.

Other links between the mandible and sphenoid include the bilateral pterygomandibular raphe and pterygoid muscles joining the pterygoid process to the mandible. The pterygomandibular raphe, also referred to as the pterygomandibular ligament, is a thickening of the buccopharyngeal fascia. It separates and gives origin to the buccinator muscle anteriorly and the superior constrictor of the pharynx posteriorly. The pterygomandibular raphe is attached superiorly to the pterygoid hamulus, the hook-shaped inferior extremity of the medial plate of the pterygoid process. Below, it is attached above the mylohyoid line behind the third molar tooth.

Indeed, multiple influences exist between the cranial base and the facial bones, potentially affecting the orofacial structures. The human profile and the position of the mandible have been correlated postnatally with the basicranial shape.[13] Furthermore, facial morphology is more related to variation of the lateral part of the basicranium than to flexion occurring in the midline.[14] Epigenetic factors play a significant role in this process. This role is largely fulfilled by several orofacial functions that start as early as the first weeks of development. It is hypothesized that, around 8 weeks of development, early mandibular movement participates in the differentiation of the primary mandible from Meckel's cartilage.[15]

Orofacial functions

Consideration of orofacial function is of great significance in the understanding and treatment of any orofacial disorder or malocclusion. To a large extent, orofacial function, interconnected with the musculoskeletal apparatus in a complex system, contributes to the formation of the oral cavity and viscerocranium. Deglutition, sucking, ventilation, facial expression, mastication and speech are the sequential events that, through dynamic processes, constantly influence the growth and development of the orofacial components.

For most of these activities, the tongue plays a central and vital part. In feeding, it moves food through the oral cavity for chewing and then to the pharynx for swallowing. In respiration, its position, relative to the posterior pharyngeal wall, determines the dimensions and shape of the airway for air to flow between the palate and the posterior tongue. With the larynx, the tongue contributes to the production of sounds and speech. Finally, the tongue seems to play an important proprioceptive role that, in turn, functionally or dysfunctionally regulates all of these activities.[1]

The tongue consists of a mass of muscle covered by mucous membrane, where the papillae of the gustatory organ are located. The lingual musculature is divided into intrinsic and extrinsic muscles. The intrinsic muscles, which are totally contained inside the tongue, are the bilateral superior and inferior longitudinal, the transverse and the vertical lingual muscles. Conversely, the extrinsic muscles extend outside the tongue and consist of the genioglossus, hyoglossus, styloglossus and palatoglossus muscles. The lingual musculature matures quite early in life, transforming the tongue into a powerful growth stimulator for the surrounding structures.

At birth, the infant tongue is totally intraoral and its extrinsic muscles are short. In the infant, the tongue fills the oral cavity, contacting the soft and osseous palates, the cheeks and lower lip. Although mobile, the tongue is solidly anchored at its base on the mandible by the paired genioglossi and on the hyoid bone by the genioglossi and hyoglossi muscles. In addition, the lateral surfaces of the tongue are suspended from the soft palate by the palatoglossi and from the styloid processes of the temporal bones by the styloglossi muscles. The fibers of these muscles blend with the superior portion of the tongue.

As in other primates, the larynx of the newborn is positioned high, with the epiglottis in direct contact with the soft palate. During the first years of life, in association with the growth of the cervical spine, the hyoid bone migrates from the level of C1–C2 at birth to C3–C4 after puberty.[16] The posterior third of the tongue follows this caudal migration, consequently stretching its superior attachments. This contributes to change the orientation of the soft palate from horizontal in the infant to more vertical in the adult.[17] Although the positional changes occur mainly during the first years of life, the reciprocal influences, from the cranial base and hyoid bone acting on the tongue and soft palate, should be kept in mind, no matter the age of the patient.

Normally, at about 4 or 5 years of age, after the descent of the larynx and tongue, the tongue rests lower in the mouth.[18] At this time it forms part of the floor of the oral cavity and part of the anterior wall of the oropharynx.[1] It is contained inside the mandibular arch and the functions of swallowing, sucking, ventilation, facial expression, chewing and phonation should be performed without difficulty. Dysfunction develops when lingual mobility and function are impaired. This may be the result of somatic dysfunction affecting the cranial base, hyoid bone or mandible, or accommodation of these areas to dysfunction in more distant body areas.

Tongue-tie, or ankyloglossia, is a partial or complete adhesion of the tongue to the floor of the mouth. Because of abnormal shortness, the frenulum linguae tethers the tongue to the floor of the mouth, impairs lingual mobility and, in severe cases, prohibits its extension beyond the lower gum. Although it may present as part of several craniofacial syndromes, in most cases the child is perfectly healthy.[19] Ankyloglossia is, however, associated with up to 12.8% of serious breastfeeding problems.[20] It is also a potential etiology for speech disorders[21] and dental problems,[22] such as diastasis between the lower incisors due to the lingual pressure.[23] Furthermore, impaired lingual mobility is related to difficulty with intraoral toileting and later with the playing of wind instruments.[23] Although surgical treatment (frenuloplasty or tongue-tie division) remains debated, in specific indications it is reported to improve difficult breastfeeding and to protect the maternal nipple,[24] and to alleviate speech disorders and improve tongue mobility.[25]

Swallowing, or deglutition, is one of the first orofacial functions to appear in utero and has been observed after 11 weeks, when the child reflexively swallows amniotic fluid.[1] At birth, new habits develop with feeding, allowing the evolution of the pattern of deglutition. In the infant, sucking and swallowing are the results of a pumping action in the hyolingual complex, with a rhythmic tongue thrust, the tip of the tongue showing regularly between the alveolar processes. Musculoskeletal growth and maturation of the neuromuscular system result in the development of a more mature or adult swallowing pattern. At around 2–3 years of age, at rest and during swallowing, the apex of the tongue is normally located on the palate, behind the upper incisor teeth. When swallowing, the lips are closed, but the perioral musculature, particularly the orbicularis oris and mentalis muscles, is relaxed. Lingual pressure applied against the palate contributes to the development of a broad palate and well-developed maxillae. The tongue works as a natural orthodontic appliance 'for better or for worse'.[26]

In the cheeks, the muscular bands formed by the buccinator and superior constrictor muscles, joined together through the pterygomandibular raphe, bilaterally act to constrain the tongue within the oral cavity. Thus, functional balance or dysfunction of the cervical spine and cranial base, the sites of origin of the superior constrictor, contributes significantly to lingual posture. In addition, because the tongue is anchored on the mandible, it affects and is affected by mandibular position and growth. When mature or adult swallowing does not develop successfully, immature or atypical swallowing will continue.

Chewing forces also contribute to maxillofacial growth. First, mastication occurs purely in the sagittal plane, with the mandible moving up and down, and demonstrating propulsion and retraction. Then, progressively, an alternating unilateral chewing pattern appears, with diagonal movements of the mandible.[8] The masticatory muscles develop in response to this demand. At around 9 months of age, a child can chew soft food and keep it in their mouth; 1 year later they can chew more solid foods.[27] As such, their diet should include food that requires sufficient chewing to allow satisfactory occlusal force per chew that can, in turn, stimulate periosteal growth. Symmetric chewing is a requisite for adequate muscular stimulation of the digastric, temporal and pterygoid muscles. The traction of these muscles will, in turn, stimulate bone growth. At this time cranial balance is necessary to facilitate the establishment of symmetric masticatory patterns that are learned and practiced throughout the rest of life, making early identification and treatment of somatic dysfunction essential.

Besides swallowing and chewing, ventilation, speech and facial expression also contribute to the development and growth of the maxillofacial structures. Ventilation, as a vital function, is present from birth onwards. In the first months, the infant is normally a nasal breather. At this time, observed respiration should be unencumbered. It is imperative that airfl ow be quiet and through both nares equally. Dysfunctional nasal respiration will impact the development of the orofacial structures, potentially leading to mouth breathing.

Establishment of the route of respiration is partly under the control of the soft palate. This muscular fold, suspended from the posterior border of the bony palate, extends inferiorly and posteriorly into the oropharynx. Under normal circumstances the soft palate and tongue act in apposition to close the oropharyngeal isthmus; conversely, when the soft palate rises and contacts the posterior pharyngeal wall, the nasopharynx is closed. Thus, the position of the soft palate determines the route of respiration and regulation of airfl ow through the nose or mouth. The soft palate is united with the tongue through the palatoglossi muscles and with the pharynx through the palatopharyngei muscles. For optimal function of all of the structures that contribute to upper airway respiration, somatic dysfunction affecting the sites of origin of these muscles should be identified and treated. For optimal breathing, the cranial base, hyoid bone and mandible should be balanced. It is well established that an inferoposterior displacement of the hyoid bone and an anteroinferior positioning of the tongue are correlated with mouth breathing.[28–30]

Normally, the tongue demonstrates large movements in all three planes of space.[31] In the production of sounds and speech, the tongue must change shape and the dorsum of the tongue must contact the palate. Shortening of the base of the tongue results from anterior displacement of the hyoid bone, whereas lengthening of the base of the tongue results from its posterior displacement. By employing the activity of the lingual muscles, speech contributes to the overall function and development of the orofacial cavity.

Although the hyoid bone has no direct articulation with other skeletal structures, it is an interface between the mandible and tongue above and the upper thoracic area below. Consequently, its position and motion are influenced by changes occurring at the level of the mandible or anywhere in the thorax. A hyolingual complex – a 'kinetic chain' – may be described,[32] part of a more global oropharyngeal complex where every structure is interdependent with others as part of the system.

Physical examination and treatment

Begin by noting the relationship between the head and the remainder of the body. The skull should be centered above the spine. Note any tension in the posterior, lateral and anterior (submandibular) cervical musculature. Divide the viscerocranium into three regions: frontal, nasal and buccal. Observe the relationship between these three regions and the relative harmony between them. In newborns, the lower two regions are proportionately smaller than in older children, adolescents and adults because the paranasal sinuses are not yet developed and the teeth have not erupted.

Observe facial expression and orofacial functions such as breathing, sucking (in infants) and swallowing. Look for coordination of the tongue and orofacial musculature, the rate of sucking if the patient is a baby, and possible tongue sucking or tongue thrusting. Note the ease of swallowing without any concomitant inappropriate muscular contraction if the patient is a child. If they are old enough to respond, ask them to describe the location of the tip of their tongue during swallowing; normally it should contact the hard palate behind the upper incisors.

Observe the resting respiration. Nasal patency of airfl ow can be assessed easily with a wisp of cotton held adjacent to each nasal aperture or look for fogging with exhalation on the convex side of a cold metal spoon or a cold mirror.

Observe the midline of the face, the metopic suture, nose and symphysis menti. All of these landmarks should be aligned in a straight line

Observe the maxillae and compare size and shape: in external rotation the maxilla appears wider; in internal rotation it appears narrower.

Observe the position of the mandible. Note its relationship with the maxillae, particularly its centric position. Observe the location of the gnathion; newborns are normally retrognathic. With the infant, an open mouth posture with tongue forward may be observed with dysfunction of the cranial base, mandible or hyoid bone.

With children, observe the mouth area and the lips for symmetry and tonicity. The upper lip reflects the functional pattern of the maxillae, whereas the lower lip reflects the mandible. Look for the capacity to keep the lips closed and in soft contact. There should be no tension, in particular in the orbicularis oris or mentalis muscle, and no protrusion, retraction or pursing of the lips. Note any abnormal perioral muscle function or nervous habits such as finger and nail picking or nail biting.

Compare the nasolabial sulci for depth and obliquity. Increased sulcus depth is associated with external rotation of the ipsilateral maxilla and/or the zygoma, whereas decreased depth is associated with internal rotation of these bones.

Look inside the mouth. Assess the position and function of the tongue. Note the presence of a large frenulum linguae. If the child is old enough to voluntarily open the mouth, look at the relative position of the tongue within the oral cavity. It should be inside the mandibular arch and should not cover the lower teeth. Again, if possible, have the child slightly protract their tongue to look for the presence of dental imprints on the lateral aspects of the tongue, unilateral or bilateral, indicating lingual malposition and/or dental malalignment. With the tongue protracted, look for tongue deviation. Assess the mobility of the tongue, looking for limitation of movement. Dysfunctional tongue posture is often accompanied by decreased tone and eversion of the lower lip.

Observe the teeth as to position, dental attrition and progression of dental development according to the child's age. Observe clenching of the teeth and observe the occlusion of the teeth. The upper and lower midline between the incisors should be in alignment. Normally, the upper incisors should slightly override the lower incisors and upper molars should rest on the lower molars. Note misalignment or protrusion of the upper or lower incisors. Note any crowding of the teeth. If asymmetric crowding is present, look to see if there is ipsilateral cranial internal rotation. Note the potential association with impaired ipsilateral nasal breathing and/or dysfunctional mastication.

Observe the shape and symmetry of the palate: a lower, flattened palate with everted teeth is associated with external rotation; a high arched palate with inwardly directed teeth is associated with internal rotation.

Observe the mandible. It should appear balanced under the cheeks. If not, differentiate between asymmetry of position and asymmetry of size and shape. Asymmetry of mandibular position is associated with asymmetry of the temporal bones: external rotation of the temporal bone results in posterior displacement of the mandibular fossa; internal rotation results in anterior fossa displacement. The chin will be displaced toward the side of temporal external rotation.

If asymmetry of mandibular size and shape is noted, look for a potential cause. Structural asymmetry may result from intraosseous mandibular dysfunction, dental malalignment or asymmetric orofacial function, such as mastication occurring only on one side.

Note the consistency between orofacial findings and the cranial pattern. If they are in concordance, a cranial osteopathic approach may be indicated. Palpation for function and treatment of identified dysfunction should follow. When treating orofacial problems, don't forget to check and treat somatic dysfunction of other areas, frequently the cranial base, craniocervical junction and upper thoracic area. Cranial procedures directed at release of the global membranous strain pattern, the SBS, vault and facial bones to ensure optimal freedom of movement are anecdotally associated with facilitation of the teething process. It is also important to remember that all tooth buds are present in the maxillae and mandible, even though not yet erupted. Any finger or object placed inside the mouth of a child can act as an orthodontic device and move the teeth. Therefore, it is inappropriate to employ force when examining the patient or using osteopathic manipulation to treat children's orofacial somatic dysfunction. The earlier osteopathic treatment of orofacial dysfunction is initiated, the better. Results may be enhanced when osteopathic treatment is employed in conjunction with appropriate orthodontic treatment.

MALOCCLUSION AND OROFACIAL DYSFUNCTIONS

Dental development begins in the 3rd month of intrauterine life and ends at approximately 25 years of age. Throughout this period profound occlusal events occur, resulting in potential sources of stress for the orofacial structures. To understand the evolution of the occlusal mechanism, it is important to begin with the infant and to follow the eruption and arrangement of the teeth along the dental arches.

During the first months, the absence of teeth allows total freedom in the displacement of the mandible and the child can experiment and discover objects surrounding them by bringing everything to their mouth. The lower central incisors are normally the first to appear between 6 and 8 months of age. When the upper central incisors emerge, the first occlusal relationship appears, associated with new constraint for mandibular mobility. The upper and lower lateral incisors are almost completely erupted at around 14 months, the time when the first molars appear. Just before the end of the 2nd year of life, the central and lateral incisors and the first molars are in occlusion, the canines have erupted and the second molars are beginning to emerge. In the 2nd year of life, the 20 deciduous teeth are present, with occlusion between the incisors, canines and first molars. At the same time, the child's orofacial functions have matured and their food is becoming more solid. Mouthing (active oral interaction with the environment by sucking different objects) is still quite frequent up to 3 years of age. Several explanations – from a means of exploring their environment to proactively exposing the naive GI tract to environmental antigens – have been offered for this behavior.[33] Whatever the reason, mouthing effectively contributes to dental attrition, thereby eliminating any dysfunctional occlusal contact and facilitating functional adaptation. Smoothing of the occlusal surfaces results in proprioception important in establishing functional balance of mandibular motion patterns. Conversely, any dysfunctional occlusal contact will result in dysfunctional mandibular motion patterns and stimulate abnormal mandibular and maxillary growth.[34] It will also prevent the establishment of alternating unilateral mastication.

The teeth develop in sockets in the alveolar parts of the maxillae and mandible. They are each held in their respective socket by a periodontal ligament. This anchors the teeth solidly while still allowing micromovements. It is also the site for periodontal innervation that is of paramount importance in the development and control of orofacial praxis. Proprioceptive input from the periodontal ligament in association with proprioception from the TMJ and surrounding myofascial structures provides constant information to the CNS. This allows the individual to adjust to the challenges of mastication as well as to global postural mechanics.[35]

Deciduous teeth are small, with thin enamel coverage, allowing rapid wearing out. On the other hand, permanent teeth are the hardest of all tissues in the body. Each consists of a crown and a root, meeting at the cervical margin. Dentine forms most of the tooth, with a central pulp cavity ending in a pulp chamber and canal. The side of the tooth in contact with the lips and cheeks is the labial or buccal surface while the side in contact with the tongue is the lingual or palatal surface. When the jaws are brought together the teeth meet, or occlude; thus, dental occlusion occurs. Occlusion is qualified according to the respective positions of the teeth. A centric occlusion takes place when the relation of opposing occlusal surfaces of mandibular and maxillary teeth provides the maximum contact, or intercuspation. In such circumstances, the mandible is in centric relation to the maxillae.

Infants usually demonstrate a retrusive mandibular position. When the first teeth erupt, the relationship will tend to show a horizontal protrusion, or overjet, of upper incisors beyond the lower incisors. However, at this early age tongue thrusting will result in a functional edge-to-edge repositioning of the teeth. In the first years of life, during eruption of the deciduous teeth, changes in the orofacial osseous and myofascial structures normally allow sufficient space for the teeth to emerge. Typically, by approximately 6 years of age, there is occlusion between all deciduous teeth that already gives a good idea of the occlusal pattern of the future permanent teeth. The overjet and overbite relationship should have resolved in order to allow for freedom of mandibular diduction, which is only possible if the mandible can slide forward slightly. This sequence occurs as the result of an alternating chewing pattern, enhanced by chewing the solid foods found in the correct type of diet.

It is important for the osteopathic practitioner to observe the oral cavity and teeth in order to identify their eruptive pattern, position, occlusal contacts and any asymmetric wear that may be associated with cranial somatic dysfunction. In addition, any asymmetry of function that predisposes the child to mouth and then chew using only one side, as might occur with a neurologic impairment, a child with one handicapped upper extremity or simply a child with a torticollis, will result in asymmetric wear of the occlusive surfaces of the teeth and eventually asymmetric mandibular growth.

The permanent incisors are significantly wider than the deciduous incisors that they have replaced by approximately 8 years of age. There might be a tendency for overjet or overbite, either positive or negative. While a horizontal protrusion of upper incisors beyond the lower ones is named overjet, a vertical overlap is named overbite (Fig. 7.7.5). At this age, the child's temporary canines, the two temporary molars and the first permanent molars are in occlusion. Around 10 years of age, occlusion exists between the permanent incisors, the temporary canines and the first permanent molars. At 12 years of age, occlusion is typically present between the permanent incisors, permanent canines and first permanent molars.

In mixed dentition, if the child has developed an asymmetric pattern of chewing, with a tendency to chew only on one side, they may wear out the teeth in a way that will not allow functional and symmetric development. Unsatisfactory occlusal contact

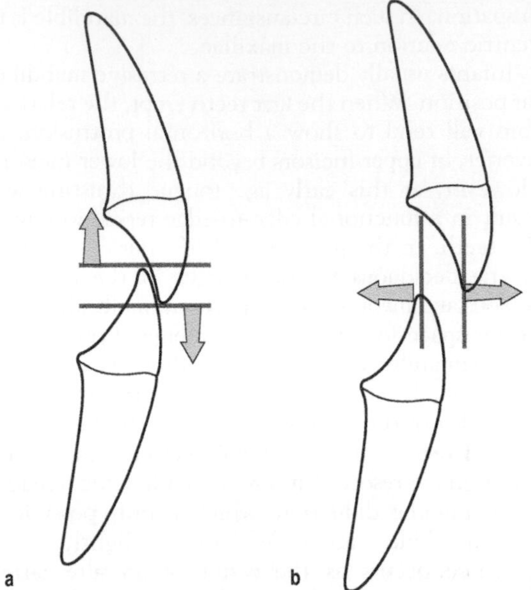

Figure 7.7.5. *Occlusal relationships: (a) overbite is the vertical overlap of the upper incisors over the lower incisors; (b) overjet is the horizontal protrusion of the upper incisors beyond the lower incisors.*

will create points of resistance that will, in turn, control and guide the movement of the mandible in asymmetric patterns. The masticatory, perioral and craniocervical muscles, as well as the highly elaborate TMJ structures, result in engrams of the repetitive dysfunctional pattern. If no change occurs, this will be the permanent pattern ingrained in the CNS. Thus, it is important to recognize asymmetric patterns and to identify and treat any underlying somatic dysfunction. Because patterns of function become fixed as the child ages, for the best therapeutic outcomes the cranial osteopathic approach should be employed at the earliest opportunity.

At the end of the 19th century, Edward Angle proposed that a definitive nomenclature was necessary in orthodontia as in anatomy.[36] He felt that the term malocclusion was far more expressive than 'irregularities of the teeth' to describe not only the relationship between the maxillary and mandibular arches, but also of the individual teeth to one another. As a result, a classification was born, referred to as Angle's classification.

Angle's classification is based on the mesiodistal relationship of the permanent molars. In dentistry, distal means away from the median sagittal plane of the face, following the curvature of the dental arch, while mesial means proximal. Three classes of dental arrangement are described. Class I identifies the normal relationship of the jaws, where the mesiobuccal cusp of the maxillary first molar occludes in the buccal groove of the mandibular first molar. In the individual with normal dentition and centric occlusion, the lower incisors bite against the lingual surfaces of the upper incisors, the crowns of the lower incisors being covered in their superior third. In addition, from the canine teeth backwards, each lower tooth is slightly in front of its upper fellow. Classes II and III categorize variations of malocclusion. In Class II, all the lower teeth occlude distal to normal, wherein the distobuccal cusp of the maxillary first molar occludes in the buccal groove of the mandibular first molar. In addition, this class is further subdivided into Division 1, labioversion of maxillary incisor teeth, and Division 2, linguoversion of maxillary central incisors. This may occur unilaterally of bilaterally. Class II is the most frequently encountered type of malocclusion. In Class III, all the lower teeth occlude mesial to normal, wherein the mesiobuccal cusp of the maxillary first molar occludes in the embrasure between the mandibular first and second permanent molars. Class III may further be classified as a unilateral condition.

The origin of malocclusion is highly debated, again with multifactorial origins proposed. Besides the genetic aspect of malocclusion, in particular for Class III,[37] malocclusal patterns are felt to result from an imbalance between intrinsic forces such as from the tongue and lips and extrinsic forces such as stressful orofacial habits. A large number of studies have considered the influence of epigenetic factors such as the orofacial functions of deglutition, sucking, ventilation, mastication and phonation (see below). In fact, it is more the orofacial dysfunctions and parafunctions or orofacial habits that are the source of malocclusion. Edward Angle said: 'Orthodontic treatments are very unlikely to succeed, if the functional disorders are still going on.'[38]

Class II malocclusion represents a heterogeneous collection of conditions with malocclusion that may be the result of purely skeletal or combined skeletal and dental origin; they are, however, more often purely dental in nature.[39] The teeth and alveolar bone constitute an interface between opposing forces and pressures, primarily from muscular function – the perioral musculature of the lips and cheeks on the one hand and intraoral forces from the tongue on the other. Pressures are applied to the teeth with varying distribution according to the oral function involved.[40] Under appropriate circumstances these pressures should affect the teeth from multiple, yet balanced, directions. When dysfunction results in chronically repeated patterns of activity, limiting the directions that these muscular pressures are applied to the teeth, dental malocclusion can be the result.

The development of Class II malocclusion has also been correlated with non-nutritive sucking habits such as thumb sucking.[41–45] In the early years of life the premaxillae may be easily pushed forward by non-nutritive sucking, pushing the upper incisors along with them. Thumb sucking creates an anterior opening between the dental arches, which facilitates the forward displacement of the tongue that occurs during tongue thrusting. It consequently results in dysfunctional forward placement of the tongue. This will, in turn, promote maxillary prognathism because, with every deglutition, which occurs approximately 1500 times per day, the tip of the tongue will move forward between the teeth, applying pressure to the premaxillae and upper incisors, pushing them forward.

For similar reasons, the sucking of a pacifier is also commonly associated with malocclusion, followed by the practice of sucking fingers.[46] Prolonged pacifier habits result in changes to the dental arches with a prevalence of posterior cross-bite and increased amount of overjet.[47] Until the age of 2–3 years the risk of developing a dysfunctional occlusion may be reduced proportionally to the reduction of time that the child uses the pacifier, and under these circumstances the dental arches should be regularly evaluated.[48] Significant maxillary prognathism has also been correlated with persistent digit sucking habits.[48,49] Among other sucking habits, a trend toward association of bottle feeding with the need for orthodontic treatment has been found.[50] On the other hand, breastfeeding seems to have a positive effect on orofacial morphogenesis,[51,52] with a protective effect for the development of posterior cross-bite in deciduous dentition.[45]

Not only the mode of feeding but also the type of food is associated with malocclusion. There are suggestions that changes in diet and food processing are associated with variations in facial size and shape.[53] The prevalence of occlusal disorders in subjects born in the 1950s has been found to be lower than in individuals born in the 1990s. It is thought that this is probably because of dietary habits resulting from the increased consumption of processed foods.[54] At the same time, there is an increased prevalence of allergies that result in mouth breathing. There is a 3% incidence of mouth breathers in individuals born in the 1950s and 21% in those born in the 1990s.[54]

When mouth breathing is associated with nasal obstruction, it results in an inferior position of the mandible. In addition, the tongue is maintained lower in the oral cavity (Fig. 7.7.6). This posture is associated with compensations in the perioral musculature, such as hypotonicity, as well as compensations at the level of the vertebral spine. Mouth breathers tend to assume an extended or forward head posture.

Respiratory dysfunctions are also associated with malocclusion. Premature molar eruption is often present in chronic mouth breathers. Mandibular growth is affected, with resulting anterior mandibular rotation[29] and an increase of the mandibular angle.[30] Thus, the vertical dimension of the lower face is increased, with resultant open bite.[29] The term 'adenoidal facies' (long faces) describes infants with an open mouth, a short upper lip and prominent and crowded anterior teeth. Lip hypotonicity – decreased tonicity of the orbicularis oris muscle – is typically found in patients with Class II, Division 1 malocclusion.[55] In this presentation, hypotonicity of the orbicularis oris muscle is balanced by compensatory contraction in the mentalis muscles. It is this aspect that can be observed in patients with 'adenoidal facies' syndrome. In addition, the maxillae are narrow and the palate high arched with concomittant increase in the mandibular angle; thus the face appears longer.[56] These individuals also demonstrate a lack of development of the masseter muscles as well as of the maxillary bones.[57]

Alternatively, hypertonic and bulbous masseter muscles with reduced facial height are correlated with a tendency to clench the teeth.[57] These findings are commonly identified in association with cranial somatic dysfunction involving the temporal bones and/or TMJs. The cranial concept lends itself well to the understanding of functional orofacial disorders. Children who have dysfunctional extension of the SBS will present with a long narrow head. The resultant internal rotation of the maxillae is associated with a palate that is narrow and high arched. This orofacial cranial pattern fails to provide sufficient space for the teeth in the dental arches, predisposing the child to dental crowding. In young children, Class II malocclusion may be found in association with an intraosseous dysfunction between the premaxilla and the maxilla. The premaxilla can be pushed forward or backward as the result of stress patterns occurring during intrauterine life or at the time of delivery. Postpartum behaviors, such as thumb sucking, can also push the premaxilla forward, while a fall forward striking the face, particularly the

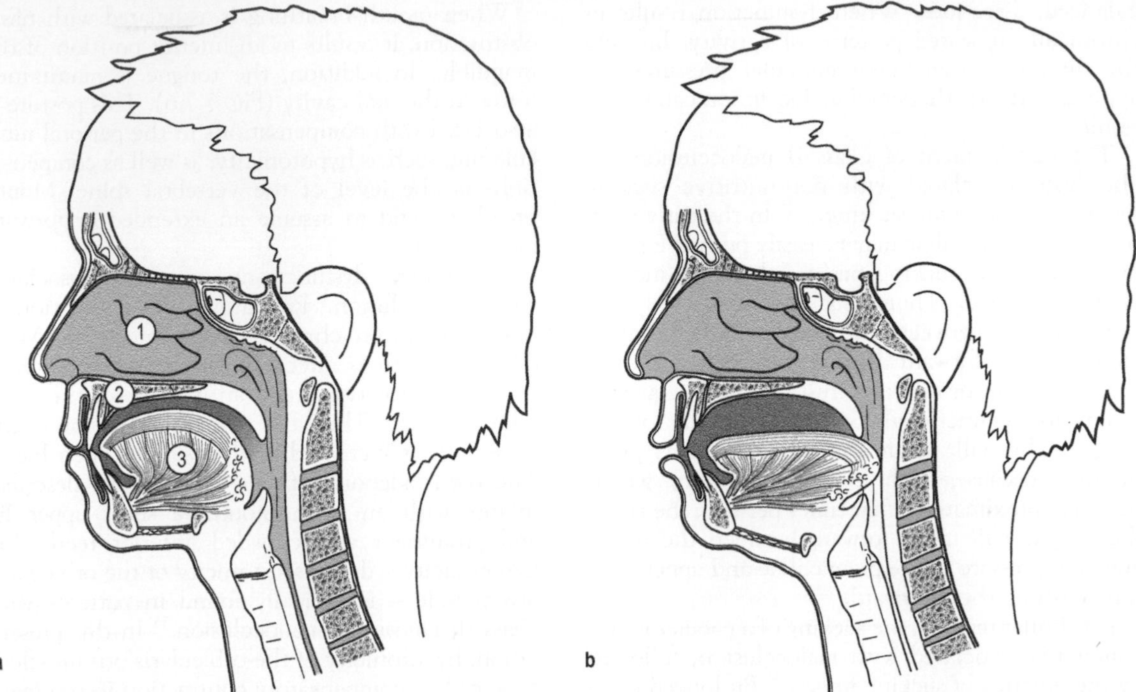

Figure 7.7.6. *The position of the tongue. (a) Functional position: note the lips are closed, the dorsum of the tongue is molding the palate, the oropharynx is patent. (b) Dysfunctional position: note the absence of labial contact, the displacement of the tongue posteroinferiorly and the decrease of the lumen of the oropharynx. 1. nasal cavity; 2. hard palate; 3. tongue.*

upper incisors, will push the premaxilla in a posterior direction.

Cranial maxillary dysfunction can be the beginning of a sequence of events that act to reinforce each other. Maxillary dysfunction can reduce nasal patency and predispose to mouth breathing. It can affect the dental arch with potential consequences for occlusion. Maxillary dysfunction can also trigger a compensatory pattern in the position and development of the mandible.

The mandible itself may demonstrate several types of dysfunction. Similar to maxillary dysfunction, mandibular dysfunction may result from strains or traumas. It can also occur as accommodation to internal or external rotation dysfunction of the temporal bones. Temporal bone dysfunction may be unilateral or bilateral, with the mandible moving anteriorly on the side of temporal internal rotation or posteriorly on the side of temporal external rotation. The resultant mandibular displacement will, in turn, affect occlusion.

In fact, any facial strain or trauma may impact the symmetry of the occlusal pattern. The area of the nasion – the junction between the frontonasal and internasal sutures – as well as the frontomaxillary sutures, may suffer compression from intrauterine pressures or as the result of a difficult delivery. The nasal bones should be attentively evaluated. With the maxillae, they are suspended from the frontal bone and as such will demonstrate restriction of movement following any trauma of the frontal bone. Furthermore, an impact on the frontal bone may result in a decrease in the vertical height of the maxillae with potential intraosseous dysfunction and resultant compromise of nasal respiration. Discrepancy in size between the maxilla and mandible may result from insufficient growth of these structures, potentially producing overjet or overbite.

Positioning of the child during the first months of life influences the growth pattern of the cranial bones. Non-synostotic plagiocephaly is associated with chronic sleep position and is most often visible in the first months of life.[58] It has also been shown that when a child sleeps in the same position for months, changes in the dental arches are observed.[59] Deformation of the face, however, because the growth of the viscerocranium continues later in life than the growth of the neurocranium, is not commonly observable by the non-trained examiner before several years of age. Facial asymmetries are, however, frequently associated with plagiocephalies.[60–62] With asymmetric occipital deformation, compensatory changes may occur in the maxillae, with resultant mandibular asymmetry.[63]

The relationship between the neurocranium, cranial base and viscerocranium has been studied extensively. An increase in anterior facial height is observed in subjects maintaining a forward-bent head position; a decrease is associated with a backward-bent head posture.[64,65] Changes in the position of the hyoid bone are observed in Class II malocclusion where the hyoid bone is higher and more forward relative to the mandible.[66] The posture of the cervical spine changes in response to changes in the occlusal plane as well as to imbalance between right and left masticatory muscles.[35] Modifications of the cranial base are linked to Class III malocclusion where a decrease in the angle between the clivus (surface from the dorsum sellae of the body of the sphenoid to the foramen magnum) and the cribriform plate of the ethmoid has been observed.[13]

Physical examination and treatment

The child's occlusal pattern should be assessed. If abnormal occlusion or malocclusion is identified, the somatic dysfunction that may be responsible should be sought out and treated. The etiology of malocclusion is multifactorial and osteopathic procedures may be employed when cranial somatic dysfunction contributing to the establishment of the malocclusive pattern is present. To be effective, these procedures should be employed at the earliest possible age. Cranial manipulation is in no way intended to be a replacement for standard orthodontic treatment. However, orthodontic treatments are less likely to be fully successful if somatic dysfunction affecting the child's occlusal pattern persists.

When examining the child with malocclusion, the principles of examination discussed above in 'Oral cavity and orofacial functions' apply. In addition, when looking for contributory somatic dysfunction, the practitioner should pay attention to the standing postural mechanics and their impact, particularly on the upper thoracic and occipitoatlantal areas. Even in cases where orthodontic treatment has been initiated, the child's posture should be addressed. The identification and treatment of dysfunctional postural mechanics resulting in functional balance of the orofacial complex will accelerate the effect of the orthodontic treatment. Furthermore, orthodontic treatment in itself serves as a source of stress, affecting the overall mechanics of the body. Thus, the release of existing dysfunctional mechanics will provide comfort to the child, making the orthodontic process more tolerable, as well as facilitating the effect of the orthodontic procedure.

With the child seated, it is appropriate to observe the occlusal pattern. Have the child actively open their mouth while observing for displacement of the symphysis menti. This motion normally should follow a straight vertical path, without a distorted pattern. Next, have the child move their mandible laterally to the right and left sides to compare ease of movement and degree of displacement bilaterally. If appropriate, give the child some chewing gum to observe the presence or absence of an alternating masticatory pattern. Observe and note the presence of a dominant side to the masticatory pattern. Check the presence of immature swallowing by observing and asking the child to describe the location of the tip of their tongue within their mouth during swallowing. Assess the musculature of the lips and cheeks by placing your thumbs inside the child's mouth, such that their palmar surfaces are in contact with the inside of the cheeks. Ask the child to close their mouth and swallow, and with your thumbs appreciate the strength of contraction of the buccinator muscles.

Next, with the child lying supine, palpate the clavicles, sternum and hyoid bone, assessing their myofascial attachments. Go on to assess the myofascial structures of the upper thoracic and cervical spine for somatic dysfunction, noting the relationship between the occiput and atlas. Palpate the myofascial structures of the skull, paying attention to the orofacial muscles and TMJ area for dysfunctional asymmetric tension. Check the TMJs and proceed with tests of listening. Evaluate the cranial base, looking for patterns of predominant cranial flexion or extension, as well as torsion, sidebending–rotation, compression and strain patterns. By placing one hand on the frontal bone with the index and middle fingers controlling the greater wings of the sphenoid and the other hand cradling the mandible, note the balance between the mandible and greater wings of the sphenoid. Listen to the different bones of the skull that may be involved in the malocclusion, paying particular attention to the temporal bones, sphenoid, frontal bones and maxillae, looking for intra- and interosseous cranial somatic dysfunctions. Treat all identified somatic dysfunction using indirect principles. Intraosseous molding may be considered if the child is young enough.

All of these relationships are often reciprocal and illustrate the integration of all parts of the body, local and distant, into a united system. Osteopathic treatment may be employed to address the somatic dysfunction that is found in association with orofacial dysfunction. When indirect principles of treatment are respectfully employed, these procedures may be used to treat from the very youngest patient on through adolescence. The earlier the dysfunction is recognized, the younger the patient and the more plastic the tissues, the greater the possibility to affect the structure and to re-establish satisfactory functional patterns, thereby activating the body's inherent ability to heal itself.

Patient education and advice to caregivers

Involve the parents or caregivers; empower them to help the child to succeed in dealing with the dysfunction. Take the time to explain to the child why it is necessary to breathe through the nose and eat slowly. Encourage the child to promote correct function, such as nasal breathing and learning how to blow their nose. Encourage the child to practice activities that promote breathing, such as singing with good articulation of the words.

Young children with dysfunctional tongue mechanics or with minor cases of ankyloglossia can perform exercises to mobilize the tongue and to stretch the frenulum as much as possible. Encourage the parents or caregivers to correct the child when there is mispronunciation. It may appear to be cute, but is actually dysfunctional. The child should repeat incorrectly pronounced words as correctly as possible to improve tongue mobility. Infants can be encouraged to play sound-making games by repeating sounds that cause the tongue to make a clicking noise against the palate.

Teach effi ient swallowing without tongue thrusting by instructing the child to consciously keep their tongue in their mouth and to learn to swallow with the tip of their tongue resting against the palate behind their upper incisors. To practice this, the child can hold a small piece of food between the tongue and palate while attempting to swallow several times. This exercise should be repeated until the act of swallowing with the tip of the tongue resting against the palate becomes automatic.

Insist on alternate unilateral mastication and that the child takes suffi cient time to chew their food thoroughly. Those children who are old enough should be encouraged to eat food that is as unrefined as possible. Soft refi ned junk food often does not require sufficient chewing.

Caution the parent or caregiver to watch for functional asymmetries that are associated with repetitive asymmetrical activities, such as unilateral bottle feeding or thumb sucking. Instruct the parent or caregiver and the patient, when old enough to understand, to avoid these activities or perform them in a fashion that alternates sides.

REFERENCES

1. Williams PL (ed). Gray's anatomy, 38th edn. Edinburgh: Churchill Livingstone; 1995.
2. Gruber DP, Brockmeyer D. Pediatric skull base surgery. 1. Embryology and developmental anatomy. Pediatr Neurosurg 2003;38(1):2–8.
3. Vacher C, Sakka M, Dauge MC. Incisive suture (fissure) in the human fetus: radiographic and histologic study. Cleft Palate Craniofac J 2001;38(4):330–6.
4. Cadenat H, Boutault F, Dupui D. Prémaxillaire et croissance faciale 68 ans après. Rev Stomatol Chir Maxillofac 1992; 93(6):393–9.
5. Reid SE, Broad MT, Dickson M, McDonald SW. The anatomy of buccinator – insights from functional casts of the oral vestibule. Arch Oral Biol 2003;48(11):787–95.
6. Inoue N, Sakashita R, Kamegai T. Reduction of masseter muscle activity in bottle-fed babies. Early Hum Dev 1995; 42(3):185–93.
7. Raymond JL. Approche fonctionnelle de l'allaitement et malocclusions. Rev Orthop Dento-Faciale 2000;34:379–402.
8. Gaspard M. Acquisition et exercice de la fonction masticatrice chez l'enfant et l'adolescent. Rev Orthop Dento-Faciale 2001;35(3):349–403.
9. Smartt JM Jr, Low DW, Bartlett SP. The pediatric mandible: I. A primer on growth and development. Plast Reconstr Surg 2005;116(1):14e–23e.
10. Couly G, Guilbert F, Cernea P, Bertrand JC. A propos de l'articulation temporo-mandibulaire du nouveau-né. Les relations oto-méniscales. Rev Stomatol Chir Maxillofac 1976;77(4):673–84.
11. Kurihara S, Enlow DH, Rangel RD. Remodeling reversals in anterior parts of the human mandible and maxilla. Angle Orthod 1980;50(2):98–106.
12. Kreiborg S, Moller E, Bjork A. Skeletal and functional craniofacial adaptations in plagiocephaly. J Craniofac Genet Dev Biol Suppl 1985;1:199–210.
13. Moss ML, Greenberg SN. Post-natal growth of the human skull base. Angle Orthod 1955;25:77–84.
14. Bastir M, Rosas A. Facial heights: evolutionary relevance of postnatal ontogeny for facial orientation and skull morphology in humans and chimpanzees. J Hum Evol 2004;47(5): 359–81.
15. Lee SK, Kim YS, Oh HS, Yang KH, Kim EC, Chi JG. Prenatal development of the human mandible. Anat Rec 2001;263(3):314–25.
16. Laitman JT, Crelin ES. Developmental change in the upper respiratory system of human infants. Perinatol Neonatol 1980;4:15–22
17. Talmant J, Renaudin S, Renaud P. Développement de l'oropharynx: évolution de la paroi ventrale du pharynx. Rev Orthop Dento-Faciale 1998;32:207–33.
18. Laitman JT, Heimbuch RC, Crelin ES. Developmental change in a basicranial line and its relationship to the upper respiratory system in living primates. Am J Anat 1978;152: 467–82.

19. Martinot VL, Manouvrier S, Anastassov Y, Ribiere J, Pellerin PN. Orodigitofacial syndromes type I and II: clinical and surgical studies. Cleft Palate Craniofac J 1994;31(5): 401–8.
20. Ballard JL, Auer CE, Khoury JC. Ankyloglossia: assessment, incidence, and effect of frenuloplasty on the breastfeeding dyad. Pediatrics 2002;110(5):e63.
21. Messner AH, Lalakea ML. The effect of ankyloglossia on speech in children. Otolaryngol Head Neck Surg 2002; 127(6):539–45.
22. Wright JE. Tongue-tie. J Paediatr Child Health 1995;31(4): 276–8.
23. Lalakea ML, Messner AH. Ankyloglossia: does it matter? Pediatr Clin North Am 2003;50(2):381–97.
24. Wallace H, Clarke S. Tongue tie division in infants with breast feeding diffi culties. Int J Pediatr Otorhinolaryngol 2006;70(7):1257–61.
25. Lalakea ML, Messner AH. Ankyloglossia: the adolescent and adult perspective. Otolaryngol Head Neck Surg 2003;128(5): 746–52.
26. Couly G. La langue, appareil naturel d'orthopédie dento-faciale 'pour le meilleur et pour le pire'. Rev Orthop Dento-Faciale. 1989;23(1):9–17.
27. Carruth BR, Skinner JD. Feeding behaviors and other motor development in healthy children (2–24 months). J Am Coll Nutr 2002;21(2):88–96.
28. Behlfelt K, Linder-Aronson S, Neander P. Posture of the head, the hyoid bone, and the tongue in children with and without enlarged tonsils. Eur J Orthod 1990;12(4): 458–67.
29. Principato JJ. Upper airway obstruction and craniofacial morphology. Otolaryngol Head Neck Surg 1991;104(6): 881–90.
30. Finkelstein Y, Wexler D, Berger G, Nachmany A, Shapiro-Feinberg M, Ophir D. Anatomical basis of sleep-related breathing abnormalities in children with nasal obstruction. Arch Otolaryngol Head Neck Surg 2000;126(5):593–600.
31. Abd-el-Malek S. The part played by the tongue in mastication and deglutition. J Anat 1955;89(2):250–4.
32. Hiiemae KM, Palmer JB. Tongue movements in feeding and speech. Crit Rev Oral Biol Med 2003;14(6):413–29.
33. Fessler DM, Abrams ET. Infant mouthing behavior: the immunocalibration hypothesis. Med Hypotheses 2004;63(6): 925–32.
34. Thurow RC. Deciduous dentition and the establishment of functional occlusal patterns. In: Atlas of orthodontic principles. Philadelphia: Mosby; 1977:171–85.
35. Shimazaki T, Motoyoshi M, Hosoi K, Namura S. The effect of occlusal alteration and masticatory imbalance on the cervical spine. Eur J Orthod 2003;25(5):457–63.
36. Angle EH. Classifi cation of malocclusion. Dental Cosmos 1899:248–64.
37. Singh GD. Morphologic determinants in the etiology of class III malocclusions: a review. Clin Anat 1999;12(5): 382–405.
38. Angle E. Treatment of malocclusion of the teeth. Angle's system, 7th edn. Philadelphia: S.S. White Dental Manufacturing Company, 1907. Quoted by Mew JR. The postural basis of malocclusion: a philosophical overview. Am J Orthod Dentofacial Orthop 2004;126(6):729–38.
39. Johnston FE, Hufham HP Jr, Moreschi AF, Terry GP. Skeletal maturation and cephalofacial development. Angle Orthod 1965;35:1–11.
40. Ruan WH, Chen MD, Gu ZY, Lu Y, Su JM, Guo Q. Muscular forces exerted on the normal deciduous dentition. Angle Orthod 2005;75(5):785–90.
41. Brauer JS, Holt TV. Tongue thrust classifi cation. Angle Orthod 1965;35:106–12.
42. Subtelny JD, Subtelny JD. Oral habits – studies in form, function, and therapy. Angle Orthod 1973;43(4):349–83.
43. Pancherz H, Zieber K, Hoyer B. Cephalometric characteristics of Class II division 1 and Class II division 2 malocclusions: a comparative study in children. Angle Orthod 1997;67(2):111–20.
44. Warren JJ, Bishara SE, Steinbock KL, Yonezu T, Nowak AJ. Effects of oral habits' duration on dental characteristics in the primary dentition. J Am Dent Assoc 2001;132(12):1685–93; quiz 1726.
45. Viggiano D, Fasano D, Monaco G, Strohmenger L. Breast feeding, bottle feeding, and non-nutritive sucking; effects on occlusion in deciduous dentition. Arch Dis Child 2004; 89(12):1121–3.
46. Tomita NE, Bijella VT, Franco LJ. Relação entre hábitos bucais e má oclusão em pré-escolares. Rev Saude Publica 2000;34(3):299–303.
47. Warren JJ, Bishara SE. Duration of nutritive and nonnutritive sucking behaviors and their effects on the dental arches in the primary dentition. Am J Orthod Dentofacial Orthop 2002;121(4):347–56.
48. Larsson E. Sucking, chewing, and feeding habits and the development of crossbite: a longitudinal study of girls from birth to 3 years of age. Angle Orthod 2001;71(2): 116–9.
49. Moore MB, McDonald JP. A cephalometric evaluation of patients presenting with persistent digit sucking habits. Br J Orthod 1997;24(1):17–23.
50. Meyers A, Hertzberg J. Bottle-feeding and malocclusion: is there an association? Am J Orthod Dentofacial Orthop 1988; 93(2):149–52.
51. Labbok MH, Hendershot GE. Does breast-feeding protect against malocclusion? An analysis of the 1981 Child Health Supplement to the National Health Interview Survey. Am J Prev Med 1987;3(4):227–32.
52. Neiva FC, Cattoni DM, Ramos JL, Issler H. Early weaning: implications to oral motor development. J Pediatr (Rio J) 2003;79(1):7–12.
53. Lieberman DE, Krovitz GE, Yates FW, Devlin M, St Claire M. Effects of food processing on masticatory strain and craniofacial growth in a retrognathic face. J Hum Evol 2004; 46(6):655–77.
54. Marinelli A, Alarashi M, Defraia E, Antonini A, Tollaro I. Tooth wear in the mixed dentition: a comparative study between children born in the 1950s and the 1990s. Angle Orthod 2005;75(3):340–3.
55. Jung MH, Yang WS, Nahm DS. Effects of upper lip closing force on craniofacial structures. Am J Orthod Dentofacial Orthop 2003;123(1):58–63.
56. Rappai M, Collop N, Kemp S, deShazo R. The nose and sleep-disordered breathing: what we know and what we do not know. Chest 2003;124(6):2309–23.
57. Mew JR, Meredith GW. Middle ear effusion: an orthodontic perspective. J Laryngol Otol 1992;106(1):7–13.
58. Kane AA, Mitchell LE, Craven KP, Marsh JL. Observations on a recent increase in plagiocephaly without synostosis. Pediatrics 1996;97(6 Pt 1):877–85.
59. Huang CS, Cheng HC, Lin WY, Liou JW, Chen YR. Skull morphology affected by different sleep positions in infancy. Cleft Palate Craniofac J 1995;32:413–9.
60. Kawamoto HK. Torticollis versus plagiocephaly. In: Marchac D (ed). Cranio-facial surgery: International Society for CranioMaxilloFacial Surgery. New York: Springer Verlag; 1987:105–9.

61. Kelly KM, Littlefield TR, Pomatto JK, Ripley CE, Beals SP, Joganic EF. Importance of early recognition and treatment of deformational plagiocephaly with orthotic cranioplasty. Cleft Palate Craniofac J 1999;36(2):127–30.
62. Biggs WS. Diagnosis and management of positional head deformity. Am Fam Physician 2003;67(9):1953–6.
63. Björk A, Björk L. Artificial deformation and cranio-facial asymmetry in ancient Peruvians. J Dent Res 1964;43(3): 353–62.
64. Solow B, Tallgreen A. Head posture and craniofacial morphology. Am J Physiol Anthropol 1976;44:417–36.
65. Solow B, Siersbaek-Nielsen S. Growth changes in head posture related to craniofacial development. Am J Orthod 1986;89:132–40.
66. Sloan RF, Bench RW, Mulick JF, Ricketts RM, Brummett SW, Westover JL. The application of cephalometrics to cinefluorography: comparative analysis of hyoid movement patterns during deglutition in Class I and Class II orthodontic patients. Angle Orthod 1967;37(1):26–34.

INDEX